Surgery of the Foot

Surgery of the Foot

Kent K. Wu, M.D.
Department of Orthopaedic Surgery
Henry Ford Hospital
Detroit, Michigan

Lea & Febiger   *1986*   **Philadelphia**

Lea & Febiger
600 Washington Square
Philadelphia, PA   19106-4198
U.S.A.
(215) 922-1330

Library of Congress Cataloging-in-Publication Data

Wu, Kent K.
  Surgery of the foot.

  Includes bibliographies and index.
  1. Foot—Surgery. I. Title. [DNLM: 1. Foot—surgery.
WE 880 W959s]
RD563.W823   1986   617'.585   85-19849
ISBN 0-8121-0995-3

PRINTED IN THE UNITED STATES OF AMERICA

Print No.   4   3   2   1

DEDICATION

Dedicated to my teacher, Dr. C. Leslie Mitchell, who popularized the Mitchell's bunionectomy, and taught two generations of orthopaedic surgeons with patience, dignity, compassion, and exceptional competence; and to my past, present, and future orthopaedic residents, whose youthful energy and enthusiasm, intellectual curiosity, and constant pursuit of the uncompromised truth are an unending inspiration to me.

FOREWORD

The multiple demands for functional adaptation made on the human foot exceed those of any part of the body, with the exception of the brain. These include adapting to the weight, age, type of shoeing, occupational and recreational requirements, and thermal and moisture variations of an individual, and to various standing and walking surfaces.

The foot is subject to laceration, contusion, ligamentous sprain and rupture, fracture, penetrating wounds, extremes of thermal changes, and toxic insect and snake bites. In addition, pathologic changes are imposed on the foot by congenital abnormalities, bacterial and fungal infections, dermatologic lesions, allergies, chemical burns, metabolic manifestations, arthritis, diabetes, peripheral vascular pathologic conditions, sympathetic dystrophies, neuropathies, myopathies, and developmental lesions and tumors. Last but not least, there are those abnormalities of iatrogenic origin.

The identification of a given patient's foot problem and the charting of a course of treatment designed to meet that individual's functional requirements are the focus of *Surgery of the Foot* by Dr. Wu. Dr. Wu, as an active senior member of the orthopaedic staff, has been able to draw upon years of clinical material provided by the orthopaedic and support medical staff of the Henry Ford Hospital. His text represents a thorough evaluation of disorders of the foot with appropriate surgical and nonsurgical methods of treatment; hundreds of line drawings, photographs, photomicrographs, radiographs, radioisotope scans, CT scans, and arteriograms are included. The author encourages the reader to individualize the treatment methods by presenting lists of indications and contraindications and a variety of applicable operative and nonoperative procedures. An exhaustive atlas of common, unusual, and rare foot disorders is included, along with a discussion of the clinical manifestations and the radiographic photomicrographic evidence of these conditions.

Dr. Wu also provides an extensive and up-to-date bibliography with each chapter, which allows the reader an opportunity for further study.

Written by a single author, *Surgery of the Foot* has the continuity and lack of contradiction and repetition that provides ease in reading. The discussion does not impose dogmatic plans of therapy on the reader, but rather presents a choice based on multiple factors to be assessed by the physician.

The book is the result of a tremendous amount of work to the advantage of potential patients, the physician reader, and to the credit of the author. The text, will take its place as a valuable addition to the understanding and care of the human foot and as an authoritative reference for the practitioner and the student.

Surgery of the Foot is dedicated to Dr. C. Leslie Mitchell and to the orthopaedic residents who have worked with Dr. Wu over the years. Dr. Mitchell was the revered Chief of Orthopaedics at the Henry Ford Hospital for many years and was an officer of a number of national orthopaedic organizations. He is rightfully ranked with the famous orthopaedic surgeons of our country, and remains a beloved member of the greater Detroit orthopaedic community and a cherished personal friend. Let us remember that we can see further because we stand on the shoulders of those who have preceded us!

William H. Blodgett, M.D.
Past President, American Orthopaedic Foot Society
Clinical Professor of Orthopaedic Surgery, Wayne State University School of Medicine
Detroit, Michigan

PREFACE

The importance of having strong and asymptomatic feet is vividly described by the old saying that when your feet hurt, you hurt all over. Unfortunately, foot pain is a common human suffering in industrialized societies, and formal training in the broad field of foot surgery is often inadequate in a significant number of orthopaedic residency programs. I was fortunate indeed to be trained by the internationally renowned orthopaedic surgeon Dr. C. Leslie Mitchell, who popularized the Mitchell's bunionectomy and had vast experience in the field of foot surgery. My good fortune was further enhanced by the timing of Dr. Mitchell's retirement from Henry Ford Hospital, which took place shortly before my return to the same institution from the U.S. Army. Having inherited Dr. Mitchell's busy foot-surgery practice, I was obliged to devote a large amount of time and energy to taking care of patients with foot problems, in addition to teaching orthopaedic residents at Henry Ford Hospital and medical students from University of Michigan Medical School, Wayne State University School of Medicine, and Michigan State University College of Medicine in the diagnosis and treatment of foot disorders. Having personally seen and treated tens of thousands of patients with various congenital and acquired foot problems and having performed thousands of foot operations at our medical center during the past 20 years, I have discovered some of the best methods of treating a vast variety of foot disorders that orthopaedic and podiatric surgeons enounter in their daily medical practice. For the sake of completeness, however, the incidence, clinical symptoms and signs, roentgenographic manifestations, pathologic anatomy, nonsurgical and surgical treatments of each foot disorder are discussed in detail in this book. In addition, the various surgical procedures available for treating each foot disorder are illustrated by detailed drawings, and my preferred surgical procedures are shown by series of drawings presented in a step-by-step manner. Furthermore, an extensive list of pertinent and up-to-date references is provided at the end of each chapter to give readers easy access to more detailed information if they so desire.

I give my sincere thanks to the many orthopaedic and podiatric surgeons from Michigan and neighboring states for referring many difficult and challenging cases to me. I am indebted to Drs. C. Leslie Mitchell, Harold M. Frost, Edwin R. Guise, and Henry H. Sprague for permitting me to use their personal cases in this book. I am grateful to Drs. Gerald Fine, Julius M. Ohorodnik, and Jacob Chason of the Department of Pathology, Henry Ford Hospital, for providing definitive tissue diagnoses of various foot diseases; and Drs. William R. Eyler, William A. Reynolds, and Roushdy S. Boulos from the Department of Radiology for the proper interpretation of many abnormal foot roentgenograms. I am also grateful to Jay Knipstein for his superb drawings, which are seen throughout this book, and to Walter Harlan and James Latif for making the numerous clinical, radiographic, and photomicrographic pictures. Finally, I am obliged to my secretary, Mrs. Justine Frankfurth, who not only tirelessly and meticulously typed the whole manuscript, but who also skillfully managed the office of my busy orthopaedic practice at the same time.

Kent K. Wu, M.D.

Detroit, Michigan

CONTENTS

Contents

1 GENERAL CONSIDERATIONS OF FOOT SURGERY

DIAGNOSIS OF FOOT PROBLEMS

History Taking

A. Biographic data: patient's age, sex, race, occupation, nationality.

B. Chief complaint: main reason for the patient's seeking medical attention.

C. History of present illness: date and mode of onset of symptom; its location, duration, and severity; relationship to other symptoms and activities; exacerbation and remission; previous medical and surgical treatments of present illness.

D. Past medical history: all past illnesses, operations, injuries, and medications.

E. Family history: determine whether the patient's blood relatives have the same disease; heredity may play a significant role in the pathogenesis of certain foot problems such as hallux valgus, flatfoot, tarsal coalition, clawfoot, clubfoot, and others.

F. System review: a thorough review of the past and present status of each body system may reveal the correct diagnosis and determine the proper method to employ in treating the patient's foot problem.

G. Social history: patient's psychologic status, expectations, secondary gain, law suit, or marital problems can materially influence the method of treatment to be adopted.

H. Personal habits: smoking, drinking, eating, sleeping, and use of narcotics and barbiturates should be noted.

I. Occupational history: exposure to irritating, toxic, and carcinogenic agents as well as physical and mental pressures of occupation may contribute to the patient's physical and psychologic problems.

General Inspection

A. Mental status: patient's state of alertness, orientation, and mentality should be carefully noted. Multiplicity of complaints, tension, nail biting, profuse sweating, emotional lability, apathy, restlessness, and

2   *Surgery of the Foot*

listlessness all suggest the presence of emotional disturbances.

B. Posture: abnormalities of the spine and extremities may give the examiner clues as to the true etiology of the foot problem.

C. Body movements: look for involuntary movements such as tics in tense and emotional persons; convulsive movement manifested by violent muscle contractions caused by epilepsy, uremia, and drug intoxication; and tremors brought about by alcohol intoxication, thyrotoxicosis, multiple sclerosis, parkinsonism, hysteria, and nervous tension.

D. Gait: pay attention to antalgic, ataxic, slapping, spastic, scissoring, and ahtetoid gaits, which may be the main cause of the patient's foot problem.

E. Shoes: note bulges, creases, and scuff marks of the shoe's upper and the wear and deformity of the sole and heel, which frequently can pinpoint the exact location of a particular foot problem.

F. Speech: certain defects in speech may be suggestive of neurologic impairment such as can occur after a stroke or in multiple sclerosis, two conditions that may have related foot problems.

G. General status of the body: obesity, cachexia, abnormal distribution of fat, body stature, and temperature should be noted.

Physical Examination

If the foot problem is in any way related to diseases of the knee, hip, back, and other parts of the body, the affected body part or system should be carefully evaluated in conjunction with the examination of the foot. Because the foot consists of skin, muscles, tendons, bones, joints, nerves, blood vessels, and lymphatics, a thorough examination of the foot

should include a careful evaluation of each of these structures.

A. Skin: look for edema, swelling, ecchymosis, petechiae, hair distribution, distention of cutaneous veins, redness, warmth, thickening and deformities of nails, and callosities.

B. Muscles and tendons: check the power, bulk, excursion, continuity, tenderness, swelling, fasciculation, and crepitation of the following muscle groups and their associated tendons:
1. Dorsiflexors of the toes: extensor hallucis longus, extensor digitorum longus and brevis, and lumbricals and interossei (proximal and distal interphalangeal joints) (PIP and DIP joints).
2. Plantar flexors of the toes: flexor hallucis longus, flexor digitorum longus, quadratus plantae, flexor digitorum brevis, flexor hallucis brevis, flexor digiti minimi brevis, and lumbricals and interossei (metatarsophalangeal joints) (M-P joints).
3. Adductors and abductors of toes: abductor hallucis, adductor hallucis, abductor digiti minimi, and interossei.
4. Plantar flexors of the foot: gastrocnemius, soleus, posterior tibialis, flexor digitorum longus, flexor hallucis longus, peroneus longus, peroneus brevis, and plantaris.
5. Dorsiflexors of the foot: tibialis anterior, extensor hallucis longus, extensor digitorum longus, and peroneus tertius.
6. Supinators of the foot: tibialis anterior, extensor hallucis longus, flexor hallucis longus, flexor digitorum longus, and tibialis posterior.
7. Pronators of the foot: peroneus longus, peroneus brevis, peroneus tertius, and extensor digitorum longus.

C. Bones: look for tenderness, overgrowths (exostoses), alignment, deformities, and crepitation of phalanges, sesamoids, metatarsals, and tarsals (cuneiforms, cuboid, navicular, calcaneus, and talus).

D. Joints: pay attention to alignments; tenderness; effusion; warmth; synovial thickening; instability; osteophyte formation; crepitation, and passive and active range of motion of I-P, M-P, tarsometatarsal, and intertarsal joints.

E. Nerves: evaluate sensation, motor function, deep tendon reflexes, pathologic reflexes, two-point discrimination, position and vibratory senses, as well as pattern of perspiration of the foot and the involved extremity or extremities.

F. Blood vessels and lymphatics: detect the pulse of the dorsalis pedis and posterior tibial arteries; assess skin temperature; watch for varicosity; red streaks of lymphangitis; enlarged regional lymph nodes; dilated superficial veins; swelling and cyanosis associated with venous thrombosis; redness, swelling, and heat associated with thrombophlebitis; and cold foot to palpation, blanch of foot on elevation, and red or reddish-purple discoloration of the foot on dependency in association with advanced arterial deficiency.

Roentgenographic Examination

At least three views of the foot (Anteroposterior, lateral, and oblique) should be employed. When indicated, special views such as the sesamoid view of the sesamoids of the great toe and axial views of the calcaneus to see the medial and posterior articulations of the subtalar joint should also be ordered. CT scan, bone scan, and arteriography are sometimes needed when the routine radiographs do not provide the information needed for diagnosis and treatment. Look for abnormalities of bones and joints and their surrounding soft tissue, and try to correlate the radiographic findings with those of the physical examination.

Laboratory Analysis

Because infectious, metabolic, inflammatory, and neoplastic diseases can also affect the foot, a selected group of laboratory studies can be valuable in confirming the diagnosis of the foot disorders. For examples, rheumatoid factor for rheumatoid arthritis, hyperuricemia for gout, typical electrophoretic pattern for myeloma, and identification of the bacterium that causes infection provide positive identifications of the various disease processes that can manifest themselves in the foot.

PRINCIPLES OF NONSURGICAL TREATMENT OF FOOT PROBLEMS

Like many other diseases, genetic and environmental factors are usually the causes of all foot problems. Because wearing improperly fitted shoes over a long period of time is responsible for a wide spectrum and the majority of foot problems encountered in clinical practice, obviously the most logical thing to do is to make the shoes fit the feet. Unfortunately, fashions, customs, ignorance, and social reasons (e.g., dress codes of some companies) prevent many people, particularly women, from wearing more physiologic shoes. As a matter of fact, many female patients with foot problems have complained to me that they have tried to buy comfortable shoes from many shoe stores and cannot find them because they simply do not carry comfortable women's shoes. A simple solution to their problems is to go to a men's shoe store where unisex and comfortable boys' shoes may be purchased, which will save them a substantial amount of money at the same time. Because shoes and their modifications, padding, and other foot devices are routinely employed in the treatment of various foot problems, a good knowledge of shoes and their modifications and the proper application of padding and foot devices to relieve pain are absolutely essential in the nonsurgical treatment of foot problems.

The Construction of the Shoe

The two main parts of a shoe (Figure 1–1) are the shoe's upper and the sole (with or

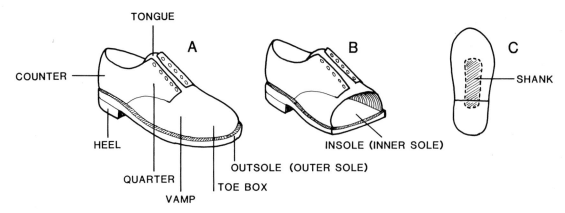

Figure 1-1. Various parts of a shoe.

without heel). The shoe's upper consists of the toe box (foremost part of the shoe that contains the toes), the vamp (the widest portion of a shoe immediately behind the toe box), the counter (the portion of shoe that surrounds the heel), the quarter (the portion of the shoe that is between the vamp and the counter), and the tongue (the tongue-like flap under the shoe lacing). The sole of the shoe includes the outsole (the outer sole in contact with the ground), the insole (the portion of the sole inside the shoe in contact with the plantar surface of the foot), the heel (the elevated portion of the sole that is under the calcaneus), and the shank (a steel or rigid plastic plate that extends from the heel into the sole to maintain rigidity and thus prevent deformity of the shoe).

A. Lasts: wooden models on which shoes are

fashioned (Figure 1-2). Consequently, lasts determine the sizes and shapes of the shoes to be produced. A list of different last shoes follows.

1. Regular (conventional) last: most commonly worn shoe in which the anterior one half of the shoe shows a slight medial deviation.
2. Straight last: anterior one half of the shoe shows neither medial nor lateral deviation.
3. Reverse (out-flare) last: anterior one half of the shoe shows a lateral deviation, like putting a shoe on the wrong foot.
4. Inflare last: anterior one half of the shoe shows a significant medial deviation.
5. Combination last: shoe that does not conform to the standard length and width measurements of regular shoes. For example, a person with a narrow

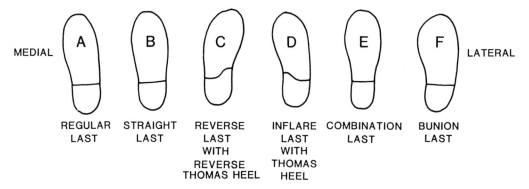

Figure 1-2. Various last shoes.

heel and wide forefoot needs a pair of combination last shoes to accommodate their feet.

6. Bunion last: anterior one half of the shoe is more roomy and has a medial enlargement to accommodate the bony prominence of the first metatarsal head (the bunion).

B. Sizing: width of a shoe increases circumferentially at the ball by 6.4 mm per one full size increase (e.g., A to B), and each size increase is equal to 8.4-mm increase in length (e.g., 7 to 8).

Narrowest   Width of shoes   Widest

AAA
$$\frac{A\ B\ C\ D\ E}{\text{Increasing width}}$$
EEE

$$\frac{\text{Length of shoes}}{5\ 6\ 7\ 8\ 9\ 10\ 11\ 12\ 13}$$
Increasing length

Alterations of the Shoe

A. Modifications of the heel (Figure 1–3) include:

1. Thomas heel: a 12.7-mm advancement of the anteromedial aspect of the heel that helps to invert the calcaneus and to support the longitudinal arch.
2. Reverse Thomas heel: a 12.7-mm advancement on the anterolateral aspect of the heel that helps to evert the calcaneus and to support the lateral border of the foot.
3. Flare heel: bottom of the heel in contact with the ground is wider than the top of the heel, which is in contact with the posterior portion of the sole. Flare heel increases the base of support and tends to decrease stress on the heel, ankle, and subtalar joints.
4. Sponge rubber heel: elastic and shock-absorbing nature helps to decrease stress on the heel, ankle, and subtalar joints, and tends to assist plantar flexion of the foot during walking.

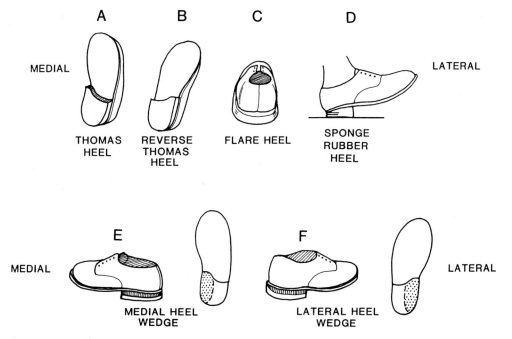

Figure 1–3. Different modifications of the heel.

5. Medial heel wedge: a 3.2-mm to 6.4-mm wedge inserted between the sole and the heel along their common medial border to invert the calcaneus under the talus.
6. Lateral heel wedge: a 3.2-mm to 6.4-mm wedge inserted between the sole and the heel along their common lateral border to evert the calcaneus under the talus.

B. Modifications of the sole (outsole) (Figure 1–4) follow:
1. Metatarsal bar: straight or curved bar fixed to the sole to shift weight from the metatarsal heads to their necks and shafts.
2. Ripple sole: rubber sole with transverse, parallel, and wave-like ridges built into the entire bottom surface of the sole. These ridges become deformed on weight-bearing and thus relieve stress on the foot.
3. Elongated shank: stiff and long shank that extends from the heel to the toe box to provide rigidity for the outsole.
4. Rocker sole: anterior portion of the outsole has a rocker-bottom configuration that limits weight-bearing in the forepart of the foot and facilitates plantar flexion of the foot during walking, especially in patients with a stiff or fused ankle joint.
5. Medial sole wedge: a 3.2-mm to 4.8-mm wedge inserted into the anteromedial border of the sole to invert the forefoot and to shift weight to the lateral border of the sole.
6. Lateral sole wedge: a 3.2-mm to 4.8-mm wedge inserted into the anterola-

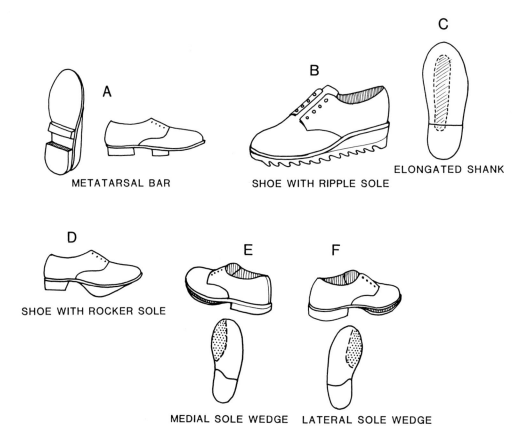

METATARSAL BAR   SHOE WITH RIPPLE SOLE   ELONGATED SHANK

SHOE WITH ROCKER SOLE

MEDIAL SOLE WEDGE   LATERAL SOLE WEDGE

Figure 1–4. Different modifications of the sole.

teral border of the sole to evert the forefoot and to shift weight to the medial border of the sole.

C. Modifications of the insole (Figure 1–5) follow:

1. Metatarsal pads (Figure 1–5A and B): commercially available triangular pads with a flat surface on one side and a convex surface on the other. They can be glued to the forepart of the insole to shift weight from the painful metatarsal heads to the asymptomatic metatarsal necks and shafts.

2. Longitudinal arch pads (Figure 1–5C and D): commercially available triangular pads with a flat surface on one side and a bulge on the other. They can be glued to the midportion along the medial border of the insole under the longitudinal arch of the foot.

3. Shoe inserts with built-in arch support and metatarsal pad (Figure 1–5E and F): commercially available shoe inserts intended to provide arch support and relief of painful stress on the metatarsal heads.

NOTE: Although the aforementioned metatarsal pads, longitudinal arch pads, and shoe inserts with built-in arch support and metatarsal pad are inexpensive and readily available, they are not effective in relieving stressful foot symptoms due to the tremendous biologic variations of patients with foot problems that demand individual attention instead of the assembly line-type of remedy.

4. Custom-made arch supports molded from casts of patients' feet:

a. Rigid arch supports (Figure 1–6A–E). Although Whitman and Shaffer plates made of stainless steel and hard plastic inserts made of heat-molded plastics and thermoplastics are more effective in relieving pain than the commercially stocked arch supports, they are not as desirable as the lighter, more comfortable, and more precisely molded semi-rigid and soft arch supports.

b. Semi-rigid and soft arch supports (Figure 1–6F–I). These devices are made of rubber, cork, leather, and polyethylene foam (plastazote) in various combinations. The softness of polyethylene foam allows it to be molded precisely to conform to both major and minor deformities of the foot. The use of these total contact plastazote shoe inserts can be significantly prolonged by incorporating cork-rubber into their under surfaces. Because semi-rigid and soft arch supports are 6.4 mm or more in thickness, extra-depth shoes or custom-molded (space) shoes (Figure 1–7A–C) are needed to accommodate these arch supports.

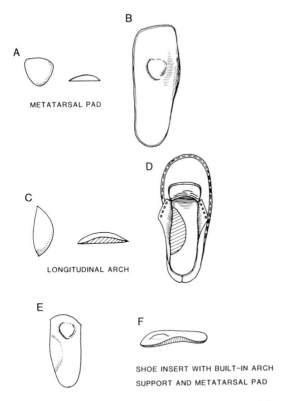

Figure 1–5. Various modifications of the insole and **B,** use of a metatarsal pad. **C** and **D,** application of a longitudinal arch pad. **E** and **F,** a commercially available shoe insert with built-in arch support and metatarsal pad.

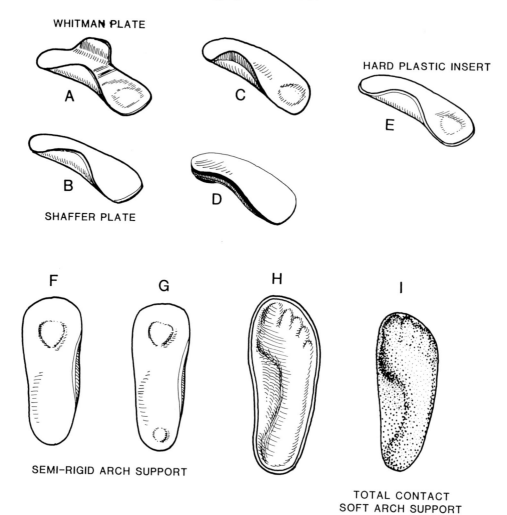

WHITMAN PLATE

HARD PLASTIC INSERT

SHAFFER PLATE

SEMI-RIGID ARCH SUPPORT

TOTAL CONTACT
SOFT ARCH SUPPORT

Figure 1–6. Custom-made rigid, semi-rigid, and soft arch supports. **A–E,** a Whitman plate, a Shaffer plate, and three hard-plastic shoe inserts. **F,** a semi-rigid arch support with a bulge proximal to the metatarsal heads to relieve metatarsalgia. **G,** another semi-rigid arch support with a metatarsal bulge to relieve metatarsalgia and a depression in the heel region to relieve a painful heel. **H** and **I,** two total contact soft arch supports made of plastazote, the useful life of which can be significantly prolonged by incorporating cork-rubber into their under surfaces.

D. Padding: used to shift weight-bearing stresses from painful, open, infected, draining, and hypersensitive areas to painless and relatively healthy areas; to maximize the total weight-bearing area so to minimize the pressure per unit area; to separate painful areas that make contact (e.g., painful interdigital clavus); to provide passive structural support during weight-bearing (e.g., arch support); and to enable deformed parts of the foot to contribute to their weight-bearing function (e.g., hammered and clawed toes). Practically speaking, the padding material should be inexpensive, readily available, durable, and easy to use. I have found the 6.4-mm adhesive-backed sponge rubber, which contains numerous enclosed air bubbles and is resistant to permanent deformity with use, ideal for padding purposes. These sponge rubber pads can be applied directly to the foot or to the shoe.

1. Direct application of sponge rubber pads to the foot (Figure 1–8): method of

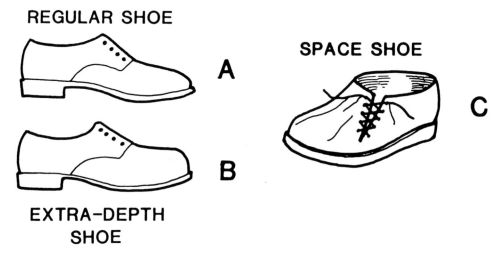

REGULAR SHOE

A

B

EXTRA-DEPTH SHOE

SPACE SHOE

C

Figure 1–7. **A,** a regular shoe; **B,** an extra-depth shoe; **C,** a custom-molded (space) shoe. Note that the extra-depth shoe and the space shoe are more roomy in the foreparts of the shoes than the regular shoe.

padding that is easy to do and can be accurately applied to the painful areas of the foot. An adherent such as compound tincture of benzoin should be painted on the foot before the pad is applied. In addition, cloth adhesive tape is usually used to hold the pad in its proper position. Disadvantages of this method include the possibility of causing an allergic reaction and maceration of the skin, difficulty in maintaining proper hygiene of the padded foot, and the need for more frequent reapplication of the pad because of its separation from the foot. Figure 1–8 shows areas where pads have been applied to the foot to treat various painful foot problems.

2. Direct application of sponge rubber pads to the shoes (Figures 1–9—1–11): a method of padding that is more time-consuming and less precise than the direct application of pads to the foot because the foot moves in the shoe during walking and the shoe can become deformed on weight-bearing or with time, decreasing the pressure-relieving function of the pads glued to the shoes. Pads applied to the shoes, however, tend to be long-lasting, do not

usually cause skin problems, and do not interfere with hygiene. Figures 1–9 to 1–11 show the various ways of applying sponge rubber pads to the shoes to relieve pain associated with certain foot problems.

NOTE: A large, 6.4-mm sponge rubber pad takes up quite a bit of room in a shoe. Therefore, before a full-length pad is applied, a shoe one size longer and two sizes wider (e.g., going from 8B to 9D) is often required to accommodate both the sponge rubber pad and the foot.

E. Office procedures to modify shoes. Many painful foot problems can be relieved by modifying the shoes with the use of three simple and inexpensive instruments: a shoemaker's swan, a scalpel, and a coffeepot (or teapot).

1. Stretching the shoe's upper to accommodate painful forefoot sites (Figure 1–12A—D): portion of shoe leather to be stretched should first be softened by holding it close to the spout of a steaming tea- or coffeepot. When the leather is sufficiently softened, the shoemaker's swan is used to stretch the involved area to the desired dimen-

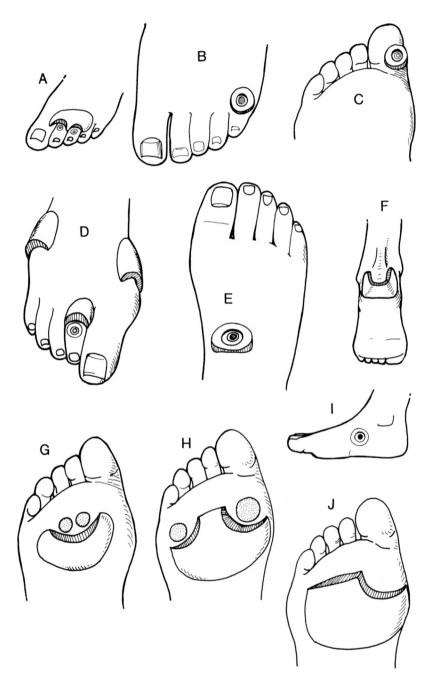

Figure 1–8. Direct application of pads to the foot to relieve various painful foot problems. **A,** corns on the dorsal aspect of the second and third toes; **B,** corn on the dorsolateral aspect of the fifth toe; **C,** corn on the medioplantar aspect of the great toe; **D,** corn on the dorsal aspect of the second toe and painful bunion and bunionette; **E,** painful callosity over the tarsometatarsal exostosis; **F,** painful pump bump; **G,** callosities under the second and third metatarsal heads; **H,** callosities under the medial sesamoid and fifth metatarsal head; **I,** callosity over the accessory navicular (prehallux deformity); **J,** padding for hallux rigidus.

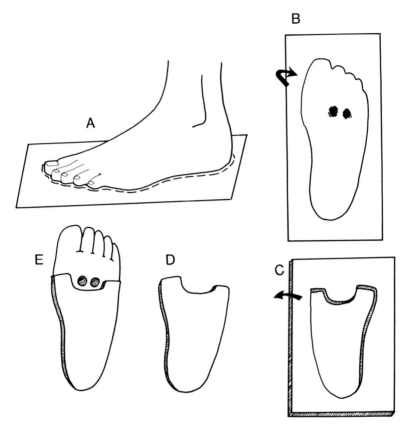

Figure 1–9. Steps taken when making a sponge rubber pad for the shoe to relieve a particular, painful foot problem. **A,** after painful callosities have been painted with lipstick, the patient stands on a piece of drawing paper. The outline of the foot is then traced. **B,** the footprint is cut out and a relief area is cut from the lipstick-stained area. The resulting paper template is inserted into the shoe to ensure a proper fit. **C,** the paper template is turned 180° and is traced on the wax paper of the adhesive-backed rubber sponge sheet. **D,** cut out sponge rubber pad with adherent wax paper. **E,** sponge rubber pad is placed on the sole of the foot to ensure that it provides relief in the painful area.

sions to accommodate the deformed toes or other parts of the foot. Shoe stretching is fairly effective in relieving pain of a symptomatic bunion, corns on the dorsal aspect of the PIP joints or hammer toes and claw toes, bunionette, corns on the dorsolateral aspect of the PIP joint of the fifth toe, dorsal exostoses of the first metatarsal head, and the like. If the shoemaker's swan is not available, the same objectives can also be achieved by making cruciate cuts in the vamp and toe box to relieve shoe pressure on the underlying painful parts of the foot (Figure 1–13A—B). When these same painful areas become open or infected, the shoe leather over them should be removed with a scalpel to eliminate all pressure and to facilitate the care of these open wounds (Figure 1–13C).

2. Modification of the shoe counter to relieve painful retrocalcaneal bursitis (pump bump) (Figure 1–14): a U-shaped cut can be made with a scalpel in the posterior aspect of the counter to remove pressure from the symptomatic pump bump. To prevent separation of the posterior seam, the margins of the cut should be stitched either by a shoe repair shop or a brace shop.

3. Making a postoperative shoe (Figure 1–

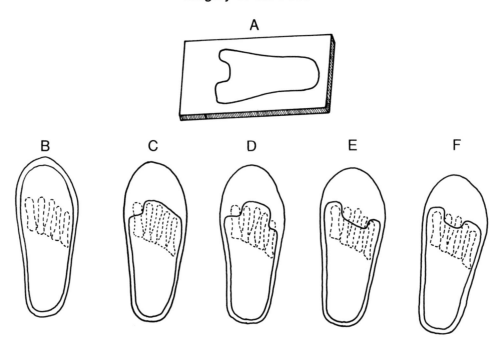

Figure 1–10. Different sponge rubber pads applied to the insoles of shoes to relieve pain associated with various foot problems. **A,** outline of a predetermined sponge rubber pad traced on a sponge rubber sheet. **B,** complete sole insert to relieve pain in multiple areas on the sole of the foot. **C,** insert for relief of sesamoiditis and hallux rigidus. **D,** insert for relief of metatarsalgia of the first and the fifth metatarsal head regions. **E,** insert for relief of pain of the three middle metatarsal heads. **F,** insert to relieve metatarsalgia of the second and third metatarsal head regions.

15): a wide variety of shoes to be worn after forefoot surgery can be made by removing the anterior portion of the vamp and the entire toe box of an old shoe and then splitting the entire tongue longitudinally at its midline. If the surgery is confined to the fifth metatarsal head and toe, only a portion of the lateral aspect of the vamp and the toe box needs to be removed.

4. Modification of the shoe to accommodate a swollen foot: the upper of an old shoe is split longitudinally from its tongue to the toe box along its midline (Figure 1–13D).

F. Commercially available devices. A great variety of the so-called foot aids is available in drug stores, department stores, supermarkets, and discount houses. The advantages of these foot devices are that they are readily available; easy to use, with pictures and instructions printed on the wrapping materials and packages; usually low in price; and relatively free of serious complications associated with their usage. The drawbacks of these foot aids include their limited and temporary relief of painful foot problems; inability to meet the tremendous biologic and pathologic variations of the affected feet; and difficulties in fitting into a patient's regular shoes, especially when the foot devices are bulky. A select list of commercially available foot devices follows.

1. Corn and callosity pads (Figure 1–16): donut-shaped and adhesive-backed pads of different sizes that can be applied directly over painful corns and callosities.

2. Hallux valgus splint, arch cuff, latex bunion shield, and plastic heel cup (Figure 1–17): hallux valgus splint (Figure 1–17A) adducts the great toe and is used as a postoperative hallux valgus night splint. Arch cuff (Figure

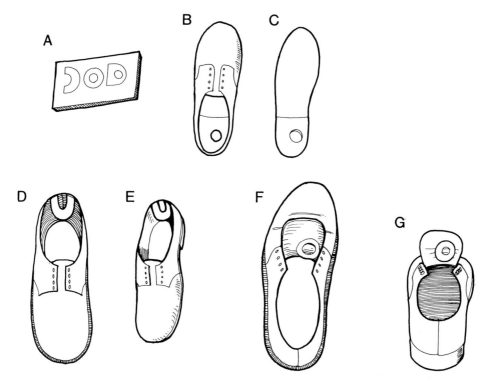

Figure 1–11. Different sponge rubber pads that can be glued to various parts of a shoe to provide pain relief. **A,** three different sponge rubber pads traced on a sponge rubber sheet. **B** and **C,** sponge rubber heel pad to relieve pain from a calcaneal spur or plantar fasciitis. **D** and **E,** U-shaped sponge rubber pad glued to the inner surface of the counter of a shoe to provide pain relief for a symptomatic pump bump. **F** and **G,** donut-shaped sponge rubber pad applied to the tongue of a shoe to relieve the pain caused by a tarsometatarsal exostosis.

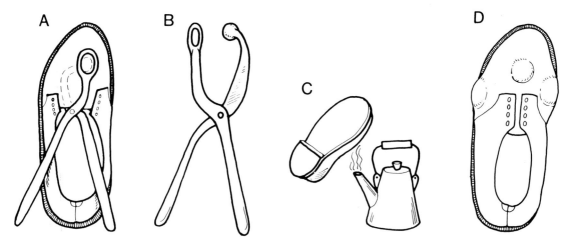

Figure 1–12. Stretching of the upper portion of the shoe with a shoemaker's swan. **A,** midportion of the toe box is stretched by using a shoemaker's swan to accommodate a hammer toe with a painful corn over the dorsal aspect of its PIP joint. **B,** shoemaker's swan. **C,** shoe leather is softened by steam from a teapot in preparation for stretching with a shoemaker's swan. **D,** left shoe with its upper already stretched for symptomatic relief of a bunionette (left), hammer toe (middle), and bunion (right).

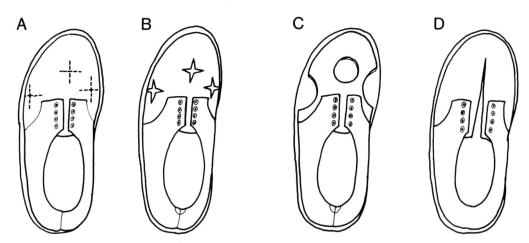

Figure 1–13. **A** and **B,** cruciate cuts made in the vamp and toe box of a shoe to accommodate symptomatic bunionette, corns, and bunion. **C,** leather was cut out to accommodate open, infected, or draining bunionette, corns, and bunion. **D,** tongue, vamp, and the toe box of a shoe can also be split longitudinally to accommodate a swollen foot.

1–17B and C) consists of a metatarsal pad imbedded in a complete cuff of elastic webbing and is used in the relief of metatarsalgia. Latex bunion shield (Figure 1–17D) acts as a bumper to protect the enlarged and painful first metartarsal head (the bunion). Heel cup (Figure 1–17E) reduces the amount of flattening of the heel pad on weight-bearing and can provide pain relief from calcaneal spur and plantar fasciitis.

3. Latex hammer toe shield, adhesive-backed foam strips, toe crest, toecaps, and hammer toe shield with callosity cushion (Figure 1–18): latex hammer toe shield (Figure 1–18A) has two relief pads situated immediately proximal and distal to the painful corn over the dorsal aspect of the PIP joint, thus protecting the painful corn from shoe pressure. Adhesive-backed foam strips (Figure 1–18B) can be applied directly over painful corns or bursae to act as pain relief pads. A toe crest (Figure 1–18C) enables hammer toes to function more effectively by providing a fulcrum, thus reducing pressure on the metatarsal heads and the tips of the corresponding toes. Toe caps, (Figure 1–18D) completely cover the toes and are used for symptomatic pain relief of ingrown toenails and painful corns. A hammer toe shield (Figure 1–18E) with callosity cushion has two elastic slings that hold the hammer toes down and a foam cushion that pads the painful

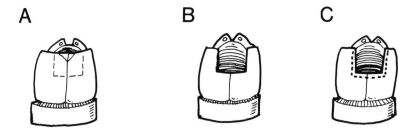

Figure 1–14. Modification of the shoe counter to relieve pain from pump bump. **A,** portion of the shoe counter to be removed is marked. **B,** marked portion is removed. **C,** margins of the U-shaped cut are stitched to prevent separation of the posterior seam.

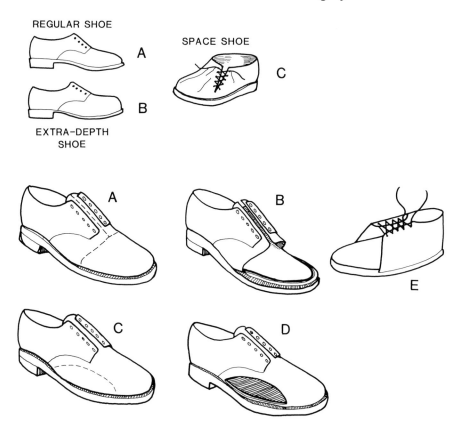

Figure 1–15. Steps taken to make a shoe to be worn postoperatively. **A,** a T-shaped incision is marked across the vamp and the central portion of the tongue. **B,** office-made postoperative shoe with all the toes exposed. The longitudinal split in the tongue accommodates foot swelling. **C,** a curved incision mark is made on the lateral aspect of the upper portion of the shoe. **D,** with the marked portion removed, the shoe is ready to be worn after bunionette or fifth toe surgery. **E,** commercially available postoperative shoe.

metatarsal heads that frequently accompany hammer toes.

4. Toe separator comb, class ring-shaped hammer toe shields, and individual toe separator (Figure 1–19): toe separator combs (Figure 1–19A) keep the toes separated and are useful in relieving painful interdigital soft corns and symptomatic overlapping and underlapping toes. Class ring-shaped hammer toe shields (Figure 1–19B and D) have slings to go around the toes and to prevent the shoes from rubbing against the painful corns of the dorsal aspects of the hammer toes. Individual toe separators (Figure 1–19C) hold the two

adjacent toes apart and are helpful in treating painful interdigital corns.

TYPICAL LOCATIONS OF FOOT PROBLEMS

Because most painful foot problems are caused by the interactions between improperly fitted shoes and the various anatomic structures of the foot, their locations are typical and predictable (Figure 1–20). A list of typical sites of painful foot problems follows.

A. Dorsal callosities: over the dorsal aspect of the PIP joints of the second and third toes and the dorsolateral aspect of the PIP joint of the fifth toe.

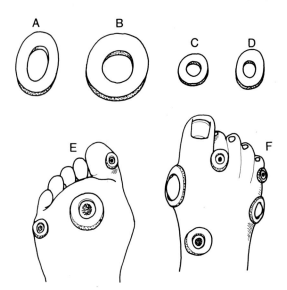

B. Bunion: dorsomedial aspect of the first metatarsal head.

C. Exostosis: dorsal aspect of the first metatarsal head and the tarsometatarsal joint.

D. Hammer toe: second toe.

E. Curling toe: third and fifth toes.

F. Overlapping toe: second and fifth toes.

G. Soft corn: fourth webspace.

H. Morton's neuroma: proximal to the third webspace.

I. Bunionette (tailor's bunion): dorsolateral aspect of the fifth metatarsal head.

J. Freiberg's disease: second metatarsal head.

Figure 1–16. Corn and callosity pads of various sizes can be used to relieve pain from corns on dorsal aspects of toes, bunion, bunionette, plantar callosities, and tarsometatarsal exostosis.

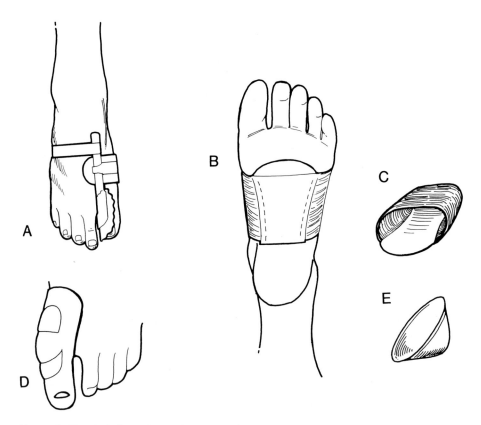

Figure 1–17. A, hallux valgus splint; **B** and **C,** arch cuff; **D,** latex bunion shield; **E,** heel cup.

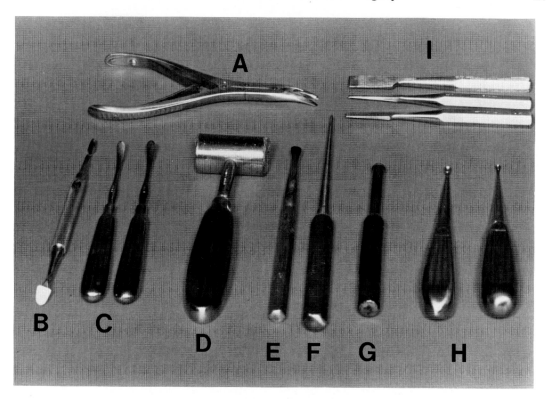

Figure 1–21. Instruments for use during foot surgery. **A,** rongeur; **B,** bone rasp; **C,** joker retractors; **D,** mallet; **E,** small periosteal elevator; **F,** bone awl; **G,** bone impactor; **H,** curets; **I,** Micro-osteotomes.

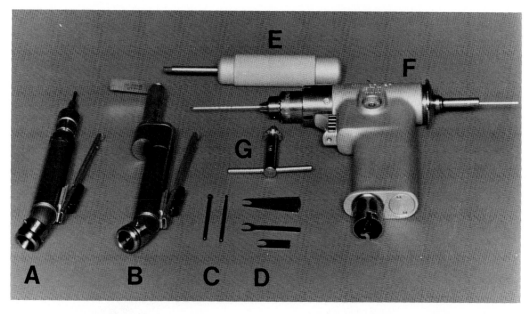

Figure 1–22. Air-powered instruments for use during foot surgery. **A,** air-powered bur; **B,** microsaw equipped with blade; **C,** two different burs; **D,** microsaw blades; **E,** wrench for tightening or loosening the microsaw blades; **F,** drill fitted with a K-wire; **G,** Jacob chuck key.

use of a microsaw is awkward, danger-ous, and impractical.

F. Air-powered burs: useful in removing ar-ticular cartilage, making slots for receiving bone grafts in performing arthrodesis pro-cedures, and grinding off unwanted bone.

SKIN INCISIONS OF FOOT SURGERY

The skin incisions in the dorsal, lateral, me-dial, and plantar aspects of the foot are illus-trated in Figure 1–23.

A. Tendons of the extensor hallucis longus and brevis, the base of the proximal pha-lanx and M-P joint of the great toe, and the distal portion of the first metatarsal. Typical use: bunion operations.

B. Lateral aspects of the base of the proxi-mal phalanx, the M-P joint, and the distal portion of the metatarsal of the great toe; conjoined tendon of the flexor hallucis brevis and adductor hallucis; the lateral sesamoid; the base of the proximal pha-

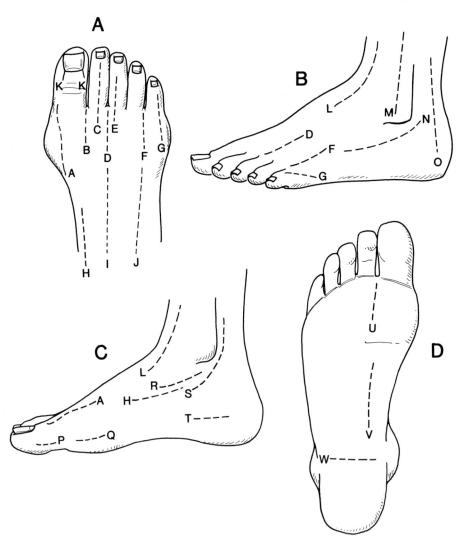

Figure 1–23. Various skin incisions. **A,** on the dorsal aspect; **B,** on the lateral aspect; **C,** on the medial aspect; **D,** on the plantar aspect.

lanx, the M-P joint, and the tendons of the extensor digitorum longus and brevis of the second toe; and the distal portion of the second metatarsal. Typical use: release of a conjoined tendon of the adductor hallucis and flexor hallucis brevis, and lateral sesamoidectomy in McBride's bunionectomy.

C. Distal, middle, and proximal phalanges and the tendons of the extensor digitorum longus and brevis of the second toe; the DIP, PIP, and M-P joints of the second toe; and the distal portion of the second metatarsal. Typical use: arthrodesis of the DIP and PIP joints, Z-plasty of the extensor tendon, and capsulotomy of the M-P joint.

D. M-P joints, the tendons of the extensor hallucis longus and brevis, and the bases of the proximal phalanges of the second and third toes; and the distal portions of the second and third metatarsals. Typical use: resection of the M-P joints of the second and third toes in rheumatoid arthritis.

E. M-P and PIP joints, the proximal phalanx, the base of the middle phalanx, and the tendons of the extensor digitorum longus and brevis of the third toe; the head and neck of the third metatarsal. Typical use: arthrodesis of the PIP joint, capsulotomy of the M-P joint, and Z-plasty of the extensor tendon.

F. M-P joints, the tendons of the extensor hallucis longus and brevis, and the base of the proximal phalanges of the fourth and fifth toes; and the distal portions of the fourth and fifth metatarsals. Typical use: resection of the M-P joints of the fourth and fifth toes in rheumatoid arthritis, and excision of Morton's neuroma.

G. Proximal phalanx, the M-P and PIP joints, the base of the middle phalanx, and the tendons of the extensor digitorum longus and brevis of the fifth toe; and the head and neck of the fifth metatarsal. Typical use: proximal phalangectomy of the fifth toe and excision of tailor's bunion.

H. Base of the first metatarsal; the first metatarsocuneiform, naviculocuneiform, and talonavicular joints; the first cuneiform; the navicular; the head of the talus; and the tendons of the extensor hallucis longus and tibialis anterior. Typical use: exostectomy of the first metatarsocuneiform joint and fusion of the medial aspect of the talonavicular joint in triple arthrodesis.

I. Proximal portions of the second and third metatarsals, the tendons of the extensor digitorum longus, the dorsal interosseous muscles, the second and third metatarsocuneiform and naviculocuneiform joints, and the second and third cuneiforms. Typical use: open reduction of fracture of the second and third metatarsals or dislocation of the second and third tarsometatarsal joints in Lisfranc's dislocation.

J. Proximal portions of the fourth and fifth metatarsals; the dorsal interosseous muscles; the tendons of the extensor digitorum longus, peroneus tertius, peroneus brevis, and extensor hallucis brevis; the metatarsocuboid joints; and the cuboid bone. Typical use: open reduction of fracture of the fourth and fifth metatarsals or dislocation of the metatarsocuboid joints in Lisfranc's dislocation.

K. Nail and nailbed of the great toe. Typical use: treatment of ingrown toenail.

L. Tendons of the extensor hallucis longus and extensor digitorum longus, the dorsalis pedis artery, and the anterior aspect of ankle joint. Typical use: exposure of the anterior aspect of the ankle joint.

M. Distal portion of the fibula and lateral malleolus. Typical use: open reduction of fracture of the lateral malleolus.

N. Tendons of the peroneus longus and brevis; the lateral aspect of the talus, calcaneus, and navicular; the superior surface of the cuboid; the posterior talocalcaneal joint; the calcaneocuboid joint, and the lateral aspect of the talonavicular joint; the sinus tarsi; and the extensor digitorum brevis. Typical use: triple arthrodesis.

O. Calcaneal tendon, the tendon of the peroneus longus and brevis, and the posterolateral aspect of the calcaneus. Typical use: excision of pump bump and lengthening of the calcaneal tendon.

P. Medial aspect of the base of the distal phalanx and DIP of the great toe. Typical use: exostectomy of the medioplantar base of the distal phalanx of the great toe.

Q. Medial tendon of the flexor hallucis brevis, the medial sesamoid, the medial sesamoidometatarsal joint, and the medio-inferior aspect of the M-P joint of the great toe. Typical use: medial sesamoidectomy.

R. Medial subtalar joint, the sustentaculum tali, and the medio-inferior aspect of the head of the talus. Typical use: exposure of the medial talocalcaneal joint and open reduction of fracture of the calcaneus.

S. Tarsal tunnel and all its contents, which include the flexor retinaculum (laciniate ligament); the tendons of the posterior tibialis, flexor digitorum longus, and flexor hallucis longus, the posterior tibial artery and vein; and the posterior tibial nerve. Typical use: tarsal tunnel release.

T. Medio-inferior aspect of the calcaneus; origins of the plantar fascia, abductor hallucis, flexor digitorum brevis, and abductor digiti quinti. Typical use: release of plantar fascia and excision of a calcaneal spur.

U. Lateral sesamoid and conjoined tendons of the adductor hallucis and flexor hallucis brevis. Typical use: excision of hypertrophied and degenerative lateral sesamoid.

V. Plantar fascia. Typical use: excision of plantar fibromatosis.

W. Inferior aspect of the calcaneus; and the origins of the plantar fascia, abductor hallucis, flexor digitorum brevis, and abductor digiti quinti. Typical use: release of origins of the plantar fascia, abductor hallucis, flexor digitorum brevis, and abductor digiti quinti; and excision of a painful calcaneal spur.

REFERENCES

1. Action, R.K.: Surgical anatomy of the foot. J. Bone Joint Surg. [Am], *49:*555, 1967.
2. American Academy of Orthopaedic Surgeons: Joint Motion. Method of Measuring and Recording. American Academy Chicago, Orthopaedic Surgeons, 1965.
3. Baker, L.D.: The foot and ankle—symptoms, pathology and diagnosis. Instr. Course Lect., *3:*8, 1947.
4. Bankart, A.S.B.: The treatment of minor maladies of the foot. Lancet, *1:*249, 1935.
5. Banks, S.W., and Laufman, H.: An Atlas of Surgical Exposures of the Extremities. Philadelphia, W.B. Saunders, 1953.
6. Basmajian, J.R., and Stecko, G.: The role of muscles in arch support of the foot. J. Bone Joint Surg. [Am.], *45:*1184, 1963.
7. Bateman, J.E.: Pitfalls in foot surgery. Orthop. Clin. North Am., *7:*751, 1976.
8. Bateman, J.E.: Foot Science. Philadelphia, W.B. Saunders, 1976.
9. Bizarro, A.H.: On sesamoid and supernumerary bones of the limbs. J. Anat., *55:*256, 1921.
10. Bojsen-Moller, F.: Anatomy of forefoot, normal and pathologic. Clin. Orthop., *142:*10, 1979.
11. Bruce, J., and Walmsley, R.: Some observations on the arches of the foot and flat foot. Lancet, *2:*656, 1938.
12. Carleton, F.J.: Shoes and Feet. West Chester, PA, Charles H. Andress, 1940.
13. Dickson, F.D., and Diveley, R.L.: Functional Disorders of the Foot. 3rd Ed. Philadelphia, J.B. Lippincott, 1953.
14. Diveley, R.L.: Foot appliances and shoe alterations. *In* American Academy of Orthopaedic Surgeons: Orthopaedic Appliances Atlas. Vol. 1, Ann Arbor, J.W. Edwards, 1952, pp. 439–478.
15. Dwight, T.: A Clinical Atlas: Variations of the Bones of the Hands and Feet. Philadelphia, J.B. Lippincott, 1907.
16. Ehrlich, M.G.: Foot disorders in infants and children. Curr. Probl. Pediatr., *4:*3, 1974.
17. Elftman, H.: A cinematic study of the distribution of

pressure in the human foot. Anat. Rec., *59:*481, 1934.

18. Ellis, T.S.: The Human Foot: Its Form and Structure, Functions and Clothing. London, J. & A. Churchill, 1889.
19. Freiberger, R.H., Hersh, A., and Harrison, M.O.: Roentgen examination of the deformed foot. Semin. Roentgenol., *5:*341, 1970.
20. Gamble, F.O., and Yale, I.: Clinical Roentgenology of the Foot. Baltimore, Williams & Wilkins, 1966.
21. Gardner, E., Gray, D.J., and O'Rahilly, R.: The prenatal development of the skeleton and joints of the human foot. J. Bone Joint Surg. [Am.], *41:*847, 1959.
22. Giannestras, N.J. (ed.): Static deformities of the foot. Clin. Orthop., *70:*1, 1970.
23. Giannestras, N.J.: Foot Disorders. 2nd Ed., Philadelphia, Lea & Febiger, 1973.
24. Goldstein, L.A., and Dickerson, R.C.: Atlas of Orthopaedic Surgery. St. Louis, C.V. Mosby, 1974.
25. Grundy, M., Tosh, P. A., McLeish, R.D., and Smidt, L.: An investigaton of the centres of pressure under the foot during walking. J. Bone Joint Surg. [Br.], *57:*98, 1975.
26. Harty, M.: The position of the foot in walking. Lancet, *2:*275, 1953.
27. Hauser, E.D.W.: Diseases of the Foot. Philadelphia, W.B. Saunders, 1939.
28. Hanorth, B.: Dynamic posture in relation to the foot. Clin. Orthop., *16:*74, 1960.
29. Henry, A.K.: Extensive Exposure. 2nd Ed. Baltimore, Williams & Wilkins, 1957.
30. Hertzman, C.A.: Use of plastazote in foot disabilities. Am. J. Phys. Med., *52:*289, 1973.
31. Hicks, J.H.: The mechanics of the foot. I. The joints. J. Anat., *87:*345, 1953.
32. Hicks, J.H.: The mechanics of the foot. II. The plantar aponeurosis and the arch. J. Anat., *88:*25, 1954.
33. Hiss, J.H.: Functional foot disorders. Los Angeles, Los Angeles University Press, 1937.
34. Hoerr, N.D., Pyle, S.L., and Francis, C.C.: Radiographic Atlas of Skeletal Development of the Foot and Ankle. Springfield, IL, Charles C Thomas, 1962.
35. Hoffmann, P.: Conclusions drawn from comparative study of the feet of barefooted and shoe-wearing people. Am. J. Orthop. Surg., *3:*105, 1905.
36. Hutton, W.C., and Dhanendran, M.: A study of the distribution of load under normal foot during walking. Int. Orthop., *3:*153, 1979.
37. Jahss, M.H.: Shoes and Shoe Modifications. *In* American Academy of Orthopaedic Surgeons: Atlas of Orthotics. Biomechanical Principles and Application. St. Louis, C.V. Mosby, 1975, pp. 267–279.
38. Jahss, M.H.: Disorders of the Foot. Philadelphia, W.B. Saunders, 1982.
39. Johnston, O.: Further studies of the inheritance of hand and foot anomalies. Clin. Orthop., *8:*146, 1956.
40. Jones, F.W.: Structure and Function as Seen In the Foot. 2nd Ed., London, Tindall & Cox, 1949.
41. Kaplan, E.B.: Surgical approach to the plantar digital nerves. Bull. Hosp. Jt. Dis. Orthop. Inst. *11:*96, 1950.
42. Kelikian, H.: Hallux Valgus, Allied Deformities of the Forefoot and Metatarsalgia. Philadelphia, W.B. Saunders, 1965.
43. Klenerman, L.: The Foot and Its Disorders. London, Blackwell Scientific Publications, 1976.
44. Lake, N.: The Foot. London, Tindall & Cox, 1952.

45. Lam, S.F., and Hodgson, A.R.: A comparison of foot forms among the non-shoe and shoe-wearing Chinese population. J. Bone Joint Surg. [Am.], *40:*1058, 1958.
46. Lambrinudi, C.: Discussion on painful feet. Proc. R. Soc. Lond. [Med.], *36:*47, 1942.
47. Lewin, P.: The Foot and Ankle. Philadelphia, Lea & Febiger, 1959.
48. Lovell, W.W., and Winter, R.: Pediatric Orthopaedics. Philadelphia, J.B. Lippincott, 1978.
49. Mann, R.A.: Biomechanics of the foot. *In* Atlas of Orthotics: Biomechanical Principles and Application. Edited by American Academy of Orthopaedic Surgeons. St. Louis, C.V. Mosby, 1975.
50. Mann, R.A. (ed.): Duvries' Surgery of Foot. 4th Ed. St. Louis, C.V. Mosby, 1978.
51. McMahan, J., and Schwab, D.: Shoes and Modifications for Pedorthic Practice. Atlanta, Rapid Printers, 1975.
52. Milgram, J.E.: Office measures for relief of the painful foot. J. Bone Joint Surg. [Am.], *46:*1095, 1964.
53. Miller, W.E.: Operative incision involving the foot. Orthop. Clin. North Am., *7:*785, 1976.
54. Morris, J.M.: Biomechanics of the foot and ankle. Clin. Orthop., *122:*10, 1977.
55. Morton, D.: The Human Foot. New York, Columbia University Press, 1948.
56. Murray, M.P., Drongert, A.B., and Kory, R.C.: Walking patterns of normal men. J. Bone Joint Surg. [Am.], *46:*335, 1964.
57. Nicola, T.: Atlas of Surgical Approaches to Bones and Joints. New York, MacMillan, 1945.
58. O'Rahilly, R., Gardner, E., and Gray, D.J.: The skeletal development of the foot. Clin. Orthop., *16:*7, 1960.
59. Perry, J.: The mechanics of walking: A clinical interpretation. Phys. Ther., *47:*778, 1967.
60. Richie, G.W., and Keim, H.H.: Major foot deformities. Their classifation and x-ray analysis. J. Can. Assoc. Radiol., *19:*155, 1968.
61. Roche, A.F., and Sunderland, S.: Multiple ossification centers in the epiphysis of the long bones of human hand and foot. J. Bone Joint Surg. [Br.], *41:*375, 1959.
62. Rossi, W.A.: The Sex Life of Foot and Shoe. London, Routlege and Keeganpaul, 1977.
63. Schuster, O.N.: Foot Orthopaedics. 2nd Ed. Albany, J.B. Lyon, 1939.
64. Schwartz, R.P., Heath, A.L., Morgan, D.W., and Towns, R.C.: A quantitative analysis of recorded variables in the walking pattern of "normal" adults. J. Bone Joint Surg. [Am.], *46:*324, 1964.
65. Scott, J.R., Hulton, W.C., and Stohes, I.A.F.: Forces under the foot. J. Bone Joint Surg. [Br.], *55:*335, 1973.
66. Shands, A.R., Jr.: The accessory bones of the foot. South. Med. Surg., *93:*326, 1931.
67. Steggerda, M.: Inheritance of short metatarsals. J. Hered., *33:*233, 1942.
68. Steindler, A.: The pathomechanics of the static disabilities of the foot and ankle. Instr. Course Lect., *9:*327, 1952.
69. Stokes, I.A.F., Hutton, W.C., and Stott, J.R.R.: Forces acting on the metatarsals during normal walking. J. Anat., *129:*579, 1979.
70. Stott, J.R.R., Hutton, W.C., and Stokes, I.A.F.: Forces under the foot. J. Bone Joint Surg. [Br.], *55:*335, 1973.
71. Tachdjian, M.O.: Pediatric Orthopaedics. Philadel-

phia, W.B. Saunders, 1972.

72. Trolle, D.: Accessory Bones of the Human Foot. Copenhagen, Munksgaard, 1948.

73. Urist, M.R. (ed.): AOFS surgery of the foot. Clin. Orthop., *85*:1, 1972.

74. Vinning, P.: Variation of the digital skeleton of the foot. Clin. Orthop., *16*:26, 1960.

75. Walsham, W.J., and Hughes, W.K.: Deformities of the Human Foot. New York, William Wood, 1895.

76. Wickstrom, J., and Williams, R.A.: Shoe corrections and orthopaedic foot supports. Clin. Orthop., *70*:30, 1970.

77. Wood-Jones, F.: Structure and Function as Seen in the Foot. Baltimore, Williams & Wilkins, 1944.

78. Zimbler, S., and Craig, C.: Foot deformities. Orthop. Clin. North Am., *7*:331, 1976.

2 SURGERY OF THE GREAT TOE

HALLUX VALGUS

Incidence

Hallux valgus is undoubtedly one of the more common foot problems in shoe-wearing people. Its two apparent deformities are lateral deviation of the great toe at the M-P joint and the presence of a bony prominence on the medial aspect of the first metatarsal head (the bunion). Although congenital hallux valgus does occur, the condition is usually acquired. The most common cause of hallux valgus is the wearing of improperly fitted shoes, especially ones with high heels and narrow, pointed toe boxes, which may explain why the majority of patients who undergo different bunion operations are women. It is of interest that before the introduction of European and American styles of shoes in Japan, hallux valgus was virtually nonexistent. Kato and Watanabe (1981) noted that with the popularity of western footwear, an increasing number of Japanese patients have developed or are developing hallux valgus deformity. Similarly, Lam and Hodgson (1958) found that 33% of the shoe-wearing Chinese people in Hong Kong had some degree of hallux valgus and only 1.9% of the unshod people in the same city had the same deformity. It should be noted that hallux valgus has a strong familial tend-

ency, probably being inherited in an autosomally dominant manner with incomplete penetrance. It should be emphasized, however, that the intrinsic ability of certain feet to resist permanent deformities caused by wearing improperly fitted shoes may explain the fact that some people simply do not develop hallux valgus in spite of constant and prolonged use of unphysiologic shoes. It has been estimated that between 15 and 20% of patients with hallux valgus have pathologic conditions associated with their second toes, most commonly, a hammer toe deformity. In addition, two thirds of patients undergoing surgical treatment of hallux valgus have a positive family history of the condition. A list of the various direct and indirect causes of hallux valgus follows.

A. Improperly fitted shoes, especially narrow and high-heeled shoes, which force the great toe into a valgus position.

B. Hereditary factor, manifested in its strong family tendency and occasional occurrence in identical twins.

C. Metatarsus primus varus increases the space between the first and second metatarsal heads and favors the development of hallux valgus.

D. Obliquity of the first metatarsocuneiform articulation produces metatarsus primus varus, which in turn favors the development of hallux valgus.

E. Pes planus, pes planovalgus, and pes equinovalgus can all cause the foot to pronate and the forefoot to abduct with weight-bearing, which may bring about the hallux valgus deformity.

F. Muscle imbalance due to neuromuscular diseases, such as poliomyelitis, cerebral palsy, spinal cord tumors, and myelodysplasia, can produce hallux valgus.

G. Extension of the posterior tibialis tendon to the flexor hallucis brevis and the oblique part of the adductor hallucis, which Kaplan (1955) found only in cadavers' feet with hallux valgus and not in those with normal-looking feet.

H. Excision of the medial sesamoid with disruption of the medial conjoined tendon, which allows the adductor hallucis and the lateral head of the flexor hallucis brevis to pull the great toe into a valgus position.

I. Polydactyly of the great toe (either partial or complete duplication of the distal phalanx of the great toe) forces the principal great toe into a valgus position.

J. Fused or unfused os intermetatarseum between the bases of the first and second metatarsals, which forces the first metatarsal into a varus position and favors the development of hallux valgus.

K. Congenital hallux valgus (hallux valgus interphalangeus), which is usually caused by an anomaly of the proximal and distal phalanges of the great toe.

L. Inflammatory and metabolic diseases, such

as rheumatoid arthritis, gout, and psoriasis, can cause synovitis and articular destruction of the M-P joint of the great toe, and can eventually lead to hallux valgus deformity.

M. Amputation of the second toe or an unstable second toe allows the shoe to push the great toe toward the third toe, producing hallux valgus.

N. A round first metatarsal head is less resistant to a valgus-deforming force exerted by a narrow and pointed shoe than a flat first metatarsal head.

O. A hypermobile first metatarsal allows itself to pronate on weight-bearing and can force the big toe into a valgus position.

P. An excessively long great toe subjects itself to bear more deforming force from the narrow shoes and results in a hallux valgus deformity.

Clinical Symptoms and Signs

The most common complaint of patients with hallux valgus is a burning pain in their bunions, which are frequently tender, red, and somewhat swollen. A fluid-filled adventitious bursa often can also be found over the medial bony prominence of the first metatarsal head. When aspiration or constant rubbing of the shoe has caused the fluid-filled bursa to become infected, purulent discharge can be expressed from the sinus tract of the infected bursa. Rarely, the infected bursa can spread infection to the underlying first metatarsal head region, which produces osteomyelitis that can produce persistent and chronic purulent discharge.

In hallux valgus, the great toe is not only laterally deviated, but also is internally rotated along its longitudinal axis, resulting in the nail of the great toe facing medially. This pronation increases pressure on the medioplantar aspect of the base of the distal phalanx of the great toe and frequently produces a painful corn in that region.

Because the two sesamoid bones of the flexor hallucis brevis articulate with the first metatarsal head and are embedded in the medial and lateral tendons of the flexor hallucis brevis, which is firmly attached to the plantar aspect of the base of the proximal phalanx of the great toe, internal rotation of the proximal phalanx naturally carries the two sesamoid bones laterally and the abductor hallucis in a more plantar direction (Figure 2–1). As a result, the medial and lateral sesamoidometatarsal joints can become subluxed or frankly dislocated, and the medial sesamoid can even become temporarily incarcerated beneath the bony ridge under the first metatarsal head known as the crista, which separates the two sesamoidometatarsal joints. A painful corn may then be produced under the dislocated medial sesamoid (Figure 2–2).

When the great toe is greatly deviated laterally, it touches the third toe and pushes the second toe upward to cause it to overlap the great toe in the form of a hammer toe. This hammered second toe frequently has a painful corn over the dorsal aspect of its PIP joint and a painful callosity under the second metatarsal head. In addition, p̶ toe in hallux valgus can con̶ velopment of ingrown toenail ̶ aspect of the toenail of the grea̶ concentrated shoe pressure. If arthr̶ developed in the M-P joint of the great̶ then pain, joint line tenderness, limited joi̶ motion, joint swelling, palpable osteophytes on the dorsal aspect of the first metatarsal head, and crepitation may be present.

Roentgenographic Manifestations

Roentgenographic evaluation of hallux valgus should include at least standing anteroposterior, lateral, and oblique views of the foot; an axial view of the sesamoids (sesamoid view of the great toe) can provide additional useful information. A list of the various abnormal radiographic features of hallux valgus follows (Figure 2-3):

A. Lateral deviation of the great toe, which increases the first M-P angle.

B. Internal rotation of the great toe with the shadow of its toenail facing medially.

A

IN NORMAL HALLUX

B

IN HALLUX VALGUS

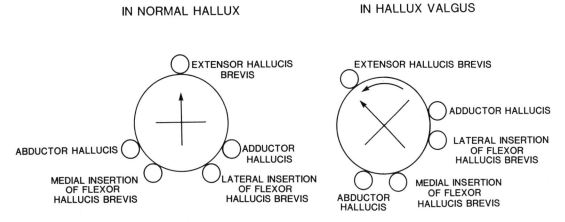

Figure 2–1. Muscle insertions at the base of proximal phalanx of the great toe. **A,** in normal hallux, the extensor hallucis brevis is in balance with the flexor hallucis brevis, and the abductor hallucis with adductor hallucis. **B,** in hallux valgus, the balance is upset and the great toe is internally rotated, carrying the abductor hallucis and medial head of the flexor hallucis brevis into a more plantar direction, and the adductor hallucis and the lateral head of the flexor hallucis brevis into a more dorsal direction.

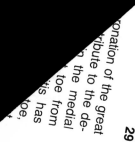

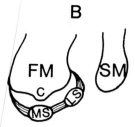

B

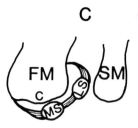

C

First Metatarsal
Second Metatarsal
C– Crista
MS– Medial Sesamoid
LM– Lateral Sesamoid

Figure 2–2. Normal and abnormal sesamoidometatarsal joints of the great toe. **A,** normal position of the medial and lateral sesamoidometatarsal joints of the great toe, which are separated from each other by the crista. **B,** with internal rotation of the great toe in hallux valgus, the medial sesamoid is incarcerated under the crista and can produce a painful corn under the medial sesamoid. Note the lateral sesamoidometatarsal joint is dislocated. **C,** when severe hallux valgus has been present for a long time, the crista is completely worn down and both the medial and lateral sesamoidometatarsal joints are dislocated laterally.

C. Prominence of the medial aspect of the first metatarsal head with lateral subluxation of the first M-P joint.

D. Medial deviation of the first metatarsal (metatarsus primus varus) in association with an increase of the first intermetatarsal angle.

E. Lateral migration of the medial and lateral sesamoid bones of the great toe with subluxation or frank dislocation of the medial and lateral sesamoidometatarsal joints in association with various degrees of wear of the crista on the undersurface of the first metatarsal head.

F. Obliquity of the first metatarsocuneiform joint.

G. When the hallux valgus is associated with a hammered second toe, hyperextension of the M-P joint and hyperflexion of the PIP joint of the second toe will be present; the second toe can overlap the great toe.

H. When degenerative arthritis has developed in the M-P joint of the great toe, joint narrowing, subchrondral osteosclerosis, osteophyte formation at the joint margins, and joint effusion may be present.

Pathologic Anatomy

In addition to the obvious deformities previously mentioned in the two preceding sections, soft tissue changes of hallux valgus include:

A. Stretching and plantar migration of the abductor hallucis.

B. Lateral migration of the medial and lateral heads of the flexor hallucis brevis muscle.

C. Stretching of the medial joint capsule and the medial collateral ligament of the M-P joint of the great toe.

D. Contracture of the lateral joint capsule and lateral collateral ligament of the M-P joint of the great toe as well as the conjoined tendon of the adductor hallucis and the lateral head of the flexor hallucis brevis.

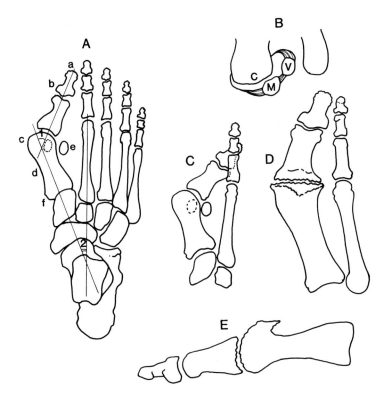

Figure 2–3. Various deformities associated with hallux valgus. **A,** a. pronation of the great toe makes the medial one half of the base of the distal phalanx appear to be narrower than that of its lateral portion; b. lateral deviation of the great toe; c. exostosis on the medial aspect of the first metatarsal head (the bunion); d. metatarsus primus varus; e. lateral migration of both medial and lateral sesamoids; f. obliquity of the first metatarsocuneiform joint (angle 1: greatly increased first M-P angle in hallux valgus; angle 2: greatly increased first intermetatarsal angle in hallux valgus). **B,** both the medial and lateral sesamoidometatarsal joints are laterally dislocated and the crista is completely worn down. **C,** in severe hallux valgus, the second toe overlaps the great toe. **D,** when arthritis of the M-P joint of the great toe is associated with hallux valgus, joint irregularity and narrowing, and osteophyte formation at the joint margins are evident. **E,** lateral view of the same toe shown in *D* again shows M-P joint irregularity and narrowing and a large exostosis on the dorsal aspect of the first metatarsal head.

E. Shortening of the extensor hallucis longus and brevis and the flexor hallucis longus.

F. The slow and progressive stretching of the medial joint capsule of the great toe produces an erosive groove in the medial aspect of the first metatarsal head, known commonly as the sagittal groove.

Nonsurgical Treatment

A. Shoe modifications: extra-depth, space, and bunion last shoes and shoes with their uppers properly stretched over the bunion area with a shoemaker's swan can provide significant pain relief from the painful bunion resulting from shoe pressure (Figures 1–2, 1–7, 1–12).

B. Padding: padding of the painful bunion with a soft foam rubber pad or other padding materials (Figure 1–8).

C. Custom-made arch support with medial bunion flange (Figure 1–6).

D. Commercially available foot aids: may include a donut-shaped bunion pad, latex bunion shield, and bunion splint (Figures 1–16 and 1–17).

Surgical Treatment

In spite of the fact that over 100 surgical procedures have been described in treating hallux valgus, they can be grouped into a number of major types. It should be emphasized, however, that the presence or absence of arthritis in the M-P joint of the great toe is the most important factor that determines the type of surgical procedure to be used.

A. Hallux valgus without arthritis in the M-P joint (Figure 2–4A—H):
    1. Soft tissue release and tightening around the M-P joint of the great toe: tightening of the abductor hallucis and medial joint capsule and transfer of the

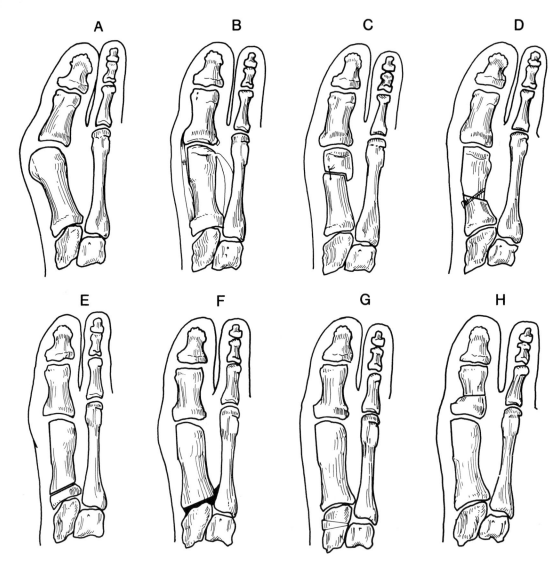

Figure 2–4. Surgical procedures for hallux valgus without arthritis in the M-P joint. **A,** hallux valgus with no arthritis in the M-P joint. **B,** soft tissue release and tightening around the M-P joint of the great toe. **C,** step-cut distal osteotomy of the first metatarsal. **D,** shaft osteotomy of the first metatarsal. **E,** proximal osteotomy of the first metatarsal. **F,** arthrodesis of the first metatarsocuneiform joint. **G,** open-wedge valgus osteotomy of the first cuneiform. **H,** varus osteotomy of the proximal phalanx of the great toe.

conjoined tendon of the adductor hallucis and the lateral head of the flexor hallucis brevis to the lateral aspect of the first metatarsal head are useful in treating young patients with hallux valgus and immature bones (Figure 2–4B).

2. Distal osteotomy of the first metatarsal: the surgical procedure that I prefer when treating hallux valgus (Figure 2–4C).

3. Osteotomy of the shaft of the first metatarsal (Figure 2–4D): may involve a longer healing time than with the proximal and distal osteotomies.

4. Proximal osteotomy of the first metatarsal (Figure 2–4E): good for hallux valgus with a short first metatarsal and a wide first intermetatarsal angle.

5. Arthrodesis of the first metatarsocuneiform joint and the adjacent bases of the first and second metatarsals (Figure 2–4F): permanent loss of motion of the first metatarsocuneiform joint.

6. Open-wedge valgus osteotomy of the first cuneiform (Figure 2–4G): more difficult to determine the intraoperative correction of the hallux valgus deformity due to the relatively longer distance between the first cuneiform and the great toe.

7. Varus osteotomy of the proximal phalanx of the great toe (Figure 2–4H): does not correct metatarsus primus varus.

B. Hallux valgus with arthritis in the M-P joint (Figure 2–5A—E):

1. Resection of the base of the proximal phalanx of the great toe (Figure 2–5B): decreases the weight-bearing function of the great toe.

2. Arthrodesis of the first M-P joint (Figure 2–5C): enhances the weight-bearing function of the great toe but interferes with fashion-minded female patients in wearing shoes with different heights of heels.

3. Partial resection of the first metatarsal head with interposition of the medial joint capsule into the M-P joint of the great toe (Figure 2–5D): a compromise between items 1 and 2.

4. Insertion of a Silastic prosthesis into the resected M-P joint of the great toe (Figure 2–5E): advantages include preservation of the length and M-P joint motion of the great toe, but possible disadvantages include inflammation, infection, and stem breakage of the prosthesis.

The above-mentioned surgical procedures can be used in various combinations to treat different painful foot problems involving the first ray. For example, resection of the base of the proximal phalanx of the great toe can be combined with proximal osteotomy of the first metatarsal in treating a foot with a wide first intermetatarsal angle and severe degenerative arthritis of the M-P joint of the great toe. It should be mentioned that I was fortunate enough to train with Dr. C. Leslie Mtichell, who popularized the Mitchell's bunionectomy for correction of hallux valgus. Having personally performed approximately 200 standard Mitchell's bunionectomies and 200 modified Mitchell's bunionectomies, which I devised, I am convinced that the modified Mitchell's bunionectomy is a better way of performing a distal osteotomy of the first metatarsal than that of the standard Mitchell's bunionectomy. Our records indicate that close to 2000 standard Mitchell's bunionectomies have been performed at our medical center to date, and the occasional complications of this procedure include delayed union, non-union, dorsal and medial displacement or both, and aseptic necrosis of the first metatarsal head that underwent osteotomy: postoperative infection; necrosis of the medial skin flap; and hallux rigidus. Properly performed Mitchell's bunionectomies, however, can be expected to yield an 80 to 85% good to excellent result (see Table 2–1), which may explain its popularity, given its ability to correct virtually all of the deformities associated with hallux valgus.

A. Lateral displacement osteotomy of the first

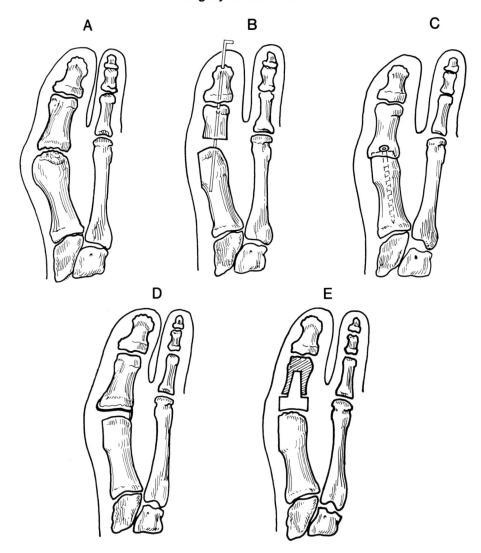

Figure 2–5. Surgical procedures for hallux valgus with arthritis in the M-P joint. **A,** foot with hallux valgus and arthritis in the M-P joint of the great toe. **B,** resection of the base of the proximal phalanx of the great toe. **C,** arthrodesis of the M-P joint of the great toe. **D,** partial resection of the first metatarsal head with interposition of the medial joint capsule into the M-P joint of the great toe. **E,** insertion of a Silastic prosthesis into the resected M-P joint of the great toe.

metatarsal head reduces the distance between the first and second metatarsal heads and relaxes the adductor hallucis and the lateral head of the flexor hallucis brevis. The result is the reduction of the hallux primus varus and hallux valgus deformities as well as the realignment of the subluxed medial and lateral sesamoidometatarsal articulations.

B. The plantar angulation osteotomy of the

distal portion of the first metatarsal restores the weight-bearing function of the great toe and tends to relieve metatarsalgia of the lesser toes.

C. By removing less bone from the dorsal aspect of the double osteotomy site, when the metatarsal head that has undergone osteotomy is laterally displaced, the extra bone on the dorsal aspect of the bony ledge naturally forces the great toe to su-

Table 2–1. Clinical Analysis of 100 Consecutive Cases of Standard Mitchell's Bunionectomy Performed by the Author

Age	14–76 Years	(Average 39.5 Years)	
Sex	14 Males (14%)	85 Females (86%)	M:F = 1:6
First intermetatarsal angle	Preoperative 10–28° (Average 14.4°)	Postoperative 2–10° (Average 5.6°)	Normal Below 9°
First Metatarsophalangeal angle	Preoperative 15–47° (Average 28.9)	Postoperative 0–25° (Average 8.6)	Normal Below 15°
Plantar angulation	–5–28°		
Relative shortening of the first metatarsal	1–8.5 mm (Average 3.7 mm)		
Overall results	Excellent and good 85 (85%)	Fair and poor 15 (15%)	
Complications	Dorsal angulation	2	
	Medial angulation	3	
	Degenerative arthritis of M-P joint with hallux rigidus	3	
	Exostosis at osteotomy site	1	
	Recurrence of hallux valgus (average 22.3°)	5	
	Keloid formation at incision site	2	
	Osteomyelitis	0	
	Aseptic necrosis	0	
Subjective evaluation	1. Symptomatic relief of pain 2. Ability to wear any kind of shoes 3. Cosmetic appearance 4. Activity 5. Occupation		
Objective evaluation	1. Motion of M-P joint 2. Joint tenderness and crepitation 3. Painful plantar callosity 4. Recurrence of hallux valgus and rotational deformity 5. Exostosis 6. Keloid at incisional site		
Criteria for determining the final results	1. *Excellent:* both patient and author are totally satisfied with results. 2. *Good:* patient has no pain or specific complaints but slight recurrence of hallux valgus, rotational deformity, or limitation of joint motion detected by examination (objective findings). 3. *Fair:* moderate recurrence of hallux valgus, exostosis formation, significant metatarsalgia, slight to moderate degenerative changes of M-P joint, plus tenderness and limitation of motion of same joint. 4. *Poor:* significant degenerative changes of M-P joint, hallux rigidus, severe recurrence of hallux valgus, severe metatarsalgia, aseptic necrosis, and dorsal and medial displacement of repaired metatarsal head.		

pinate, thus correcting the internal rotational deformity of the great toe.

D. Plication of the medial joint capsule and tightening of the abductor hallucis restore these two important anatomic structures to their proper tension and lengths.

When a hammered second toe with subluxation or dislocation of its M-P joint is associated with hallux valgus, it should be corrected simultaneously with the hallux valgus to prevent postoperative recurrence of hallux valgus due to the loss of lateral support of the great toe normally provided by the normal second toe. In addition, it is a popular misconception that when the first metatarsal is shorter than the second, Mitchell's bunionectomy is contraindicated. The truth is that many of my patients who underwent Mitchell's bunionectomies had their first metatarsals that were shorter than their corresponding second metatarsals. Most patients had good to excellent long-term results because the carefully performed plantar angulation osteotomy had adequately compensated for the original and surgically induced relative shortening of the first metatarsals. However, significant arthritis of the M-P joint of the great toe, extremely short first metatarsals, and a wide first intermetatarsal angle are the three main contraindications of Mitchell's bunionectomy.

An attempt to minimize the possible complications of the bunionectomy procedure, the modified Mitchell's bunionectomy is based on the sound surgical principle of maximal preservation of the vascular supply to the soft tissues and bone at the operative site, minimal stripping of soft tissues from the operated bone, and maximal reduction of the intraoperative time to minimize the chances of soft tissue and bone necrosis; postoperative infection; and displacement, delayed union, and non-union of the operated first metatarsal head.

The modified Mitchell's bunionectomy procedure includes the following steps (Figures 2–6—2–9):

1. Make a slightly curved longitudinal incision over the dorsomedial aspect of the great toe, extending from the proximal phalanx to the midportion of the first metatarsal (Figure 2–6B).

2. Incise the skin and subcutaneous tissue down to the M-P joint capsule of the great toe (Figure 2–6C).

3. Incise the M-P joint of the great toe longitudinally to expose the medial exostosis (the bunion) and the neck of the first metatarsal (Figure 2–6D).

4. Remove the exostosis along its sagittal groove with a microsaw and smooth the peripheral sharp edges with a small bone rasp (Figure 2–7A).

5. While protecting the sesamoids with a Joker retractor, drill two holes through the distal portion of the first metatarsal, with the distal hole emerging from the plantar side where the articular cartilage of the first metatarsal head ends, and the proximal hole about 12.7 mm to 19.1 mm proximal and 6.4 mm lateral to the distal hole (Figure 2–7B).

6. Inserting a straight Keith needle through the distal hole to serve as a guide, make the distal partial osteotomy cut about 3 to 4 mm proximal to the distal hole and at a right angle to the longitudinal axis of the first metatarsal to the desired depth (e.g., a more shallow cut for a foot with a wider first intermetatarsal angle, and a more shallow dorsal cut than its plantar cut to correct the internal rotational deformity of the great toe), and mark the oblique proximal osteotomy cut with a 10 to 15° plantar inclination or a higher angulation when the first metatarsal is fairly short or when severe metatarsalgia is present in the lesser toes due to their excessively flexed position in a planar direction. To minimize the unnecessary shortening of the first metatarsal, the two parallel cuts on the dorsal aspect of the

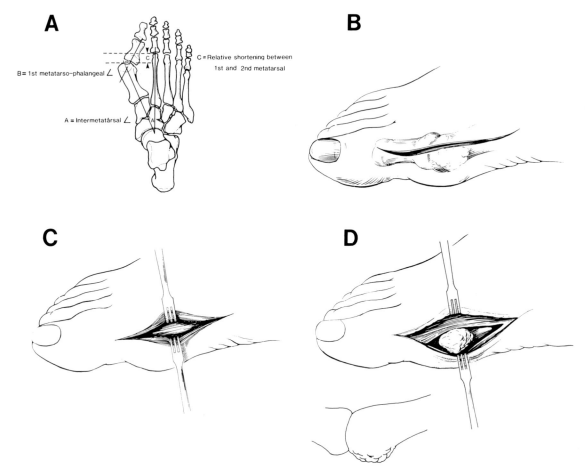

Figure 2–6. Modified Mitchell's bunionectomy. **A,** foot with hallux valgus showing the first intermetatarsal angle A, first M-P angle B, and the relative shortening between the first and second metatarsals (C). **B,** skin incision on the dorsomedial aspect of the great toe. **C,** incise the skin and subcutaneous tissue to expose the dorsomedial aspect of the M-P joint of the great toe. **D,** incise the dorsomedial aspect of the M-P joint capsule to expose the exostosis (the bunion) and the neck of the first metatarsal.

first metatarsal are only 1 to 2 mm apart (Figure 2–7C).

7. Perform the proximal osteotomy by carefully following the lines marked on the dorsal and medial aspects of the distal portion of the first metatarsal in a dorsoplantar direction (Figure 2–7D).

8. Remove the unwanted bone from the medial aspect of the osteotomy site with a small rongeur and displace the cut first metatarsal head laterally to engage its lateral bony ledge on the lateral aspect of the neck of the first metatarsal. Next, pass two size-O Mersilene sutures through the proximal hole by carrying them through the hole with a straight Keith needle and by pulling out their two free ends with a small mosquito hemostat. Then pass another size-O Mersilene suture with another straight Keith needle through the distal hole and pull out a small suture loop with a hemostat. The two sutures through the proximal hole are passed through the single suture loop, which is drawn upward by pulling on the Keith needle and

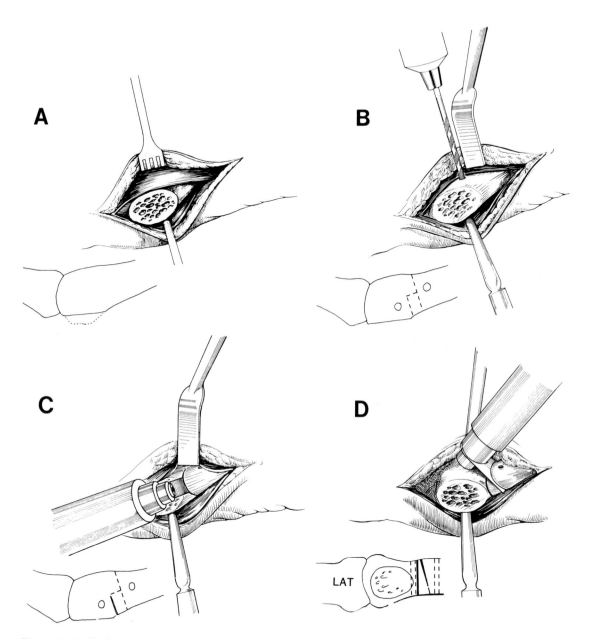

Figure 2–7. Modified Mitchell's bunionectomy (continued). **A,** remove the exostosis along its sagittal groove with a microsaw and smooth the peripheral sharp edges with a small bone rasp. **B,** drill two holes through the distal portion of the first metatarsal, with the distal hole emerging on the plantar side where the articular cartilage of the first metatarsal head ends and the proximal hole about 12.7 mm to 19.1 mm proximal and 6.4 mm lateral to the distal hole. **C,** by inserting a straight Keith needle through the distal hole as a guide, perform the distal partial osteotomy cut at right angle to the longitudinal axis of the first metatarsal to the desired depth. Then mark the oblique proximal osteotomy cut with a 10 to 15° plantar angulation on the medial aspect of the first metatarsal neck. **D,** perform the proximal osteotomy with a microsaw by carefully following the lines marked on the dorsal and medial aspects of the first metatarsal neck in a dorsoplantar direction.

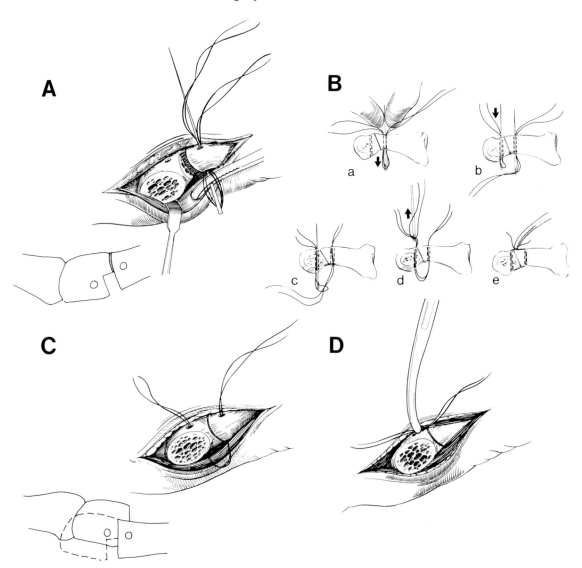

Figure 2–8. Modified Mitchell's bunionectomy (continued). **A–C,** remove the unwanted bone on the medial aspect of the osteotomy site, displace the repaired first metatarsal head laterally, and pass the two sutures through the two drilled holes by using two straight Keith needles. **D,** holding the raw-bone surfaces of the osteotomy site in intimate contact, tie the first knot snuggly and hold it with a mosquito hemostat while the second square knot is tied and cinched. Five to six square knots are usually tied for each suture to prevent slippage.

the two free ends of the single suture to pull the two sutures through the distal hole to the dorsal aspect of the first metatarsal head (Figure 2–8A—C).

9. By holding the two raw-bone surfaces at the osteotomy site in intimate contact, the two sutures individually are tied tightly over

the dorsal aspect of the first metatarsal neck by holding the first knot down with a mosquito hemostat before the second square knot is tightened, using a total of five to six square knots to prevent slippage (Figure 2–8D).

10. Remove the bony prominence on the

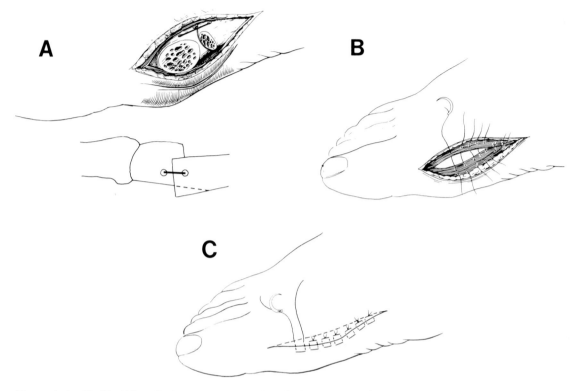

Figure 2–9. Modified Mitchell's bunionectomy (continued). **A,** remove the bony prominence on the medial aspect of the fixed osteotomy site with a microsaw **B,** close the redundant joint capsule tightly in a vest-over-pants manner. **C,** close the skin in a regular manner.

medial aspect of the fixed osteotomy site with a microsaw (Figure 2–9A).

11. Close the joint capsule tightly by overlapping the redundant joint capsule in a "vest over pants" manner, and close the skin and subcutaneous tissue in a regular manner (Figures 2–9B and C).

12. Upon completion of the operation, three padded tongue blades placed on the dorsal, medial, and plantar aspects of the great toe are incorporated into a bulky compression dressing and the foot is elevated on two pillows during the first two postoperative days. Subsequently, if everything is in order, a plaster ankle boot is applied over the compression dressing with three tongue blades, and the patient is sent home. The skin sutures are re-

moved 12 to 14 days after the operation and a short walking cast, with a great toe spica and with the great toe in neutral alignment with the lesser toes, is applied. The patient is then evaluated at 2-week intervals, and the cast is usually removed 6 to 8 weeks after surgery, when the osteotomy site is usually solidly united. Patients are advised to wear soft and wide shoes and to go back to wearing their regular shoes gradually.

The superiority of the modified Mitchell's bunionectomy over the standard Mitchell's bunionectomy has been borne out by the success of approximately 200 modified Mitchell's bunionectomies, the majority of which were accomplished in significantly shorter operative time than that of the standard procedure, cases of non-union, delayed union, displacement, and aseptic necrosis of the repaired first metatarsal head have yet to be encountered.

A videotape of the modified Mitchell's bunionectomy has been prepared for the American Academy of Orthopaedic Surgeons, which provides a visual step-by-step guide to the entire procedure.

Simple bunionectomy (removal of the bony prominence on the medial aspect of the first metatarsal head) is occasionally performed on an elderly patient who has a localized and painful bunion deformity and has difficulty finding shoes that fit properly. Simple bunionectomy does not correct hallux valgus, metatarsus primus varus, pronation of the great toe, and subluxation of the sesamoidometatarsal joints, although it does improve the cosmetic appearance of the foot and makes shoe fitting easier. In contrast with other bunion operations, simple bunionectomy can be easily performed under local anesthesia and has a short intraoperative time, a short period of postoperative disability, and infrequent soft tissue complications. The contraindications for simple bunionectomy include severe arthritis of the M-P joint of the great toe, severe hallux valgus deformity of over 50°, poor circulation of the foot, the presence of infection or skin ulceration, severe diabetes mellitus, and overlapping of the severely hammered second toe over the great toe. When hallux valgus is over 50°, simple bunionectomy may make the M-P joint of the great toe so unstable that the great toe can easily become dislocated laterally, making the hallux valgus deformity worse.

REFERENCES

Hallux Valgus

1. Akin, O.F.: The treatment of hallux valgus—an operative procedure and its results. Med. Sentinel, *33:*678, 1925.
2. Allan, F.G.: Hallux valgus and rigidus. Br. Med. J., *1:*579, 1940.
3. Allen, T.R., et al.: The assessment of adolescent hallux valgus before and after first metatarsal osteotomy—clinical and walkway studies. Int. Orthop., *5:*111, 1981.
4. Anderson, R.L.: Hallux valgus: Report of end re-
sults. South Med. Surg., *91:*74, 1929.
5. Armstrong, W.P., Jr.: Treatment of hallux valgus (bunion). Am. J. Surg., *36:*332, 1937.
6. Artz, T., and Rogers, S.C.: Osteotomy for correction of hallux valgus. Clin. Orthop., *88:*50, 1972.
7. Auerbach, A.M.: Review of distal metatarsal osteotomies for hallux valgus in the young. Clin. Orthop., *70:*148, 1970.
8. Austin, D.W., and Leventen, F.O.: A new osteotomy for hallux valgus: A horizontally directed "V" displacement osteotomy of the metatarsal head for hallux valgus and primus varus. Clin. Orthop., *157:*25, 1981.
9. Bargman, J., Corless, J., Gross, A.F., and Lange, F.: A review of surgical procedures for hallux valgus. Foot Ankle, *1:*39, 1980.
10. Barker, A.E.: An operation for hallux valgus. Lancet, *1:*655, 1884.
11. Batchelor, J.S.: Hallux valgus. Acta Orthop. Belg., *38:*217, 1972.
12. Bateman, J.E., and Colwill, J.C.: Modified Joplin sling procedure for splay foot using peroneus tertius. Instr. Course Lect., *21:*288, 1972.
13. Bingham, R.: The Stone operation for hallux valgus. Clin. Orthop., *17:*366, 1960.
14. Bleck, E.E.: Spastic abductor hallucis. Dev. Med. Child Neurol., *9:*602, 1967.
15. Bonney, G., and MacNab, J.: Hallux valgus and hallux rigidus—critical survey of operative results. J. Bone Joint Surg. [Br.] *34:*366, 1952.
16. Booley, B.J., and Berryman, D.B.: Wilson's osteotomy of the first metatarsal for hallux valgus in the adolescent and the young adult. Aust. N.Z. J. Surg., *43:*255, 1973.
17. Borovoy, M., and Mendelsohn, E.S.: Wedge osteotomies for correction of hallux abducto valgus with case histories. J. Foot Surg., *18:*47, 1979.
18. Bourdillon, J.: Butler's operation for hallux valgus. J. Bone Joint Surg. [Br.], *40:*346, 1958.
19. Brahms, M.A.: Hallux valgus—the Akin procedure. Clin. Orthop., *157:*47, 1981.
20. Breck, I.W.: The classic. A conservative operation for bunions by Earl Duwain McBride, M.D. (1891–1975). Clin. Orthop., *157:*2, 1981.
21. Brindley, H.H.: Mobilization and transfer of the intrinsics of the great toe for hallux valgus. Clin. Orthop., *165:*144, 1982.
22. Butson, A.R.: A modification of the Lapidus operation for hallux valgus. J. Bone Joint Surg. [Br.], *62:*350, 1980.
23. Butterworth, R.D., and Clay, B.R.: A bunion operation. Va. Med., *90:*10, 1963.
24. Carr, C.R., and Boyd, B. M.: Correctional osteotomy for metatarsus primus varus and hallux valgus. J. Bone Joint Surg. [Am.], *50:*1353, 1968.
25. Cholmeley, J.A.: Hallux valgus in adolescents. Proc. R. Soc. Lond. [Med.], *51:*903, 1958.
26. Clark, J.J.: Hallux valgus and hallux varus. Lancet, *1:*609, 1900.
27. Colloff, B., and Weitz, E.M.: Surgery in hallux valgus. Clin. Orthop., *164:*312, 1982.
28. Corless, J.R.: A modification of the Mitchell procedure. J. Bone Joint Surg. [Br.], *58:*138, 1976.
29. Cotton, F.J.: Foot statistics and surgery. Trans. N. Engl. Surg. Soc., *18:*181, 1935.

30. Creer, W.S.: The hallux valgus complex. Br. Med. J., *2:*5, 1938.
31. Davis, G.F.: Cure for hallux valgus: The interdigital incision. Surg. Clin. North Am., *1:*651, 1917.
32. Daw, S.W.: An unusual type of hallux valgus (two cases). Br. Med. J., *2:*580, 1935.
33. Dewar, F.P., and Rathburn, J.B.: Oblique transposition osteotomy of the first metatarsal for adolescent hallux valgus. J. Bone Joint Surg. [Br.], *35:*663, 1973.
34. Dintcho, A.: Procedures to correct hallux abducto valgus and metatarsus primus adductus. J. Foot Surg., *15:*15, 1976.
35. Donick, I.I., et al.: An approach for hallux valgus surgery—fifteen-year review: Part I. J. Foot Surg., *19:*113, 1980.
36. Donick, I.I., et al. An approach for hallux valgus surgery—Fifteen-year review: Part II. J. Foot Surg., *19:*171, 1980.
37. Donovan, J.C.: Results of bunion correction using Mitchell osteotomy. J. Foot Surg., *21:*181, 1982.
38. Dovey, H.: The treatment of hallux valgus by distal osteotomy of the 1st metatarsal. Acta Orthop. Scand., *40:*402, 1969.
39. Dubois, G.A., and Knowles, K.G.: The Stone operation: A clinical review of seven years' experience. Orthop. Clin. North Am., *7:*799, 1976.
40. Durman, D.C.: Hallux valgus. J. Bone Joint Surg. [Am.], *39:*221, 1957.
41. Ellis, V.H.: A method of correcting metatarsus primus varus: A preliminary report. J. Bone Joint Surg. [Br.], *33:*415, 1951.
42. Fitzgerald, W.: Hallux valgus. J. Bone Joint Surg. [Br.], *32:*139, 1950.
43. Fuld, J.E.: Surgical treatment of hallux valgus and its complications. Am. Med., *14:*536, 1917.
44. Funk, Jr., F.J., and Wells, R.E.: Bunionectomy: With distal osteotomy. Clin. Orthop., *85:*71, 1972.
45. Galland, W.I., and Jordan, H.H.: Hallux valgus. Surg. Gynecol. Obstet., *66:*95, 1938.
46. Ganel, A., Chechick, A., and Farine, I.: Chevron osteotomy. Clin. Orthop., *154:*300, 1981.
47. Gardner, R.C.: Improving operative technique and postoperative course of McBride bunionectomy. Orthop. Rev., *2:*35, 1973.
48. Gibson, J., and Piggott, H.: Osteotomy of the neck of the first metatarsal in the treatment of hallux valgus: A follow-up study of eighty-two feet. J. Bone Joint Surg. [Br.], *44:*349, 1962.
49. Gilmore, G.H., and Bush, L.F.: Hallux valgus. Surg. Gynecol. Obstet., *104:*524, 1957.
50. Girdleston, G.R., and Spooner, H.J.: A new operation for hallux valgus and hallux rigidus. J. Bone Joint Surg., *19:*30, 1937.
51. Glynn, M.K., Dunlop, J.B., and Fitzpatrick, D.: The Mitchell distal metatarsal osteotomy for hallux valgus. J. Bone Joint Surg. [Br.], *62:*188–191, 1980.
52. Golden, G.N., Hallux valgus, the osteotomy operation. Br. Med. J., *1:*1361, 1961.
53. Goldfarb, W.L., et al.: The tear-drop capsulectomy and capsulorrhaphy: A new approach in aiding the soft tissue repair of hallux abducto valgus. J. Foot Surg., *19:*199, 1980.
54. Goldner, J.L.: Hallux valgus and hallux flexus associated with cerebral palsy: Analysis and treatment. Clin. Orthop., *157:*98, 1981.
55. Goldner, J.L., and Gaines, R.W.: Adult and juvenile hallux valgus: Analysis and treatment. Orthop. Clin. North Am., *7:*863, 1976.
56. Gottschalk, F.A., Beighton, P.H., and Solomon, L.: The prevalence of hallux valgus in three South African populations. S. Afr. Med. J., *60:*655, 1981.
57. Gottschalk, F.A., Sallis, J.G., Beighton, P.H., and Solomon, L.: A comparison of the prevalence of hallux valgus in three South African populations. S. Afr. Med. J., *57:*355, 1980.
58. Haines, R.W., and McDougall, A.: The Anatomy of hallux valgus. J. Bone Joint Surg. [Br.], *36:*272, 1954.
59. Hammond, G.: Mitchell osteotomy-bunionectomy for hallux valgus and metatarsus primus varus. Instr. Course Lect., *21:*1972.
60. Hansen, C.E.: Hallux valgus treated by the McBride operation. Acta Orthop. Scand., *45:*788, 1974.
61. Hardy, R.H., and Clapham, J.C.R.: Hallux valgus. Predisposing and anatomical causes. Lancet, *1:*1170, 1952.
62. Hauser, E.D.W.: Hallux valgus, hammer toe and contracted toes. Surg. Clin. North Am., *21:*169, 1944.
63. Hawkins, F.B.: Acquired hallux valgus: Cause, prevention and correction. Clin. Orthop., *76:*169, 1971.
64. Hawkins, F.B., Mitchell, C.L., and Hedrick, D.W.: Correction of hallux valgus by metatarsal osteotomy. J. Bone Joint Surg., *27:*387, 1945.
65. Helal, B.: Surgery for adolescent hallux valgus. Clin. Orthop., *157:*50, 1981.
66. Helal, B., Gupta, S.K., and Gotaseni, P.: Surgery for adolescent hallux valgus. Acta Orthop. Scand., *48:*271, 295, 1974.
67. Heller, E.P.: Congenital bilateral hallux valgus. Arch. Surg., *88:*798, 1928.
68. Henry, A.P.J., and Waugh, W.: The use of footprints in assessing the results of operations for hallux valgus: A comparison of Keller's operation and arthrodesis. J. Bone Joint Surg. [Br.], *57:*478, 1975.
69. Hiss, J.M.: Hallux valgus: Its causes and simplified treatment. Am. J. Surg., *11:*50, 1931.
70. Holstein, A.: Hallux valgus—an acquired deformity of the foot in cerebral palsy. Foot Ankle, *1:*33, 1980.
71. Houghton, G.R., and Dickson, R.A.: Hallux valgus in the younger patients. The structural abnormality. J. Bone Joint Surg. [Br.], *61:*176, 1979.
72. Hulbert, K.F.: Compression clamp for arthrodesis of the first metatarsophalangeal joint. Lancet, *1:*597, 1955.
73. Hutton, W.C., and Dhanendran, M.: The mechanics of normal and hallux valgus feet. A quantitative study. Clin. Orthop., *157:*7, 1981.
74. Iida, M., and Basmajian, J.V.: Electromyography of hallux valgus. Clin. Orthop., *101:*220, 1974.
75. Inman, V.T.: Hallux valgus: A review of etiology factors. Orthop. Clin. North Am., *5:*59, 1974.
76. Jahss, M.H.: The sesamoids of the hallux. Clin. Orthop., *157:*88, 1981.
77. Jahss, M.H.: Hallux valgus: Further considerations—the first metatarsal head. Foot Ankle, *2:*1, 1981.
78. Jahss, M.H.: Hallux valgus surgery. Foot Ankle, *1:*305, 1981.

79. Jamieson, E.S.: Hallux valgus. J. Bone Joint Surg. [Br.], *34:*328, 1952.
80. Johnson, K.A., Cofield, R.H., and Morrey, B.F.: Chevron osteotomy for hallux valgus. Clin. Orthop., *142:*44, 1979.
81. Johnson, P.H.: The bunion. J. Arkansas Med. Soc., *78:*235, 1981.
82. Johnston, O.: Further studies of the inheritance of hand and foot anomalies. Clin. Orthop., *8:*146, 1956.
83. Jones, A.R.: Hallux valgus in the adolescent. Proc. R. Soc. Med., *41:*392, 1948.
84. Joplin, R.J.: Sling procedure for the correction of splay foot, metatarsus varus primus, and hallux valgus. J. Bone Joint Surg. [Am.], *32:*779, 1950.
85. Joplin, R.J.: Some common foot disorders amenable to surgery. Instr. Course Lect., *15:*144, 1958.
86. Joplin, R.J.: Sling procedure in the teen-ager. Instr. Course Lect., *21:*1972.
87. Jordon, H.H., and Brodsky, A.E.: Keller operation for hallux valgus and hallux rigidus. Arch. Surg., *62:*586, 1951.
88. Juvara, E.: Nouveau procedure pour la cure radicale du "hallux valgus." Nouv. Presse Med., *40:*395, 1919.
89. Kaplan, E.B.: The tibialis posterior muscle in relation to hallux valgus. Bull. Hosp. Joint Dis. Orthop. Inst., *16:*88, 1955.
90. Kato, T., and Watanabe, S.: The etiology of hallux valgus in Japan. Clin. Orthop., *157:*78, 1981.
91. Keizer, D.P.R.: Hallux valgus. Lancet, *1:*1305, 1952.
92. Kelikian, H.: Hallux Valgus, Allied Deformities of the Forefoot and Metatarsalgia. Philadelphia, W.B. Saunders, 1965.
93. Keller, W.L.: The surgical treatment of bunion and hallux valgus. N.Y. State J. Med., *80:*741, 1904.
94. Khoury, C.: Hallux valgus. Int. Surg., *17:*840, 1952.
95. Kleinberg, S.: Operative cure of hallux valgus and bunions. Am. J. Surg., *15:*75, 1932.
96. Kromann-Andersen, C., and Frandsen, P.A.: Oblique displacement osteotomy according to Crawford Adams for hallux valgus. Acta Orthop. Scand., *53:*477, 1982.
97. Lam, S.F., and Hodgson, A.R.: A comparison of foot forms among the non-shoe and shoe-wearing Chinese population. J. Bone Joint Surg. [Am.], *40:*1058, 1958.
98. Lapidus, P.W.: The operative correction of the metarsus primus varus in hallux valgus. Surg. Gynecol. Obstet., *58:*183, 1934.
99. Lapidus, P.W.: Quarter of a century experience with operative correction of metatarsus primus varus in hallux valgus. Bull. Hosp. Joint Dis. Orthop. Inst., *17:*404, 1956.
100. Lapidus, P.W.: The author's bunion operation from 1931 to 1959. Clin. Orthop., *16:*119, 1960.
101. Lennon, W.P.: Hallux valgus. Med. J. Aust., *2:*225, 1972.
102. Levine, M.A.: An operative technique for hallux valgus. J. Bone Joint Surg., *20:*932, 1938.
103. Lewis, R.J., and Feffer, H.L.: Modified chevron osteotomy of the first metatarsal. Clin. Orthop., *157:*105, 1981.
104. Lindgren, U., and Turan, I.: A new operation for hallux valgus. Clin. Orthop., *175:*179, 1983.

105. Ludloff, K.: Die beseitigung des hallux valgus durch die schraege planto-dorsale osteotomie des metatarsus I (erfahrungen und erfolge). Arch. Klin. Chir., *110:*364, 1918.
106. Lundberg, B.J., and Sulja, T.: Skeletal parameters in hallux valgus foot. Acta Orthop. Scand., *43:*576, 1972.
107. MacLennan, R.: Prevalence of hallux valgus in a neolithic New Guinea population. Lancet, *1:*1398, 1966.
108. Mann, R.A., and Coughlin, M.J.: Hallux valgus—etiology, anatomy, treatment and surgical considerations. Clin. Orthop., *157:*31, 1981.
109. Markheim, H.R., and Phillips, P.: Surgical treatment of bunions. Surg. Clin. North Am., *49:*1491, 1969.
110. Martorell, J.M.: Hallux disorder and metatarsal alignment. Clin. Orthop., *157:*14, 1981.
111. Mau, C., and Lauber, H.T.: Die operative behandlung des hallux valgus (nachuntersuchungen). Dtsch. Z. Chir., *197:*363, 1926.
112. Mayo, C.H.: The surgical treatment of bunions. Ann. Surg., *48:*300, 1908.
113. Mayo, C.H.: The surgical treatment of bunions. Minn. Med., *3:*326, 1920.
114. McBride, E.D.: A conservative operation for bunions. J. Bone Joint Surg., *10:*735, 1928.
115. McBride, E.D.: The conservative operation for bunions. J.A.M.A., *105:*1164, 1935.
116. McBride, E.D.: The McBride bunion hallux valgus operation. Refinements in the successive surgical step of the operation. J. Bone Joint Surg. [Am.], *49:*129, 1942.
117. McBride, E.D.: Hallux valgus bunion deformity. Instr. Course Lec., *9:*334, 1982.
118. McBride, E.D.: Hallux valgus bunion deformity: Its treatment in mild, moderate and severe stages. Int. Surg., *21:*99, 1954.
119. McBride, E.D.: Surgical treatment of hallux valgus bunions. Am. J. Orthop. Surg., *5:*44, 1953.
120. McBride, E.D.: The McBride bunion hallux valgus operation. J. Bone Joint Surg. [Am.], *49:*1675, 1967.
121. McElvenny, R.T., and Thompson, F.R.: A clinical study of one hundred patients subjected to simple exostosectomy for the relief of bunion pain. J. Bone Joint Surg., *22:*942, 1940.
122. McKeever, D.C.: Arthrodesis of the first metatarsophalangeal joint for hallux valgus, hallux rigidus and metatarsus primus varus. J. Bone Joint Surg. [Am.], *34:*129, 1952.
123. Merkel, K.D., Katoh, Y., Johnson, Jr., E.W., and Chad, F.Y.: Mitchell osteotomy for hallux valgus: Long-term follow-up and gait analysis. Foot Ankle, *3:*189, 1983.
124. Mikhail, I.K.: Bunion, hallux valgus and metatarsus primus varus. Surg. Gynecol. Obstet., *111:*637, 1960.
125. Miller, J.W.: Distal first metatarsal displacement osteotomy: Its place in the scheme of bunion surgery. J. Bone Joint Surg. [Am.], *56:*923, 1974.
126. Mitchell, C.L., et al., Osteotomy-bunionectomy for hallux valgus. J. Bone Joint Surg. [Am.], *40:*41, 1958.
127. Mizuno, S., Sima, Y., and Yamazaki, K.: Detorsion osteotomy of the first metatarsal bone in hallux valgus. J. Jpn. Orthop. Assoc., *30:*105, 1956.
128. Mygind, H.: Operation for hallux valgus. Report of

the Danish Orthopedic Association. J. Bone Joint Surg. [Br.], *34:*529, 1982.

129. Peabody, C.W.: The surgical cure of hallux valgus. J. Bone Joint Surg., *13:*273, 1931.
130. Pelet, D.: Osteotomy and fixation for hallux valgus. Clin. Orthop., *157:*42, 1981.
131. Piggott, H.H.: The natural history of hallux valgus in adolescents and early adult life. J. Bone Joint Surg. [Am.], *42:*749, 1960.
132. Raymakers, R., and Waugh, W.: The treatment of metatarsalgia with hallux valgus. J. Bone Joint Surg. [Br.], *53:*684, 1971.
133. Reikeras, O.: Metatarsal osteotomy for relief of hallux valgus. Arch. Orthop. Trauma. Surg., *99:*209, 1982.
134. Rix, R.: Modified Mayo operation for hallux valgus and bunion—a comparison with the Keller procedure. J. Bone Joint Surg. [Am.], *50:*1368, 1968.
135. Roberts, P.W.: An operation for hallux valgus. J.A.M.A., *80:*540, 1923.
136. Robinson, H.A.: Bunion, its causes and cure. Surg. Gynecol. Obstet, *27:*343, 1918.
137. Rosenbaum-de-Bristo, S.: The first metatarso-sesamoid joint. Int. Orthop., *6:*61, 1982.
138. Roth, P.B.: Hallux valgus: A note on operative technique. Br. Med. J., *1:*443, 1931.
139. Sandelin, T.: Operative treatment of hallux valgus. J.A.M.A., *80:*736, 1923.
140. Scranton, Jr., P.E.: Adolescent bunions: Diagnosis and management. Pediatr. Ann., *11:*518, 1982.
141. Scranton, Jr., P.E.: Principles in bunion surgery. J. Bone Joint Surg. [Am.], *65:*1026, 1983.
142. Shapiro, F., and Heller, L.: The Mitchell distal metatarsal osteotomy in the treatment of hallux valgus. Clin. Orthop., *107:*225, 1975.
143. Shepherd, B.D., and Giutronich, L.: Correction of hallux valgus. Med. J. Aust., *1:*131, 1982.
144. Shimazaki, K., and Takebe, K.: Investigations on the origin of hallux valgus by electromyographic analysis. Kobe J. Med. Sci., *27:*139, 1981.
145. Shine, I.B.: Incidence of hallux valgus in a partially shoe-wearing community. Br. Med. J., *1:*1648, 1965.
146. Silver, C.M., Simon, S.D., and Litchman, H.M.: Calcaneal osteotomy for valgus and varus deformities of the foot. Further experience. Int. Surg., *58:*24, 1973.
147. Silver, D.: The operative treatment of hallux valgus. J. Bone Joint Surg., *5:*225, 1923.
148. Simmonds, F.A., and Menelaus, M.B.: Hallux valgus in adolescents. J. Bone Joint Surg. [Br.], *42:*261, 1960.
149. Smith, S.E., and Meyer, T.L., Jr.: End result study of Stone bunionectomies. Clin. Orthop., *109:*144, 1975.
150. Soren, A.: Surgical correction of hallux valgus. Surgery, *71:*44, 1972.
151. Soren, A.: Surgical correction of hallux valgus. Arch. Orthop. Trauma. Surg., *96:*53, 1980.
152. Stamm, T.T.: Surgical treatment of hallux valgus. Guy's Hosp. Rep., *106:*273, 1957.
153. Stanley, L.L., and Breck, L.W.: Bunions, J. Bone Joint Surg., *17:*961, 1936.
154. Stein, H.C.: Hallux valgus. Surg. Gynecol. Obstet., *66:*889, 1938.
155. Stokes, I.A., Hutton, W.C., Stott, J.R., and Lowe, L.W.: Forces under the hallux valgus foot before and after surgery. Clin. Orthop., *142:*64, 1979.
156. Swanson, A.B.: Implant arthroplasty for the great toe. Clin. Orthop., *86:*74, 1972.
157. Syms, P.: Bunion, its aetiology, anatomy and operative treatment. N.Y. State J. Med., *66:*448, 1897.
158. Szaboky, G.T., and Raghaven, V.C.: Modification of Mitchell's lateral displacement angulation osteotomy. J. Bone Joint Surg. [Am.], *51:*1430, 1969.
159. Tangen, O.: Hallux valgus. Treatment by distal wedge osteotomy of first metatarsal (Hohmann-Thomasen). Acta Chir. Scand., *137:*151, 1971.
160. Trethowan, J.: Hallux valgus. In A System of Surgery. C.C. Choyce (ed.). New York, P.B. Hoeber, 1923, p. 1046.
161. Truslow, W.: Metatarsus primus varus or hallux valgus. J. Bone Joint Surg., *7:*98, 1925.
162. Wattling, W.O., and Cox, K.L.: Double osteotomies for structural correction of hallux abducto valgus. J. Foot Surg., *15:*61, 1976.
163. Waugh, W.: Mitchell's operation for hallux valgus. Proc. R. Soc. Lond. [Med.], *56:*159, 1963.
164. Wheeler, P.H.: Os intermetatarseum and hallux valgus. Am. J. Surg., *18:*341, 1932.
165. Wilson, D.W.: Treatment of hallux valgus and bunions. Br. J. Hosp. Med., *24:*548, 1980.
166. Wilson, J.N.: Oblique displacement osteotomy of hallux valgus. J. Bone Joint Surg. [Br.], *45:*552, 1963.
167. Young, J.K.: The etiology of hallux valgus or os intermetatarseum. Am. J. Orthop. Surg., *7:*336, 1909.
168. Young, J.K.: A new operation for adolescent hallux valgus. Univ. Penn. Med. Bull., *23:*459, 1910.

HALLUX RIGIDUS

Incidence

Hallux rigidus is caused by degenerative arthrosis of the first M-P joint, which shows a predilection for young male adults and some familial tendency. It is also known as metatarsus primus elevatus, hallux flexus, hallux limitus, hallux nonentensus, and dorsal bunion. Many factors directly or indirectly contribute to the development of hallux rigidus:

A. Acute trauma of the M-P joint of the great toe, which includes fracture, dislocation, and compression (jamming) injury.

B. Chronic trauma of the M-P joint of the great toe in people such as dancers and football and soccer kickers, whose professions put the M-P joints of their great toes in constant jeopardy of injury.

C. Dorsal hyperextension of the first metatarsal.

D. Excessively long first metatarsal.

E. Pronated (planovalgus) foot.

F. Osteochondritis dissecans of the first metatarsal head.

G. Hypermobile first metatarsal.

H. Epiphysitis of the proximal phalanx of the great toe.

I. Flat head of the first metatarsal.

J. Hallux valgus.

K. Inflammatory and metabolic diseases such as rheumatoid arthritis, gout, psoriatic arthritis, and ankylosing spondylitis.

L. Bunion or other M-P joint surgery of the great toe.

M. Genetic factors.

N. Obesity.

Clinical Symptoms and Signs

Hallux rigidus is second only to hallux valgus in causing painful and disabling deformity of the great toe, but it is significantly more disabling than hallux valgus. Patients with hallux rigidus usually complain of pain and swelling of the M-P joints of their great toes, particularly with prolonged standing and walking. Examination of the great toe often reveals an enlarged M-P joint; dorsal and dorsomedial exostosis of the first metatarsal head and sometimes the dorsal aspect of the base of the proximal phalanx; tenderness and pain with active and passive motion of the M-P joint; limited range of motion of the M-P joint with maximal limitation in extension, crepitations, and effusion of the M-P joint; tender bursitis over the dorsal exostosis; hypermobile interphalangeal joint; and painful callosities under the central metatarsal heads. Examination of the shoe frequently reveals that the vamp on the dorsum of the shoe has an oblique crease instead of the transverse crease of ordinary shoes. The sole of the same shoe also usually shows excessive wear on the lateral aspect of the sole and heel. For a patient with hallux rigidus weight is borne during barefoot walking on the outer fifth metatarsal. Then the great toe actively flexes its interphalangeal joint and the lesser toes also flex their M-P, PIP, and DIP joints, while the foot actively inverts and adducts the forefoot without moving the M-P joint of the great toe.

Roentgenographic Manifestations

Radiographic examination of a foot with hallux rigidus usually shows osteoarthritic changes of its M-P joint, which can include joint narrowing and irregularity; joint effusion; subchondral osteosclerosis; loose bodies; osteophyte formation on the dorsal aspect of the first metatarsal head and frequently also the dorsal aspect of the base of the proximal phalanx; hyperextension of the first metatarsal; flexion of the great toe at its M-P joint; and enlargement and arithritic changes of the medial and lateral sesamoids with narrowing of the sesamoidometatarsal joints (Figure 2–10).

Pathologic Anatomy

In hallux rigidus, the M-P joint capsule of the great toe commonly becomes thickened, and there is gross and microscopic evidence of chronic synovitis. When hallux rigidus has been present for a long time, contracture of the plantar joint capsule and collateral ligaments of the M-P joint of the great toe and flexor hallucis brevis is frequently present. In addition, thinning, fissuring, and erosion of the articular surfaces with exposure of the subchondral bone in differing degrees can usually be found in the M-P joint and often in the sesamoidometatarsal joints.

Nonsurgical Treatment

A. Shoe modifications: stiffening of the sole by means of an elongated shank or a

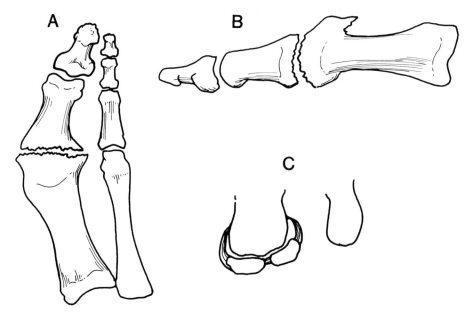

Figure 2–10. Various roentgenographic abnormalities associated with hallux rigidus. **A,** irregularity and narrowing of the M-P joint of the great toe. **B,** osteophyte formation on the dorsal aspect of the first metatarsal head in addition to irregularity and narrowing of the M-P joint of the great toe. **C,** enlargement of both the medial and lateral sesamoids in association with arthritic changes of the medial and lateral sesamoidometatarsal joints.

thicker leather sole (triple sole), stretching of the shoe vamp over the metatarsal exostosis, a metatarsal bar, a metatarsal pad, a rocker-bottom sole, or an arch support help to relieve symptoms of hallux rigidus (Figures 1–4—1–6 and 1–12).

B. Padding: padding of the foot and shoe with pressure relief areas cut out of the pad under the first metatarsal head (Figures 1–8 and 1–10).

C. Commercially available foot aids: donut-shaped pads to be placed over the dorsal exostosis, an arch support, and a metatarsal pad can also be used (Figures 1–16—1–18).

Surgical Treatment

A. Cheilectomy of the M-P joint of the great toe (Figure 2–11B): author's preferred surgical treatment of hallux rigidus by which all the osteophytes are removed from the M-P joint and the first metatarsal head is carefully and smoothly reshaped into a semispherical configuration. These changes are designed to improve range of motion, decrease pain, preserve stability, and minimize postoperative morbidity of the M-P joint of the great toe.

B. Excision of the proximal portion of the proximal phalanx of the great toe (Figure 2–11C): although it does give pain relief, this procedure results in a weaker great toe with reduced weight-bearing function, shortening, the possibility of developing a hallux extensus due to loss of flexor hallucis brevis function, and aggravation of metatarsalgia of the lesser toes.

C. Partial resection of the first metatarsal head with interposition of the medial joint capsule into the M-P joint of the great toe (Figure 2–11D): medial joint capsule is used to resurface the arthritic M-P joint after part of the first metatarsal head has been removed.

D. Insertion of a Silastic prosthesis into the resected M-P joint of the great toe (Figure

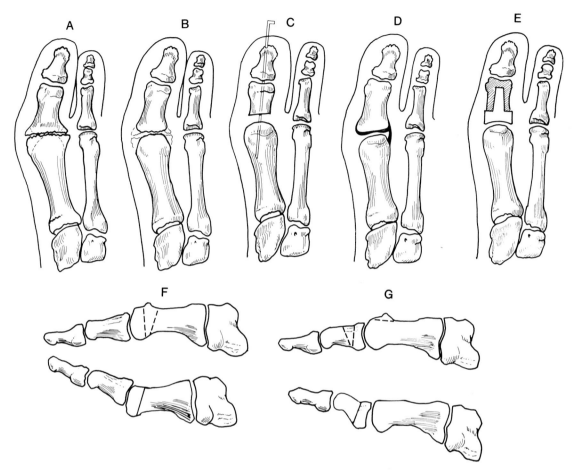

Figure 2–11. Various surgical procedures for treating hallux rigidus. **A,** hallux rigidus as evidenced by the irregularity, narrowing, and osteophyte formation of the M-P joint of the great toe. **B,** cheilectomy of the M-P joint of the great toe. **C,** resection of the proximal portion of the proximal phalanx of the great toe. **D,** partial resection of the head of the first metatarsal with interposition of the medial joint capsule into the M-P joint of the great toe. **E,** insertion of a Silastic prosthesis after the base of the proximal phalanx of the great toe is removed. **F,** close-wedge dorsal angulation osteotomy of the first metatarsal with simultaneous removal of its dorsal exostosis. **G,** close-wedge dorsal angulation osteotomy of the proximal phalanx of the great toe with removal of exostosis on the dorsal aspect of the first metatarsal head.

2–11E): although this procedure does. preserve the length of the great toe and motion at its M-P joint, postoperative swelling, infection, and breakage of the prosthesis are some of the possible complications.

E. Arthrodesis of the M-P joint of the great toe (Figure 2–5C): M-P joint should be fused at 15 to 20° of dorsiflexion and about 10° of valgus position of the great toe. This arthrodesis enhances the weight-bearing function of the great toe in addition to complete pain relief of its previously symptomatic M-P joint. Drawbacks include inability to wear shoes with various heel heights, the possibility of developing a painful non-union of the M-P joint, and symptomatic arthrosis of the interphalangeal joint of the great toe.

F. Dorsal wedge cuneiform osteotomy of the head of the first metatarsal (Figure 2–11F): increases the dorsiflexion of the great toe and thus lessens the weight-bearing pressure on its M-P joint. This procedure is useful in treating young patients with hallux rigidus and mild arthritis of the M-P joints of their great toes.

G. Dorsal wedge osteotomy of the proximal phalanx of the great toe (Figure 2–11G): increases the dorsiflexion of the great toe and decreases the weight-bearing pressure on its painful M-P joint. Useful technique for treating hallux rigidus in young patients with mild arthritis of the M-P joint of the great toes.

Cheilectomy of the M-P joint of the great toe includes the following steps (Figure 2–12):

1. Make a longitudinal and slightly curved skin incision over the dorsomedial aspect of the M-P joint of the great toe (Figure 2–12A).

2. Longitudinally incise the underlying M-P joint capsule and expose its dorsal, medial, and lateral aspects by means of sharp dissection. Remove all exostoses around the joint with a small sharp osteotome. The metatarsal head and base of the proximal phalanx that have undergone osteophytectomy are carefully smoothed with a small bone rasp, and the joint capsule and skin are closed in a regular manner (Figures 2–12B and C).

3. On the second or third postoperative day, gentle active and passive motion of the M-P joint is started to maintain the improved range of motion gained by the

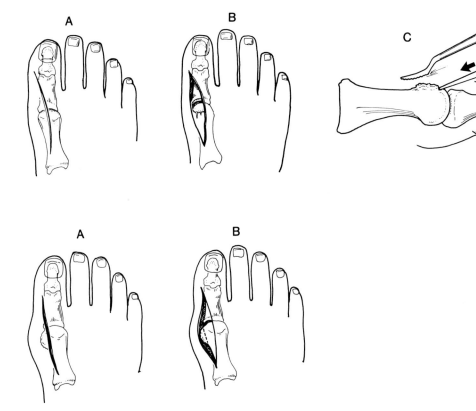

Figure 2–12. Cheilectomy of the M-P joint of the great toe. **A,** skin incision. **B,** incision of the M-P joint capsule and removal of the dorsal and medial exostoses of the first metatarsal head. **C,** smoothing of all rough bone edges after osteophytectomy with a small bone rasp before closing the joint capsule and skin.

cheilectomy. Exercises are continued for several days until desired results are achieved.

Resection of the proximal portion of the proximal phalanx of the great toe includes the following steps (Figure 2–13):

1. Make a slightly curved longitudinal skin incision over the dorsomedial aspect of the great toe, extending from the distal portion of the proximal phalanx to the neck of the first metatarsal (Figure 2–13A).

2. Longitudinally incise the dorsal aspect of the M-P joint capsule and expose the proximal one half of the proximal phalanx as well as the dorsal and medial aspects of the first metatarsal head. By placing two Joker retractors under the midportion of the proximal phalanx to protect the underlying flexor hallucis longus tendon and neurovascular bundles, osteotomy of the proximal phalanx is performed with a microsaw (Figure 2–13B).

3. Remove the proximal one half of the proximal phalanx by detaching its joint capsule, collateral ligaments, and the insertions of extensor and flexor hallucis brevis. Excise the dorsal exostosis of the first metatarsal head with a sharp osteo-

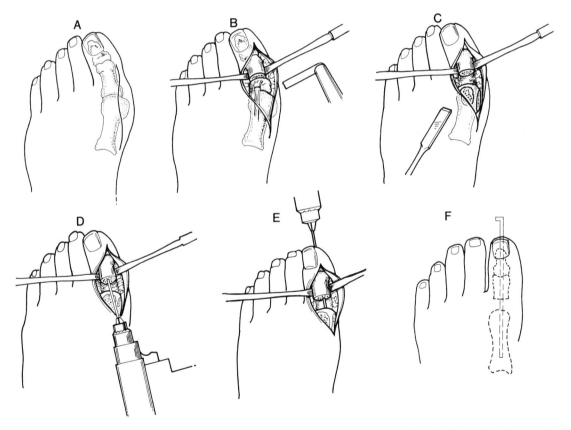

Figure 2–13. Resection of the proximal portion of the proximal phalanx of the great toe. **A,** skin incision. **B,** capsular incision plus exposure of the proximal phalanx and the head of the first metatarsal, and osteotomy of the proximal phalanx with a microsaw. **C,** removal of the dorsal and medial exostoses of the first metatarsal head. **D,** driving the K-wire from the distal portion of the proximal phalanx through the distal phalanx to emerge from the tip of the great toe. **E,** driving the same wire in a retrograde manner into the first metatarsal. **F,** bending the end of the wire and closure of the joint capsule and the skin in a regular manner.

88. Wishart, J.: Arthrodesis of the first metatarsophalangeal joint for hallux valgus and rigidus. J. Bone
Joint Surg. [Br.], *35:*494, 1953.
89. Wrighton, J.D.: A ten-year review of Keller's operation: Review of Keller's operation at the Princess
Elizabeth Orthopaedic Hospital, Exeter. Clin. Orthop., *89:*207, 1972.
90. Zadik, F.R.: Arthrodesis of the great toe. Br. Med. J.,
*2:*1573, 1960.

HALLUX VARUS

Incidence

The two principal forms of hallux varus are
congenital and acquired hallux varus. The
congenital form is usually present at birth or
soon after and can be associated with
metatarsus primus varus or more commonly
with adductovarus deformity of the forefoot and
equinovarus deformity of the entire foot. Preaxial polydactyly of the foot can also be associated with congenital hallux varus, which
shows bilateral involvement in about one third
of cases with no sex predilection. There are
three main types of congenital hallux varus:

A. Primary type, which is not associated with
   other congenital anomalies. This type is
   caused by a supernumerary toe anlage on
   the medial side of the foot that has undergone developmental arrest to produce a
   tight fibrous or cartilaginous band extending from the medial aspect of the great toe
   to the base of the first metatarsal, which
   pulls the great toe into a varus position.

B. Associated with other congenital deformities of the forepart of the foot, such as
   metatarsus varus, marked shortening and
   broadening of the first metatarsal, and accessory bones or toes (accessory hallux,
   metatarsal, and toe).

C. Associated with developmental affections
   of the skeleton, such as diatrophic dwarfism.

In contrast, there are many factors that are
responsible for the development of the acquired form of hallux varus:

A. Complication of the Silver or McBride bunion operation in which the conjoined tendon is detached from the lateral base of
   the proximal phalanx of the great toe favoring subsequent development of hallux
   varus.

B. Muscle imbalance between a stronger abductor hallucis and a weaker adductor hallucis, which can take several forms:
   1. A paralyzed adductor hallucis against a
      weak, normal, or spastic abductor hal-
      lucis.
   2. A weak adductor hallucis against a
      normal or spastic abductor hallucis.
   3. A normal adductor hallucis against a
      spastic abductor hallucis.

C. Infection of the M-P joint of the great toe.

D. Gout of the M-P joint of the great toe.

E. Malunion of fractures about the M-P joint
   of the great toe.

F. Rupture of the adductor hallucis caused
   by synovitis or rheumatoid arthritis.

G. Resection of too much bone from the medial aspect of the metatarsal head, creating a medial instability of the M-P joint and
   favoring the development of hallux varus.

H. Medial displacement of the medial sesamoid bone.

I. Improper application of a cast after Mitchell bunionectomy, which causes medial
   displacement of the affected first metatarsal head.

Clinical Symptoms and Signs

The most obvious deformity of hallux varus
is medial deviation of the great toe with a wide
separation between the great and second toes.

In addition, the great toe is also laterally rotated along its longitudinal axis with the toenail facing laterally (Figure 2–14). Passive lateral deviation of the great toe is usually met with resistance from the contracted soft tissues on the medial aspect of the M-P joint of the great toe. The patient is often unable to adduct the great toe toward the second toe actively. Painful callosity on the dorsal aspect of the interphalangeal joint of the great toe is another common clinical finding, and patients frequently complain of the ugly appearance of their great toes and inability to wear shoes comfortably. When degenerative arthritis has developed in the M-P joint of the great toe, crepitations, osteophyte formation, painful and limited joint motion, and joint tenderness and effusion may all be present. When hallux extensus is associated with hallux varus, the extensor hallucis longus becomes contracted and the great toe is both medially deviated and hyperextended at its M-P joint, resulting in severe restriction of the active and passive plantar flexion of the great toe at the M-P joint.

Roentgenographic Manifestations

The standing anteroposterior view of the foot usually shows medial deviation of the great toe at the M-P joint, and the shadow of the toenail may appear to be laterally displaced due to supination of the great toe. An axial view of the sesamoids may also show medial deviation of both the medial and lateral sesamoid bones (Figure 2–15). When hallux extensus is associated with hallux varus, hyperextension of the great toe at its M-P joint may be seen on the lateral view. When arthritic changes have occurred in the M-P joint of the great toe, joint irregularity and narrowing, osteophyte formation at the joint margins, joint effusion, and subchrondral osteosclerosis are present.

Pathologic Anatomy

The external rotation and medial deviation of the great toe in hallux varus favor the contracture of the medial joint capsule and medial collateral ligament of the M-P joint of the great toe. Similarly, the abductor hallucis and the medial head of the flexor hallucis brevis become contracted and rotated in a dorsal direction. On the contrary, the same deformities of the great toe cause the lateral joint capsule and lateral collateral ligament of the M-P joint to become stretched, and the adductor hallucis and the lateral head of the flexor hallucis brevis also rotate in a more plantar direction. When hallux extensus is also present, the dorsal capsule of the M-P joint of the great toe is contracted and the extensor hallucis

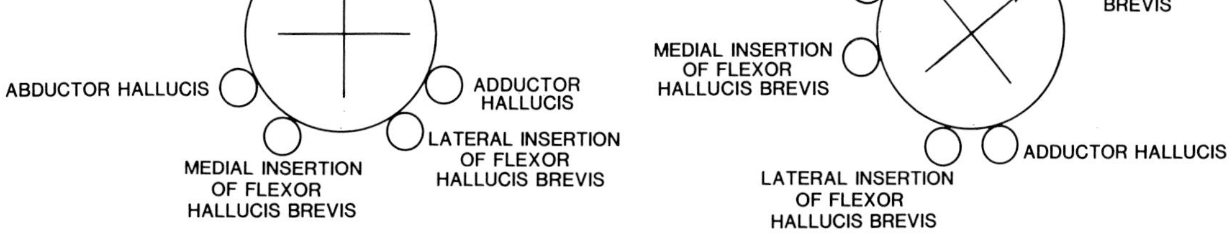

A

IN NORMAL HALLUX

B

IN HALLUX VARUS

Figure 2–14. Rotational deformity of hallux varus. **A,** in normal hallux, the great toe is in a neutral position. **B,** in hallux varus, the great toe is externally rotated along its longitudinal axis, displacing the insertions of the extensor hallucis brevis, adductor hallucis, and the lateral head of the flexor hallucis brevis into a more plantar position, and the abductor hallucis and medial head of the flexor hallucis brevis into a more dorsal position.

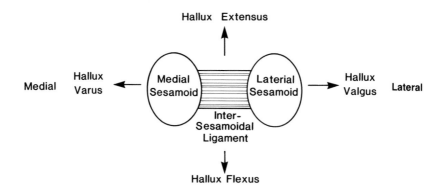

Figure 2–15. Various displacements of the sesamoids of the great toe: distal displacement in hallux extensus; proximal displacement in hallux flexus; medial displacement in hallux varus; lateral displacement in hallux valgus.

longus likewise becomes shortened, whereas the plantar capsule of the same M-P joint becomes correspondingly stretched. If degenerative arthritis has occurred in the M-P joint of the great toe, then deterioration of the articular surfaces, synovial proliferation, and thickening of the joint capsule may be present.

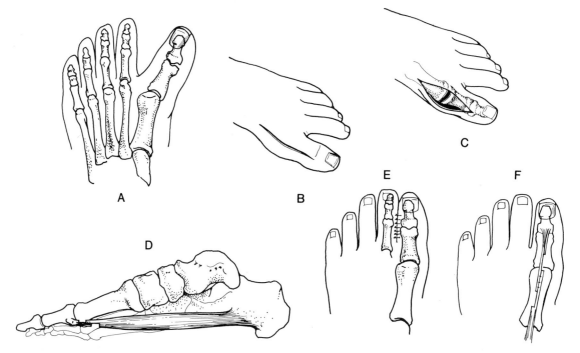

Figure 2–16. Surgical treatment of hallux varus with or without hallux extensus. **A,** hallux varus without arthritis of the M-P joint. **B,** skin incision. **C,** medial capsulotomy of the M-P joint. **D,** tendon lengthening of the contracted abductor hallucis. **E,** syndactylization of the great and second toes for additional stability of the great toe. **F,** Z-plasty lengthening of the extensor hallucis longus in combination with dorsal and medial capsulotomies and lengthening or tenotomy of the abductor hallucis in treating hallux varus extensus.

Nonsurgical Treatment

A. Shoe modifications: extra-depth and space shoes can be prescribed to accommodate the deformed great toe and the painful callosity on the dorsal aspect of the interphalangeal joint (Figure 1–7).

B. Padding and taping of the great toe: padding the painful exostosis on the dorsal aspect of the interphalangeal joint and taping of the great toe to the second toe can provide some symptomatic pain relief (Figure 1–8).

C. Commercially available foot aids: donut-shaped pad for the exostosis on the dorsal aspect of the interphalangeal joint of the great toe, and putting the great toe and the second toe into a large and soft toe cap can also provide pain relief for the painful dorsal callosity of the great toe while keeping the deformed great toe in a more anatomic position (Figures 1–16 and 1–18).

Surgical Treatment

A. Congenital hallux varus
  1. McElvenny (1941) operation: includes excision of accessory bones; medial sesamoidectomy and capsulotomy; release of medial fibrous band; passing the extensor hallucis brevis tendon through a drilled hole of the first metatarsal neck, wrapping it around the extensor hallucis longus, passing it through the dorsal capsule, and finally anchoring it to the metatarsal; transfixing the M-P joint with a K-wire; and partial syndactylization of the first and second toes. (Readers are urged to read McElvenny's original article to become familiar with this complex operation.)
  2. Farmer (1958) operation: includes the use of a Y-shaped dorsal or plantar skin flap between the first and second toe; curving the skin incision medially across the M-P joint; moving the big toe next to the second toe to unite the two dig-

its; excising the accessory phalanx and hypertrophied soft tissue; moving the Y-shaped flap medially to cover the medial skin defect; and finally covering any area still exposed with full-thickness skin graft. (Readers are advised to read Farmer's original article for complete information.)

B. Acquired hallux varus
  1. In the absence of metatarsus primus varus on in the presence of minimal metatarsus primus varus: perform adductor lengthening or tenotomy and medial capsulotomy, and maintain correction with a small K-wire through the

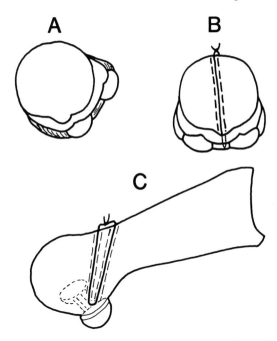

Figure 2–17. Reduction of the dislocated medial and lateral sesamoidometatarsal joints in hallux varus. **A,** both the medial and lateral sesamoidometatarsal joints are dislocated medially. **B,** hold the medial and lateral sesamoids in their anatomic position by passing a stout suture through the intersesamoidal ligament and through two holes drilled in the crista to emerge on the dorsal aspect of the first metatarsal neck, where the free suture ends are tied tightly. **C,** lateral view of the first metatarsal showing the two sesamoid bones held in their anatomic site by passing a suture through the intersesamoidal ligament and two oblique drilled holes through the head and neck of the first metatarsal before the two ends of the suture are tied on the dorsal aspect of the first metatarsal.

M-P joint of the great toe (Figure 2–16A—D).

2. Hallux extensus associated with hallux varus (hallux varus extensus): in addition to abductor lengthening or tenotomy and medial capsulotomy, also perform lengthening of extensor hallucis longus and dorsal capsulotomy of the M-P joint of the great toe (Figure 2–16A—F).

3. Associated with medial displacement of the sesamoids: in addition to abductor lengthening or tenotomy and medial capsulotomy, realign the sesamoidometatarsal articulation and hold them to the first metatarsal with sutures through drilled holes in the distal portion of the first metatarsal (Figure 2–17).

4. Significant degenerative changes in the M-P joint of the great toe: perform an arthroplasty or an arthrodesis procedure (Figure 2–18).

5. Due to traumatic rupture of adductor hallucis: join together the first and second toes (Figure 2–16E).

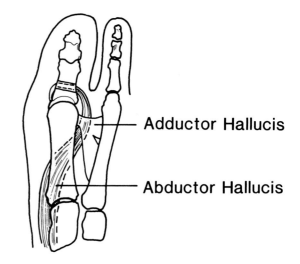

Adductor Hallucis

Abductor Hallucis

Figure 2–19. Transfer of the abductor hallucis under the first metatarsal shaft and the flexor hallucis brevis and adductor hallucis to the lateral aspect of the proximal phalanx of the great toe where it is fixed to the proximal phalanx through a drilled hole. This transferred abductor hallucis can now actively pull the great toe toward the second toe, thus preventing recurrence of hallux varus.

6. Associated with excessive resection of the medial one half of the first metatarsal head: in addition to medial soft tissue release, transfer the tendon of

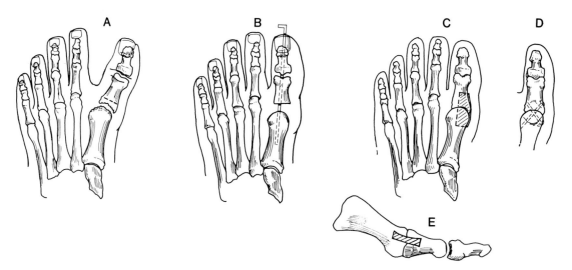

Figure 2–18. Various surgical methods for treating hallux varus associated with significant arthritis of the M-P joint. **A,** hallux varus and arthritis of the M-P joint of the great toe. **B,** resection of the proximal portion of the proximal phalanx of the great toe. The great toe is held in a corrected position with a K-wire through the M-P joint. **C,** arthrodesis of the M-P joint of the great toe with an inlay bone graft. **D,** arthrodesis of the M-P joint of the great toe with two screws across the joint after the articular cartilage has been completely removed with a fine air-powered burr. **E,** lateral view of *C* showing that the two ends of the bone graft are purposely made thicker than its central portion to resist the separation of the fusional site.

the abductor hallucis to the lateral aspect of the proximal phalanx of the great toe, and fix it to the proximal phalanx through a drilled hole. Alternative methods are to transfer the extensor hallucis longus tendon and fix it to the lateral side of the proximal phalanx of the great toe through a drilled hole, or simply to perform an arthrodesis of the M-P joint (Figures 2–18C—E, 2–19).

REFERENCES

Hallux Varus

1. Albitsky, B.A.: Bilateral hallux varus. Vestn. Khir., *70:*50, 1950.
2. Christian, J.C., Cho, K.S., Franken, E.A., and Thompson, B.H.: Dominant preaxial brachydactyly with hallux varus and thumb abduction. Am. J. Hum. Genet., *24:*694, 1972.
3. Clarke, J.J.: Hallux valgus and hallux varus. Lancet, *1:*609, 1900.
4. Farmer, A.W.: Congenital hallux varus. Am. J. Surg., *95:*274, 1958.
5. Haas, S.L.: An operation for correction of hallux varus. J. Bone Joint Surg., *20:*705, 1938.
6. Hawkins, F.B.: Acquired hallux varus: Cause, prevention and correction. Clin. Orthop., *76:*169, 1971.
7. Howitz, M.T.: An unusual hallux varus deformity and its surgical correction. J. Bone Joint Surg., *19:*828, 1937.
8. Jahss, M.H.: Spontaneous hallux varus: Relation to poliomyelitis and congenital absence of fibular sesamoid. Foot Ankle, *3:*224, 1983.
9. Kelikian, H., Clayton, L., and Loseff, H.: Surgical syndactylism of the toes. Clin. Orthop., *19:*208, 1961.
10. Kimizuka, M., and Miyanaga, Y.: The treatment of acquired hallux varus after the McBride procedure. J. Foot Surg., *19:*135, 1980.
11. Kleiner, B.C., and Holmes, L.B.: Hallux varus and preaxial polysyndactyly in brothers. Am. J. Med. Genet., *6:*113, 1980.
12. Lasserre, C.: Polysyndactylia of great toe with hallux varus. Rev. D'Orthop., *33:*133, 1947.
13. McElvenny, R.T.: Hallux varus. Bull Northwestern Med School, *15:*277, 1941.
14. Miller, J.W.: Acquired hallux varus: A preventable and correctable disorder. J. Bone Joint Surg. [Am.], *57:*183, 1975.
15. Myginal, H.B.: Surgical correction of congenital hallux varus. Nord. Med., *49:*914, 1953.
16. Pavasars, R.: Hallux varus; Rare deformity of toes. Arch. Orthop. Trauma Surg., *44:*333, 1950.
17. Rutte, E.: Bilateral congenital hallux varus. Z. Orthop., *80:*144, 1950.
18. Skoblin, A.P.: Case of unusual congenital abnormality of the foot. Ortop. Travmatol. Protez., *1:*84, 1955.
19. Sloane, D.: Congenital hallux varus. J. Bone Joint Surg. *17:*209, 1935.
20. Thomson, S.A.: Hallux varus and metatarsus varus. Clin. Orthop., *16:*109, 1960.
21. Wood, W.A.: Acquired hallux varus: A new corrective procedure. J. Foot Surg., *20:*194, 1981.

HALLUX EXTENSUS (ELEVATUS)

Incidence

The balance of the M-P joint of the great toe in the dorsal and plantar direction is maintained by two sets of muscles, the extensor hallucis longus and brevis acting on its dorsal side and the flexor hallucis longus and brevis on its plantar side. These muscles insert to the dorsal and plantar bases of the proximal and distal phalanges of the great toe, respectively (Figure 2–20). Whenever the pull of the extensor hallucis longus and brevis exceeds the counterbalancing force exerted by the flexor hallucis longus and brevis, a hallux extensus deformity may develop. A list of the various possible causes of hallux extensus follows:

A. Laceration of the flexor hallucis longus.

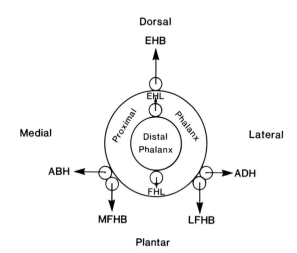

Figure 2–20. Forces acting on the bases of the proximal and distal phalanges of the great toe. Dorsiflexion: extensor hallucis brevis (EHB) and longus (EHL); plantar flexion: flexor hallucis brevis (FHB) and longus (FHL); abduction: abductor hallucis (ABH); adduction: adductor hallucis (ADH). LFHB and MFHB: lateral and medial FHB.

B. Paralysis of the flexor hallucis longus and brevis in poliomyelitis.

C. Complication of Keller's bunionectomy, during which the insertions of the flexor hallucis brevis are routinely eliminated from the base of the proximal phalanx of the great toe.

D. Complication of medial and lateral sesamoidectomies of the great toe.

E. Complication of McBride or Silver's bunion operations, which may result in hallux varus extensus.

F. Trauma, inflammatory and neuromuscular diseases, clubfoot, and the like can produce clawfoot deformity in which the M-P joint of the great toe is hyperextended and the interphalangeal joint of the same toe is hyperflexed.

G. Complication of Mitchell's bunionectomy in which the operated first metatarsal head heals in a dorsally displaced position.

H. Complete detachment of both heads of the flexor hallucis brevis from their insertions at the base of the proximal phalanx of the great toe caused by pyarthrosis of the M-P joint and osteomyelitis of the proximal phalanx. Such a situation occurred in a 55-year-old man with polyarteritis nodosa who was treated by the author.

I. Rheumatoid arthritis can occasionally produce an unusual deformity of the great toe called hallux extensus interphalangeus, in which the proximal phalanx of the great toe is in a neutral or slightly flexed position while the distal phalanx is in a hyperextended position.

Loss of function of the flexor hallucis longus commonly results in hyperextension of the M-P joint of the great toe, whereas loss of flexor hallucis brevis function may cause both hyperextension of the M-P joint and hyper-flexion of the interphalangeal joint of the great toe.

Clinical Symptoms and Signs

Patients with hallux extensus usually complain of the ugly appearance of their deformed great toes and inability to wear shoes comfortably. Examination usually reveals hyperextension deformity of the great toe at the M-P joint with the extensor hallucis longus tendon bowstrung across the M-P joint. Both active and passive plantar flexion of the great toe at the M-P joint is significantly decreased. When hyperextension of the M-P joint is associated with flexion contracture of the interphalangeal joint of the great toe, active and passive extension of the interphalangeal joint is greatly restricted. A painful corn may also be present on the dorsal aspect of the interphalangeal joint of the great toe. When hallux varus extensus is present, the great toe is both hyperextended and medially deviated at the M-P joint. When hallux extensus interphalangeus caused by rheumatoid arthritis is present, the M-P joint of the great toe is generally in a neutral or a slightly flexed position, but the interphalangeal joint is hyperextended in association with possible crepitation, tenderness, swelling, and osteophyte formation.

Roentgenographic Manifestations

In hallux extensus, the standing lateral view of the foot usually shows hyperextension of the proximal phalanx of the great toe at the M-P joint with dorsal subluxation or even frank dorsal dislocation of the great toe. Both the medial and lateral sesamoid bones are distally displaced. When hallux extensus is associated with a clawfoot deformity, hyperextension of the proximal phalanx at the M-P joint and hyperflexion of the distal phalanx at the interphalangeal joint of the great toe occur. When hallux varus extensus is present, an anteroposterior standing view of the foot also shows medial deviation of the great toe at the M-P joint. When hallux extensus interphalangeus is caused by rheumatoid arthritis, in addition to hyperextension of the distal phalanx at the interphalangeal joint of the great toe, arthritic changes such as joint irregularity and narrowing may also be noted in the same joint.

Pathologic Anatomy

In hallux extensus, the sesamoids move distally and may lie in front of the first metatarsal head. This distal displacement of the sesamoid is accompanied by stretching of both the flexor hallucis brevis and the plantar joint capsule of the M-P joint of the great toe. Dorsal subluxation and dislocation of the great toe cause the dorsal joint capsule and medial and lateral collateral ligaments of the M-P joint, as well as the extensor hallucis longus and brevis, to become contracted. This contraction results in restriction of the active and passive plantar flexion of the great toe at the M-P joint. When hallux varus extensus is present, in addition to the aforementioned contracted structures, the abductor hallucis and the medial joint capsule of the M-P joint of the great toe likewise become contracted. When rheumatoid arthritis has produced hallux extensus interphalangeus, in addition to the contracted medial and lateral collateral ligaments and dorsal joint capsule of the interphalangeal joint of the great toe, synovial proliferation and articular destruction by the synovial ingrowths also occur.

Nonsurgical Treatment

A. Shoe modifications: extra-depth, space, and combination last shoes with roomy toe boxes to accommodate the deformed great toe and corn on the dorsal aspect of the same toe can provide pain relief (Figures 1–2 and 1–7).

B. Padding and taping of the great toe: taping the deformed great toe to the normal second toe and padding the painful corn on the dorsal aspect of the great toe can give symptomatic relief (Figure 1–8).

C. Commercially available foot aids: donut-shaped pads for a painful corn on the dorsal aspect of the great toe and putting the

deformed great toe and the normal second toe into a large and soft toe cap are helpful (Figures 1–16 and 1–18).

Surgical Treatment

A. Repair acute laceration of the flexor hallucis longus to prevent subsequent development of hallux extensus.

B. Hallux extensus with a relatively normal interphalangeal joint of the great toe: perform Z-plasty lengthening of the extensor hallucis longus and capsulotomy of the M-P joint of the great toe. Hold the M-P joint in a neutral position with a small smooth K-wire (Figure 2–21A and C—G).

C. With flexion contracture of the interphalangeal joint of the great toe: perform an arthrodesis of the interphalangeal joint by removing its opposing articular surfaces with a microsaw, keeping them in intimate contact with a longitudinal and an oblique K-wire; perform a capsulotomy of the M-P joint of the great toe; and transfer the extensor hallucis longus to the neck of the first metatarsal followed by holding the M-P joint in a neutral position with a small smooth K-wire (Figures 2–21H and I and 2–22).

D. Caused by pyarthrosis of the M-P joint, rupture of the flexor hallucis brevis, and osteomyelitis of the proximal phalanx of the great toe: perform a proximal phalangectomy and debridement of the M-P joint of the great toe, followed by splinting the great toe in a neutral position and the use of appropriate antibiotics (Figure 2–23).

E. Secondary to previous infection or trauma resulting in arthritis of the M-P joint of the great toe: resect the proximal portion of the proximal phalanx of the great toe (Figure 2–18B) or perform an arthrodesis of the M-P joint of the great toe (Figure 2–18C—E).

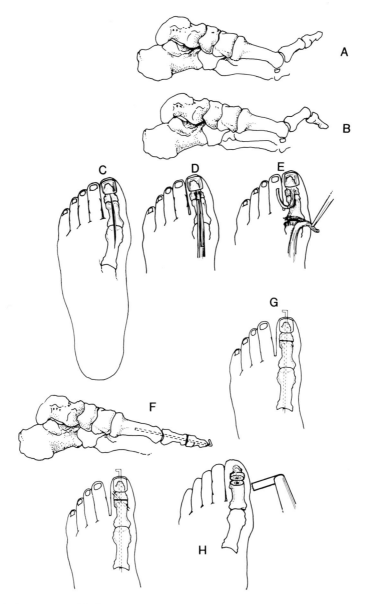

Figure 2–21. Surgical treatment of hallux extensus. **A,** hallux extensus with the interphalangeal joint of the great toe in a neutral position. **B,** hallux extensus with flexion contracture of the interphalangeal joint of the great toe. **C,** longitudinal skin incision on the dorsal aspect of the great toe to expose the underlying extensor hallucis longus. **D,** extensor hallucis longus split longitudinally into two equal parts. **E,** two ends of the tendon are separated and the dorsal capsulotomy is performed. The split extensor hallucis longus is then sutured in a lengthened position. **F** and **G,** hallux extensus has been corrected and a K-wire is used to hold the M-P joint in a neutral position. **H,** resection of the articular surfaces of the interphalangeal joint of the great toe with a microsaw. **I,** completion of the fusion of the interphalangeal joint by fixing the joint with a longitudinal and an oblique K-wire.

F. Secondary to Keller's bunionectomy: fuse the remaining M-P joint with a bone graft, or perform lengthening of the extensor hallucis longus and capsulotomy of the M-P joint. Hold the M-P joint in a neutral position by using a smooth K-wire with or without syndactylization of the great and second toes (Figure 2–16E).

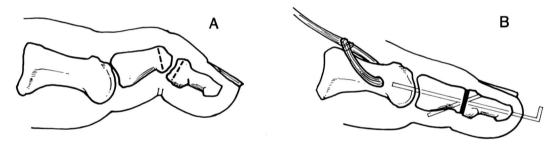

Figure 2–22. Surgical treatment of hallux extensus with flexion contracture in the interphalangeal joint of the great toe. **A,** resection of the joint surfaces of the interphalangeal joint of the great toe. **B,** transfer of the extensor hallucis longus to the neck of the first metatarsal and fusion of the interphalangeal joint with two K-wires. The M-P joint is held in a neutral position with the same longitudinal wire used in fusing the interphalangeal joint.

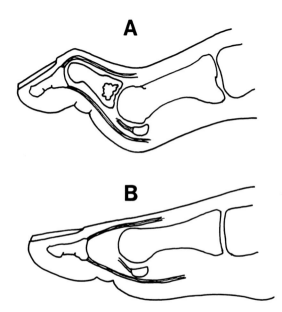

Figure 2–23. Surgical treatment of hallux extensus caused by pyarthrosis of the M-P joint, rupture of the flexor hallucis brevis, and osteomyelitis of the proximal phalanx of the great toe. **A,** hallux extensus associated with rupture of the flexor hallucis brevis and osteomyelitis of the proximal phalanx. **B,** proximal phalanx has been removed and the deformity of the hallux extensus has been corrected.

G. Brought about by a healed and dorsally displaced first metatarsal head (an occasional complication of Mitchell's bunionectomy): perform a carefully planned plantar angulation osteotomy of the first metatarsal.

H. Associated with hallux varus (hallux varus extensus): perform abductor lengthening or tenotomy; medial and dorsal capsulotomies of the M-P joint of the great toe; Z-plasty lengthening of the extensor hallucis longus, and hold the M-P joint in a neutral position with a small smooth K-wire, with or without syndactylization of the great and second toes (Figures 2–16A—F).

I. Hallux extensus interphalangeus secondary to rheumatoid arthritis: fuse the interphalangeal joint of the great toe and transfer the extensor hallucis longus to the neck of the first metatarsal (Figure 2–22B).

REFERENCES

Hallux Extensus (Elevatus)

1. Jahss, M.H.: Disorders of the The Foot. Philadelphia, W.B. Saunders, 1982, pp. 603–604.
2. Kelikian, H.: Hallux Valgus, Allied Deformities of The Forefoot and Metatarsalgia. Philadelphia, W.B. Saunders, 1965, p. 443.
3. Mann, R.A. (ed.): DuVries' Surgery of the Foot. 4th Ed. St. Louis, C.V. Mosby, 1978. pp. 269–273.

HALLUX FLEXUS

Incidence

Hallux flexus is a relatively uncommon deformity of the great toe in which the great toe is plantarly flexed at the M-P joint. Several causes are either directly or indirectly responsible for the pathogenesis of hallux flexus:

A. Muscle imbalance between the stronger

flexors and the weaker extensors of the great toe caused by both upper and lower motor neuron lesions.

B. An associated deformity of a dorsal bunion.

C. Rupture of the extensor hallux longus caused by rheumatoid tenosynovitis.

D. Previous laceration of the extensor hallucis longus and brevis.

E. Congenital talipes planovalgus with a rocker-bottom deformity.

F. Scarring and flexion contracture of the flexor hallucis longus secondary to trauma to the foot and ankle region.

G. Hallux rigidus in which the large dorsal exostosis on the first metatarsal head forces the proximal phalanx of the great toe into a flexed position.

Clinical Symptoms and Signs

The typical deformity of hallux flexus is plantar flexion of the great toe at the M-P joint. This flexion deformity of the great toe causes concentration of pressure at the plantar aspect of the distal portion of the great toe during weight-bearing activities, and may produce a painful callosity in that region. When hallux flexus has been present for some time, active and passive dorsiflexion of the great toe at the M-P joint is restricted. When degenerative arthritis is present in the M-P joint of the great toe, pain, crepitation, tenderness, swelling, limited range of motion, and dorsal osteophyte formation are possible clinical findings.

Roentgenographic Manifestations

The standing lateral view of the foot usually shows flexion of the proximal phalanx of the great toe at the M-P joint, and the medial and lateral sesamoids are also somewhat proximally displaced. When arthritis has developed in the M-P joint of the great toe, joint

irregularity and narrowing, subchrondral osteosclerosis, and osteophyte formation at joint margins may be present.

Pathologic Anatomy

When hallux flexus has been present for a considerable length of time, the plantar joint capsule and collateral ligaments of the M-P joint of the great toe become contracted; the flexor hallux longus and brevis also become proportionally shortened. This plantar soft tissue contracture is responsible for the restricted active and passive dorsiflexion of the great toe at the M-P joint. When arthritis has developed in the M-P joint of the great toe, degeneration of the articular cartilage, patchy exposure of the subchondral bone, gross and microscopic evidence of chronic synovitis, and osteophyte formation on the dorsal aspect of the M-P joint may be present.

Nonsurgical Treatment

A. Shoe modifications: a roomy shoe fitted with a soft, custom-made total contact insole can distribute weight-bearing pressure over the entire plantar surface of the foot, and can provide relief for the symptomatic and deformed great toe (Figures 1–6 and 1–7).

B. Padding and taping of the great toe: donut-shaped pads applied to the painful callosity on the plantar surface of the great toe and taping the deformed great toe to the normal second toe can give symptomatic relief (Figure 1–8).

C. Commercially available foot aids: application of a donut-shaped pad and putting the big toe in a soft toe cap or both the great toe and the second toe into a large toe cap to hold the great toe in a more physiologic position are helpful (Figures 1–16 and 1–18).

Surgical Treatment

A. Acute rupture or laceration of the extensor hallucis longus: primarily repair the dam-

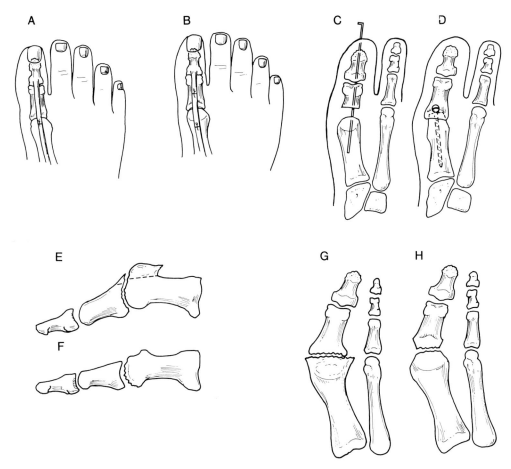

Figure 2–24. Various surgical procedures for treating hallux flexus. **A,** primary end-to-end repair of acutely ruptured extensor hallucis longus tendon. **B,** tendon graft obtained from extensor digitorum longus of the fourth or fifth toe is used to bridge the gap caused by a neglected rupture of the extensor hallucis longus tendon. **C,** resection of the proximal portion of the proximal phalanx of the great toe. **D,** arthrodesis of the M-P joint of the great toe. **E–H,** cheilectomy of the M-P joint of the great toe.

aged extensor hallucis longus (Figure 2–24A).

B. Neglected rupture or laceration of the tendon of the extensor hallucis longus with myostatic contracture of the extensor hallucis longus: repair the ruptured extensor hallucis longus with a tendon graft obtained from the extensor digitorum longus of the fourth or fifth toe (Figure 2–24B).

C. Hallux flexus associated with severe degenerative arthritis of the M-P joint of the great toe: resect the proximal portion of

the proximal phalanx or perform an arthrodesis of the M-P joint of the great toe (Figure 2–24C and D).

D. Associated with dorsal bunion: discussed in detail in the next section.

E. Associated with hallux rigidus: perform a cheilectomy of the M-P joint of the great toe (Figure 2–24E—H).

F. Caused by muscle imbalance between the stronger flexors and the weaker exten-

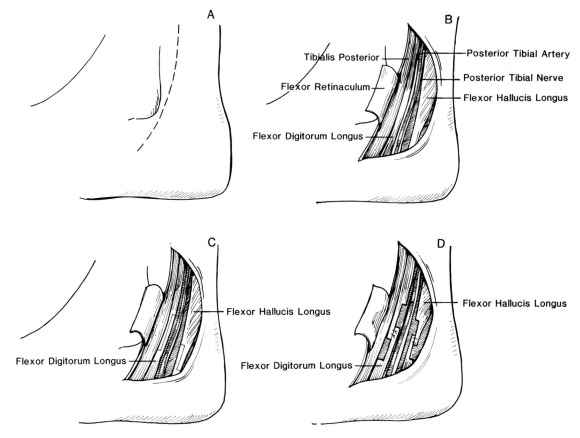

Figure 2–25. Z-plasty lengthening of the flexor tendons in the ankle region. **A,** slightly curved longitudinal skin incision behind the medial malleolus. **B,** flexor retinaculum longitudinally incised to expose the underlying flexor tendons and neurovascular structures. **C,** Z-plasty lengthening performed on the tendons of the flexor hallucis longus and flexor digitorum longus. **D,** ends of the tendons of the flexor hallucis longus and flexor digitorum longus sutured in a lengthened position to compensate for their myostatic contracture.

sors: weaken the stronger flexors by tenotomy of Z-plasty lengthening.

G. Secondary to congenital talipes planovalgus with a rocker-bottom deformity: perform various soft tissue and bone procedures to correct the primary deformities; the secondary hallux flexus will correct itself, provided no fixed flexion contracture has occurred in the M-P joint of the great toe.

H. Caused by trauma-induced scarring and flexion contracture of the flexor hallucis longus in the foot and ankle region: frequently both the flexor hallucis longus and the flexor digitorum longus are scarred

down and shortened. Tenolysis and Z-plasty lengthening of both tendons either in the foot or ankle region are usually required to correct hallux flexus and flexion contracture of the lesser toes (Figures 2–25A—2–26D). When fixed contracture is also present in the M-P and interphalangeal joints of the toes, it should also be corrected by various soft tissue and bone procedures.

REFERENCES

Hallux Flexus

1. Davies-Colley, N.: Contraction of the metatarsophalangeal joint of the great toe (hallux flexus). Br. Med. J., *1:*728, 1887.

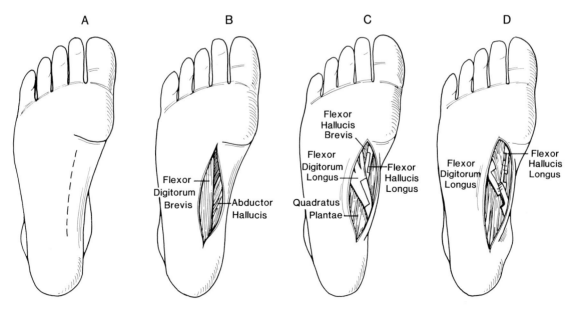

Figure 2–26. Lengthening of flexor tendons through a longitudinal plantar incision. **A,** longitudinal skin incision is made along the midportion of the plantar arch. **B,** after longitudinally splitting the plantar fascia, develop the interval between the flexor digitorum brevis and the abductor hallucis. **C,** after retracting the medial and lateral plantar nerves, identify, isolate, and perform Z-plasty on the tendons of the flexor hallucis longus and the flexor digitorum longus. **D,** free ends of the flexor hallucis longus and the flexor digitorum longus tendons are sutured together in a lengthened manner to relieve their myostatic contracture.

2. Galimberti, A., and Marabelli, A.: Hallux flexus and its treatment. Osp. Ital. Chir., *15:*417, 1966.
3. Goldner, J.L.: Hallux valgus and hallux flexus associated with cerebral palsy: Analysis and treatment. Clin. Orthop., *157:*98, 1981.
4. Jahss, M.H.: Disorders of The Foot. Philadelphia. W.B. Saunders, 1982, p. 618.
5. Kingreen, O.: Zur aetiologies des hallux flexus. Zbl. Chir., *60:*2116, 1933.
6. Lucero, B., and Forneri, O.C.: Surgical treatment of poliomyelitic "hallux flexus." Arch. Argent. Pediatr., *63:*362, 1965.
7. Mann, R.A. (ed.): DuVries' Surgery of The Foot. 4th Ed. St. Louis, C.V. Mosby, 1978, pp. 268–269.
8. Mau, H.: Compartment syndromes of the lower extremities. Z. Orthop., *120:*202, 1982.
9. Newmark, D.B.: Bilateral severe hallux flexus and abductus resulting from cerebral palsy. J. Foot Surg., *18:*121, 1979.
10. Schede, F.: Hallux valgus, hallux flexus and fussenkung. Zt. Orthop., *48:*569, 1927.

DORSAL BUNION

Incidence

The term dorsal bunion, by itself, means a bony prominence on the dorsal aspect of the M-P joint of the great toe. This deformity can be caused by dorsiflexion of the first metatarsal accompanied by plantar flexion or subluxation of the proximal phalanx of the great toe; a large exostosis on the dorsal aspect of the first metatarsal head (dorsal exostosis of the great toe); large osteophytes on the dorsal aspect of the M-P joint of the great toe (hallux rigidus); or simply plantar flexion of the great toe at the M-P joint (hallux flexus), with or without dorsal exostosis on the first metatarsal head. This section deals only with dorsal bunion caused by dorsiflexion of the first metatarsal at its first metatarsocuneiform joint associated with plantar flexion of the great toe at the M-P joint; a prominent bump on the dorsal aspect of the first metatarsal head is also present, caused by both plantar subluxation of the great toe at the M-P joint and an osteocartilaginous excrescence on the dorsal aspect of the first metatarsal head. The causes of this specific kind of dorsal bunion are various combinations of muscle imbalance and are discussed in the following sections.

The most common cause of dorsal bunion is a muscle imbalance between the peroneus longus and the tibialis anterior, which can take three forms:

1. A paralyzed peroneus longus against a weak, normal, or spastic tibialis anterior.

2. A weak peroneus longus against a normal or spastic tibialis anterior.

3. A normal peroneus longus against a spastic tibialis anterior.

This imbalance between the peroneus longus and the tibialis anterior can be caused by a variety of the upper or lower motor neuron diseases, and can also result from transfer of the peroneus longus muscle to different places, such as in transfer of the peroneus longus to the calf to improve plantar flexion of the ankle or in transfer of the same muscle to the tibialis anterior to improve dorsiflexion of the ankle. When the peroneus longus is weak, paralyzed, or absent, the first metatarsal is dorsiflexed by the much stronger tibialis anterior, and the great toe must become actively plantar flexed to establish a point of weight-bearing for the forefoot to assist push-off in walking. With time, soft tissue contracture causes the dorsiflexion of the first metatarsal at the first metatarsocuneiform joint and flexion of the great toe at the M-P joint to become fixed. The dorsal bunion deformity then becomes well established.

The second and less common cause of dorsal bunion is brought about by paralysis of all muscles controlling the foot, except for the triceps surae muscle (gastrocnemius and soleus) with variable strength and the strong long toe flexors, which are constantly used to stabilize the foot in weight-bearing and sustain push-off in walking. Consequently, the almost constant plantar flexion of the great toe causes the plantar capsule of the M-P joint of the great toe to become contracted. The first metatarsal head gradually becomes upwardly displaced to accommodate the plantar flexion of

the great toe, resulting in a typical dorsal bunion deformity.

Finally, weak extensors of the great toe in the presence of strong flexors of the same toe result in primary plantar flexion deformity of the great toe at its M-P joint and secondary dorsiflexion of the first metatarsal at its metatarsocuneiform joint.

Clinical Symptoms and Signs

The most prominent feature of dorsal bunion is the bony bump on the dorsal aspect of the first metatarsal head, associated with dorsiflexion of the first metatarsal at the metatarsocuneiform joint and plantar flexion of the great toe at the M-P joint. Shoe wearing can produce a painful adventitious bursa over the exostosis on the first metatarsal head, associated with localized pain, tenderness, swelling, and redness. Excessive pressure on the plantar aspect of the distal portion of the great toe can also produce a painful callosity. When flexion contracture has developed in the M-P joint of the great toe, active and passive dorsiflexion of the great toe at the M-P joint will be significantly restricted. In addition, when arthritic changes have occurred in the M-P joint of the great toe, joint pain, tenderness, effusion, and osteophyte formation at the M-P joint margins are present. When dorsal bunion has been present for a long time, similar arthritic changes may also be noted in the first metatarsocuneiform joint.

Roentgenographic Manifestations

In the evaluation of dorsal bunion, the standing lateral view usually shows abnormal extension of the first metatarsal at its metatarsocuneiform joint, plantar flexion of the proximal phalanx of the great toe at its M-P joint, proximal displacement of the medial and lateral sesamoids, and exostosis on the dorsal aspect of the first metatarsal head. When arthritic changes have taken place in the M-P joint of the great toe and the first metatarsocuneiform joint, joint narrowing and irregularity, osteophyte formation at joint margins, joint effusion, and subchrondral osteosclerosis may be present.

Pathologic Anatomy

In dorsal bunion, dorsiflexion of the first metatarsal at its metatarsocuneiform joint causes the dorsal joint capsule and the tarsometatarsal ligament to become contracted.

Similarly, flexion of the great toe at the M-P joint causes the plantar joint capsule to become contracted. In addition, the flexor hallucis brevis and longus also undergo adaptive shortening, and the two sesamoids show proximal migration because of the flexion of the great toe at its M-P joint and contracture of the flexor hallucis brevis, the two tendons

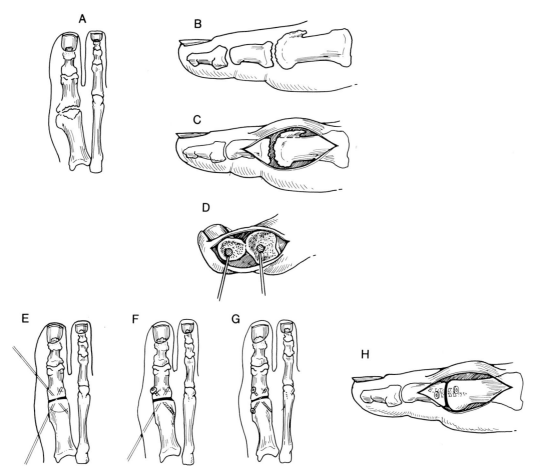

Figure 2–27. Surgical technique for fusing the M-P joint of the great toe. **A** and **B,** anteroposterior and lateral views show severe arthritis of the M-P joint of the great toe. **C,** expose the M-P joint of the great toe and remove the exostosis on the dorsal aspect of the first metatarsal head. **D,** cutting the dorsal, medial, and plantar M-P joint capsule and its medial collateral ligament, as well as the tendon of the abductor hallucis, the M-P joint is opened like a book to expose its arthritic articular surfaces. With an air-powered burr, degenerated articular cartilage is removed completely down to the bleeding subchondral bone. **E,** by holding the two raw bone surfaces in intimate contact, with the great toe in 15 to 20° extension and 10° valgus deviation at the M-P joint, transfix the M-P joint with two K-wires. **F,** after confirming the correct position of the transfixed M-P joint and the two K-wires, withdraw one of the two K-wires and insert an A-O miniscrew of appropriate length into the hole made by the K-wire; sink the screw head into the bone. **G,** withdraw the second K-wire and insert another screw of proper length into the hole made by the second K-wire; similarly, sink the screw head into the bone. **H,** lateral view of the same foot shows two screws have been driven across the M-P joint of the great toe to hold the two raw bone surfaces in intimate contact so to maximize the chances of achieving a solid bony union in a reasonable period of time.

of which contain the two sesamoids. When degenerative arthritis has developed in the metatarsocuneiform and M-P joints of the great toe, fissure and erosion of the articular cartilage with exposure of subchrondral bone, synovial proliferation, fibrosis of the joint capsule, and osteocartilaginous overgrowth at the joint margins may occur.

Nonsurgical Treatment

A. Shoe modifications: extra-depth and space shoes with wide vamps and roomy toe boxes are useful in accommodating the deformed first metatarsal and great toe and the associated dorsal bunion. Stretching of the shoe upper with a shoemaker's swan to accommodate the dorsal bony prominence of the great toe is also beneficial (Figures 1–7 and 1–12).

B. Padding and taping of the great toe: when flexion contracture of the M-P joint of the great toe is not yet fixed, taping the great toe to the second toe can temporarily and partially correct the deformity of dorsal bunion. Padding of the symptomatic dorsal bony prominence and the painful plantar callosity of the great toe can also provide pain relief (Figure 1–8).

C. Commercially available foot aids: use of donut-shaped pads and soft toe caps can also give symptomatic relief (Figures 1–16 and 1–18).

Surgical Treatment

The main surgical principle in treating dorsal bunion or any other foot problems is that every effort should be made to correct all the deformities, which in the case of dorsal bunion, include the following necessary corrections:

A. Elimination of the overpowering and deforming force of the tibialis anterior muscle. Transfer of the tibialis anterior to the tibialis posterior or to the dorsal aspect of

the middle of the foot removes its direct pull on the first metatarsal completely.

B. Correction of the dorsal angulation of the first metatarsal. Plantar angulation osteotomy at the base of the first metatarsal; fusion of the first metatarsocuneiform and perhaps also the cuneiform-navicular joints in plantar flexion, especially when there are arthritic changes in these joints; and transfer of the flexor hallucis brevis, abductor hallucis, and adductor hallucis to the dorsal aspect of the first metatarsal neck to depress the dorsiflexed first metatarsal when the foot is still supple and not fixed, are the surgical options.

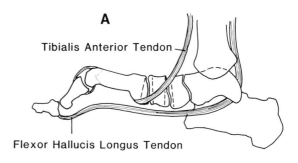

A

Tibialis Anterior Tendon

Flexor Hallucis Longus Tendon

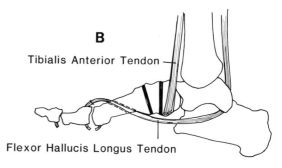

B

Tibialis Anterior Tendon

Flexor Hallucis Longus Tendon

Figure 2–28. Surgical correction of a severe and fixed dorsal bunion deformity. **A,** lateral view shows dorsiflexion deformity at the metatarsocuneiform and cuneiform-navicular joints, and flexion deformity of the proximal phalanx at the M-P joint. Dotted lines, bone to be removed in preparation for subsequent metatarsocuneiform and cuneiform-navicular fusion. **B,** dorsal bunion deformity has been fully corrected after proximal transfer of the tibialis anterior tendon to the navicular, fusion of the metatarsocuneiform and cuneiform-navicular joints, plantar capsulotomy of the M-P joint of the great toe, and transfer of the flexor hallucis longus through an oblique drilled hole of the first metatarsal to the dorsal capsule of the M-P joint of the great toe.

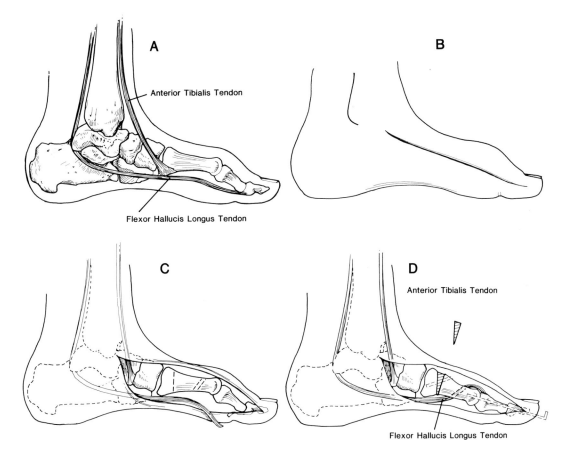

Figure 2–29. Surgical correction of a moderate dorsal bunion deformity. **A,** lateral view shows dorsiflexion of the first metatarsal at the metatarsocuneiform joint and plantar flexion at the M-P joint of the great toe. **B,** medial longitudinal incision. **C,** tenotomy of the flexor hallucis longus near its insertion. Osteotomy of the first metatarsal at its base and drilling of the oblique hole through the first metatarsal are complete. **D,** completion of the proximal transfer of the tibialis anterior tendon to the navicular, open-wedge plantar angulation osteotomy of the first metatarsal, transfer of the flexor hallucis longus through the oblique hole of the first metatarsal to the dorsal capsule of the M-P joint of the great toe, capsulotomy of the plantar capsule of the M-P joint of the great toe, and fixation of the M-P joint of the great toe in a neutral position with a smooth small K-wire results in a nice correction of the original dorsal bunion deformity.

C. Removal of the dorsal exostosis on the first metatarsal head.

D. Correction of the flexion deformity of the great toe at the M-P joint. Plantar capsulotomy of the M-P joint of the great toe to release the contracted plantar capsule, and transfer of the flexor hallucis longus through an obliquely drilled hole through the first metatarsal to the dorsal capsule of the M-P joint of the great toe, helping to depress the first metatarsal and extend the M-P joint of the great toe, are the commonly used surgical procedures.

E. Arthrodesis (Figure 2–27), various arthroplasties, and cheilectomy of the M-P joint of the great toe are the different surgical options when significant arthritic changes are present in the M-P joint of the great toe.

The three surgical procedures that can be used to treat dorsal bunions are discussed in the following section.

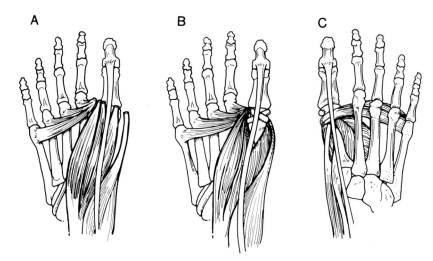

Figure 2–30. Surgical correction of a supple foot with a mild to moderate dorsal bunion deformity that is not yet fixed. **A,** plantar view shows that both sesamoids have been removed. Ends of the tendons (left to right) are: transverse head of the adductor hallucis, oblique head of the adductor hallucis, lateral head of the flexor hallucis brevis, medial head of the flexor hallucis brevis, and the abductor hallucis. **B,** another plantar view shows the tendons of the adductor hallucis and lateral head of the flexor hallucis brevis have been wrapped around the dorsal aspect of the neck of the first metatarsal from the lateral side, and the tendons of the abductor hallucis and medial head of the flexor hallucis brevis are wrapped around the dorsal aspect of the neck of first metatarsal neck from the medial side. These tendons are to be sutured to the periosteum and to each other to convert them into depressors of the first metatarsal. **C,** dorsal view shows the tendons of the adductor hallucis and lateral head of the flexor hallucis brevis coming from the lateral side and the tendons of the abductor hallucis and medial head of the flexus hallucis brevis from the medial side have been sutured to the dorsal aspect of the first metatarsal neck in a criss-crossing manner.

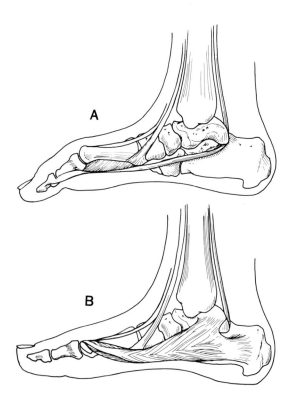

A. Transfer the tibialis anterior tendon to the navicular, perform plantar capsulotomy of the M-P joint of the great toe, fuse the first metatarsocuneiform and cuneiform-navicular joints, and transfer the flexor hallucis longus through a hole drilled on an oblique angle to the dorsal joint capsule of the M-P joint of the great toe (Figure 2–28).

B. Transfer the tibialis anterior tendon to the navicular, perform plantar angulation osteotomy at the base of the first metatarsal with a wedge-shaped bone graft, transfer the flexor hallucis longus through a hole

←———————————————————

Figure 2–31. Lateral views of the foot before and after transfer of intrinsic muscles of the great toe to the dorsal aspect of the first metatarsal neck. **A,** hyperextension of the first metatarsal at the first metatarsocuneiform joint, and a plantar flexion deformity of the great toe at the M-P joint. **B,** correction of the typical deformities of dorsal bunion after the intrinsic muscles of the great toe have been transferred to the dorsal aspect of the first metatarsal neck.

drilled at an oblique angle to the dorsal capsule of the M-P joint of the great toe, perform capsulotomy of the plantar capsule of the M-P joint of the great toe, and hold the great toe in a neutral position with a small smooth K-wire through the M-P joint of the great toe (Figure 2–29).

C. When the foot with dorsal bunion is supple and not yet fixed, excise the medial and lateral sesamoids of the great toe, transfer the flexor hallucis brevis and abductor and adductor hallucis to the dorsal aspect of the neck of the first metatarsal to depress the first metatarsal, perform plantar capsulotomy of the M-P joint of the great toe (but keep the adductor hallucis insertion intact in the presence of hallux varus), and preserve the abductor hallucis insertion intact in the presence of hallux valgus to provide dynamic correction of the associated varus or valgus deformity of the great toe (Figures 2–30 and 2–31).

REFERENCES

Dorsal Bunion

1. Hammond, G.: Elevation of the first metatarsal bone with hallux equinus. Surgery, *13:*240, 1943.
2. Inman, V.T. (ed.): DuVries' Surgery of The Foot. 3rd Ed. St. Louis, C.V. Mosby, 1973, pp. 232–234.
3. Lapidus, P.W.: "Dorsal bunion": Its mechanics and operative correction. J. Bone Joint Surg. *22:*627, 1940.
4. McKay, D.W.: Dorsal bunion in children. J. Bone Joint Surg. [Am.], *65:*975, 1983.
5. Tachdjian, M.O.: Pediatric Orthopedics. Philadelphia, W.B. Saunders, 1972, pp. 994–995.
6. Turek, S.L.: Orthopaedics: Principles and Their Application. 3rd Ed. Philadelphia, J.B. Lippincott, 1977, pp. 1283–1284.

HALLUX VALGUS INTERPHALANGEUS

Incidence

Hallux valgus interphalangeus is a relatively uncommon form of hallux valgus in which the deformity occurs between the proximal and distal phalanges of the great toe; it is frequently congenital in origin. Acquired hallux valgus interphalangeus can be caused by traumatic arrest of growth of one of the phalangeal epiphyses, malunited fracture of one of the phalanges, rheumatoid arthritis, arthrogryposis multiplex congenita, previous surgery on the great toe, neurotrophic diseases with foot involvement, and others. The congenital form of the disorder is present at birth or shortly thereafter, whereas the acquired form usually makes its appearance later in life because it takes a certain amount of time for the deformity to develop and to become clinically apparent. It should also be noted that bilateral involvement of hallux valgus interphalangeus tends to be more common in the congenital form than in the acquired form.

Clinical Symptoms and Signs

Although the great toe in hallux valgus interphalangeus grossly appears to be in a simple valgus position, close scrutiny reveals that the deformity occurs only in the interphalangeal joint instead of the M-P joint of the great toe, as in regular hallux valgus. In addition, the typical bony prominence on the medial aspect of the first metatarsal head (the bunion) is conspicuously absent. The lateral deviation of the great toe at its interphalangeal joint causes the lateral aspect of the distal portion of the great toe to press on the medial aspect of the distal portion of the second toe, and can produce two painful kissing corns in the first interdigital space. The same laterally deviated great toe can also displace the second toe upward. This displacement can cause it to overlap the great toe, producing a hammer toe deformity of the second toe with its associated painful corn on its dorsal aspect and callosity under its metatarsal head from the dorsal subluxation of the proximal phalanx of the second toe at its M-P joint. Similarly, the laterally deviated great toe can also overlap the second toe and internally rotate along its longitudinal axis, with its toenail facing medially at the same time. When arthritic changes occur in the interphalangeal joint of the great toe, pain, tenderness, swelling, crepitation, loss of joint motion, swelling, and osteophyte formation at joint margins may be present.

Roentgenographic Manifestations

The anteroposterior view of a foot with hallux valgus interphalangeus usually shows lateral deviation of the distal phalanx of the great toe at its interphalangeal joint, which is caused by deformity of the proximal or distal phalanges or both. In an immature foot with open epiphyses, the medial one half of the epiphysis of the distal phalanx of the great toe can be significantly thicker than its corresponding lateral portion, causing the distal phalanx to deviate toward the second toe. The common deformities of the regular hallux valgus, such as metatarsus primus varus, hallux valgus at its M-P joint, lateral migration of the two sesamoid bones, and bony prominence on the medial aspect of the first metatarsal head are absent. When arthritis has developed in the interphalangeal joint of the great toe, joint narrowing and irregularity, osteophyte formation at joint margins, subchondral osteosclerosis, and periarticular soft tissue swelling may be noted.

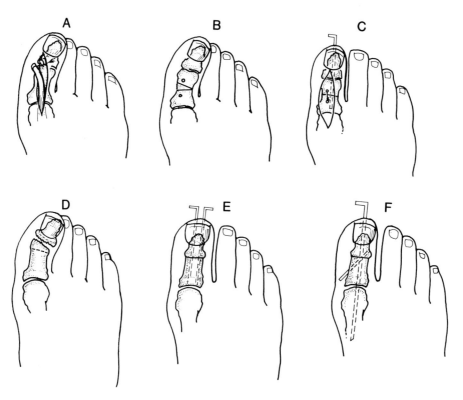

Figure 2–32.   Surgical treatment of hallux valgus interphalangeus. **A,** make a longitudinal skin incision on the dorsal aspect of the great toe from the level of the base of the distal phalanx to the level of the first metatarsal head. Cut the extensor hallucis longus tendon near its insertion to the dorsal aspect of the distal phalanx in preparation for arthrodesis of the interphalangeal joint of the great toe. **B,** in performing a varus osteotomy of the great toe, use the same skin incision but only retract the extensor hallucis longus tendon laterally. Drill two holes through the proximal and distal portions of the proximal phalanx before performing the varus osteotomy of the proximal phalanx. **C,** by using the lateral cortex of the proximal phalanx as a hinge, close the osteotomy site and thread a size O suture through the two drilled holes by means of the two, straight Keith needle method fully described in modified Mitchell's bunionectomy before tying it snugly to keep the raw bone surfaces in intimate contact. Drive a small smooth K-wire from the tip of the toe through the distal phalanx across the osteotomy site into the proximal portion of the proximal phalanx to get a firmer fixation of the osteotomy site. **D,** after retracting the severed extensor hallucis longus tendon, the arthritic interphalangeal joint is resected with a microsaw to remove more bone from the medial side than the lateral side; the fused great toe will then be straight. **E,** fuse the resected interphalangeal joint of the great toe in a neutral position with two small smooth K-wires. **F,** an alternative fusional technique is to run a K-wire from the tip of the distal phalanx to the first metatarsal, and transfix the interphalangeal joint with an oblique K-wire to secure the fusional site.

Pathologic Anatomy

Lateral deviation of the distal phalanx of the great toe favors contracture of the lateral joint capsule and the collateral ligament of the interphalangeal joint of the great toe. When arthritis has developed in the same interphalangeal joint, articular cartilage degeneration, synovial proliferation, and periarticular soft tissue fibrosis may also be present.

Nonsurgical Treatment

A. Shoe modifications: a comfortable shoe with wide vamp and roomy toe box reduces the shoe pressure on the deformed great toe. If the great toe is overlapped by the second toe, stretching of the shoe leather over the high-riding second toe by using a shoemaker's swan can give significant symptomatic relief to the painful and deformed second toe (Figures 1–7 and 1–12).

B. Padding of the toes: Foam rubber pads between the great and second toe and on the dorsal aspect of the second toe can provide pain relief for the painful interdigital corns and the hard corn on the dorsal aspect of the second toe that are sometimes associated with hallux valgus interphalangeus (Figure 1–8).

C. Commercially available foot aids: donut-shaped pads, toe separators, and soft toe caps are useful devices in relieving painful soft and hard corns (Figures 1–16, 1–18, and 1–19).

Surgical Treatment

A. Hallux valgus interphalangeus in the absence of significant arthritis of the interphalangeal joint of the great toe. Perform a carefully measured varus osteotomy of the proximal phalanx of the great toe to compensate for the valgus deformity at the interphalangeal joint (Figure 2–32B and C).

B. Hallux valgus interphalangeus in the presence of significant arthritis of the interphalangeal joint of the great toe. Resect the interphalangeal joint with removal of more bone from the medial side of the joint to correct its valgus deformity. Fuse the resected joint in a neutral position (Figure 2–32A, D—F).

REFERENCES

Hallux Valgus Interphalangeus

1. Akin, O.F.: The treatment of hallux valgus—a new operative procedure and its results. Med. Sentinel, *33:*678, 1925.
2. Barnett, C.H.: Valgus deviation of the distal phalanx of the great toe. J. Anat., *4:*265, 1905.
3. Colloff, B., and Weitz, E.M.: Proximal phalangeal osteotomy in hallux valgus. Clin. Orthop., *54:*105, 1967.
4. Daw, S.W.: An unusual type of hallux valgus (two cases). Br. Med. J., *2:*580, 1935.
5. Edmonson, A.S., and Crenshaw, A.H.: Campbell's Operative Orthopaedics. 6th Ed. St. Louis, C.V. Mosby, 1980, pp. 1728–1729.
6. Giannestras, N.J.: Foot Disorders. 2nd Ed. Philadelphia, Lea & Febiger, 1973, p. 403.
7. Gutzeit, R.: Über hallux valgus in interphalangeus. Verh. Dtsch. Ges. Chir., *43:*62, 1914.
8. Jahss, M.H.: Disorders of the Foot. Philadelphia, W.B. Saunders, 1982, pp. 583–584.
9. Kelikian, H.: Hallux Valgus, Allied Deformities of the Forefoot and Metatarsalgia. Philadelphia, W.B. Saunders, 1965, p. 54.
10. Levitsky, D.R., Digilio, J., Kander, R., and Rubin, B.: Rigid compression screw fixation of first proximal phalanx osteotomy for hallux abducto valgus. J. Foot Surg., *21:*65, 1982.
11. Seelenfreund, M., Fried, A., and Tikva, P.: Correction of hallux valgus deformity by basal phalanx osteotomy of the big toe. J. Bone Joint Surg. [Am.], *55:*1411, 1973.
12. Silberman, F.S.: Proximal phalangeal osteotomy for the correction of hallux valgus. Clin. Orthop., *85:*98, 1972.
13. Tachdjian, M.O.: Pediatric Orthopedics. Philadelphia, W.B. Saunders, 1972, p. 1427.
14. Theander, G., and Danielsson, L.G.: Ossification anomaly associated with interphalangeal hallux valgus. Acta Radiol., *23:*301, 1982.

INGROWN TOENAIL (ONYCHOCRYPTOSIS)

Incidence

Ingrown toenail is a common, painful foot problem in shoe-wearing people. To gain a better understanding of this disease entity, a good knowledge of the normal anatomy of the nail and its associated soft tissues is of vital importance (Figure 2–33). The toenail is made of hard keratin and can be divided into three layers: the dorsal nail plate derived from the the upper nail root matrix, the intermediate nail (the main nail body) from the lower nail root matrix, and the relatively thin ventral nail plate from the nail bed. In practice, however, the distal and exposed part of the nail is commonly called the nail body, and the proximal and hidden portion of the nail is called the nail root, which is covered by a proximal skin fold and is embedded in the nail matrix that is responsible for longitudinal growth of the nail. The thin membrane that extends from the proximal skin fold for a short distance over the nail is the eponychium. The proximal nail fold is divided into a dorsal root and a ventral floor by the nail root proximally, and by the flanking borders of the nail laterally. Slightly distal to the eponychium is a semicircular, whitish area called lunula, the whitish color of which is due to the fact that the soft tissues under the lunula are less vascular and are not firmly attached to the nail. The surrounding area is vascular and is also firmly attached to the nail, giving it a pinkish color. The thickened horny zone under the distal free edge of the nail is called hyponychium. The nail bed consists of all the soft tissues immediately under the nail plate (nail body). The nail bed is surrounded on each side and proximally by

a fold of skin called nail wall, and the nail rests in a depression called nail groove (or nail sulcus and nail furrow). Although the proximal nail bed (the nail matrix) is mainly responsible for the growth of the nail, the most superficial layer of the nail (the dorsal nail plate) may originate, at least in part, from the proximal nail wall.

There are many intrinsic and extrinsic factors that directly and indirectly contribute to the pathogenesis of ingrown toenail:

A. Abnormal convexity of the nail.

B. Dorsally turned tip of the distal phalanx.

C. Narrow, tight, and high-heeled shoes.

D. Shoes made of synthetic material that interferes with proper ventilation of the foot.

E. Tight socks and socks made of synthetic material that impairs the proper ventilation of the foot.

F. Improper pedicure.

G. Poor foot hygiene.

H. Hyperhidrosis of the foot.

I. Faulty foot balance and foot deformities

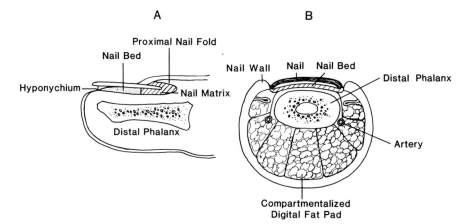

Figure 2–33. Longitudinal and cross-sectional views through the distal phalanx of the great toe show the anatomy of a nail and its associated bone and soft tissue structures.

(e.g., hallux valgus favors development of ingrown toenail on the medial side of the great toenail due to excessive pronation of the great toe).

J. Abnormal intrauterine position may be responsible for the occasional development of congenital ingrown toenail.

The persistent and excessive pressure between the nail edge and the soft tissue of the nail wall and groove eventually leads to pressure necrosis of the soft tissue. The opportunistic fungal and bacterial flora of the skin of the foot invade the open wound and produce local inflammatory and infectious processes accompanied by pain, tenderness, purulent discharge, and granulation tissue formation under the nail at the distal portion of the nail groove. The exuberant granulation tissue and the swollen and edematous nail wall interfere with proper drainage and encourage the growth of more granulation tissue. Further growth impedes the drainage of the infected area in a vicious cycle, resulting in subungual abscess formation with possible proximal extension under the edge of the nail, which can lead to the development of osteomyelitis of the distal phalanx of the great toe with chronic purulent discharge. It should be mentioned that ingrown toenail involves the lateral edge of the great toenail more commonly than that of the medial side, perhaps due to more pressure and poorer ventilation between the lateral edge of the great toenail and the adjacent side of the second toe than those of the corresponding medial side. In addition, ingrown toenail can occasionally involve the nails of the lesser toes.

Clinical Symptoms and Signs

Ingrown toenail is in reality a form of skin infection along the anteromedial or anterolateral nail edge accompanied by redness, warmth, swelling, pain, tenderness, purulent discharge, and chronic edematous granulation tissue that usually completely surround the offending nail edge. In advanced cases, much of the toenail can become separated from its nail bed by subungual abscess formation, which can also extend in a proximal direction under the edge of the nail. When the subungual suppuration has spread to the distal phalanx of the great toe, the resulting osteomyelitis can produce chronic purulent discharge for a long time. An ingrown toenail can also cause cellulitis, lymphangitis, and lymphadenitis of the lower extremity, manifested clinically by erythema, swelling, pain, warmth, tenderness, red streaking along the lymphatic drainage system, and enlarged regional lymph nodes. Ingrown toenail should be differentiated from a painful calloused nail groove, which is a small corn in the nail sulcus caused by the chronic irritation of an incurvating nail edge with no skin ulceration, infection, redness, swelling, granulation tissue, and purulent discharge that commonly accompany ingrown toenail. Removal of the offending nail edge usually gives immediate pain relief.

Roentgenographic Manifestations

The only visible radiologic evidence of ingrown toenail is the soft tissue swelling around the ingrown toenail. When a large subungual abscess has caused the nail to become widely separated from its nail bed, the distance between the distal phalanx of the great toe and the toenail is significantly increased. When an ingrown toenail has produced osteomyelitis of the distal phalanx of the great toe, localized or diffuse bone destruction and sometimes a periosteal reaction are present.

Pathologic Anatomy

Depending on how long the ingrown toenail has been present and the extent of its soft tissue and bone involvement, ingrown toenail can show a wide spectrum of acute, subacute, and chronic inflammatory tissue changes, including infiltration of acute and chronic inflammatory cells such as polymorphonuclear leukocytes, histiocytes, plasma cells, and lymphocytes; tissue necrosis; thrombosis of small blood vessels; fibrosis; devitalized bone fragments with empty lacunae; and reactive and reparative new bone formation.

Nonsurgical Treatment

A. Shoe modifications: shoes with a wide toe box, open shoes, and postoperative shoes can remove the pressure from the inflamed and painful great toe (Figures 1–7 and 1–15).

B. Local treatment: a pledget of cotton soaked with an antiseptic solution can be used to pack under the offending nail tip to free it from the underlying and surrounding in-

flamed tissue to allow the offending nail corner to grow out. The nail can then be trimmed squarely across at a level beyond the nail groove to prevent recurrence. In addition, warm soaks, topical antiseptic application, frequent clean and sterile dressing changes, and cauterization of the exuberant granulation tissue with silver nitrate sticks can all promote drainage and reduce the growth of granulation tissue. When an ingrown toenail is thick and rigid (e.g., onychocryptosis associated with on-

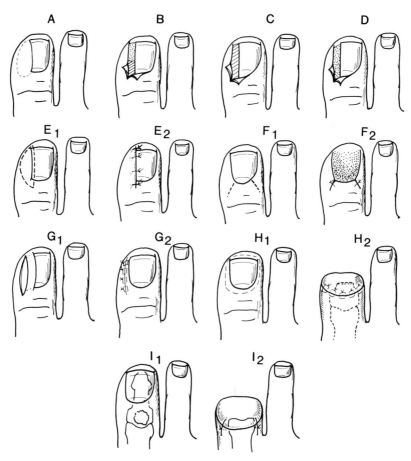

Figure 2–34. Various surgical procedures used in treating ingrown toenail. **A,** great toe with an ingrown toenail on its medial side. **B,** avulsion of the medial border of the nail plus matricetomy of its proximal medial corner. **C,** simple avulsion of the medial border of the nail. **D,** avulsion of the medial border of the nail plus removal of the nail bed and matrix under the removed strip of nail. **E1** and **E2,** excision of the strip of the offending nail, the affected nail groove and nail wall, and associated nail bed and matrix down to the bone of the distal phalanx. The remaining skin edge is then sutured to the nail edge. **F1** and **F2,** simple excision of the entire toenail. **G1** and **G2,** excision of an elliptical piece of skin next to the ingrown toenail and closure of the resulting defect to restore the previously obliterated nail groove and to promote drainage. **H1** and **H2,** complete excision of the nail, the nail bed and matrix, and the distal portion of the distal phalanx of the great toe. **I1** and **I2,** complete excision of the nail, the nail bed and matrix, and the distal phalanx of the great toe to treat osteomyelitis in the excised distal phalanx caused by an ingrown toenail.

ychogryposis or onychomycosis), the nail may have to be filed down at its central one third to increase pliability and flexibility so that the offending corner of the nail may be easily elevated with cotton pledget or plastic insert.

C. Antibiotic therapy: when ingrown toenail is associated with spreading cellulitis, lymphangitis, or lymphadenitis, systemic administration of appropriate antibiotics based on the results of culture and sensitivity should be instituted in combination with the aforementioned local treatment and shoe modifications.

D. Commercially available foot aids: soft toe caps can cushion the painful ingrown toenail from shoe pressure and thus provide symptomatic relief (Figure 1–18).

Surgical Treatment

Various surgical procedures are used to treat ingrown toenail (Figure 2–34).

A. Medial partial onychectomy and matricectomy: remove the medial border of the toenail and resect the nail matrix under the removed strip of nail. This is a commonly used procedure (Figure 2–34B).

B. Medial partial onychectomy plus complete removal of the nail bed and matrix under the removed strip of nail (Figure 2–34C).

C. Simple medial onychectomy: remove only the medial border of the nail. Procedure is useful in draining a subungual abscess (Figure 2–34D).

D. Wedge resection of the nail edge including all hypertrophied skin and soft tissue along the edge of the nail down to the underlying bone of the distal phalanx (Figure 2–34E1 and E2).

E. Simple complete onychectomy: remove the entire toenail (Figure 2–34F1 and F2).

F. Elliptical resection of soft tissue next to the nail wall to restore the previously obliterated nail sulcus and to promote drainage: gives a good cosmetic result but is ineffective in draining subungual abscess (Figure 2–34G1 and G2).

G. Complete onychectomy and matricectomy plus distal hemiphalangectomy of the distal phalanx of the great toe: has a low recurrence rate, but results in a shorter great toe (Figure 2–34H1 and H2).

H. Complete onychectomy and matricectomy plus distal phalangectomy of the great toe for ingrown toenail associated with osteomyelitis of the distal phalanx: completely eliminates the infection, but results in a significantly shorter great toe (Figure 2–34I1 and I2).

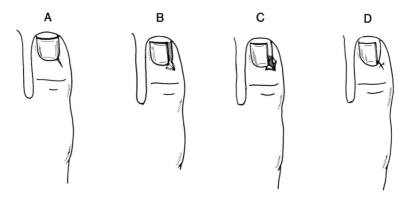

Figure 2–35. Conservative excision of an ingrown toenail. **A,** make a short oblique skin incision at the proximal and medial corner of the toenail. **B,** remove a narrow strip of nail from the medial border of the nail. **C,** excise the nail matrix from the proximal aspect of the operated site. **D,** close the skin incision.

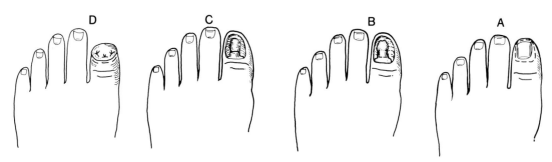

Figure 2–36. Radical excision of a toenail. **A,** make a skin incision completely around the toenail. **B,** remove the nail, the nail walls, the proximal nail fold, and the nail bed and matrix. **C,** excise the distal portion of the distal phalanx of the great toe. **D,** close the resultant skin flap over the partially amputated distal phalanx to the proximal skin edge.

I. Chemosurgical matricectomy: after nail avulsion, cauterize the nail bed and nail matrix with 80% phenol solution or 10% sodium hydroxide solution, which should be neutralized with 3% acetic acid solution. Reported series show chemosurgical matricectomy can achieve good results.

Various steps are used in performing three different surgical procedures in the treatment of ingrown toenail.

A. Avulsion of the medial border of the nail plus excision of the corresponding nail matrix (Figure 2–35).

B. Complete excision of the nail, nail bed, and nail matrix (Figure 2–36).

C. Complete excision of the nail, the two flanking nail folds, and the entire nail matrix (Figure 2–37).

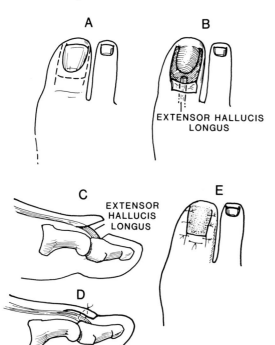

Figure 2–37. Radical excision of a toenail with preservation of the central nail bed. **A,** make an H-shaped incision around the medial, lateral, and proximal aspects of the nail. **B** and **C,** remove both nail grooves and the entire nail matrix down to the bone of the distal phalanx of the great toe, but preserve the insertion of the extensor hallucis longus tendon. **D** and **E,** close the wound by suturing the medial and lateral skin edges to the nail bed and the proximal skin edge to the extensor hallucis longus tendon.

REFERENCES

Ingrown Toenail (Onychocryptosis)

1. Andrew, T.A.: Ingrowing toenails: An evaluation of two treatments. Br. Med. J., *284:*118, 1982.
2. Andrew, T.A., and Wallace, W.A.: Nail bed ablation—excise or cauterise? A controlled study. Br. Med. J., *1:*1539, 1979.
3. Austin, R.T.: A method of excision of the germinal matrix. Proc. R. Soc. Lond. [Med.], *63:*757, 1970.
4. Bailey, F.B., and Evans, D.M.: Ingrowing toenails in infancy. Br. Med. J., *2:*737, 1978.
5. Baran, R., and Bureau, H.: Surgical management of some conditions in and about nails. J. Dermatol. Surg. Oncol., *2:*308, 1976.
6. Bartlett, R.W.: A conservative operation for the cure of so-called ingrown toenail. J.A.M.A., *108:*1257, 1937.
7. Bentley, P.B., and Coll., I.: Ingrowing toenail of infancy. Int. J. Dermatol., *32:*115, 1983.
8. Birrer, R.B., and Rausher, H.: Office podiatry. Am. Fam. Physician, *25:*141, 1982.

9. Boll, O.F.: Surgical correction of ingrowing nails. J. Am. Podiatry Assoc., *35:*8, 1945.
10. Bose, B.: A technique for excision of nail fold for ingrowing toenail. Surg. Gynecol. Obstet., *132:*511, 1971.
11. Brearley, R.: Treatment of ingrowing toenails. Lancet, *2:*122, 1958.
12. Brereton, R.J.: Simple old surgery for juvenile embedded toenails. Z. Kinderchri., *30:*285, 1980.
13. Brown, F.C.: Chemocautery for ingrown toenails. J. Dermatol. Surg. Oncol., *7:*331, 1981.
14. Bryant, A.R.: Ingrowing toenail. Aust. Fam. Physician, *11:*407, 1982.
15. Cameron, P.F.: Ingrowing toenails: An evaulation of two treatments. Br. Med. J., *283:*821, 1981.
16. Chambers, D.G.: Ingrown toe-nails. Med. J. Aust., *1:*608, 1968.
17. Clarke, D.G., and Dillinger, K.A.: The surgical treatment of ingrown toenail. Surgery, *21:*919, 1947.
18. Dixon, G.L., Jr.: Treatment of ingrown toenail. Foot Ankle, *3:*254, 1983.
19. Dubois, J.P.: The treatment of ingrown nails. Nouv. Presse Med., *31:*1938, 1954.
20. Eibel, P.: Unguis incarnatus complicated by glomus tumour. Can. Med. Assoc. J., *93:*811, 1965.
21. Fosnaugh, R.P.: Surgery of the nail. In Skin Surgery. E. Epstein and E. Epstein Jr. (eds.). Springfield, IL, Charles C Thomas, 1978, pp. 725–755.
22. Fowler, A.W.: Excision of the germinal matrix; a unified treatment for embedded toenail and onychogryposis. Br. J. Surg., *45:*382, 1958.
23. Gabriel, S.S., Dallos, V., and Stevenson, D.L.: The ingrowing toenail: A modified segmental matrix excision operation. Br. J. Surg., *66:*285, 1979.
24. Gallocher, J.: The phenol (alcohol method of nail matrix sterilization. N.Z. Med. J., *86:*140, 1977.
25. Gibbs, R.C.: Foot notes: Treatment of the uncomplicated ingrown toenail. J. Dermatol. Surg. Oncol., *4:*438, 1978.
26. Graham, H.F.: Ingrown toenail. Am. J. Surg., *6:*411, 1929.
27. Heifetz, C.J.: Ingrown toe-nail. Am. J. Surg., *38:*298, 1937.
28. Heifetz, C.J.: Operative management of ingrown toenail. J. Miss. State Med. Assoc., *42:*213, 1945.
29. Hendricks, W.M.: Congenital ingrown toenails. Cutis, *24:*393, 1979.
30. Herold, H.Z., and Daniel, D.: Radical wedge resection in the treatment of ingrowing toe nail. Int. Surg., *49:*558, 1968.
31. Ilfeld, F.W., and August, W.: Treatment of ingrown toenail with plastic insert. Orthop. Clin. North Am., *5:*95, 1974.
32. Jansey, F.: Etiologic therapy of ingrowing toe nail. Q. Bull. Northwestern Univ. Med. School, *29:*358, 1955.
33. Jarrett, A., and Spearman, R.J.C.: The histochemistry of the human nail. Arch. Dermatol., *94:*652, 1966.
34. Kaushal, S.P., and Raibard, A.: Ingrowing toenails. Am. Fam. Physician, *15:*134, 1977.
35. Keyes, E.L.: The surgical treatment of ingrown toenails. J.A.M.A., *102:*1458, 1934.
36. Kopell, H.P., Winokur, J., and Thompson, W.A.L.: Ingrown toe-nail. New Concept. N.Y. State J. Med., *66:*1215, 1966.
37. Lapidus, P.W.: Complete and permanent removal of toenail in onychogryposis and surgical osteoma. Am. J. Surg., *19:*92, 1933.
38. Lapidus, P.W.: The ingrown toenail. Bull. Hosp. Jt. Dis. Orthop. Inst., *33:*181, 1972.
39. Lathrop, R.G.: Ingrowing toenails: Causes and treatment. Cutis, *20:*119, 1977.
40. Lewis, B.L.: The histology of the nail and perionychial tissue. Thesis, University of Minnesota, Graduate School, 1953.
41. Lloyd-Davies, R.W., and Brill, G.C.: The aetiology and out-patient management of ingrowing toenails. Br. J. Surg., *50:*592, 1963.
42. McGlamry, E.D.: Management of painful toes from distorted toenails. J. Dermatol. Surg. Oncol., *5:*554, 1979.
43. McKay, I.: Nail elevator. Lancet, *1:*864, 1973.
44. Mogensen, P.: Ingrowing toenail: Follow-up on 64 patients treated by labiomatricectomy. Acta Orthop. Scand., *42:*94, 1971.
45. Morley, J.S.: The surgical approach to ingrowing toenail. Aust. Fam. Physician, *10:*283, 1981.
46. Murray, W.R.: Onychocryptosis: Principles of nonoperative and operative care. Clin. Orthop., *142:*96, 1979.
47. Murray, W.R., and Bedi, B.S.: The surgical management of ingrowing toenail. Br. J. Surg., *62:*409, 1975.
48. Murray, W.R., and Robb, J.E.: Soft-tissue resection for ingrowing toenails. J. Dermatol. Surg. Oncol., *7:*157, 1981.
49. Newman, R.W.: A simplified treatment of ingrown toenail. Surg. Gynec. Obstet., *89:*638, 1949.
50. Ney, G.C.: An operation for ingrowing toenails. J.A.M.A., *80:*374, 1923.
51. Palmer, B.V., and Jones, A.: Ingrowing toenails: The results of treatment. Br. J. Surg., *66:*575, 1979.
52. Pardo-Castello, V., and Pardo, O.A.: Diseases of The Nails. 3rd Ed. Springfield, Charles C Thomas, 1960.
53. Rees, R.W.M.: Radical surgery for embedded or deformed great toenails. Proc. R. Soc. Lond. [Med.], *57:*355, 1964.
54. Robb, J.E.: Surgical treatment of ingrowing toenails in infancy and childhood. Z. Kinderchir., *36:*63, 1982.
55. Ross, W.R.: Treatment of the ingrown toenail and a new anesthetic method. Surg. Clin. North Am., *49:*1499, 1969.
56. Sadr., B., and Schenck, R.R.: Ingrowing nail of a transplanted toe. Hand, *14:*337, 1982.
57. Samman, P.D.: The Nails in Disease. London, William Heinemann Medical Book Ltd., 1965.
58. Scott, P.H.: Ingrown toenails. Med. J. Aust, *1:*47, 1963.
59. Scranton, P.E., Jr.: The management of superficial disorder of the forefoot. Foot Ankle, *2:*238, 1982.
60. Shepherdson, A.: Nail matrix phenolization: A preferred alternative to surgical excision. Practitioner, *219:*725, 1977.
61. Siegle, R.J., and Swanson, N.A.: Nail surgery: A review. J. Dermatol. Surg. Oncol., *8:*659, 1982.
62. Sweetman, K.F.: Ingrowing toenails. Br. Med. J., *2:*765, 1967.
63. Synder, M., and Hansen, R.: Ingrowing toenails. Fact or fancy (unguis incarnatus onychocryptosis). Ariz. Med., *38:*759, 1981.
64. Tarara, E.L.: Ingrown toenail: A problem among the aged. Postgrad. Med., *47:*199, 1970.
65. Thompson, T.C., and Terwilliger, C.: The terminal

Syme operation for ingrown toenail. Surg. Clin. North Am., *31:*575, 1951.

66. Townsend, A.C., and Scott, P.J.: Ingrowing toenail and onychogryposis. J. Bone Joint Surg. [Br.], *48:*354, 1966.

67. Travers, G.R., and Ammon, R.G.: The sodium chemical matricectomy procedure. J. Am. Podiatry Assoc., *70:*476, 1980.

68. Vandenbos, K.Q., and Bowers, W.F.: Ingrown toenail: A result of weight bearing on soft tissue. U.S. Armed Forces Med. J., *10:*1168, 1959.

69. Wallace, W.A.: Gutter treatment for ingrowing toenails. Br. Med. J., *2:*670, 1979.

70. White, C.J., and Laipply, T.C.: Diseases of the nails: 792 cases. Ind. Med. Surg., *27:*325, 1958.

71. Whitehead, J.S.: Ingrowing toenail. Aust. Fam. Physician, *11:*436, 1982.

72. Wilson, T.E.: The treatment of ingrowing toenails. Med. J. Aust., *2:*33, 1944.

73. Winograd, A.M.: A modification in the technic of operation for ingrown toe-nail. J.A.M.A., *92:*229, 1929.

74. Yale, J.F.: Phenol-alcohol technique for correction of infected ingrown toenail. J. Am. Podiatry Assoc., *64:*46, 1974.

75. Zadik, F.R.: Obliteration of the nail bed of the great toe without shortening the terminal phalanx. J. Bone Joint Surg. [Br.], *32:*66, 1950.

76. Zaias, N.: Onychomycosis. Arch. Dermatol., *105:*263, 1972.

77. Zaias, N.: The Nail in Health and Disease. New York, Spectrum Publications, 1980.

78. Zechel, G.: The fallacy of the ingrown nail. Surg. Gynecol. Obstet., *131:*117, 1970.

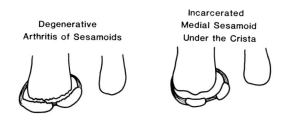

Degenerative Arthritis of Sesamoids

Incarcerated Medial Sesamoid Under the Crista

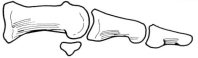

Exostosis on Plantar Surface of the Medial Sesamoid

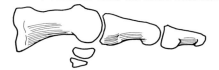

Accessory Sesamoid Under the Medial Sesamoid

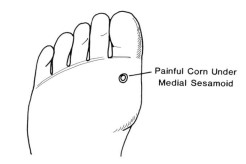

Painful Corn Under Medial Sesamoid

Figure 2–38. Various diseases and anomalies of the sesamoids of the great toe.

DISEASES OF THE SESAMOIDS OF THE GREAT TOE

Incidence

The medial and lateral sesamoids of the great toe are two pea-sized bones that are embedded in the medial and lateral heads of the flexor hallucis brevis muscle, and form the medial and lateral sesamoidometatarsal joints with the undersurface of the first metatarsal head. By providing a fulcrum for the flexor hallucis brevis to act, the two sesamoids strengthen the muscle pull of the flexor hallucis brevis. Quite a few anomalies and diseases affect these sesamoids and are briefly discussed (Figures 2–38—2–40).

A. Absence of one or both sesamoids.

B. Bipartite, tripartite, and multipartite sesamoids: produced by failure to fuse the multicentric ossification centers, and occur in about 10% of the population, of which bilateral involvement accounts for approximately 85% of cases (Figure 2–40).

C. Displacement of the sesamoids: laterally in hallux valgus, medially in hallux varus, distally in hallux extensus, and proximally in hallux flexus.

D. Degeneration of the sesamoids and arthritis of the sesamoidometatarsal joints: caused by hallux rigidus, osteoarthritis, rheumatoid arthritis, gouty arthritis, pseudogout, ankylosing spondylitis, and psoriatic arthritis (Figure 2–38).

Osteomyelitis of the Medial Sesamoid

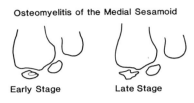

Early Stage   Late Stage

Osteochondrosis (Aseptic Necrosis) of the Laterial Sesamoid

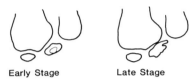

Early Stage   Late Stage

Figure 2–39. Osteomyelitis and osteochondrosis (osteochondritis) of the sesamoids in their early and late stages.

Bipartite Medial Sesamoid

Medial 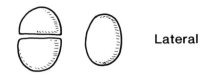 Lateral

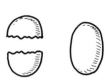

Fractured Medial Sesamoid

E. Exostoses: on the sides or the undersurface of the sesamoids (Figure 2–38).

F. Traumatic injuries of the sesamoids: fracture, dislocation, wide separation of the two sesamoids caused by rupture of the intersesamoid ligament, and gunshot wound (Figure 2–40).

G. Osteomyelitis of the sesamoids: puncture wound, septicemia, and diabetes mellitus are some of the causes. Causative microorganisms are usually Staphylococcus or Pseudomonas (Figure 2–39).

H. Osteochondritis of the sesamoids (Ilfeld's disease): usually affects adolescent girls and young women and shows predilection for the medial sesamoid (Figure 2–39).

I. Tumors of the sesamoids: a greatly enlarged lateral sesamoid caused by an intraosseous hemangioma has been observed.

J. Accessory ossicle under the sesamoids (Figure 2–38).

K. Subhallux sesamoid: large sesamoid located between the plantar aspect of the

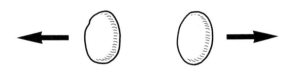

Rupture of Intersesamoid Ligament

Figure 2–40. Bipartite sesamoid, fractured sesamoid, and rupture of the intersesamoid ligament.

interphalangeal joint and the flexor hallucis longus tendon of the great toe (see Figure 2–44).

Clinical Symptoms and Signs

The clinical symptoms and signs of various diseases of the sesamoids naturally depend on the nature of these diseases.

A. Displacement of the sesamoids: usually associated with deformities of the great toe such as hallux valgus, varus, extensus, and flexus.

B. Degeneration of the sesamoids and the different arthritides that involve the sesamoidometatarsal joints: can cause pain,

swelling, tenderness, and crepitation under the first metatarsal head region.

C. Exostosis or accessory ossicle under the sesamoids and incarcerated sesamoid directly under the crista of the first metatarsal head: often produce a painful callosity under these abnormal sesamoids due to their prominent position on the plantar aspect of the foot.

D. Traumatic injuries of the sesamoids: fracture, dislocation, and diastasis of the interconnected sesamoids, usually brought about by acute trauma: commonly accompanied by pain, swelling, ecchymosis, tenderness, and inability to bear full weight on the injured sesamoids under the first metatarsal head.

E. Osteomyelitis of the sesamoids: chronic cases have only pain and tenderness, but acute cases may have typical symptoms and signs of acute infection such as erythema, pain, induration, tenderness, sinus tract with purulent discharge, and fever.

F. Osteochondritis (osteochondrosis) of the sesamoids: ordinarily accompanied by pain and tenderness in the affected region.

G. Tumors of the sesamoids: frequently cause pain, tenderness, and enlargement of the affected sesamoids.

H. Subhallux sesamoid: may produce a painful corn on the plantar aspect of the interphalangeal joint of the great toe.

Roentgenographic Manifestations

Radiologic evaluation of the sesamoid bones of the great toe should always include the sesamoid (axial) view in addition to the routine anteroposterior, lateral, and oblique views. The advantages of the axial view include isolation of the sesamoids from their adjacent first metatarsal head and excellent visualization of the medial and lateral sesamoidometatarsal joints. Radiologic abnormalities of the sesa-

moids naturally depend on the intrinsic pathologic processes. A brief discussion of the abnormal roentgenographic manifestations of the sesamoids of the great toe (Figures 2–38—2–40) follows.

A. Absence of one or both sesamoids: quite obvious on routine radiographs.

B. Bipartite, tripartitie, and multipartite sesamoids: medial bipartite, tripartite, or multipartite sesamoid is approximately 10 times more frequent than that of the lateral sesamoid. In comparison with a normal sesamoid, a bipartite or multipartite sesamoid tends to undergo premature degeneration. In addition, the differences between a bipartite sesamoid and a fractured sesamoid include the following points (Figure 2–40):
1. A bipartite sesamoid is usually bigger than a fractured normal sesamoid in the same person.
2. A bipartite sesamoid has smooth edges. A fractured sesamoid tends to show wider separation and jagged edges.
3. A bipartite sesamoid is usually asymptomatic, whereas a fractured sesamoid is almost always symptomatic.
4. Arthrographic study of the sesamoidometatarsal joints may show penetration of the radiopaque dye into the fracture site, whereas the space in a bipartite sesamoid is occupied by fibrous or fibrocartilaginous tissue that is impermeable to the dye.

C. Displacement of the sesamoids in association with different deformities of the great toe: quite evident when compared with the radiographs of a normal foot or a normal opposite foot of the same patient.

D. Degeneration and different arthritides of the sesamoids: include enlargement, osteophyte formation, bone erosion and eburnation, periosteal elevation, narrowing of the sesamoidometatarsal joints, flattening and mushroom-shaped deformities,

subluxation and dislocation of the sesamoidometatarsal articulations, and erosion of the crista under the first metatarsal head (Figure 2–38).

E. Exostoses of the sesamoids: found on their sides or undersurface (Figure 2–38).

F. Traumatic injuries of the sesamoids: include fracture, dislocation, and wide separation of the previously closely paired sesamoids due to rupture of the intersesamoidal ligament (Figure 2–40).

G. Osteomyelitis of the sesamoids: can produce cystic changes, narrowing of the joint space, fragmentation, sclerosis, soft tissue swelling around the infected sesamoid, and bony ankylosis of the sesamoidometatarsal joints (Figure 2–39).

H. Osteochondritis of the sesamoids: can show cystic changes, fragmentation, osteosclerosis, and other deformities of the affected sesamoids (Figure 2–39).

I. Tumors of the sesamoids: commonly produce destruction and enlargement of the involved sesamoids.

J. Accessory ossicle under the sesamoid: small piece of bone with an irregular configuration that does not have any bony connection with its adjacent sesamoid (Figure 2–38).

K. Subhallux (interphalangeal) sesamoid: best visualized on the lateral view of the great toe, and is directly under the plantar aspect of the interphalangeal joint of the great toe (see Figure 2–44).

Pathologic Anatomy

A. Absence of one or both sesamoid: does not seem to alter the anatomy or function of the flexor hallucis brevis muscle.

B. Bipartite, tripartite, and multipartite sesamoids: contain fibrous or fibrocartilaginous tissue that tightly binds the different fragments of bone of the internally subdivided sesamoid bones.

C. Displacement of the sesamoids: associated with contracture and stretching of different muscles connected with the great toe, e.g., lateral displacement of the sesamoids in hallux valgus associated with contracture of adductor hallucis and lateral head of flexor hallucis brevis muscle; distal displacement in hallux extensus with stretching of both heads of the flexor hallucis brevis muscle; and proximal displacement in hallux flexus with contracture of both heads of the flexor hallucis brevis muscle.

D. Degeneration and arthritides of the sesamoids: cause degeneration and erosion of the articular cartilage and subchondral bone, synovial proliferation, fibrosis, infiltration of acute and chronic inflammatory cells, and deposition of urate and calcium pyrophosphate crystals.

E. Exostoses of the sesamoids: bony outgrowths attached to the nonarticular surface of the sesamoids and covered by hyaline cartilage or fibrocartilage.

F. Traumatic injuries of the sesamoids: include fracture and rupture of ligaments and tendons associated with the sesamoids.

G. Osteomyelitis of the sesamoids: causes bone and cartilage destruction, synovial proliferation, purulent discharge, production of granulation tissue, and bone and soft tissue necrosis accompanied by many inflammatory cells.

H. Osteochondritis of the sesamoids: shows foci of necrosis, degeneration of articular cartilage, fragmentation of bone, cystic changes, chondroid metaplasia, and new bone formation, resulting in marked deformity of the affected sesamoids.

I. Tumors of the sesamoids: usually produce destruction of the host bone by the tumor tissue, which has its typical histologic appearance.

J. Accessory ossicle under the sesamoids: small piece of bone with no distinctive gross or microscopic features.

K. Subhallux sesamoid: small roundish bone between the plantar aspect of the interphalangeal joint capsule of the great toe and the tendon of the flexor hallucis longus.

Nonsurgical Treatment

A. Shoe modifications: total contact insoles, metatarsal bars, metatarsal pads, and arch supports, which either distribute the body weight over the entire sole or shift weight away from the symptomatic sesamoid area, can provide relief for painful sesamoid diseases (Figures 1–4—1–6).

B. Padding of the foot or shoe: thick and soft pads with a relief area cut out of the sesamoid region, applied to the foot directly or to the insole of the shoe, can give pain relief to the symptomatic area (Figures 1–8 and 1–10).

C. Commercially available foot aids: donut-shaped pads can relieve painful callosity under the diseased sesamoid. Various other soft plantar pads may also be helpful (Figures 1–16—1–18).

Surgical Treatment

Sesamoidectomy is usually used in treating diseases of the sesamoids with severe symptoms that do not respond to nonsurgical treatment. These diseases include different arthritides, fracture, osteomyelitis, gunshot wound, tumors, osteochondritis, and exostoses of the sesamoids. When a subhallux sesamoid has produced a painful corn on the plantar aspect of the interphalangeal joint of the great toe, excision of this sesamoid is usually followed by the disappearance of the plantar corn. When treating a painful corn caused by an accessory ossicle under the sesamoid, however, only the accessory ossicle need be removed. In addition, the use of appropriate antibiotics based on the results of culture and sensitivity may be required to combat osteomyelitis of the sesamoids, especially the ones with extension of infection into the surrounding soft tissues. A discussion of the surgical techniques for different sesamoidectomies follows.

A. Medial sesamoidectomy requires the following steps (Figure 2–41):
   1. Make a longitudinal skin incision along the medioplantar border of the M-P joint of the great toe.
   2. After palpating and locating the medial sesamoid with the index finger, make

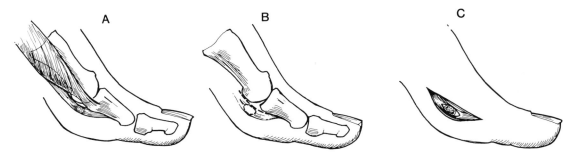

Figure 2–41. Surgical technique for medial sesamoidectomy. **A,** medial view of the great toe shows the relationship between the medial sesamoid and the M-P joint of the great toe. **B,** incision is made on the medioplantar aspect of the M-P joint of the great toe. **C,** medial sesamoid is exposed and then can be removed by detaching all soft tissue attachments.

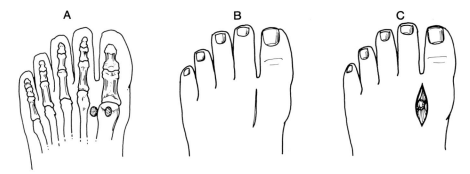

Figure 2–42. Lateral sesamoidectomy through a dorsal incision. **A,** dorsal view shows lateral displacement of both sesamoids. **B,** dorsal longitudinal skin incision between the first and second metatarsal heads and necks. **C,** after incising the dorsal fascia, the lateral sesamoid should be identified and then excised by detaching it from its soft tissue.

a longitudinal incision through the medial aspect of the medial sesamoidometatarsal joint and expose the medial aspect of the medial sesamoid by sharp dissection.

3. By grasping the medial sesamoid with a small towel clip, the medial sesamoid is removed by sharp dissection after detaching it from the tendon of the medial head of the flexor hallucis brevis muscle and the intersesamoidal ligament.

4. Close the medial sesamoidometatarsal joint capsule and the skin in a regular manner.

B. Lateral sesamoidectomy can be per-

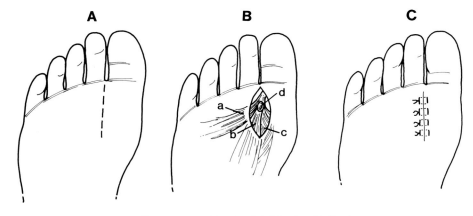

a– Transverse Head of Adductor Hallucis

b– Oblique Head of Adductor Hallucis

c– Lateral Head of Flexor Hallucis Brevis

d– Lateral Sesamoid Bone

Figure 2–43. Lateral sesamoidectomy through a plantar incision. **A,** plantar skin incision between the first and second metatarsal heads and necks. **B,** after incising the plantar fascia, the lateral sesamoid, found at the confluence of the two heads of the adductor hallucis and the lateral head of the flexor hallucis brevis, can be excised by detaching it from its soft tissue. **C,** close the soft tissues in a regular manner.

formed through a dorsal incision when the lateral sesamoid is of normal size and is also laterally displaced to the space between the first and second metatarsal necks (Figure 2–42).

1. Make a longitudinal dorsal skin incision between the first and second metatarsal heads and necks.
2. After palpating and identifying the lateral sesamoid with the index finger, shell out the lateral sesamoid by means of sharp dissection by detaching it from the lateral sesamoidometatarsal joint capsule, the tendon of the lateral head of the flexor hallucis brevis muscle, and the intersesamoidal ligament.
3. Close the skin in a regular manner.

C. Lateral sesamoidectomy through a plantar incision is the best way to remove the lateral sesamoid, especially when the bone is greatly enlarged and is still in its normal anatomic position (Figure 2–43).

1. Make a plantar longitudinal skin incision between the first and second metatarsal heads and necks.
2. After longitudinally incising the plantar fascia, identify the lateral sesamoid by palpation and shell it out by detaching it from the intersesamoidal ligament and the tendon of the lateral head of the flexor hallucis brevis muscle.
3. Close the incision in a regular manner.

D. Subhallux sesamoidectomy requires several steps (Figure 2–44).

1. Make either a longitudinal medioplantar skin incision across the interphalangeal joint of the great toe or a transverse plantar skin incision across the interphalangeal joint of the great toe.
2. By carefully retracting the flexor hallu-

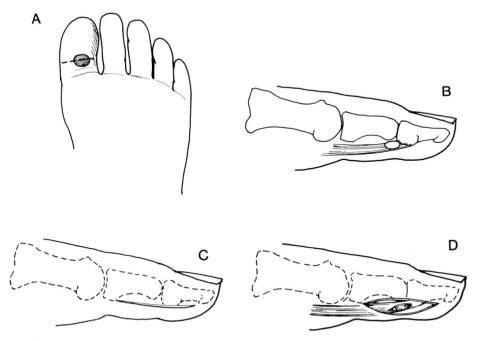

Figure 2–44. Surgical excision of the subhallux sesamoid. **A,** plantar view shows a large callus under the subhallux sesamoid, and the transverse incision used to remove the subhallux sesamoid, **B,** medial view of the great toe shows the relationship between the subhallux sesamoid, the plantar aspect of the M-P joint, and the tendon of the flexor hallucis longus muscle. **C,** longitudinal medioplantar incision can also be used to remove the subhallux sesamoid. **D,** by retracting the medial neurovascular bundle and the flexor hallucis longus tendon, the subhallux sesamoid is ready to be excised by sharp dissection.

cis longus and the neurovascular bundles, the subhallux is excised by sharp dissection.

3. Close the skin in a regular manner.

REFERENCES

Diseases of the Sesamoids of the Great Toe

1. Apley, A.G.: Open sesamoid. Proc. R. Soc. Lond. [Med.], *59:*120, 1966.
2. Bizarro, A.H.: On sesamoid and super numerary bones of the limbs. J. Anat., *55:*256, 1920.
3. Bizarro, A.H.: On the traumatology of the sesamoid structures. Ann. Surg., *74:*783, 1921.
4. Burman, M.S., and Lapidus, P.W.: The functional disturbances caused by inconstant bones and sesamoids of the foot. Arch. Surg., *22:*936, 1931.
5. Colwill, M.: Osteomyelitis of the metatarsal sesamoids. J. Bone Joint Surg. [Br.], *51:*464, 1969.
6. Enna, C.D.: Observations of the hallucal sesamoids in trauma to the denervated foot. Int. Surg., *53:*97, 1970.
7. Golding, C.: Sesamoid of hallux. J. Bone Joint Surg. [Br.], *42:*840, 1960.
8. Gordon, S.L., Evans, C., and Creer, III, R.B.: Pseudomonas osteomyelitis of the metatarsal sesamoid of the great toe. Clin. Orthop., *99:*188, 1974.
9. Hobart, M.: Fracture of the sesamoid bones of the foot. J. Bone Joint Surg., *11:*299, 1929.
10. Holly, E.W.: Radiography of the tarsal sesamoid bones. Med. Radiogr. Photogr., *31:*73, 1955.
11. Hubay, C.A.: Sesamoid bones of the hands and feet. AJR, *61:*493, 1949.
12. Ilfeld, F.W., and Rosen, V.: Osteochondritis of the first metatarsal sesamoid. Clin. Orthop., *85:*38, 1972.
13. Inge, G.A.L., and Ferguson, A.B.: Surgery of the sesamoid bones of the great toe. Arch. Surg., *27:*466, 1933.
14. Jacobs, P.: Multiple sesamoid bones of the hand and foot. Clin. Radiol., *25:*267, 1974.
15. Lapidus, P.W.: Sesamoids beneath all the metatarsal heads of both feet. J. Bone Joint Surg., *22:*1059, 1940.
16. Lapidus, P.W.: Lesions of the inconstant sesamoids of the foot. Radiology, *40:*581, 1943.
17. Leonard, M.: The sesamoids of the great toe—the pedal polemic; report of 3 cases. Clin. Orthop., *16:*295, 1960.
18. Miller, W.A., and Love, B.P.: Cartilaginous sesamoid or nodule of the interphalangeal joint of the big toe. Foot Ankle, *2:*291, 1982.
19. Parra, G.: Stress fractures of the sesamoids of the foot. Clin. Orthop., *18:*281, 1960.
20. Renander, A.: Two cases of typical osteochondropathy of the medial sesamoid of the first metatarsal. Acta Radiol. [Diagn] (Stockh), *3:*521, 1924.
21. Resnick, D., Niwayama, G., and Feingold, M.L.: The sesamoids of hands and feet. Participators in arthritis. Radiology, *123:*57, 1977.
22. Rowe, M.M.: Osteomyelitis of metatarsal sesamoid. Br. Med. J., *1:*1071, 1963.
23. Seder, J.I.: Sesamoiditis. J. Am. Podiatry Assoc., *64:*444, 1974.
24. Smith, R.: Osteitis of the metatarsal sesamoid, including a report of a case of acute pyogenic osteomyelitis. Br. J. Surg., *29:*19, 1941.
25. Speed, K.: Injuries of the great toe sesamoids. Ann. Surg., *60:*478, 1914.
26. Stanley, L.G., Evans, C., and Greer, R.B.: Pseudomonas osteomyelitis of the metatarsal sesamoid of the great toe. Clin. Orthop., *99:*188, 1974.
27. Togerson, W.R., and Hammond, G.: Osteomyelitis of the sesamoid bones of the first metatarsophalangeal joint. J. Bone Joint Surg. [Am.], *51:*1420, 1969.

PAINFUL CALLOSITY ON THE MEDIOPLANTAR ASPECT OF THE DISTAL PHALANX OF THE GREAT TOE

Incidence

Painful callosity on the medioplantar aspect of the distal phalanx of the great toe is usually caused by pronation of the great toe, which concentrates pressure on this particular area. The resulting hyperkeratosis is the common reaction of skin to any excessive and abnormal pressure. This painful corn is most commonly associated with hallux valgus, but it can also be associated with a wide variety of foot deformities with marked pronation of the forefeet, including hypermobile flatfoot, vertical talus, tarsal coalition, rocker-bottom flatfoot secondary to improper treatment of clubfoot, complication of tarsometatarsal fracture and dislocation, neurotrophic arthritis of the tarsometatarsal joints secondary to diabetes mellitus or other peripheral neuropathies, muscle imbalance secondary to upper or lower motor neuron diseases, various kinds of muscular dystrophies, rheumatoid arthritis, collagen diseases, and fractures and dislocations of the ankle, tarsal bones, and joints resulting in severe pronation of the foot.

Clinical Symptoms and Signs

In addition to the painful corn on the medioplantar aspect of the great toe about which the patient commonly complains, pronation of the great toe and flattening of the longitudinal arch of the foot are apparent on weight-bearing. Hallux valgus, eversion of the forefoot, and valgus position of the heel are other associated deformities. Examination of the shoe often reveals excessive wear on the antero-medial aspect of the sole as well as the medial aspect of the heel.

Roentgenographic Manifestations

On the anteroposterior view, the internal rotational deformity of the great toe is evidenced by the medial displacement of the nail shadow of the great toe, and by the significantly decreased width of the medial halves of the phalanges in contrast to that of the lateral halves. In the presence of a large callosity, the medioplantar base of the distal phalanx of the great toe may show a localized exostosis with associated soft tissue enlargement around the bony overgrowth caused by the large callosity, and the possible presence of an adventitious bursa between the exostosis and the callosity. In addition, many other associated deformities of the foot, such as hallux valgus; metatarsus primus varus; lateral displacement of the sesamoids; degeneration or malalignment of the tarsometatarsal and intertarsal joints, coalition of tarsal bones; vertical position of the talus; old fractures and dislocations of the ankle, tarsal bones, and joints, which contribute to the marked pronation of the great toe, can also be present.

Pathologic Anatomy

Pronation of the great toe forces the extensor hallucis longus and brevis, the abductor hallucis, and the medial head of flexor hallucis brevis into a more plantar position; the flexor hallucis longus, the adductor hallucis, and the lateral head of flexor hallucis brevis are in a more dorsal position. The excessive pressure on the medioplantar aspect of the base of the distal phalanx causes localized exostosis, atrophy of the fat pad normally present in the medioplantar aspect of the great toe, adventitious bursa formation, and thick callosity of the skin, which commonly bulges into the subcutaneous tissue and causes further atrophy of the fat pad.

Nonsurgical Treatment

A. Shoe modifications: total contact or soft and thick insoles can decrease weight-bearing pressure on the painful plantar callosity of the great toe and can provide symptomatic relief (Figures 1–6 and 1–7).

B. Padding of the foot: soft pads applied directly to the painful corn on the plantar surface of the great toe or to the insole of the shoe can give pain relief (Figures 1–8 and 1–10).

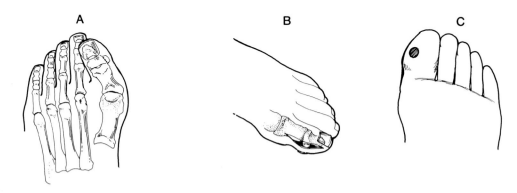

Figure 2–45. Excision of the medial corner of the base of distal phalanx of the great toe. **A,** dorsal view shows a pronated great toe. The medial corner of the base of the distal phalanx of the great toe (dotted line) will be removed. **B,** medial corner of the basal portion of the distal phalanx of the great toe is exposed through a medioplantar incision and can be removed with a microsaw or a small osteotome. **C,** plantar view of the same foot shows a corn on the medioplantar aspect of the distal phalanx of the great toe, which tends to disappear after the offending basal portion has been excised.

C. Commercially available foot aids: donut-shaped pads applied directly to the painful plantar callosity and a soft toe cap worn by the great toe are both helpful (Figures 1–16 and 1–18).

Surgical Treatment

Any surgical procedure that corrects the pronation of the great toe will automatically decrease or eliminate the callosity on the medioplantar aspect of the great toe. Excision of the medial corner of the base of the distal phalanx of the great toe, however, can also decrease the painful symptom of the plantar callosity of the great toe. This procedure can be performed under local anesthesia in the following manner (Figure 2–45):

A. Make a small longitudinal skin incision on the medioplantar aspect of the great toe at the level of the base of the distal phalanx.

B. Detach all the soft tissue attachments from the medial base of the proximal phalanx of the great toe and remove its medial corner with a microsaw.

C. Close the skin in a regular manner.

DORSAL EXOSTOSES OF THE GREAT TOE

Incidence

The three typical locations for dorsal exostoses of the great toe are the dorsal aspect of the first metatarsal head, the head of the proximal phalanx, and the terminal tuft of the distal phalanx. Because of its subungual location, the exostosis on the distal portion of the distal phalanx is commonly known as subungual exostosis, which primarily involves the great toe but can also develop in the lesser toes. The subungual exostosis differs from other exostoses of the great toe in that it does not arise in the juxta-epiphyseal area; it is thought to be caused by chronic irritation of the tuft of the distal phalanx. Subungual exostosis is usually unilateral and shows a predilection for young female patients with a male to female ratio of about 1 to 2. In contrast, exostoses on the dorsal aspects of the first metatarsal head and the head of the proximal phalanx of the great toe can be brought about by a wide spectrum of factors including different kinds of arthritis and metabolic or inflammatory diseases, fractures, dislocations, previous surgery, clawtoe deformity, dorsal bunion, hallux rigidus, upper and lower motor neuron diseases, muscular dystrophies, ruptures of various tendons of the great toe, and improperly fitted shoes. There is a wide range in age of these patients, and there does not seem to be any particular sex predilection.

Clinical Symptoms and Signs

Subungual exostosis usually projects upward and forward from the terminal tuft of the distal phalanx of the great toe, and can cause tenderness, pain, deformity and elevation of the toenail, and an inability to wear shoes comfortably. Similarly, exostoses on the metatarsal and phalangeal heads can produce painful callosities on their dorsal skin and sometimes in adventitious bursa between them and the overlying callosities. When arthritic changes have taken place in the interphalangeal and M-P joints of the great toe, pain, tenderness, limited joint motion, joint effusion and contracture, osteophyte formation at joint margins, and crepitation may be present.

Roentgenographic Manifestations

The lateral view of the great toe usually shows that the subungual exostosis projects upward and forward between the tip of the nail and the terminal tuft of the great toe. When the toenail has been elevated and separated from the nail bed by the exostosis, the distance between the distal phalanx and the toenail is significantly increased. Likewise, the exostoses on the dorsal aspects of the heads of the first metatarsal and the proximal phalanx are best demonstrated by the lateral view of the great toe. Soft tissue swelling caused by large callosity and adventitious bursa formation above these exostoses normally casts

an enlarged soft tissue shadow over the exostoses, and may occasionally contain small
radiopacities due to calcification in the adventitious bursa.

Pathologic Anatomy

The bases of all exostoses are ordinarily
continuous with the cortices of the parental
bones from which they originate. The protruding surfaces of the exostoses are usually covered by a thin hyaline cartilage or fibrocartilage, which in turn can be surrounded by an
adventitious bursa that separates the exostosis from the overlying thick callosity of the
skin. When arthritis has developed in the interphalangeal and M-P joint of the great toe,
degeneration of the articular cartilage, synovial proliferation, loose body formation, and

soft tissue contracture of the joints may be
present.

Nonsurgical Treatment

A. Shoe modifications: roomy and comfortable shoes and stretching of the shoe leather
around the great toe with a shoemaker's
swan can provide symptomatic relief for
painful dorsal exostoses of the great toe
(Figures 1–7 and 1–12).

B. Padding of the great toe: soft pads applied over the exostoses can decrease the
shoe pressure significantly on these painful dorsal exostoses (Figure 1–8).

C. Commercially available foot aids: donut-
shaped pads and soft toe caps are also

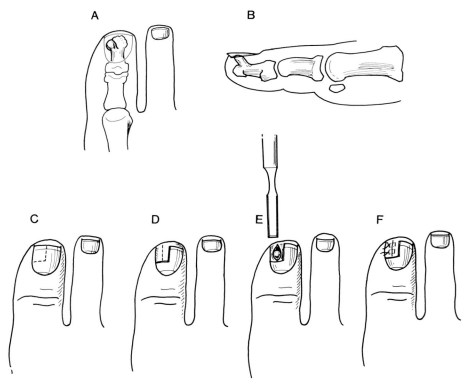

Figure 2–46. Excision of the subungual exostosis of the great toe. **A,** anteroposterior view of a great toe with an subungual exostosis. **B,** lateral view of same toe shows the subungual exostosis projecting upward and forward be-tween the tip of the nail and the terminal pulp. **C,** avulse the mediodistal corner of the toenail. **D,** make a longitudinal incision through the exposed nail bed right on top of the subungual exostosis to expose it. **E,** remove the exostosis near its base with a small curved osteotome. **F,** close the nail bed in a regular manner.

useful in providing pain relief (Figures 1–16 and 1–18).

Surgical Treatment

All dorsal exostoses can be easily removed through different dorsal incisions of the great toe under local anesthesia.

A. Excision of the subungual exostosis of the great toe (Figure 2–46).
1. Avulse the part of the toenail that covers the subungual exostosis.
2. Longitudinally incise the exposed nail bed to expose the subungual exostosis.
3. Remove the subungual exostosis near its base with a small curved osteotome.

4. Close the nail bed in a regular manner.

B. Excision of the dorsal exostosis of the head of the proximal phalanx of the great toe (Figure 2–47).
1. Make a short, longitudinal skin incision directly over the exostosis on the head of the proximal phalanx.
2. Expose the exostosis by carefully isolating and retracting the extensor hallucis longus tendon sideways.
3. Excise the exostosis near its base with a small curved osteotome.
4. Close the skin in a regular manner.

C. Excision of the dorsal exostosis on the first metatarsal head (Figure 2–48).
1. Make a longitudinal skin incision di-

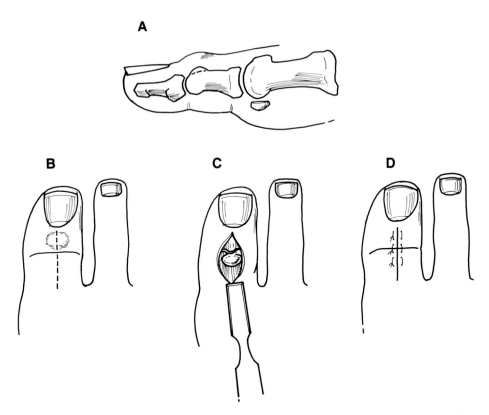

Figure 2–47. Excision of dorsal exostosis on the head of the proximal phalanx of the great toe. **A,** lateral view of the great toe shows the dorsal exostosis of the proximal phalanx and the associated soft tissue swelling. **B,** make a short longitudinal skin incision directly over the exostosis. **C,** excise the exposed exostosis near its base after retracting the extensor hallucis longus. **D,** close the skin in a regular manner.

A   B

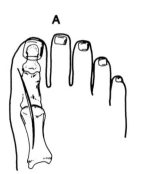
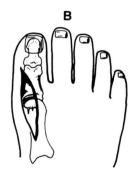
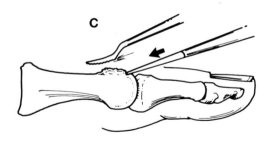

Figure 2–48. Excision of the dorsal exostosis of the first metatarsal head. **A,** make a dorsal longitudinal skin incision over the M-P joint of the great toe. **B,** by retracting the extensor hallucis longus tendon sideways, expose the exostosis. **C,** remove the exostosis near its base with a small osteotome and smooth the base with a small bone rasp before closing the skin in a regular manner.

rectly over the dorsal exostosis of the first metatarsal.

2. Expose the exostosis by retracting the extensor hallucis longus tendon sideways.

3. Excise the exostosis near its base with a small osteotome and smooth off its base with a small bone rasp.

4. Close the skin in a regular manner.

REFERENCES

Dorsal Exostoses of the Great Toe

1. Brenner, M.A., Montgomery, R.M., and Kalish, S.R.: Subungual exostosis. Cutis, *25*:518, 1980.
2. Bundl, B.J.: Subungual exostosis. Cutis, *26*:260, 1980.
3. Claustre, J., and Simon, L.: The hyperostotic foot. Rev. Rhum. Mal. Osteoartic., *49*:629, 1982.
4. Cohen, H.J.: Frank, S.B., Minkin, W., and Gibbs, R.C.: Subungual exostosis. Arch. Dermatol., *107*:431, 1973.
5. Evison, G., and Price, C.H.G.: Subungual exostosis. Br. J. Radiol., *39*:451, 1966.
6. Landon, G.C., Johnson, K.A., and Dahlin, D.C.: Subungual exostoses. J. Bone Joint Surg. [Am.], *61*:256, 1979.
7. Oliveira, A.D.S., Picoto, A.D.S., Verde, S.F., and Martins, O.: Subungual exostosis: Treatment as an office procedure. J. Dermatol. Surg. Oncol., *6*:555, 1980.
8. Pambor, M., and Neubert, H.: Tumor-like accompanying reactions of the skin in exostoses of the toes. Differential diagnosis of para- and subungual tumors. Dermatol. Monatsschr., *157*:532, 1971.
9. Sebastian, G.: Subungual exostosis of the big toe, occupational stigma of dancers. Dermatol. Monatsschr., *163*:998, 1977.
10. Stern, J.: Removal of subungual exostosis and subsequent removal of needle. J. Am. Podiatry Assoc., *60*:406, 1970.
11. Wichman, B.: Subungual exostoses and nail border problems. J. Am. Podiatry Assoc., *57*:521, 1967.
12. Zimmerman, E.H.: Subungual exostosis. Cutis, *19*:185, 1977.

3 SURGERY OF THE THREE MIDDLE TOES

HAMMER TOE

Incidence

A hammer toe is characterized by hyperextension of the M-P joint and hyperflexion of the PIP joint, with the DIP joint in either a neutral, flexed, or extended position. A hammer toe differs from a clawtoe in the following important ways:

	Hammer Toe	Clawtoe
Position of toe joints	M-P joint in extension, PIP joint in flexion, and DIP joint in either neutral, flexion, or extension	M-P joint in extension, PIP joint in flexion, and DIP joint always in flexion
Incidence of bilateral involvement	Unilateral or bilateral	Usually bilateral
Symmetry of involvement	Can be present or absent	Usually present
Association with dysfunctions of other body systems	Frequently absent	Frequently present
Association with midfoot and hindfoot deformities	Frequently absent	Frequently present

Hammer toe can be congenital or acquired. The congenital form often shows bilateral and symmetric involvement, with a high familial incidence. The acquired form has a strong predilection for the fashion-minded women who wear high-heeled, narrow, and pointed shoes, and is frequently accompanied by hallux valgus deformity. Hammer toe deformity most often involves the second toe, which is usually the longest toe and is also right next to the great toe, although the third and fourth toes less frequently can be affected. Hammer toe deformity is more often found in shoe-wearing people than in barefoot people, and usually develops slowly and insidiously with its incidence of occurrence increasing linearly with age. Having personally performed at least 1000 hammer toe operations, experience indicates that the female to male ratio of patients who have undergone surgical correction of their painful hammer toes is at least 20 to 1, which provides strong support for my contention that the majority of acquired hammer toes are caused by wearing improperly fitted shoes over a long time. It should be mentioned that an excessively short first metatarsal can produce an associated hammer toe of the second toe due to transfer of increased weight-bearing to the second metatarsal ray.

Clinical Symptoms and Signs

The typical painful sites of a hammer toe include a painful corn on the dorsal aspect of the PIP joint and a painful callosity under the corresponding metatarsal head caused by hyperextension of the M-P joint and hyperflexion of the PIP joint. When the DIP joint of a hammer toe is also in flexion, an end corn may be present at the tip of the toe. In addition, an adventitious bursa can be interposed between the dorsal aspect of the PIP joint and the calloused dorsal skin. When a hammered second toe is associated with hallux valgus, the second toe frequently overlaps the great toe in various degrees, and the great toe can even touch the third toe. When a hammered second toe is associated with a curled third toe, the second toe often overrides the third toe to varying extent. The plantarly displaced metatarsal heads frequently become quite superficial and palpable under the calloused plantar skin, and have caused marked atrophy of the protective fat pad commonly present under any normal metatarsal heads. Active and passive flexion of the M-P joint and extension of the PIP joint of a fixed hammer toe are markedly reduced, and the extensor digitorum longus tendon becomes taut and prominent when the M-P joint of a hammer toe is passively plantar-flexed. Examination of the shoes of these patients often reveals bulges on the toe boxes corresponding to the exact sites inside the shoes occupied by these offending hammer toes. Chronic shoe irritation of the skin and its associated bursa over the PIP joint of a hammer toe can produce ulceration and purulent discharge;

which can lead to pyarthrosis of the underlying PIP joint with possible further extension of infection to involve the proximal and middle phalanges from which chronic discharge may be produced.

Roentgenographic Manifestations

The lateral view of a hammer toe typically shows hyperextension of the M-P joint and hyperflexion of the PIP joint with the base of the proximal phalanx frequently dorsally subluxed and sometimes even frankly dislocated. When a hammer toe has been present for a long time, degenerative changes of the articular surfaces of the PIP and M-P joints, such as narrowing and irregularity, subchondral osteosclerosis, and marginal osteophyte formation, can become quite apparent on routine radiographs. When a hammered second toe overlaps a great toe with hallux valgus, the phalanges of the second and the great toes cross each other. To identify a particular metatarsal head that has produced a painful plantar callosity, a lead marker, such as the letter O, can be accurately taped to the plantar callus, and a standing anteroposterior view of the foot can then be taken to pinpoint the callus-producing metatarsal head.

Pathologic Anatomy

In a fixed hammer toe, flexion contracture of the PIP joint is accompanied by contracture of its plantar joint capsule and collateral ligaments; hyperextension of the M-P joint also causes contracture of the dorsal joint capsule and collateral ligaments. Dorsal subluxation or dislocation of the M-P joint carried the insertion of the dorsal interosseous muscle to the dorsal aspect of the axis of rotation of the M-P joint, which changes its function from a flexor of the M-P joint to an extensor of the same joint. The deformities of the PIP and M-P joints cause both the extensor digitorum longus and the flexor digitorum longus muscles to become adaptively shortened. When arthritic changes have occurred in the PIP and M-P joints of a hammer toe, degeneration of the articular cartilage, synovial proliferation, osteophyte formation at the joint margins, and fibrosis of the para-articular soft tissues may be present. Frequently, the small adventitious bursa between the painful corn and the bony prominence on the dorsal aspect of the PIP joint becomes inflamed and filled with a straw-colored fluid that can become frankly purulent when an infection is present. In addition, atrophy of the fat pad under the plantarly displaced metatarsal head deprives the metatarsal head of its cushioning effect and enables the condyles of the metatarsal head to come close to the painful plantar callosity.

Nonsurgical Treatment

A. Shoe modifications: roomy, extradepth, and space shoes, and stretching of toe boxes with a shoemaker's swan to accommodate the cock-up hammer toe, as well as padding of the insoles, arch supports, metatarsal bars and pads, and rocker-bottom soles to relieve the painful plantar callosity are useful (Figures 1–4—1–7, 1–9, 1–10, 1–12, and 1–13).

B. Padding of the foot: soft pads applied di-

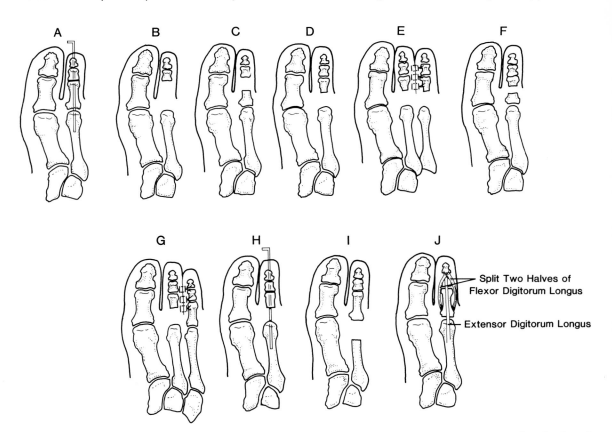

Figure 3–1. Various surgical procedures for correcting hammer toe. **A,** fusion of PIP joint, Z-plasty lengthening of the extensor digitorum longus, dorsal capsulotomy of the M-P joint, and reduction and fixation of the M-P joint in a neutral position with a small K-wire. **B,** proximal phalangectomy. **C,** excision of the distal portion of the proximal phalanx. **D,** excision of the proximal portion of the proximal phalanx. **E,** excision of the proximal portions of the proximal phalanges and syndactylization of the two adjacent toes. **F,** diaphysectomy of the proximal phalanx. **G,** excision of the proximal portion of the proximal phalanx and syndactylization of the operated toe to its normal adjacent toe. **H,** resection of the proximal one half of the proximal phalanx and fusion of its PIP joint followed by K-wire fixation across the M-P joint. **I,** excision of the metatarsal head. **J,** transfer of the two split ends of the flexor digitorum longus tendon to the tip of the extensor digitorum longus tendon, with the toe held in slight plantar flexion.

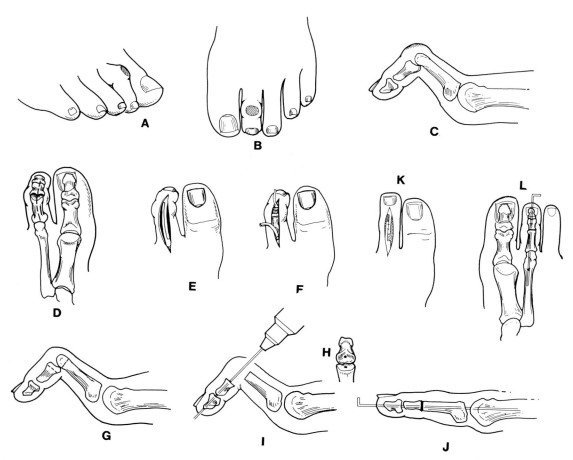

Figure 3-2. The author's preferred surgical technique for treating hammer toes. 3–2A—C, different views of a hammer toe (also see Figure 3-3A). 3–2D, dorsal skin incision extending from the level of the middle phalanx to the metatarsal head region (also see Figure 3–3B). 3–2E, Z-plasty of the extensor digitorum longus tendon (also see Figure 3–3C and D). 3–2F and G, removal of the head of the proximal phalanx and the articular cartilage on the base of the middle phalanx with a microsaw followed by performing a dorsal capsulotomy of the M-P joint (also see Figure 3–3E). 3–2H—L, making two matching holes through the centers of the base of the middle phalanx and the head of the proximal phalanx, driving a small smooth K-wire through the middle and distal phalanges to emerge at the tip of the toe, and then driving the same K-wire retrograde through the center of the proximal phalanx into the distal portion of the corresponding metatarsal. The lengthened extensor digitorum longus tendon is then approximated and the skin is closed (also see Figure 3–3F). Postoperative management: K-wire is usually left in place for 5 to 6 weeks for the fusion of the PIP joint to take place and for the subluxed or dislocated M-P joint to heal in its reduced position.

rectly to the dorsal and end corns and plantar callosity of a hammer toe can give symptomatic relief (Figure 1–8).

C. Commercially available foot aids: donut-shaped pads, an arch cuff, a hammer toe shield, a toecrest, a hammer toe shield with callosity cushion, and class ring-shaped or latex hammer toe shields are useful ap-

pliances for giving pain relief (Figures 1–16—1–19).

Surgical Treatment

The surgical repair of any hammer toe should correct the hyperextension deformity of the M-P joint, the flexion deformity of the PIP joint, the subluxed or dislocated M-P joint, and all the contracted tendons. A list of sur-

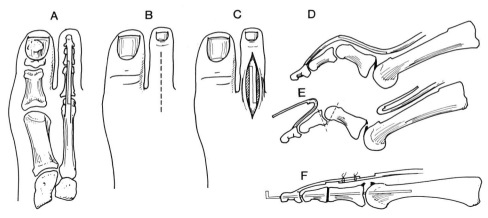

Figure 3–3. See legend to Figure 3–2.

gical procedures for correcting hammer toe deformities follows (Figures 3–1—3–3).

A. Fusion of the PIP joint in a neutral position, Z-plasty lengthening of the extensor digitorum longus, dorsal capsulotomy of the M-P joint, reduction of subluxation or dislocation of the M-P joint by cutting the joint capsule and collateral ligaments (and dorsal interosseous tendon if necessary), and fixation of the whole toe in a neutral position with a small smooth K-wire that is driven from the tip of the toe through the phalanges into the distal portion of the corresponding metatarsal to maintain the correction for approximately 5 to 6 weeks to ensure permanent correction. This is the author's preferred method of treating hammer toes (Figures 3–1A, 3–2, and 3–3).

B. Proximal phalangectomy: although it does correct the hammer toe deformity to a certain extent, it creates an unstable, flail, and deformed toe that can contribute to the development of hallux valgus when the unstable toe is the second toe (Figure 3–1B).

C. Excision of the distal portion of the proximal phalanx: does not correct the deformity of the M-P joint such as hyperextension and dorsal subluxation or dislocation (Figure 3–1C).

D. Excision of the proximal portion of the proximal phalanx: creates an unstable M-P joint that can become dislocated and can also encourage the development of hallux valgus when the operated hammer toe is the second toe (Figure 3–1D).

E. Excision of the proximal portions of the proximal phalanges and syndactylization of the two adjacent toes: provides some stability for the M-P joints and tends to prevent subsequent deformity (Figure 3–1E).

F. Diaphysectomy of the proximal phalanx: does not correct the deformity of the M-P joint such as hyperextension and subluxation or dislocation (Figure 3–1F).

G. Excision of the proximal portion of the proximal phalanx and syndactylization of the operated toe to its normal adjacent toe: normal toe provides stability for the toe with proximal hemiphalangectomy of its proximal phalanx (Figure 3–1G).

H. Resection of the proximal one half of the proximal phalanx, fusion of the PIP joint, and K-wire fixation across the M-P joint: although the K-wire does provide temporary stability of the M-P joint, the absence of the proximal one half of the proximal phalanx may make the toe vulnerable to subsequent subluxation or dislocation at the M-P joint (Figure 3–1H).

I. Excision of the metatarsal head: usually causes gradual proximal migration and cock-up deformity of the corresponding toe, and with time tends to transfer the painful plantar callosity to the adjacent toe (Figure 3–1I).

J. Transfer of the two split ends of the flexor digitorum longus tendon to the tip of the extensor digitorum longus tendon with the toe held in slight plantar flexion: useful only in a supple and flexible hammer toe and will not correct a fixed hammer toe (Figure 3–1J).

REFERENCES

Hammer Toe

1. Borg, I.: Operation for hammer-toe. Acta Chir. Scand., *100:*619, 1950.
2. Cahill, B.R., and Connor, D.E.: A long-term follow-up on proximal phalangectomy for hammertoes. Clin. Orthop., *86:*191, 1972.
3. Ellis, T.S.: Hallux valgus and hammer toe. Lancet, *1:*1155, 1899.
4. Ely, I.W.: Hammertoe, Surg. Clin. North Am., *6:*133, 1926.
5. Glassmon, F., and Wolin, I.: Phalangectomy for toe deformities. Surg. Clin. North Am., *29:*275, 1949.
6. Haward, W.: Hammer-toe and hallux valgus and rigidus. Lancet, *2:*240, 1900.
7. Higgs, S.L.: "Hammer-toe." Postgrad. Med. J., *6:*130, 1931.
8. Lapidus, P.W.: Operation for correction of hammertoe. J. Bone Joint Surg., *21:*977, 1939.
9. McConnell, B.E.: Correction of hammer toe deformity, a 10 year review of subperiosteal waist resection of proximal phalanx. Orthop. Rev., *8:*65, 1979.
10. Merrill, W.J.: Conservative operative treatment of hammertoe. Am. J. Orthop. Surg., *10:*262, 1912.
11. Meznik, V.F.: On the technique of hammer-toe operation. Wien. Med. Wochenschr., *112:*108, 1962.
12. Michele, A.A., and Krueger, F.J.: Operative correction for hammertoe. Milit. Med., *103:*52, 1948.
13. Mladick, R.A.: Correction of hammertoe surgery deformity by Z-plasty and bone graft. Ann. Plast. Surg., *4:*224, 1980.
14. Newman, R.J., and Fitton, J.M.: An evaluation of operative procedures in the treatment of hammertoe. Acta Orthop. Scand., *50:*709, 1979.
15. O'Neil, J.: An arthroplastic operation for hammertoe. J.A.M.A., *57:*1207, 1911.
16. Scheck, M.: Degenerative changes in the metatarsophalangeal joints after surgical correction of severe hammer toe deformities. A complication associated with avascular necrosis in three cases. J. Bone Joint Surg. [Am.], *50:*727, 1968.
17. Scheck, M.: Etiology of acquired hammertoe deformity. Clin. Orthop., *123:*63, 1977.
18. Selig, S.: Hammertoe: A new procedure for its correction. Surg. Gynecol. Obstet., *72:*101, 1941.
19. Soule, R.E.: Operation for the cure of hammertoe. N.Y. State J. Med., *91:*649, 1910.
20. Taylor, R.G.: An operative procedure for the treatment of hammer toe and claw toe. J. Bone Joint Surg., *22:*608, 1940.
21. Trethowan, W.H.: The treatment of hammertoe. Lancet, *1:*1257, 1925.
22. Wee, G.C., and Tucker, G.L.: An improved procedure for the surgical correction of hammer toe. Mo. Med., *67:*43, 1970.
23. Young, C.S.: An operation for the correction of hammer toe and claw toe. J. Bone Joint Surg., *20:*715, 1938.
24. Zimmerman, E.: Hammer-toe operating experiences and successes. Beitr. Orthop. Traumatol., *13:*654, 1966.

CLAWTOES AND PES CAVUS (THE CLAWFOOT DEFORMITY)

Incidence

Clawtoe deformity is characterized by hyperextension of the M-P joints, hyperflexion of the PIP and DIP joints, bilateral and symmetric involvement, association with disorders of other body systems, and frequent presence of midfoot and hindfoot deformities. When clawtoe deformity is associated with cavus deformity of the foot, the term clawfoot is often used to describe the deformities of the whole foot. Many causes can produce clawtoes and cavus feet.

A. Primary (idiopathic) pes cavus.

B. Secondary pes cavus.
   1. Neurologic diseases.
      a. Spinocerebellar hereditary degeneration.
      b. Poliomyelitis.
      c. Diastematomyelia.
      d. Spinal cord tumors.
      e. Cerebral palsy.
      f. Friedreich's ataxia.
      g. Charcot-Marie-Tooth disease.
      h. Myelodysplasia.
      i. Discogenic disease of the spine.
      j. Multiple sclerosis.

k. Spinal cord injuries.
l. Polyneuritis.
m. Peripheral nerve injuries.
2. Crush injury and fractures and dislocations of the lower leg and foot.
3. Various myopathies and muscular dystrophies.
4. Talipes equinovarus.
5. Congenital lymphedema.
6. Infection of the foot and congenital syphilis.
7. Frost bite of the foot and immersion foot.
8. Sudeck's atrophy.
9. Hysteria-induced pes cavus.

On a clinical basis, the deformity of pes cavus can be of different degrees.

A. First degree: visible only when the affected foot is relaxed.

B. Second degree: associated with fixed equinus and pronation deformity of the first metatarsal and the great toe.

C. Third degree: associated with equinus deformity of all five metatarsals and some varus deformity of the calcaneus.

D. Fourth degree: definite structural bone changes are present at the apex of the cavus deformity, which usually centers about the inner cuneiform, and is frequently accompanied by a significant amount of varus deformity of the calcaneus.

E. Fifth degree: firmly fixed and extremely prominent cavus deformity of the foot is present with its apex at the midtarsal and distal tarsal areas, accompanied by dorsal dislocation of the M-P joints, marked flexion contracture of the PIP and DIP joints, painful corns over the dorsal aspect of PIP joints, painful callosities under the metatarsal heads, marked contracture of the plantar fascia and its associated intrinsic plantar muscles, and severe varus deformity of the calcaneus.

It is commonly thought that neuromuscular diseases affect the foot primarily and the toes secondarily, and produce clawtoes and cavus feet by means of muscle imbalance. For example, in the presence of a weak or paralyzed anterior tibialis muscle, the extensor hallucis longus and extensor digitorum longus muscles are used constantly to dorsiflex the foot, particularly when the heel cord is tight, producing clawing of the toes that is most pronounced at the beginning of swing phase. On the other hand, in the presence of a weak or paralyzed triceps surae muscle, the flexor hallucis longus and flexor digitorum longus muscles are used to plantar flex the foot, causing clawing of the toes that is present during the stance phase and tends to increase at the point of push-off when all the toes exert maximal pressure on the ground. It should be noted that the long toe extensors primarily extend the M-P joints and to a lesser extent the PIP and DIP joints, and the long toe flexors mainly flex the DIP joint. In contrast, the interosseous muscles principally flex the M-P joints and extend the PIP and DIP joints. Consequently, weakness or paralysis of the interosseous muscles in the presence of overactive long toe flexors and extensors creates a perfect set-up for the development of clawtoes. It should also be noted that there are several different types of pes cavus.

A. Simple pes cavus: plantar flexion deformity of the forefoot is equal in its medial and lateral columns, with its heel in either a neutral position or only a few degrees of valgus.

B. Pes cavovarus: only the medial column of the forefoot is plantar flexed with the first metatarsal rigidly and noticeably plantar flexed and pronated. The fifth metatarsal is still in a normal and flexible position, and is associated with either dynamic or fixed varus deformity of the heel.

C. Pes calcaneocavus: fixed equinus position of the forefoot and the calcaneal position of the hindfoot are usually produced by paralysis of the triceps surae muscle.

D. Pes equinovarus: inverted and adducted forefoot and the inverted and equinus hindfoot are the typical deformities of a clubfoot (talipes equinovarus).

Clinical Symptoms and Signs

Patients with clawtoes and cavus feet frequently complain of a general fatigue and discomfort of their feet; pain under the metatarsal heads, especially the balls of the feet; difficulty in obtaining comfortable shoes to wear, particularly when the foot deformities are asymmetric; and a relatively high incidence of falls and sprained ankles due to decreased total area of foot contact with the ground and awkward gait. Examination often reveals hyperextension with subluxation or dislocation of the M-P joints; fixed flexion contracture of the PIP and DIP joints, with painful corns on the dorsal aspect of the PIP joints and the tips of the toes; painful callosities under the metatarsal heads, especially under the first metatarsal head, accompanied by marked atrophy of the plantar fat pads under the metatarsal heads; increased heights of both the longitudinal and transverse arches of the feet; contracture of the plantar fascia, abductor hallucis, flexor digitorum brevis, and abductor digiti quinti; and varus deformity of the heels. Examination of the shoes frequently shows wearing down of the outer borders of the shoes and the area of the soles under the first metatarsal heads, and bulging and distortion of the fronts of the shoes due to dropping of the forefeet and clawing of the toes.

A useful test to determine the flexibility of the hindfoot is the so-called "standing lateral block test." To perform the test, a 1-in. wooden block is placed under the fourth and fifth metatarsals and the lateral one half of the heel to make the three medial metatarsals pronate. If the hindfoot varus is corrected by this test, the hindfoot varus deformity is still flexible and will resolve with correction of the forefoot deformities. If the hindfoot varus is

not corrected by this test the correction of the cavus foot deformities should include both forefoot and hindfoot procedures.

Because a wide variety of neuromuscular diseases can cause cavus foot deformity, a wide spectrum of neurologic symptoms and signs, such as motor and sensory deficits, reflex changes, muscle atrophy, and bladder and bowel disturbances, may accompany cavus foot deformity; these symptoms can be demonstrated by abnormal electromyographic and impaired nerve conduction velocity studies.

Roentgenographic Manifestations

The clawfoot deformity makes the foot bones appear to be somewhat shortened on the anteroposterior radiograph. The lateral view usually shows hyperextension and subluxation or dislocation of the M-P joints, hyperflexion of the PIP and DIP joints, and plantar flexion of the forefoot, producing a high longitudinal arch of the foot. Axial views of the calcaneus frequently show varus deformity of the calcaneus. In addition, depending on the particular type of pes cavus, the calcaneus can be in a neutral, varus, equinus, or calcaneal position. Ordinarily, on the lateral view of a normal foot, the longitudinal axis of the talus coincides with that of the first metatarsal. In contrast, in a cavus foot, the longitudinal axis of the talus forms an angle (the so-called Meary's angle or first metatarsal-talar angle) with that of the first metatarsal; the size of this angle is proportional to the severity of the pes cavus deformity. In addition, the cavus deformity of the foot can also be determined by the first metatarsal-calcaneal angle (also known as the Hibbs' angle) formed by the longitudinal axis of the calcaneus with that of the first metatarsal (Figure 3–4).

As a rule of thumb, if the first metatarsal-calcaneal angle is less than 150°, pes cavus is present. It should be noted that the first metatarsal-talar angle (the Meary's angle) is useful in identifying the apex of the cavus deformity of the foot, which is usually the place where osteotomy or fusion is performed (Figure 3–5). When the clawfoot deformity is

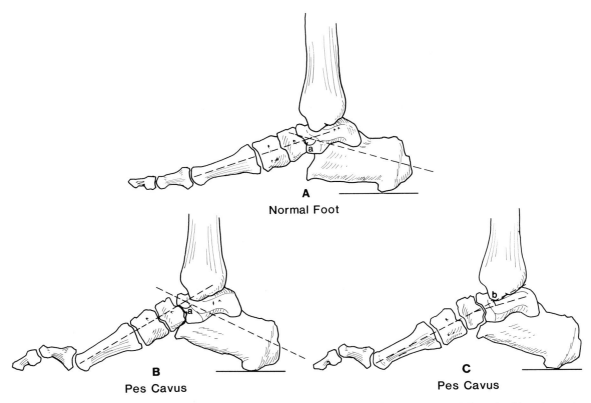

A
Normal Foot

B
Pes Cavus

C
Pes Cavus

Figure 3–4. Hibbs' and Meary's angles in a normal foot and in pes cavus. **A,** in a normal foot, the Meary's angle is usually 0° and the Hibbs' angle is usually greater than 150°. **B,** in pes cavus, the Hibbs' angle is less than 150°. **C,** in pes cavus, the Meary's angle is greater than 0°.

caused by various neurologic diseases, radiography of the spine, myelography, and CT scans of the spinal column are helpful in identifying the spinal anomalies or diseases that have produced the clawfoot deformity.

Pathologic Anatomy

In a clawfoot deformity, the hyperextension and subluxation or dislocation of the M-P joints is accompanied by contracture of their dorsal joint capsules and collateral ligaments, interosseous muscles, extensor hallucis and digitorum longus tendons, and atrophy of plantar fat pads under the metatarsal heads. Flexion contracture of the PIP and DIP joints also occurs by contracture of their plantar joint capsules, collateral ligaments, and flexor hallucis and digitorum longus tendons. Also noted is cavus deformity by plantar flexion of the fore-

foot frequently at the metatarsotarsal joints, sometimes at cuneiform-navicular joints, or occasionally at the talonavicular joint, or by calcaneal deformity of the hindfoot, in association with contracture of the plantar intertarsal and tarsometatarsal ligaments such as the long and short plantar, plantar calcaneonavicular (spring), and plantar tarsometatarsal ligaments, as well as the plantar fascia, abductor hallucis, flexor digitorum brevis, and abductor digiti quinti. In addition, deformity of the bases of the metatarsals and tarsal bones as well as arthritic changes of the tarsometatarsal and intertarsal articulations gradually develop in the wake of the plantar soft tissue contracture. In pes calcaneocavus, the calcaneal tendon is somewhat lengthened, whereas in pes equinovarus, the calcaneal tendon is significantly shortened.

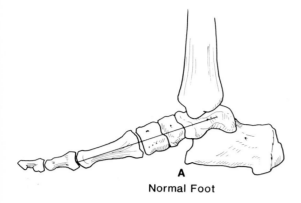

A
Normal Foot

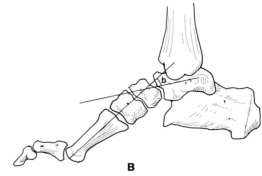

B
The Apex of the Cavus Deformity
at Talonavicular and Calcaneocuboid Joints

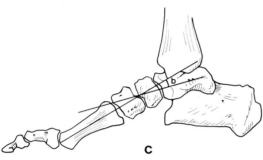

C
The Apex of the Cavus Deformity
at Cuneiformnavicular Joints

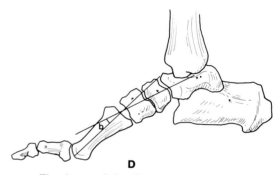

D
The Apex of the Cavus Deformity
at Tarsometatarsal Joints

Figure 3–5. Use of Meary's angle to determine the apex of the cavus deformity of the foot. **A,** normal foot has a Meary's angle of 0°. **B,** cavus foot with its apex at the talonavicular and calcaneocuboid joints. **C,** cavus foot with its apex at the cuneiform-navicular joints. **D,** cavus foot with its apex at the tarsometatarsal joints.

Nonsurgical Treatment

A. Shoe modifications: wide, extra depth, and space shoes; stretching of the toe boxes with a shoemaker's swan to accommodate the greatly deformed clawtoes; metatarsal pads and bars, arch supports, rocker-bottom soles, total contact insoles, and ankle-foot orthosis to relieve the painful plantar callosities can be helpful in providing symptomatic relief for painful clawfeet (Figures 1–4—1–7, 1–12, 1–13).

B. Padding of the toes and feet: soft pads applied to the corns on the dorsal aspects and the tips of the toes as well as to the painful plantar callosities, or to the insoles

of shoes under the painful plantar-flexed metatarsal heads, can provide pain relief (Figures 1–8—1–10).

C. Commercially available foot aids: donut-shaped corn and callosity pads, an arch cuff, a toe crest, and a hammer toe shield with callosity cushion are some of the useful aids in rendering pain relief from symptomatic clawfeet (Figures 1–16—1–18).

Surgical Treatment

Treatment of clawfoot should include correction of the clawtoes, cavus foot, and varus or occasionally calcaneal heel.

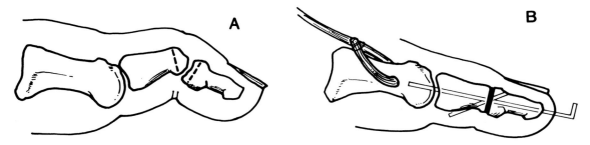

Figure 3–6. Surgical correction of a clawed great toe. **A** through a longitudinal dorsal incision, expose the extensor hallux longus and detach it from the distal phalanx. Resect part of the head of the proximal phalanx and the base of the distal phalanx with a microsaw. **B,** drill a transverse hole through the neck of the first metatarsal and pass the free end of the detached extensor hallucis longus tendon through the hole; suture it to itself. Fuse the interphalangeal joint of the great toe with longitudinal and oblique K-wires.

A. Correction of the claw toes. Reduction of the hyperextension and dorsal subluxation or dislocation of the M-P joints by performing dorsal capsulotomies; sectioning of collateral ligaments and tendons of interosseous muscles, and transfer of extensor hallucis and digitorum longus tendons to the necks of the metatarsals to assist in dorsiflexion of the forefoot; fusion of the PIP and DIP joints in a neutral position; and holding the resected PIP and DIP joints in intimate contact and the M-P joint in a neutral position with a small smooth K-wire (Figures 3–6—3–8).

B. Correction of the cavus deformity of the foot.
  1. Flexible pes cavus: strip the plantar fas-

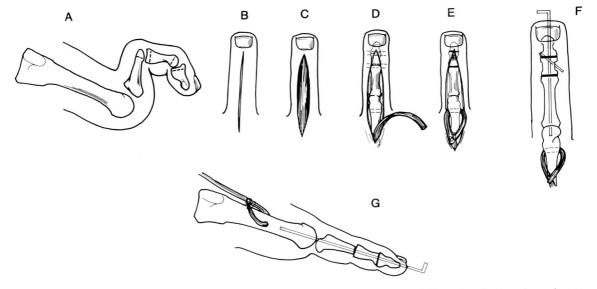

Figure 3–7. Surgical correction of clawtoe deformity of the lesser toes. **A,** lateral view of a clawtoe shows hyperextension and dislocation of the M-P joint and hyperflexion of the PIP and DIP joints. Dotted lines, amount of bone to be removed in preparation for interphalangeal fusions. **B,** longitudinal dorsal skin incision that extends from the distal phalanx to the distal portion of its corresponding metatarsal. **C,** extensor digitorum longus has been exposed. **D,** detach the extensor digitorum longus tendon from its insertion on the distal phalanx and resect the PIP and DIP joints with a microsaw. **E,** transfer the extensor digitorum longus tendon to the metatarsal neck. **F** and **G,** fuse the PIP and DIP joints with a longitudinal wire that can be accompanied by an oblique wire to secure the interphalangeal fusion further.

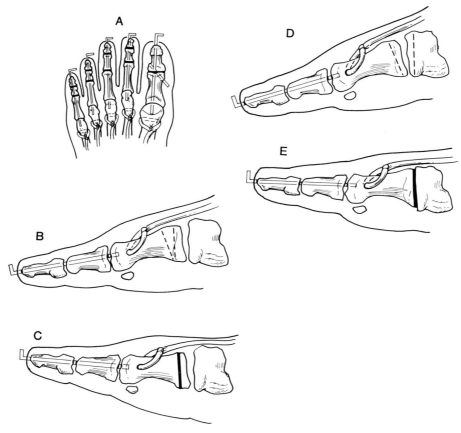

Figure 3–8. Surgical treatment of severe clawtoes in association with a second degree pes cavus with the first metatarsal in pronation and fixed equinus. **A,** fusion of the PIP and DIP joints of all five toes and transfer of all five long extensor tendons to their respective metatarsal necks. **B** and **C,** closing-wedge dorsal angulation osteotomy with the wedge based on the dorsal aspect of the base of the first metatarsal. **D** and **E,** closing-wedge dorsal angulation osteotomy with a dorsally based wedge resection of the first metatarsocuneiform joint.

cia and the origins of the abductor hallucis, flexor digitorum brevis, and abductor digiti quinti from the anteroinferior aspect of the calcaneus.

2. Fixed pes cavus with its apex at the metatarsotarsal joints: strip the plantar fascia and the abductor hallucis, flexor digitorum brevis, and abductor digiti quinti from the calcaneus. Perform multiple dorsal closing-wedge osteotomies of the bases of the metatarsals or fuse the metatarsotarsal joints in a dorsiflexed position to correct the plantar flexion deformity of the forefoot. Fusion of the metatarsotarsal joints is particu-

larly indicated when arthritic changes are present in these metatarsotarsal joints (Figures 3–9—3–11).

3. Fixed pes cavus with its apex at its cuneiform-navicular joint: strip the plantar fascia and the abductor hallucis, flexor digitorum brevis, and abductor digiti quinti from the calcaneus. Fuse the cuneiform-navicular joints in a dorsiflexed position and perform a dorsal closing-wedge osteotomy of the cuboid bone to correct the plantar flexion deformity of the forefoot. Arthrodesis of the cuneiform-navicular joints is especially indicated when arthritis has developed in

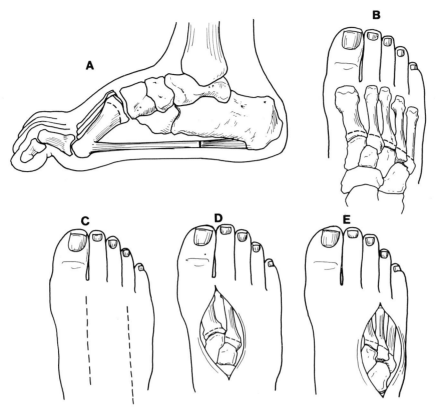

Figure 3–9. Crescentic metatarsal osteotomy to correct pes cavus with its apex at the metatarsotarsal joints. **A** and **B,** tight plantar fascia and short abductors and flexors should be released first. Circular dotted lines, osteotomy cuts to be performed. **C,** two longitudinal dorsal incisions commonly used to reach the five underlying metatarsals. **D,** osteotomy of the bases of the first and second metatarsals through the medial longitudinal dorsal incision. **E,** osteotomy of the bases of the third, fourth, and fifth metatarsals through the lateral longitudinal dorsal incision. These metatarsals can then be dorsiflexed by sliding their bases downward along the crescentic osteotomy lines.

these cuneiform-navicular joints (Figures 3–12 and 3–13).

4. Fixed pes cavus with its apex at its talonavicular and calcaneocuboid joints: strip the plantar fascia and abductor hallucis, flexor digitorum brevis, and abductor digiti quinti from the calcaneus. Fuse the talonavicular and calcaneocuboid joints in a dorsiflexed position to correct the cavus deformity of the foot. Fusion of the talonavicular and calcaneocuboid joints is particularly indicated when degenerative changes have taken place in the talonavicular or calcaneocuboid joints or both, and is frequently combined with fusion of the subtalar joint, resulting in a triple arthrodesis of the foot (Figure 3–14).

5. V-shaped dorsiflexion osteotomy of the forefoot with the apex of the V located at the navicular bone and the two arms of the V extended to the cuboid bone and the first cuneiform bone: does not shorten the foot, can correct adduction or abduction deformity of the forefoot, and achieves a low incidence of nonunion rate at the site of the osteotomy due to the large area of raw bone surfaces present at the osteotomy site (Figure 3–15).

C. Correction of the varus or occasionally

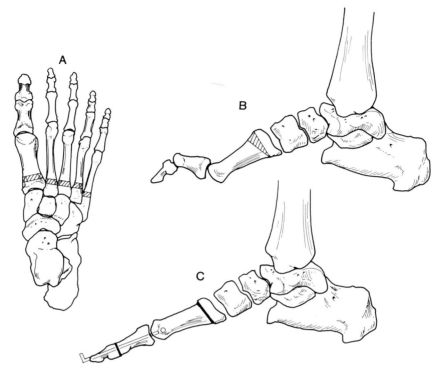

Figure 3–10. Closing-wedge dorsal angulation osteotomy with the dorsal wedges situated at the bases of the five metatarsals. **A** and **B,** the shaded areas, the dorsally based wedges to be removed. **C,** close the osteotomy sites to correct forefoot equinus deformity.

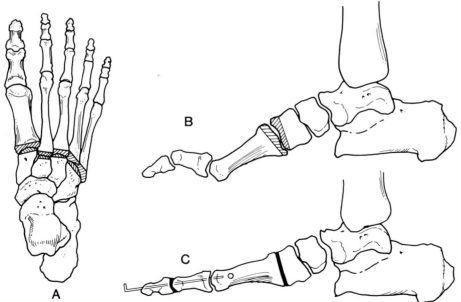

Figure 3–11. Fusion of the metatarsotarsal joints in a dorsally angulated position to correct pes cavus deformity. **A** and **B,** shaded areas, amount of bone to be removed from metatarsotarsal joint. **C,** close the osteotomy sites to correct the pes cavus deformity.

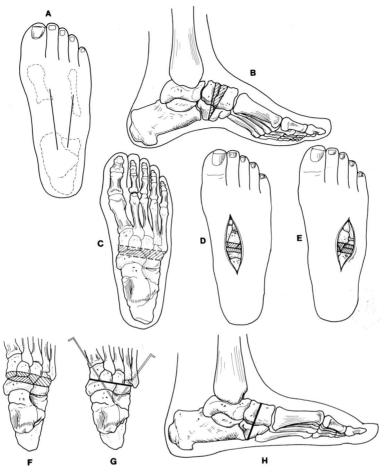

Figure 3–12. Dorsal angulation osteotomy of the forefoot by fusing the cuneiform-navicular joint and performing an osteotomy of the cuboid bone. **A,** two dorsal longitudinal incisions. **B** and **C,** dotted lines, amount of bone to be removed. **D** and **E,** resection of the cuneiform-navicular joints and osteotomy of the cuboid bone through the two dorsal longitudinal incisions. **F,** completed cuneiform-navicular joint resection and osteotomy of the cuboid. **G,** closure of the osteotomy site; fixation with two K-wires. **H,** correction of the pes cavus deformity after dorsal angulation osteotomy through the cuneiform-navicular joint and the cuboid bone.

calcaneal heel deformity of the foot.

1. Flexible varus heel deformity correctable by the standing lateral block test: will automatically correct itself after the forefoot deformity has been corrected.
2. Fixed varus heel deformity not correctable by the standing lateral block test: usually needs lateral closing-wedge osteotomy to bring the heel into a neutral position (Figure 3–16).
3. Fixed varus heel deformity associated with degenerative arthritis of the sub-

talar joint: fuse the subtalar joint by resecting more bone from its lateral aspect to bring the heel into a neutral position (Figure 3–17).
4. Fixed calcaneus heel deformity: perform a crescentic osteotomy of the calcaneus near its midportion. Rotate the inferior portion upward along the line of the crescentic osteotomy to correct the calcaneal heel deformity after the plantar fascia, abductor hallucis, flexor digitorum brevis, and abductor digiti quinti

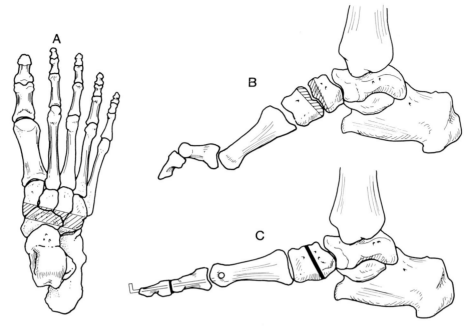

Figure 3–13. Surgical correction of pes cavus by performing cuneiform-navicular fusion and osteotomy of the cuboid bone. **A** and **B**, shaded area, amount of bone to be removed. **C**, closure of the osteotomy site corrects the pes cavus deformity.

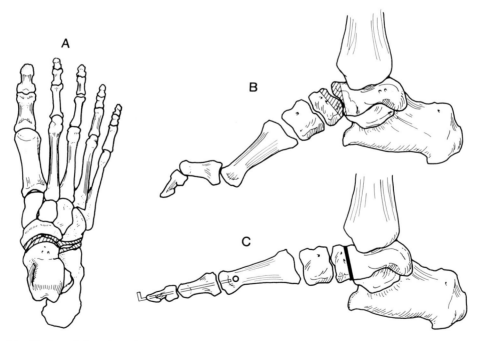

Figure 3–14. Fusion of the talonavicular and calcaneocuboid joints in treating pes cavus. **A** and **B**, shaded area, extent of the bone resection of the talonavicular and calcaneocuboid joints. **C**, pes cavus has been corrected after the osteotomy sites are closed.

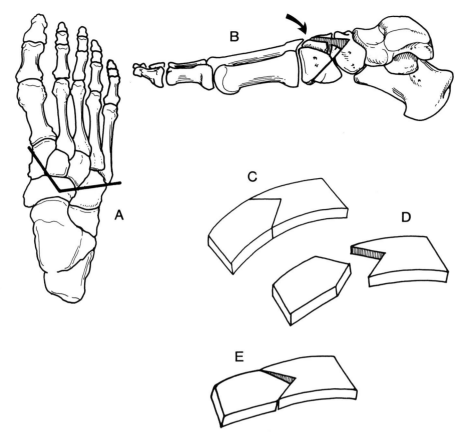

Figure 3–15. V-shaped dorsal angulation osteotomy of the forefoot. **A,** apex of the V is located at the navicular, with its two arms extending to the cuboid and the first cuneiform bones. **B,** by dorsiflexing the metatarsals to correct the pes cavus deformity, the convex portion of the V-shaped osteotomy drops below the concave portion of the same osteotomy site. **C–E,** curvature of a rectangular object can be greatly decreased or increased by manipulating the V-shaped osteotomy created at its midportion.

have been detached from the calcaneus (Figure 3–18).

REFERENCES

Clawtoes and Pes Cavus (The Clawfoot Deformity)

1. Alvik, I.: Operative treatment of pes cavus. Acta Orthop. Scand., *23:*137, 1953.
2. Barenfeld, P.A., Weseley, M.S., and Shea, J.M.: The congenital cavus foot. Clin. Orthop., *79:*119, 1971.
3. Barwell, R.: Pes planus and pes cavus; An anatomical and clinical study. Edinburgh Med. J., *3:*113, 1898.
4. Brewerton, D.A., Sandifer, P.H., and Sweetnam, D.R.: "Idiopathic" pes cavus. Br. Med. J., *1:*659, 1963.
5. Brockway, A.: Surgical correction of talipes cavus deformities. J. Bone Joint Surg., *22:*81, 1940.
6. Chuinard, E.G., and Baskin, M.S.: Correction of claw toe deformity in children. J. Bone Joint Surg. [Am.], *51:*1043, 1969.
7. Chuinard, E.G., and Baskin, M.S.: Claw-foot deformity, treatment by transfer of the long extensors into the metatarsals and fusion of the interphalangeal joints. J. Bone Joint Surg. [Am.], *55:*351, 1973.
8. Clawson, D.K.: Claw toes following tibial fracture. Clin. Orthop., *103:*47, 1974.
9. Cole, W.H.: The treatment of claw-foot. J. Bone Joint Surg., *22:*895, 1940.
10. Davies-Colley, N.: On hallux flexus, claw toe and pes cavus. Guy's Hosp. Rep., *52:*1, 1895.
11. Davis, G.G.: The treatment of hollow foot (pes cavus). Am. J. Orthop. Surg., *11:*231, 1913.
12. Dickson, F.D., and Diveley, R.L.: Operation for correction of mild claw-foot. J.A.M.A., *87:*1275, 1926.
13. Dunn. N.: Calcaneocavus and its treatment. J. Orthop. Surg., *1:*711, 1919.

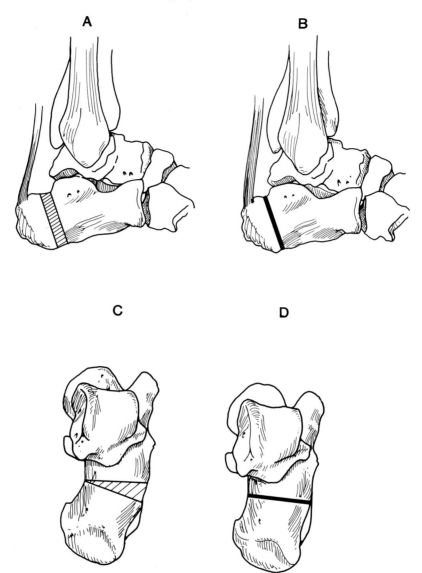

Figure 3–16. Valgus calcaneal osteotomy to correct varus deformity of the heel. **A** and **C,** shaded area, laterally based bone wedge to be removed from the calcaneus. **B** and **D,** closure of the osteotomy site results in correction of varus deformity of the heel.

14. Dwyer, F.C.: Osteotomy of the calcaneum for pes cavus. J. Bone Joint Surg. [Br.], *41:*80, 1959.
15. Dwyer, F.C.: The present status of the problem of pes cavus. Clin. Orthop., *106:*254, 1975.
16. Dyck, P.J., and Lambert, E.H.: Lower motor and primary sensory neuron disease with peroneal muscular atrophy. Arch. Neurol., *18:*603, 1968.
17. Foley, T.M.: Pes cavus, due to paralysis of the extensor muscles, dorsal flexors of the feet. South. Med. J., *17:*798, 1924.
18. Forbes, A.M.: Clawfoot, and how to relieve it. Surg. Gynecol. Obstet., *16:*81, 1913.
19. Fowler, A.W.: The surgery of fixed claw toes. J. Bone Joint Surg. [Br.], *39:*585, 1957.
20. Fowler, B., Brooks, A.L., and Parrish, T.F.: The cavovarus foot. J. Bone Joint Surg. [Am.], *41:*757, 1959.
21. Frank, G.R., and Johnson, W.N.: Extensor shift procedure in the correction of claw toe deformities in children. South. Med. J., *59:*889, 1966.
22. Garceau, G.J., and Brahms, M.A.: A preliminary study

A   **B**

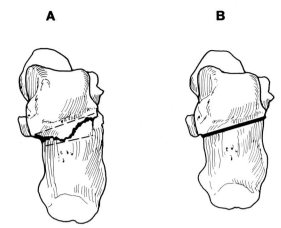

Figure 3–17. Varus deformity of the heel in association with arthritis of the subtalar joint. **A,** dotted lines, bone to be removed in preparation for subtalar fusion. **B,** raw bone surfaces have been brought into intimate contact to correct the varus heel deformity and to achieve a solid subtalar fusion.

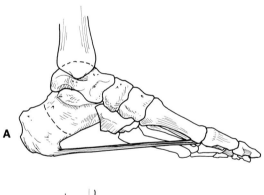

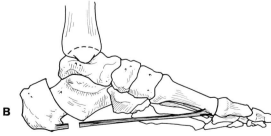

Figure 3–18. Crescentic calcaneal osteotomy for correction of a fixed calcaneal heel deformity. **A,** curved dotted line, osteotomy line. **B,** calcaneal heel deformity has been corrected after releasing the plantar fascia and short abductors and flexors, and sliding the inferior portion of the operated calcaneus upward.

of selective plantar muscle denervation for pes cavus. J. Bone Joint Surg. [Am.], *38:*553, 1956.
23. Goff, C.W.: Pes cavus of congenital syphilis. Am. J. Surg., *22:*359, 1933.
24. Heron, J.R.: Neurological syndromes associated with pes cavus. Proc. R. Soc. Lond. [Med.], *62:*270, 1969.
25. Heyman, C.H.: The operative treatment of claw-foot. J. Bone Joint Surg., *14:*335, 1932.
26. Hibbs, R.A.: An operation for clawfoot. J.A.M.A., *73:*1583, 1919.
27. Hoffman, P.: An operation for severe grades of contracted or clawed toes. Am. J. Orthop. Surg., *9:*441, 1912.
28. Irwin, C.E.: The calcaneus foot. South. Med. J., *44:*191, 1951.
29. Jacobs, J.T.: Achilles tenodesis for paralytic calcaneocavus foot. Clin. Orthop., *47:*143, 1966.
30. Jahss, M.H.: Tarsometatarsal truncated-wedge arthrodesis for pes cavus and equinovarus deformity of the fore part of the foot. J. Bone Joint Surg. [Am.], *62:*713, 1980.
31. Japas, L.M.: Surgical treatment of pes cavus by tarsal V-osteotomy. J. Bone Joint Surg. [Am.], *50:*927, 1968.
32. Jones, A.R.: Discussion on the treatment of pes cavus. Proc. R. Soc. Lond. [Med.], *20:*1117, 1927.
33. Lambrinudi, C.: An operation for claw toes. Proc. R. Soc. Lond. [Med.], *21:*239, 1927.
34. Lipscomb, P.R.: Osteotomy of calcaneus, triple arthrodesis, and tendon transfer for severe paralytic calcaneocavus deformity. J. Bone Joint Surg. [Am.], *51:*548, 1969.
35. Mayer, P.J.: Pes cavus: A diagnostic and therapeutic challenge. Orthop. Rev., *7:*105, 1978.
36. McElvenny, R.T., and Caldwell, G.D.: A new operation for correction of cavus foot. Clin. Orthop., *11:*85, 1958.
37. Mills, C.P.: The etiology and treatment oc claw foot. J. Bone Joint Surg., *6:*142, 1924.
38. Olmos, V.S.: The treatment of paralytic calcaneus. J. Bone Joint Surg., *28:*780, 1946.
39. Plowright, O.: Familial clawfoot with absent tendon-jerks and cerebral disease. Guy's Hosp. Rep., *8:*314, 1928.
40. Pyper, J.B.: The flexor-extensor transplant operation for claw toes. J. Bone Joint Surg. [Br.], *40:*428, 1958.
41. Rivera-Dominguez, M., Dibenedetto, M., Frisbie, J.H., and Rossier, A. B.: Pes cavus and claw toes deformity in patients with spinal cord injury and multiple sclerosis. Paraplegia, *16:*375, 1979.
42. Royle, N.D.: A new conception in the etiology of clawfoot and associated talipes equinus. J. Bone Joint Surg., *9:*465, 1927.
43. Rubacky, G.E.: Claw toes: An early sign of lumbar diskogenic disease. J.A.M.A., *214:*375, 1970.
44. Rugh, J.T.: An operation for the correction of plantar and adduction contraction of the foot arch. J. Bone Joint Surg., *6:*664, 1924.
45. Rugh, J.T.: The etiology of cavus and a new operation for its correction. Bull. N.Y. Acad. Med., *3:*423, 1927.
46. Sandeman, J.C.: The role of soft tissue correction of claw toes. J. Clin. Pract., *21:*489, 1967.
47. Saunders, J.T.: Etiology and treatment of clawfoot. Arch. Surg., *30:*179, 1935.

48. Scheer, G.E., and Crego, Jr., C.H.: A two-stage sta-
    bilization procedure for correction of calcaneocavus.
    J. Bone Joint Surg. [Am.], *38:*1247, 1956.
49. Schmier, A.A.: Spastic calcaneocavus foot deformity.
    Am. J. Surg., *68:*116, 1945.
50. Schnepp, K.H.: Hammer toe and clawfoot. Am. J.
    Surg., *36:*351, 1937.
51. Sherman, H.M.: The operative treatment of pes ca-
    vus. Am. J. Orthop. Surg., *2:*374, 1905.
52. Siffert, R.J., Forster, R.I., and Nachamie, B.: "Beak"
    triple arthrodesis for correction of severe cavus de-
    formity. Clin. Orthop., *45:*101, 1966.
53. Smith, A.D., and Von Lackum, H.L.: End results of
    operations for claw foot. J.A.M.A., *85:*499, 1925.
54. Spitzy, H.: Operative correction of claw-foot. Surg.
    Gynecol. Obstet., *65:*813, 1927.
55. Steindler, A.: Operative treatment of pes cavus. Surg.
    Gynecol. Obstet., *24:*612, 1917.
56. Steindler, A.: The treatment of pes cavus (hollow claw
    foot). Arch. Sugr., *2:*325, 1921.
57. Stuart, F.W.: Clawfoot—its treatment. J. Bone Joint
    Surg., *6:*360, 1924.
58. Swanson, A.B., Browne, H.S., and Coleman, J.D.:
    The cavus foot—concepts of production and treat-
    ment by metatarsal osteotomy. J. Bone Joint Surg.
    [Am.], *48:*1016, 1966.
59. Symonds, C.P., and Shaw, M.D.: Familiar claw-foot
    with absent tendon jerks. Brain, *49:*387, 1926.
60. Taylor, R.G.: An operative procedure for the treat-
    ment of hammer toe and claw toe. J. Bone Joint Surg.,
    *22:*608, 1940.
61. Taylor, R.G.: The treatment of claw toes by multiple
    transfers of flexor into extensor tendons. J. Bone Joint
    Surg. [Br.], *33:*539, 1951.
62. Thomas, W.: On the treatment of talipes cavus. Bir-
    mingham Med. Rev., *34:*1, 1893.
63. Todd, A.H.: The treatment of pes cavus. Proc. R. Soc.
    Lond. [Med.], *28:*117, 1934.
64. Tyler, J.H., and Sutherland, J.M.: The primary spino-
    cerebellar atrophies and their associated defects, with
    a study of the foot deformity. Brain, *84:*289, 1961.
65. Wang, G.J., and Shaffer, L.W.: Osteotomy of the
    metatarsal for pes cavus. South. Med. J., *70:*77, 1977.
66. Weseley, M.S., and Barenfeld, P.A.: Calcaneal os-
    teotomy for the treatment of cavus deformity. Bull.
    Hosp. Joint Dis., Orthop. Inst., *31:*93, 1970.
67. Whitman, R.: The operative treatment of paralytic
    talipes of the calcaneus type. AM. J. Med. Sci.,
    *122:*593, 1901.
68. Young, C.S.: An operation for the correction of ham-
    mertoe and claw toe. J. Bone Joint Surg., *20:*715,
    1938.

CURLY TOE

Incidence

Curly toe (also known as curled, curling, varus, or underlapping toe) is a relatively common deformity of the lesser toes. The condition can involve one or more lesser toes and can present itself in unilateral, bilateral, congenital, and acquired forms. The typical clinical presentation however, includes bilateral and symmetric involvement, high familial incidence, tendency for the deformity to become more exaggerated with growth, and predilection for the third toes. The typical deformities of a curly toe consist of flexion and medial deviation at the DIP joint and lateral rotation along its longitudinal axis with its toenail pointing laterally. The congenital form of curly toe is present at birth and is often flexible; later the deformity becomes fixed and in severe cases, the proximal interphalangeal joint can also be involved. It has been postulated that congenital curly toe is caused by hypoplasia of the intrinsic muscles of the affected toes. As time goes on, the flexion and supination deformity of the curly toe gradually brings the distal portion of the toe to lie under the adjacent medial toe. When the curly toe has established itself well under the adjacent medial toe, it causes the adjacent toe to develop a painful callosity under its metatarsal head because the underlying toe prevents the adjacent toe from performing its normal weight-bearing function, resulting in hyperextension and dorsal subluxation of the M-P joint of the adjacent toe and increased weight-bearing pressure on its plantarly dropped metatarsal head.

Clinical Symptoms and Signs

Curly toes are usually completely asymptomatic in young children, but can cause disabling discomfort in adolescent and adult life, particularly in women who wear high-heeled, narrow, and pointed shoes. The varus and external rotation deformity of a curly toe causes it to impinge upon its adjacent medial toe and can produce painful interdigital corns. In addition, a curly toe can cause its adjacent medial toe to become a hammer toe, which is characterized by hyperextension and subluxation or even dislocation of the M-P joint in association with a painful plantar callosity under its metatarsal head, and flexion deformity of the PIP joint with a painful corn on its dorsal aspect, frequently accompanied by an adventitious bursa under the cornified skin. In severe cases of curly toe, when the proximal interphalangeal joint is also involved by the flexion and external rotation deformity, a painful corn can also develop on the lateral plantar aspect of the tip of the curly toe due to concentration of weight-bearing pressure.

Roentgenographic Manifestations

The typical, abnormal radiologic findings of a curly toe include flexion and varus and external rotation deformities of the DIP joint, which result in convergence of the phalanges of the curly toe toward those of the adjacent medial toe with the shadow of the toenail facing laterally; in severe cases, the curly toe is overlapped by its adjacent medial toe. When the curly toe has caused its adjacent medial toe to become a hammer toe, the typical deformities of a hammer toe are usually apparent on a standing lateral view of the foot.

Pathologic Anatomy

In a curly toe, flexion contracture of the DIP joint is accompanied by contracture of its plantar joint capsule, collateral ligaments, and flexor digitorum longus. In severe cases, the PIP joint can also have the same soft tissue contracture. When a curly toe has caused its adjacent medial toe to become a hammer toe, the hyperextension of the M-P joint is accompanied by contracture of the dorsal joint capsule, collateral ligaments, extensor digitorum longus, and interosseous muscles; the hyperflexion of the DIP joint is associated with contracture of the plantar joint capsule, collateral ligaments, and flexor digitorum longus.

Nonsurgical Treatment

A. Shoe modifications: roomy, extra-depth, and space shoes, metatarsal pads and bars, rocker-bottom soles, total contact soft

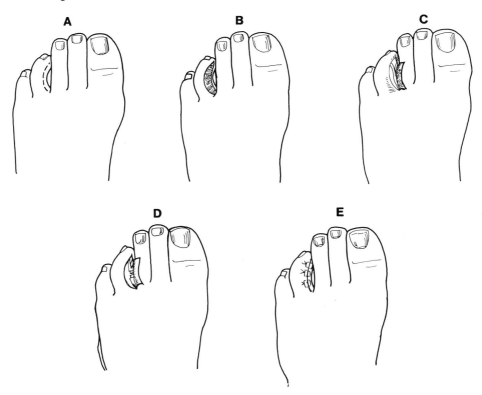

Figure 3–19. Tenotomy of the flexor digitorum longus and brevis. **A,** make a longitudinal midlateral incision on the medial aspect of the fourth toe. **B,** longitudinally incise the digital sheath. **C,** by retracting the incised digital sheath sideways, the flexor tendons are visualized. **D,** cut both the flexor digitorum longus and brevis tendons. **E,** close the skin in a regular manner.

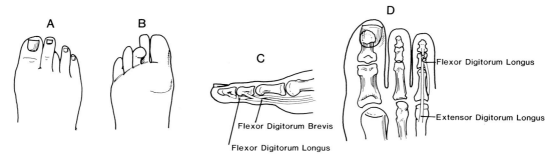

Figure 3–20. Transfer of the flexor digitorum longus to the dorsolateral aspect of the extensor hood. **A** and **B,** dorsal and plantar views of a curly third toe show its underlapping position under the second toe. **C,** cut the flexor digitorum longus tendon near its insertion through a midlateral skin incision. **D,** bring the severed flexor digitorum longus tendon around the lateral aspect of the toe and suture it to the dorsolateral aspect of the extensor hood.

arch supports, and stretching of the shoe's upper with a shoemaker's swan are helpful measures in relieving painful curly toe and its associated adjacent hammer toe (Figures 1–4—1–7, 1–12).

B. Padding of the foot and the shoe: soft pads applied directly to the painful areas of the curly toe and its associated hammer toe or to the insole of the shoe can all render pain relief to the associated corns and callosity (Figures 1–8—1–10).

C. Commercially available foot aids: corn and callosity pads, an arch cuff, a hammer toe shield, a toe crest, toe caps, a hammer toe shield with callosity cushion, and toe separators can be used to relieve the painful corns and callosities (Figures 1–16—1–19).

Surgical Treatment

The most important factor that determines what surgical procedure should be used usually depends on whether the DIP joint of the toe is still supple and flexible or has become fixed in flexion. A list of the various surgical procedures used in treating curly toes follows.

A. A curly toe with a supple and flexible DIP joint.
1. Tenotomy of the flexor digitorum longus and brevis (Figure 3–19).

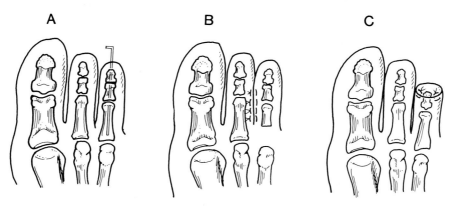

Figure 3–21. Various surgical treatments for curly toes with a fixed flexion contracture of the DIP joint. **A,** fusion of the DIP joint with a small smooth K-wire after the articular surfaces of the DIP joint have been resected. **B,** resection of the proximal portion of the proximal phalanx of the third toe and syndactylization of the second and third toes. **C,** Syme's terminal amputation through the DIP joint by removing the nail and its matrix and the underlying distal phalanx.

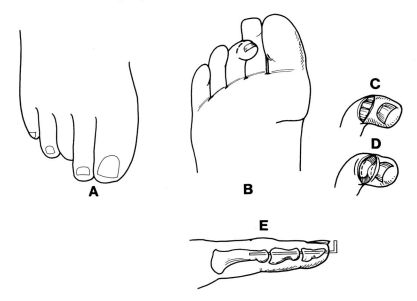

Figure 3–22. Fusion of the PIP joint for the treatment of a fixed curly toe. **A** and **B,** dorsal and plantar views of a foot with a curly third toe. **C,** make a transverse skin incision over the dorsal aspect of the DIP joint and cut the extensor digitorum longus tendon at the same level. **D,** resect the joint surfaces of the DIP joint with a small microsaw blade. **E,** fix the DIP joint in a neutral position with a small smooth K-wire.

2. Tenotomy of the flexor digitorum longus near its insertion and its transfer to the dorsal and lateral aspect of the extensor hood, especially in children with

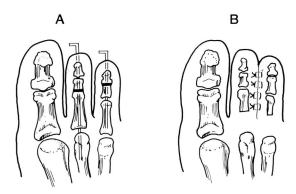

Figure 3–23. Treatment of a fixed curly toe in association with an adjacent hammer toe. **A,** fusion of the PIP joint, Z-plasty lengthening of the extensor digitorum longus tendon, dorsal M-P joint capsulotomy, and fixation of the M-P joint in a neutral position with a small smooth K-wire of the hammer toe, plus fusion of the DIP joint of the curly toe with a similar K-wire. **B,** resection of the proximal portions of the two adjacent proximal phalanges and syndactylization of the neighboring hammer toe and curly toe.

mild or moderate deformity (Figure 3–20.

B. A curly toe with a fixed flexion contracture of its DIP joint.
   1. In the absence of an associated hammer toe deformity of its adjacent medial toe (Figures 3–21 and 3–22).
      a. Fusion of the DIP joint of the curly toe (Figures 3–21A and 3–22).
      b. Proximal hemiphalangectomy of the proximal phalanx of the curly toe and syndactylization of the curly toe to its adjacent normal toe (Figure 3–21B).
      c. Syme's terminal amputation through the DIP joint for elderly patients (Figure 3–21C).
   2. In the presence of an associated hammer toe deformity of its adjacent medial toe (Figure 3–23).
      a. Fusion of PIP joint, Z-plasty lengthening of the extensor digitorum longus tendon, dorsal M-P joint capsulotomy, and fixation of the M-P

joint in a neutral position with a small smooth K-wire of the hammer toe plus fusion of the DIP joint of the curly toe with a similar K-wire (Figure 3–23A).

    b. Proximal hemiphalangectomies of the proximal phalanges of the neighboring hammer toe and curly toe, and syndactylization of the same two toes (Figure 3–23B).

REFERENCES

1. Lovell, W.W., and Winter, R.B.: Pediatric Orthopaedics. Philadelphia, J.B. Lippincott, 1978, pp. 980–981.
2. Polard, J.P., and Morrison, P.J.M.: Flexor tenotomy in the treatment of curly toes. Proc. R. Soc. Lond. [Med.], *68*:486, 1975.
3. Sharrard, W.J.W.: The surgery of deformed toes in children. Br. J. Clin. Pract., *17*:263, 1963.
4. Sweetnam, R.: Congenital curly toes. An investigation into the value of treatment. Lancet, *2*:398, 1958.
5. Taylor, R.G.: the treatment of claw toes by multiple transfers of flexor with extensor tendons. J. Bone Joint Surg. [Br.], *33*:539, 1951.
6. Watson, H.K., and Boyes, J.H.: Congenital angular deformities of the digits. J. Bone Joint Surg. [Am.], *49*:333, 1967.

MALLET TOE

Incidence

A mallet toe is characterized by flexion deformity of the DIP joint without any rotational deformity; usually one or more lesser toes are involved. The condition shows a definite predilection for shoe-wearing people, and occurs most often in the second toe, which is usually the longest digit. Although the majority of mallet toes are acquired, a congenital form does exist. A list of the different etiologic factors that cause a mallet toe follows.

A. Improperly fitted shoes: short and narrow shoes force the longest toes (usually the second toes) to become flexed at the DIP joint.

B. Traumatic rupture of the extensor digitorum longus near its insertion at the base of the distal phalanx: allows the unopposed flexor digitorum longus to pull the distal phalanx into flexion to produce a mallet toe.

C. Fusion of the PIP joint in the treatment of hammer toe: materially lengthens the toe and subjects it to the deforming force of a short and narrow shoe, resulting in flexion deformity of the DIP joint and resultant mallet toe.

D. Rheumatoid arthritis, Sudeck's atrophy, and immersion foot, can produce one or more mallet toes.

E. Congenital failure to develop the intrinsic extensor mechanism for the distal interphalangeal joint: results in a congenital mallet toe.

Clinical Symptoms and Signs

Congenital mallet toe is usually flexible and completely asymptomatic in young children. Fixed flexion contracture gradually develops in the DIP joint of both congenital and acquired mallet toes, however. A painful corn appears on the tip of the mallet toe close to the nail (an end corn) and is often accompanied by nail deformity, such as an ingrown toenail with or without infection, and by another corn on the dorsal aspect of the DIP joint (Figure 3–24). Active and passive extension of the DIP joint is usually significantly restricted. During barefoot walking, the tip of the mallet toe can be observed firmly pressing on the ground. When arthritic changes have developed in the deformed DIP joint, pain, tenderness, swelling, and osteophyte formation can be clinical findings.

Roentgenographic Manifestations

The anteroposterior view of a mallet toe often shows that it is shorter than its neighboring toes due to the 90° flexion contracture at the DIP joint. The distal phalanx is frequently overshadowed by the middle phalanx of the same toe. The lateral view of a mallet toe usually shows marked plantar angulation of the distal phalanx at its DIP joint, with the

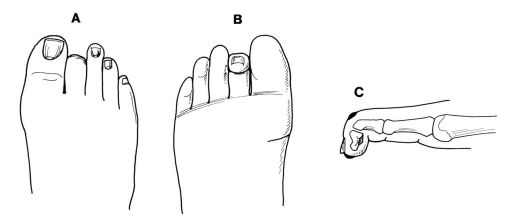

Figure 3–24. Dorsal, plantar, and lateral views of a mallet toe involving the second toe. Acute flexion contracture of the DIP joint in association with a painful corn on the dorsal aspect of the DIP joint and the tip of the same toe.

distal phalanx commonly making a 90° angle with the longitudinal axis of the middle and proximal phalanges. When degenerative arthritis has occurred in the DIP joint, joint narrowing and irregularity, subchondral osteosclerosis, and osteophyte formation at the joint margin may be present.

Pathologic Anatomy

The flexion contracture of the DIP joint of a mallet toe is usually accompanied by contracture of its plantar joint capsule, collateral ligaments, and flexor digitorum longus. When arthritis has developed in the DIP joint, degeneration of the articular cartilage, synovial proliferation, joint effusion, and para-articular soft tissue fibrosis may be present. In addition, the corn at the tip of a mallet toe tends to cause local atrophy of its underlying fat pad, and an adventitious bursa is frequently interposed between the cornified skin on the dorsal aspect of the DIP joint and the DIP joint itself. A defective intrinsic extensor mechanism for the distal interphalangeal joint may also be found in congenital mallet toe.

Nonsurgical Treatment

A. Shoe modifications: shoes with roomy toe boxes and soft shoe inserts can provide pain relief for the dorsal and plantar corns of mallet toe (Figures 1–6 and 1–7).

B. Padding of the foot and the shoe: soft pads applied directly to the painful corns or to the insole of a shoe to cushion the end corn of a mallet toe are helpful in giving symptomatic relief (Figures 1–8—1–10). Paring of the painful corns of mallet toe can also help.

C. Commercially available foot aids: corn pads, soft toe caps, and hammer toe shields can render symptomatic relief (Figures 1–16 and 1–18).

Surgical Treatment

A. Acute traumatic rupture of the extensor digitorum longus: surgical repair of the ruptured tendon.

B. A still flexible and supple DIP joint:
   1. Tenotomy of the flexor digitorum longus near its insertion (Figure 3–25A).
   2. Splitting of the flexor digitorum longus into two strips and passing them around the two sides of the mallet toe to be sutured to the top of the proximal phalanx (Figure 3–25B).

C. Fixed flexion contracture of the DIP joint:
   1. Fusion of the DIP joint through a transverse dorsal skin incision over the DIP

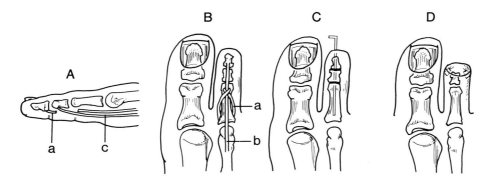

a – Flexor Digitorum Longus

b – Extensor Digitorum Longus

c – Flexor Digitorum Brevis

Figure 3–25. Various surgical treatments for a mallet toe. **A,** tenotomy of the flexor digitorum longus near its insertion. **B,** splitting of the flexor digitorum longus tendon into two equal strips and passing them around both sides of the mallet toe to be sutured to the top of the proximal phalanx. **C,** fusion of the DIP joint through a transverse dorsal skin incision over the DIP joint with a small smooth K-wire. **D,** Syme's terminal amputation through the DIP joint by removing the nail, its matrix, and the underlying distal phalanx.

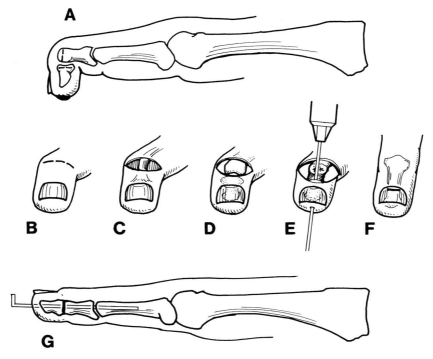

Figure 3–26. Fusion of the DIP joint for treatment of a fixed mallet toe. **A,** lateral view of a mallet toe. Amount of bone to be removed from the DIP joint in preparation for DIP joint fusion. **B,** transverse dorsal incision over the DIP joint. **C,** tenotomy of the extensor digitorum longus tendon at the level of the DIP joint. **D** and **E,** resection of the articular surfaces of the DIP joint with a small microsaw blade. **F** and **G,** completion of the DIP fusion by keeping the raw bone surfaces in intimate contact and driving a small and smooth K-wire through the center of all three phalanges.

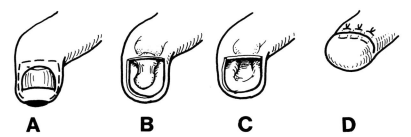

A   **B**   **C**   **D**

Figure 3–27. Syme's terminal amputation. **A,** skin incision completely surrounds the nail and its matrix. **B,** completely excise the nail and its matrix. **C,** perform a distal phalangectomy by cutting the dorsal and plantar joint capsules and collateral ligaments of the DIP joint, and severing the flexor and extensor digitorum longus tendons near the DIP joint. **D,** approximate the skin flap to the proximal incision site.

joint with a small smooth K-wire (Figures 3–25C and 3–26).

2. Syme's terminal amputation through the DIP joint in elderly patients (Figures 3–25D and 3–27).

REFERENCES

1. Brahm, M.A.: Common foot problems. J. Bone Joint Surg. [Am.], *49:*1653, 1967.
2. Buggiani, F.P., and Biggs, E.: Mallet toe. J. Am. Podiatry Assoc., *66:*321, 1976.
3. Edmonson, A.S., and Crenshaw, A.H. (eds.): Campbell's Operative Orthopaedics. 6th Ed. St. Louis, C.V. Mosby, 1980, pp. 1736–1737.
4. Inman, V.T. (ed.): DuVries' Surgery of The Foot. 3rd Ed. St. Louis, C. V. Mosby, 1973, pp. 241–249.
5. Lovell, W.W., and Winter, R.B.: Pediatric Orthopaedics. Philadelphia, J. B. Lippincott, 1978, p. 981.
6. Sharrard, W.J.W.: The surgery of deformed toes in children. Br. J. Clin. Pract., *17:*263, 1963.
7. Tachdjian, M.O.: Pediatric Orthopedics. Philadelphia, W.B. Saunders, 1972, pp. 1415.

OVERLAPPING TOE

Incidence

Overlapping toe usually involves the second and the fifth toes. The overlapping second toe is frequently acquired and is often associated with hallux valgus; the overlapping fifth toe is usually congenital, and is discussed in detail in Chapter 4. Rarely, the third or the fourth toe can also become an overlapping toe. A list of the various etiologic factors that are directly or indirectly responsible for the pathogenesis of overlapping toes follows.

A. Genetic factor: may play a role in producing congenital overlapping fifth toe.

B. Wearing high-heeled, narrow, and pointed shoes over a long time: tends to produce hallux valgus, which is frequently associated with an overlapping second toe.

C. Improper operation of the second toe: allows the iatrogenically induced unstable second toe to become dorsally subluxed or dislocated at the M-P joint and to overlap the laterally deviated great toe.

D. Fracture and dislocation of the second toe.

E. Infections of the second toe.

F. Inflammatory diseases, such as rheumatoid arthritis, Still's disease, and ankylosing spondylitis, can cause the second toe to overlap the great toe.

G. Degenerative arthritis can cause the second toe to become dorsally dislocated at the M-P joint and to overlap the great toe.

H. Metabolic disease, such as gout, can cause overlapping toes.

I. Skin disease, psoriasis for example, can produce overlapping toes.

J. The spectrum of diseases that produce hallux valgus and hammer toes discussed in preceding chapters can also bring about overlapping toes.

Clinical Symptoms and Signs

Because an overlapping toe usually involves the second toe and is frequently associated with hallux valgus, a wide spectrum of symptoms and signs of hammer toe and hallux valgus can be present in various degrees. A list of the different possible deformities and symptoms of the deformed second and great toes follows.

A. Second toe: painful corn on the dorsal aspect of the PIP joint, painful callosity under the second metatarsal head, painful end corn at the tip of the toe, hyperextension of the M-P joint, hyperflexion of the PIP joint, marked reduction of active and passive flexion of the M-P joint and extension of the PIP joint, bulge on the toe box caused by the overlapping toe, and signs of infection or inflammation of the PIP joint region.

B. Great toe: lateral deviation and pronation, painful prominence on the dorsomedial aspect of the first metatarsal head in association with a fluid-filled bursa, painful corn on the medioplantar aspect of the base of the distal phalanx, and painful callosity under the medial sesamoid.

Roentgenographic Manifestations

The anteroposterior view of the foot shows that the phalanges of the second toe overlap those of the great toe. The other radiologic abnormalities of the second toe include hyperextension and subluxation or dislocation of the M-P joint and hyperflexion of the PIP joint. Similarly, the abnormal features of the great toe consist of lateral deviation at the M-P joint, medial prominence of the first metatarsal head (the bunion) in association with soft tissue swelling, internal rotation along its longitudinal axis with its toenail facing medially, lateral migration of the medial and lateral sesamoids with subluxation or dislocation of the corre-

sponding medial and lateral sesamoidometatarsal joints, and metatarsus primus varus frequently associated with an oblique first metatarsocuneiform articulation.

Pathologic Anatomy

When the second toe overlaps the great toe, the pathologic structural changes of the second toe include hyperextension and subluxation or dislocation of the M-P joint in association with contracture of the dorsal joint capsule, collateral ligaments, extensor digitorum longus, and interossei; atrophy of the plantar fat pad under the second metatarsal head; hyperflexion of the PIP joint with contracture of its plantar joint capsule, collateral ligaments, and flexor digitorum longus and brevis; and formation of an adventitious bursa between the dorsal aspect of the PIP joint and the overlying cornified skin. In addition, the associated hallux valgus deformity is usually accompanied by plantar migration and stretching of the abductor hallucis, the medial head of the flexor hallucis brevis, the medial joint capsule, and the collateral ligament of the M-P joint; dorsal migration and contracture of the adductor hallucis, the lateral head of the flexor hallucis brevis, and the lateral joint capsule and collateral ligament of the M-P joint; lateral subluxation or even frank dislocation of the medial and lateral sesamoidometatarsal joints with possible degenerative arthritis of these two joints; formation of a sagittal groove that separates the articular surface of the first metatarsal head from the medial bony prominence (the bunion) with an adventitious bursa over the bunion; and atrophy of the fat pad under the medioplantar aspect of the base of the distal phalanx of the great toe.

Nonsurgical Treatment

A. Shoe modifications: extra-depth, space, and bunion last shoes, shoes with their uppers stretched with a shoemaker's swan, arch supports, metatarsal bars and pads, and rocker-bottom soles can provide symptomatic relief for the painful overlapping toe and its associated hallux valgus (Figures 1–2, 1–4—1–7, 1–9, 1–10, 1–12, 1–13).

B. Padding of the foot and shoe: soft pads applied directly to the painful corns, callosities, and bunions or to the insoles to cushion the painful plantar callosities can give pain relief (Figures 1–8—1–10).

C. Commercially available foot aids: donut-shaped pads, arch cuffs, hammer toe shields, toe crests, hammer toe shields with callosity cushion, latex bunion shields, and bunion pads are helpful in relieving symptomatic overlapping toe and its associated bunion (Figures 1–16—1–19).

Surgical Treatment

Although various surgical procedures for treating hammer toe and hallux valgus can all be used in treating an overlapping toe and its associated hallux valgus deformity, I prefer the following combinations of surgical procedures:

A. When the M-P joint of the great toe is relatively free of arthritic changes: reduce the dorsally subluxed or dislocated M-P joint and fuse the PIP joint of the overlapping toe by means of a small smooth K-wire, which should pass through all three digital phalanges and the distal portion of the corresponding metatarsal. Perform a Mitchell's bunionectomy on the first metatarsal to correct the hallux valgus defor-

mity. This is the method of treatment I prefer (Figure 3–28). An alternative method is to perform a proximal hemiphalangectomy of the proximal phalanx and syndactylization of the second and third toe, followed by a Mitchell's bunionectomy of the great toe.

B. When the M-P joint of the great toe has developed a significant amount of arthritic changes, the following combinations of surgical procedures can be used:
1. Reduce the dorsally subluxed or dislocated M-P joint and fuse the PIP joint of the overlapping toe by using a small smooth K-wire, which should pass through all three digital phalanges and the distal portion of the second metatarsal. Then, excise the base of the proximal phalanx of the great toe and hold the great toe in a neutral position with another small smooth K-wire. The wire should be driven from the tip of the distal phalanx through the proximal phalanx into the distal portion of the first metatarsal (Figure 3–28D).
2. Perform a proximal hemiphalangectomy of the proximal phalanx of the second toe and sew it to the third toe. Fuse the M-P joint of the great toe in about 15 to 20° dorsiflexion and 10° valgus position (Figure 3–29).

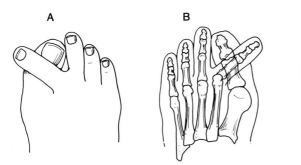
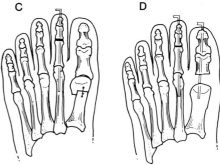

Figure 3–28. Various surgical procedures for the treatment of an overlapping second toe in association with a hallux valgus. **A,** severe overlapping second toe in association with a hallux valgus. **B,** overlapping of the phalanges of the second and great toes. **C,** fusion of the PIP joint and reduction of the subluxed or dislocated M-P joint of the second toe, plus a Mitchell's bunionectomy of the great toe. **D,** fusion of the PIP joint, reduction of the subluxed or dislocated M-P joint of the second toe with a K-wire through its M-P joint, and resection of the proximal portion of the proximal phalanx of the great toe.

A   B   C

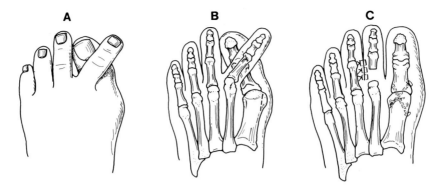

Figure 3–29. Alternative surgical procedures for correcting an overlapping second toe in association with a hallux valgus. **A** and **B**, overlapping second toe and its associated hallux valgus. **C**, excision of the proximal portion of the proximal phalanx of the second toe, syndactylization of the second and third toes, and fusion of the M-P joint of the great toe.

REFERENCES

Overlapping Toe

1. Borg, I.: Operation for hammer-toe. Acta Chir. Scand., *100:*619, 1950.
2. Cahill, B.R., and Connor, D.E.: A long-term follow-up on proximal phalangectomy for hammertoes. Clin. Orthop., *86:*191, 1972.
3. Ellis, T.S.: Hallux valgus and hammer toe. Lancet, *1:*1155, 1899.
4. Ely, I.W.: Hammertoe. Surg. Clin. North Am., *6:*133, 1926.
5. Glassmon, F., and Wolin, I.: Phalangectomy for toe deformities. Surg. Clin. North Am., *29:*275, 1949.
6. Haward, W.: Hammer-toe and hallux valgus and rigidus. Lancet, *2:*240, 1900.
7. Higgs, S.L.: "Hammer-toe." Postgrad. Med. J., *6:*130, 1931.
8. Lapidus, P.W.: Operation for correction of hammertoe. J. Bone Joint Surg., *21:*977, 1939.
9. McConnell, B.E.: Correction of hammer toe deformity, a 10 year review of subperiosteal waist resection of proximal phalanx. Orthop. Rev., *8:*65, 1979.
10. Merrill, W.J.: Conservative operative treatment of hammertoe. Am. J. Orthop. Surg., *10:*262, 1912.
11. Meznik, V.F.: On the technique of hammer-toe operation. Wien. Med. Wochenschr., *112:*108, 1962.
12. Michele, A.A., and Krueger, F.J.: Operative correction for hammertoe. Milit. Med., *103:*52, 1948.
13. Mladick, R.A.: Correction of hammertoe surgery deformity by Z-plasty and bone graft. Ann. Plast. Surg., *4:*224, 1980.
14. Newman, R.J., and Fitton, J.M.: An evaluation of operative procedures and the treatment of hammertoe. Acta Orthop. Scand., *50:*709, 1979.
15. O'Neil, J.: An arthroplastic operation for hammertoe. J.A.M.A., *57:*1207, 1911.
16. Scheck, M.: Degenerative changes in the metatarsophalangeal joints after surgical correction of severe hammer toe deformities. A complication associated with avascular necrosis in three cases. J. Bone Joint Surg. [Am.], *50:*727, 1968.
17. Scheck, M.: Etiology of acquired hammertoe deformity. Clin. Orthop., *123:*63, 1977.
18. Selig, S.: Hammertoe: A new procedure for its correction. Surg. Gynecol. Obstet., *72:*101, 1941.
19. Soule, R.E.: Operation for the cure of hammertoe. N.Y. State J. Med., *91:*649, 1910.
20. Taylor, R.G.: An operative procedure for the treatment of hammer toe and claw toe. J. Bone Joint Surg., *22:*608, 1940.
21. Trethowan, W.H.: The treatment of hammertoe. Lancet, *1:*1257, 1925.
22. Wee, G.C., and Tucker, G.L.: An improved procedure for the surgical correction of hammer toe. Mo. Med., *67:*43, 1970.
23. Young, C.S.: An operation for the correction of hammer toe and claw toe. J. Bone Joint Surg., *20:*715, 1938.
24. Zimmerman, E.: Hammer-toe operating experiences and successes. Beitr. Orthop. Traumatol., *13:*654, 1966.

SOFT AND HARD CORNS AND CALLOSITIES

Incidence

Corn (heloma or clavus) and callosity (tyloma) are areas of hyperkeratosis of the skin produced by excessive pressure from within (e.g., an osseous condyle) and without (e.g., the shoe). Although corn and callosity have virtually identical histologic findings, corn differs from callosity in its smaller size, a more localized painful site, predilection for the dorsal aspect of the toes, more pointed or prominent bony abnormality underlying a corn, and its bearing greater friction pressure or trauma. There are four basic types of corns:

A. Hard corn (heloma or clavus durum): calloused area of skin with a hard central core overlying a bony prominence or an arthritic joint of the toes. The most common site is the dorsolateral aspect of the head of the proximal phalanx of the fifth toe, which is constantly subjected to maximal pressure from the outer border of the shoe. The dorsal aspects of the PIP and DIP joints and the tips of the lesser toes are also common sites (Figure 3–30). Hard corns can be caused by numerous disorders of the foot, including hallux valgus, hallux rigidus, hallux flexus, hallux extensus, hammer toes, clawtoes, overlapping toes, curly toe, mallet toe, and many other systemic and localized diseases that produce foot deformities.

B. Soft corn (heloma molle, clavus molle, or interdigital corn): usually an area of trauma-induced hyperkeratosis in the interdigital spaces, especially the fourth webspace. Moisture and poor ventilation cause maceration and a whitish discoloration of these well-circumscribed soft corns that can be single or in a pair on the opposing surfaces of an interdigital space. Any condition that brings interdigital bony prominences into opposition can potentially produce soft corns. A list of the different causes of soft corns follows (Figure 3–31).

1. Hallux valgus, overlapping toes, curly toes, hammer toes, and mallet toes are capable of bringing bony prominences of the toes into opposition to produce soft corns.

2. Presence of a relatively short fifth metatarsal: enhances the opportunity of impingement between the medial aspect of the head of the fifth proximal phalanx and the lateral basal condyle

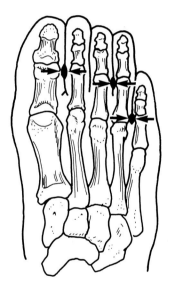

Figure 3–31. Different causes and sites of soft corns. 1. Relatively short fifth metatarsal brings the medial aspect of the head of the fifth proximal phalanx into opposition with the lateral aspect of the basal condyle of the fourth proximal phalanx to produce a soft corn in the fourth webspace; this is the most common site of soft corn. 2. Relatively short first metatarsal enhances the chances of impingement between the medial aspect of the proximal interphalangeal joint of the second toe and the lateral aspect of the interphalangeal joint of the great toe to produce a soft corn in the first interdigital space. 3. Equal length of the third and fourth metatarsals encourages the impingement between the lateral condyle of the head of the proximal phalanx of the third toe and the medial aspect of the proximal interphalangeal joint of the fourth toe to produce a soft corn in the third webspace.

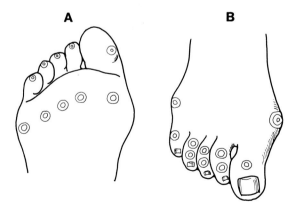

Figure 3–30. Various sites of hard corns and callosities on the forefoot. **A,** corns under the mediobasal portion of the distal phalanx of the great toe and at the tips of the four lesser toes; callosities under the medial sesamoid and the heads of the four lateral metatarsals. **B,** corns on the dorsal aspects of the interphalangeal joint of the great toe and the PIP and DIP joints of the lesser toes, and over the bunion and bunionette.

of the fourth proximal phalanx to produce a soft corn in the fourth webspace.

   3. Presence of a relatively short first
metatarsal: increases the chances of
impingement between the opposing
surfaces of the proximal interphalangeal joint of the second toe and the interphalangeal joint of the great toe to
produce a soft corn in the first interdigital space.

   4. Presence of equal length of the third
and fourth metatarsals: encourages the
impingement of the lateral condyle of
the head of the proximal phalanx of
the third toe on the medial aspect of
the proximal interphalangeal joint of the
fourth toe to produce a soft corn in the
third webspace.

C. Seed corns: multiple small corns of unknown etiology often found on the non-
weight-bearing areas of the soles of elderly persons.

D. Neurovascular corns: uncommon corns
found along the medial border of the interphalangeal joint of the great toe, under
the first and fifth metatarsals, and on the
dorsal aspect of hammer toes; there seems
to be a predilection for the feet of patients
affected by hallux rigidus. These neurovascular corns are vascular, exquisitely
tender, and tend to bleed profusely when
pared. It has been postulated that deeply
nucleated corns cause invagination of live
epithelium containing small nerve fibers and
blood vessels, which make them extremely sensitive and vascular. Electro-
cauterization is an effective method of
eliminating these painful and vascular
corns.

   Similarly, intractable plantar keratosis (callosity) can be produced by a wide variety of
etiologic factors (Figure 3–30A):

A. Varus or valgus tilt of the forefoot from
neuromuscular or other diseases: produces excessive weight-bearing pressure
on one or more areas of the forefoot, resulting in plantar callus formation.

B. Congenital or acquired bony abnormalities
such as an excessively long metatarsal,
excessive plantar flexion of a metatarsal,
hypertrophy and degeneration of the sesamoids, clawtoes, hammer toes, and malunited fractures of metatarsals: can produce concentrated pressure on a particular
plantar surface of the forefoot to produce
a plantar callosity.

C. High-heeled, narrow, and pointed shoes:
cause the great toe to go into a valgus position and the fifth toe into a varus position, accompanied by dorsal migration of
the first and fifth metatarsal heads. Excessive weight-bearing pressure on the
three central metatarsal heads results,
causing atrophy of their plantar fat pads
and formation of painful plantar callosities.

D. Puncture wounds and laceration or surgical scars on the weight-bearing portion
of the plantar surface: can produce intractable and painful plantar keratosis.

   It is of vital importance to differentiate a
plantar callus from a plantar verruca (wart),
because their treatments are quite different.
A list of the differences between plantar callus and plantar wart follows.

Plantar verruca (wart)	Plantar callus (callosity)
A. Can be proximal or distal to the meta-tarsal head, or any-where in the foot.	Usually under the metatarsal head.
B. Painful to lateral pressure and pinch.	Painful to direct pressure.
C. Irregular shape.	Conical shape.
D. Both solitary or cluster of lesions (mother and daugh-ter warts).	Usually one single lesion per each bony prominence.

E. Soft and papillary (wart-like) center.

F. Vascular (bleeding with curettage).

G. Virus is the etiologic agent.

H. Can affect both children and adults.

I. Usually responds to tissue destroying therapies such as electrical cauterization, liquid nitrogen, caustic chemicals, and irradiation.

J. Microscopic features of central hyperplasia of squamous epithelium surrounded by severe hyperkeratosis with elongated rete pegs that spread outward and upward toward the epithelial surface from its center in a

Hard and smooth center.

Avascular (no bleeding with curettage).

Bony prominence is the etiologic agent.

Primarily affects adults, particularly female adults.

Usually responds well to removal of the bony prominence.

Microscopic features of complete lack of blood vessels in the keratosis, indented epithelium in the center of the lesion, and some elongated rete pegs that extend downward into the corneum rather

wart-like fashion. Marked increase in vascularity throughout the central part of the lesion.

than upward toward the epithelial surface.

Clinical Symptoms and Signs

A soft corn is a painful, whitish, macerated, fairly circumscribed, and slightly raised area of skin, measuring 3 to 9 mm in its greatest diameter with a rubber-like texture that differs from skin lesions caused by dermatophytoses in its absence of itching and presence of considerable pain localized to the site of bony prominence. Soft corns can exist as single interdigital lesions or in pairs on the opposing surfaces of the webspaces. In contrast, a hard corn is a painful, pearly gray, hard, well-defined, and slightly raised skin lesion, measuring approximately 5 to 10 mm in its greatest diameter with a hard and conical central core; it usually appears on the exposed portion of the toes and over the bony prominences. In contrast, a plantar callosity is a painful, yellowish or pearly white, hard, well-circumscribed or ill-defined, and somewhat raised area of skin on the plantar surface of the foot, which measures about 1 to 1.5 cm in its greatest diameter with or without a hard central core. Plantar callosity is usually situated under the three central metatarsal heads.

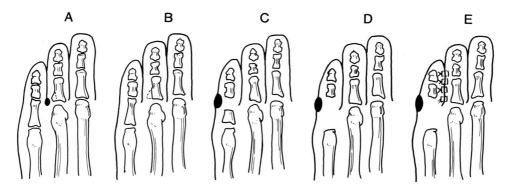

Figure 3–32. Various surgical procedures for the treatment of a soft corn in the fourth webspace. **A** and **B**, excision of the lateral basal condyle of the fourth proximal phalanx. **C**, excision of the head of the proximal phalanx of the fifth toe. **D**, proximal phalangectomy of the fifth toe. **E**, proximal phalangectomy of the fifth toe plus syndactylization of the fourth and fifth toes.

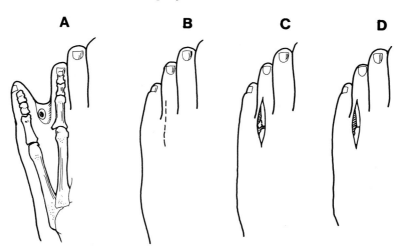

Figure 3–33. Surgical technique in the excision of the lateral basal condyle of the fourth proximal phalanx. **A,** soft corn in the fourth webspace. **B,** make a longitudinal dorsal skin incision over the lateral aspect of the M-P joint of the fourth toe. **C,** detach the lateral collateral ligament and joint capsule from the lateral base of the fourth proximal phalanx. **D,** remove the lateral basal condyle of the fourth proximal phalanx with a narrow microsaw blade. Close the skin in a regular manner.

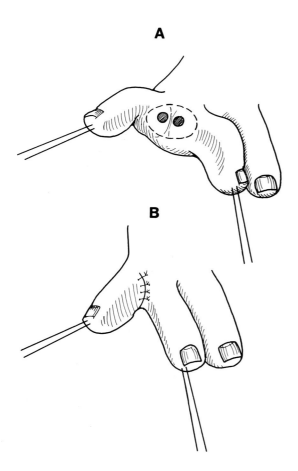

Roentgenographic Manifestations

Because corns and callosities are skin lesions, they are usually not demonstrable by routine radiographic examination, unless they are large enough to cast a superficial soft tissue shadow. The various deformities of the foot that cause these corns and calluses, however, are readily visible radiographically. To reconfirm a particular bony prominence that has produced either a corn or a callosity, a lead marker, such as the letter O, should be taped directly to the symptomatic corn or callosity. Appropriate radiographs should then be taken to identify positively the bony prominence responsible for the development of the painful corn or callosity.

Pathologic Anatomy

The typical histologic features of corns or callosity consist of hyperplasia of the epider-

Figure 3–34. Surgical treatment of two soft corns of the fourth webspace. **A,** dotted line, elliptical piece of skin containing the soft corns to be excised. **B,** approximate the two halves of the elliptical skin incision to create a syndactylization of the basal portion of the fourth and fifth toes.

A

B

C

D

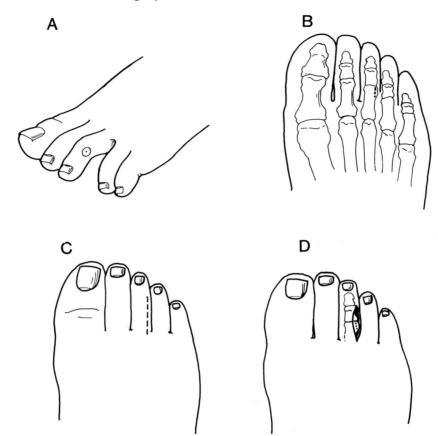

Figure 3–35. Surgical treatment of interdigital corns caused by prominent condyles of the PIP joints. **A,** painful interdigital corn over the lateral aspect of the PIP joint of the third toe. **B,** dotted line, portion of the lateral condyle of the head of the third proximal phalanx to be removed. **C,** longitudinal incision is placed on the dorsolateral aspect of the PIP joint of the third toe. **D,** expose the lateral condyle of the head of the third proximal phalanx by detaching its lateral collateral ligament and joint capsule; excise it with a narrow microsaw blade. Close skin in a regular manner.

mis, particularly the stratum corneum; an avascular center with no true blood vessels; hypertrophied and elongated rete pegs that extend down into the corneum; and deep invagination of keratinized tissue in association with atrophy of the normal plantar fat pad.

Nonsurgical Treatment

A. Shoe modifications: roomy, extra-depth, space, and bunion last shoes, stretching of the shoe uppers with a shoemaker's swan, metatarsal bars and pads, a rocker-bottom sole, and arch supports are the various means used to relieve painful corns and callosities (Figures 1–2, 1–4—1–7, 1–12).

B. Padding of the foot and shoe: soft pads of various sizes and shapes applied directly to the painful corns and callosities or to the insoles of shoes can provide symptomatic relief (Figures 1–8—1–10).

C. Commercially available foot aids: donut-shaped pads of different sizes, arch cuffs, hammer toe shields, a toe crest, toe caps, hammer toe shields with callosity cushion, and toe separators are useful aids in relieving pain (Figures 1–16—1–19).

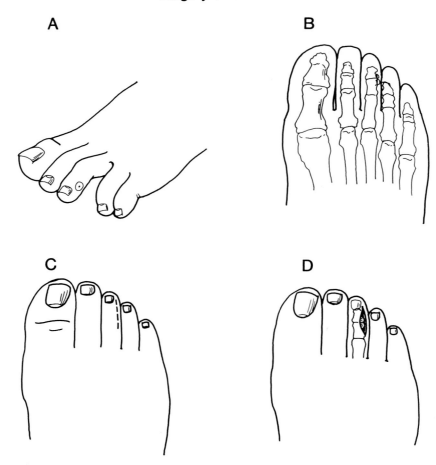

Figure 3–36. Surgical treatment of interdigital corns caused by prominent condyles of the DIP joints. **A,** painful interdigital corn over the lateral aspect of the DIP joint of the third toe. **B,** dotted line, amount of bone to be excised from the lateral aspect of the DIP joint. **C,** make a longitudinal incision over the dorsolateral aspect of the DIP joint of the third toe. **D,** expose the lateral aspect of the DIP joint by detaching its lateral collateral ligament and joint capsule. Remove the lateral condyles of the DIP joint with a narrow microsaw blade. Close the skin in a regular manner.

Surgical Treatment

The surgical treatments of the corns and callosities associated with the many deformities of the great toe and the lesser toes have been or will be discussed in detail. Only surgical treatment of interdigital corns and plantar callosities are discussed in this chapter.

A. Surgical treatment of interdigital corns (Figures 3–32—3–36).
   1. When the soft corn is in its most common and typical location, the fourth webspace.
      a. Excision of the lateral base of the proximal phalanx of the fourth toe: the author's preferred method of treating soft corn of the fourth interdigital space, provided no painful corn is over the dorsolateral aspect of the PIP joint of the fifth toe (Figures 3–32B and 3–33).
      b. Excision of the head of the proximal phalanx of the fifth toe: can take care of both soft corn of the fourth webspace and hard corn over the dorsolateral aspect of the fifth toe (Figure 3–32C).
      c. Proximal phalangectomy of the fifth

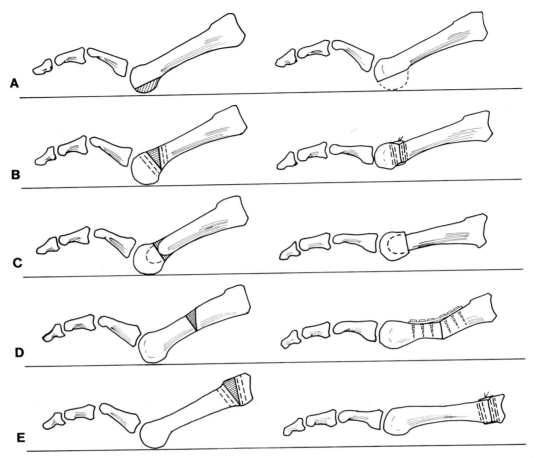

Figure 3-37. Different surgical procedures for the treatment of painful and intractable plantar callosities. **A,** plantar condylectomy of the offending metatarsal head. **B,** closing-wedge dorsal angulation osteotomy through the metatarsal neck, holding the osteotomy site together with two strong sutures through two drilled holes. **C,** shortening and telescoping the metatarsal neck into the metatarsal head. **D,** closing-wedge dorsal angulation osteotomy of the metatarsal shaft and fixation of the osteotomy site with a mini-bone plate. **E,** closing-wedge dorsal angulation osteotomy at the basal portion of the metatarsal, holding the osteotomy site together with two stout sutures through two drilled holes.

toe: takes care of both the soft corn of the fourth webspace and the hard corn over the dorsolateral aspect of the fifth toe, but it also creates a frail fifth toe that will become significantly shortened with time (Figure 3-32D).

d. Proximal phalangectomy of the fifth toe plus syndactylization of the fourth and fifth toes: cures the soft corn of the fourth webspace and the hard corn on the dorsolateral aspect of the fifth toe, and also maintains the length and stability of the fifth toe (Figure 3-32E). Syndactylization of the proximal portion of the fourth webspace can also cure soft corn (Figure 3-34).

2. When the interdigital corn is caused by prominent condyles of the PIP and DIP joints: excise the offending bony condyles (Figures 3-35 and 3-36).

B. Surgical treatment of painful and intractable plantar callosities (Figures 3-37 and 3-38).

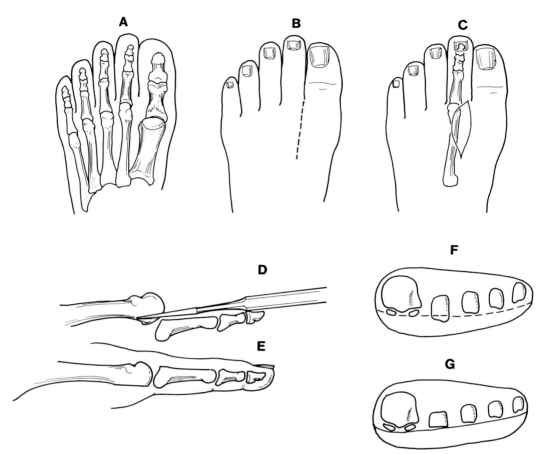

Figure 3–38. Surgical technique for plantar condylectomy of the metatarsal head. **A** and **B,** make a longitudinal skin incision over the dorsal aspect of the M-P joint of the second toe. **C,** expose the M-P joint by cutting the medial collateral ligament and medial and dorsal joint capsules. **D,** dorsally dislocate the metatarsal head and remove its offending condyle with a short, sharp osteotome. **E,** reduce the dislocated M-P joint and approximate the cut collateral ligament and joint capsules. **F** and **G,** relative positions of the second metatarsal head preoperatively and postoperatively. Plantar condylectomy has realigned the second metatarsal head with all the other metatarsal heads and has removed the concentrated weight-bearing pressure from the second metatarsal head.

1. Plantar condylectomy of the metatarsal head: easiest procedure to perform and is the method I prefer for treating intractable plantar callosity (Figures 3–37A and 3–38).
2. Dorsal angulation osteotomy of the metatarsal head with a dorsally based wedge at the metatarsal neck: may cause a stiff and cock-up deformity of the M-P joint (Figure 3–37B).
3. Shortening of the metatarsal by telescoping the metatarsal neck into the metatarsal head: may produce a stiff

and deformed M-P joint (Figure 3–37C).
4. Dorsal angulation osteotomy of the distal portion of the metatarsal through its shaft portion and fixation of the osteotomy site with a mini-bone plate: may have non-union of the osteotomy site and may need removal of the plate and screws after the osteotomy is well healed (Figure 3–37D).
5. Dorsal angulation osteotomy by taking out a dorsal wedge near the basal portion of the metatarsal: a more difficult surgical procedure to perform, espe-

cially when the second metatarsal base is involved due to its deeply and firmly held position in the three cuneiform bones (Figure 3–37E).

REFERENCES

Soft and Hard Corns and Callosities

1. Avellan, L., and Johanson, B.: Hyperkeratosis of scars in the weight-bearing areas of the foot. Acta Chir. Scand., *131:*269, 1966.
2. Durlacher, L.: A Treatise on Corns, Bunions, Disease of the Nails and the General Management of the Feet. London, Simkin, Marshall & Co., 1845.
3. Galland, W.I.: An operative treatment for corns. J.A.M.A., *100:*880, 1933.
4. Giannestras, N.J.: Shortening of the metatarsal shaft for the correction of plantar keratosis. Clin. Orthop., *4:*225, 1954.
5. Giannestras, N.J.: Shortening of the metatarsal shaft in the treatment of plantar keratosis: An end-result study. J. Bone Joint Surg. [Am.], *40:*61, 1958.
6. Giannestras, N.J.: Plantar keratosis, treatment by metatarsal shortening: Operative technique and end-result study. J. Bone Joint Surg. [Am.], *48:*72, 1966.
7. Gibbs, R.C.: Calluses, corns and warts. Am. Fam. Physician, *3:*92, 1971.
8. Gillett, H.G.D.: Incidence of interdigital clavus. A note on its location. J. Bone Joint Surg. [Br.], *56:*753, 1974.
9. Gillett, H.G.D.: Interdigital clavus: Predisposition is the key factor of soft corns. Clin. Orthop., *142:*103, 1979.
10. Kiehn, C.L., Earle, A.S., and Desprez, J.D.: Treatment of the chronic, painful metatarsal callus by a tendon transfer. Plast. Reconstr. Surg., *51:*154, 1973.
11. Lapidus, P.W.: Soft corns and their etiology and operative treatment. Med. Rec., *146:*61, 1937.
12. Lapidus, P.W.: Orthopaedic skin lesions of the soles and toes—calluses, corns, plantar warts, keratomas, neurovascular growths, onychomas. Clin. Orthop., *45:*87, 1966.
13. Macey, H.B.: The etiology and treatment of soft corns. Mayo Clin. Proc., *15:*549, 1940.
14. Mann, R.A., and DuVries, H.L.: Intractable plantar keratosis. Orthop. Clin. North Am., *41:*67, 1973.
15. McElvenny, R.T.: Corns—their etiology and treatment. Am. J. Surg., *50:*761, 1940.
16. Meltzer, L.: Surgical correction of intertriginous soft corns. J. Dermatol. Surg., *2:*135, 1976.
17. Rutledge, B.A., and Green, A.L.: Surgical treatment of plantar corns. U.S. Armed Forces Med. J., *8:*219, 1957.
18. Strach, E.H., and Cornah, M.S.: Syndactylopoiesis: A simple operation for interdigital soft corn. J. Bone Joint Surg. [Br.], *54:*530, 1972.
19. Strode, J.E.: A satisfactory operation for interdigital soft corns (clavus molle). Am. J. Surg., *119:*353, 1970.
20. Whitfield, A.: On development of callosities, corns and warts. Br. J. Dermatol., *44:*580, 1932.
21. Wolf, M.D.: Metatarsal osteotomy for the relief of painful metatarsal callosities. J. Bone Joint Surg. [Am.], *55:*1760, 1973.

4 SURGERY OF THE FIFTH TOE

CURLY FIFTH TOE ASSOCIATED WITH A PAINFUL CORN NEXT TO THE DISTAL AND LATERAL BORDER OF THE NAIL

Incidence

A curly fifth toe is a relatively common toe deformity and has a predilection for bilateral involvement and fashion-minded females whose high-heeled, narrow, and pointed shoes can sometimes force the fifth toes to undergo external rotation, flexion contracture of the DIP joints, and medial migration toward the undersurface of the fourth toes. Like the acquired curly fifth toes, the congenital curly fifth toes are usually bilateral and are often completely asymptomatic during childhood, becoming symptomatic during adult life when painful corns develop at the distal and lateral borders of the toenails of the fifth toes.

Clinical Symptoms and Signs

The most common complaint of patients with curly fifth toes concerns the painful corns near the lateral and distal border of the toenails of their fifth toes. In addition to these painful corns, examination often reveals external rotation of the fifth toe along its longitudinal axis, with its nail laterally and plantarly displaced; flexion contracture of the DIP joint with re-

striction of both active and passive dorsiflexion of the DIP joint; and displacement of the fifth toe to the undersurface of the fourth toe, which can also produce interdigital corns between the fourth and fifth toes. When the curly fifth toe has been present for a long time, flexion contracture of the PIP joint can also develop in the same toe; a painful corn can also appear on the dorsolateral aspect of its PIP joint.

Roentgenographic Manifestations

The radiologic abnormalities of a curly fifth toe include flexion deformity of the DIP joint, approximation of its terminal phalanx to those of the fourth toe, lateral displacement of the nail shadow, and overlapping of the phalanges of the fourth and fifth toes. Flexion deformity of the PIP joint may be seen in severe cases.

Pathologic Anatomy

Flexion deformity of the DIP joint of a curly fifth toe is accompanied by flexion contracture of its plantar joint capsule, collateral ligaments, and flexor digitorum longus. The painful corn on the lateral tip of the fifth toe often produces atrophy of the underlying fat pad. When flexion contracture also involves the PIP joint, its plantar joint capsule and collateral ligament will also be contracted, and a painful corn with an underlying adventitious bursa is likely to be present on the dorsolateral aspect of the PIP joint.

Nonsurgical Treatment

A. Shoe modifications: roomy, extra-depth, and space shoes as well as soft total contact insoles are helpful in relieving pain associated with symptomatic curly fifth toes (Figures 1–6 and 1–7).

B. Padding of the foot and shoe: soft pads applied directly to the painful corns or to the insoles of shoes can render symptomatic relief (Figures 1–8—1–10).

C. Commercially available foot aids: donut-shaped pads, toe caps, toe separators, and adhesive-back foam strips are useful foot aids in providing symptomatic relief for painful curly fifth toes (Figures 1–16—1–19).

Surgical Treatment

A. When the curly fifth toe is associated with painful corn on the lateral tip of the fifth toe next to the nail (Figures 4–1 and 4–2):
   1. Syme's terminal amputation of the fifth toe (Figures 4-1A and 4–2).
   2. Fusion of the DIP joint of the fifth toe through a transverse dorsal incision over the DIP joint (Figure 4–1B).
   3. Middle phalangectomy of the fifth toe and taping the fourth and fifth toes together postoperatively for the correction to take place gradually with wound healing (Figure 4–1C).

B. When the curly fifth toe is associated with a painful corn on the lateral tip of the fifth toe and on the dorsolateral aspect of the contracted PIP joint of the same toe (Figure 4–3):
   1. Excision of the head of the fifth proximal phalanx (Figure 4–3A).

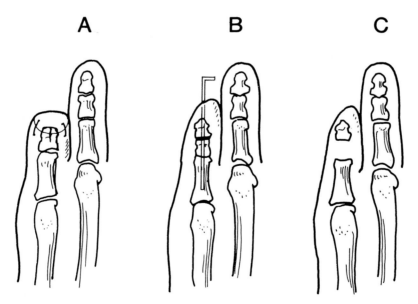

A   **B**   **C**

Figure 4–1. Surgical treatments for a curly fifth toe with a painful corn on its lateral tip next to the nail. **A,** Syme's terminal amputation by excising the nail, its matrix, and the underlying distal phalanx. **B,** fusion of the DIP joint through a transverse dorsal incision over the DIP joint by resecting the articular surfaces with a narrow microsaw blade. **C,** middle phalangectomy of the fifth toe.

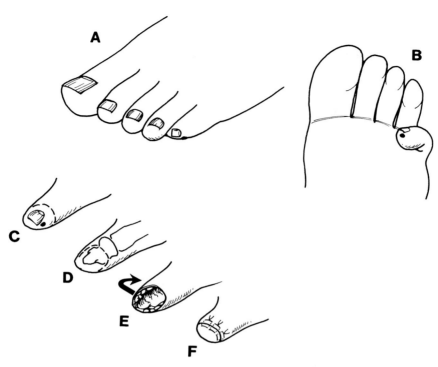

Figure 4–2. Syme's terminal amputation for the treatment of a curly fifth toe in association with a painful corn on its lateral tip. **A** and **B,** curly fifth toe with a painful corn on its lateral tip next to the nail. **C,** make a skin incision that completely surrounds the toenail and the painful corn. **D,** excise the nail, its matrix, and the painful corn. **E,** excise the distal phalanx by cutting the joint capsule and collateral ligament of the DIP joint and the flexor and extensor digitorum longus tendons near the DIP joint. **F,** close the resulting skin flap to the proximal skin incision site with horizontal mattress sutures.

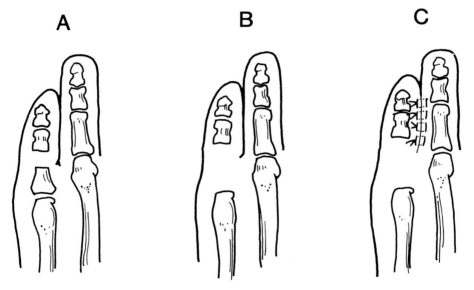

Figure 4–3. Surgical treatment of a curly fifth toe associated with a painful corn on its lateral tip and on the dorsolateral aspect of its contracted PIP joint. **A,** excision of the head of the fifth proximal phalanx. **B,** proximal phalangectomy of the fifth toe. **C,** proximal phalangectomy of the fifth toe plus syndactylization of the fourth and fifth toes.

2. Proximal phalangectomy of the fifth toe (Figure 4–3B).
3. Proximal phalangectomy of the fifth toe plus syndactylization of the fourth and fifth toes (Figure 4–3C).

REFERENCES

Curly Toe Associated with Corns

1. Lovell, W.W., and Winter, R.B.: Pediatric Orthopaedics. Philadelphia, J.B. Lippincott, 1978, pp. 980–981.
2. Polard, J.P., and Morrison, P.J.M.: Flexor tenotomy in the treatment of curly toes. Proc. R. Soc. Lond. [Med.], *68*:486, 1975.
3. Sharrard, W.J.W.: The surgery of deformed toes in children. Br. J. Clin. Pract., *17*:263, 1963.
4. Sweetnam, R.: Congenital curly toes. An investigation into the value of treatment. Lancet, *2*:398, 1958.
5. Taylor, R.G.: The treatment of claw toes by multiple transfers of flexor with extensor tendons. J. Bone Joint Surg. [Br.], *33*:539, 1951.
6. Watson, H.K., and Boyes, J.H.: Congenital angular deformities of the digits. J. Bone Joint Surg. [Am.], *49*:333, 1967.

CORN ON THE DORSOLATERAL ASPECT OF THE HEAD OF THE FIFTH PROXIMAL PHALANX

Incidence

The hard corn on the dorsolateral aspect of the head of the fifth proximal phalanx is undoubtedly one of the most common lesions of the foot. It is caused by prolonged wearing of high-heeled, narrow, and pointed shoes, which force the fifth toes into a varus and dorsal position and subject the heads of the fifth proximal phalanges to concentrated pressure from the lateral border of the shoes; this pressure results in formation of painful corns over the dorsolateral aspect of the heads of the fifth proximal phalanges. This occurrence may well explain why bilateral corns over the dorsolateral aspect of the fifth toes are almost invariably present in fashion-minded women who wear the aforementioned style of shoes. Because this corn is caused by wearing improperly fitted shoes, it should not be surprising to find that it is often associated with hallux valgus, hammer toes, other hard corns, soft corns, plantar callosities, bunionette, and Morton's neuroma.

Clinical Symptoms and Signs

The painful dorsal corn of the fifth toe is a small, yellowish or yellowish-gray, slightly raised area of hyperkeratosis of skin with a hard central core. It measures 5 to 10 mm in its greatest diameter and overlies the dorsolateral aspect of the head of the fifth proximal phalanx. The corn contains avascular keratinized skin, which can be pared with a sharp scalpel blade. An adventitious bursa is often interposed between the hard corn and the underlying bony prominence and may show signs of inflammation, such as redness, warmth, and swelling. Occasionally, the bursa may even become infected and purulent discharge through a small sinus tract is frequently present. When flexion contracture has taken place in the PIP joint of the fifth toe, active and passive extension of this joint is significantly restricted.

Roentgenographic Manifestations

When the corn on the dorsal aspect of the fifth toe is large enough, it may cast a superficial soft tissue shadow on routine radiographs. When an inflamed or infected adventitious bursa is associated with the corn, the superficial soft tissue shadow is more prominent. In addition, when the fifth toe has been subjected to relentless shoe pressure for a long time, flexion contracture and degenerative changes of its PIP joint may all appear on routine roentgenograms.

Pathologic Anatomy

The hard corn and its invaginated avascular central core usually cause marked atrophy of the subcutaneous tissue, and a richly innervated adventitious bursa containing a straw-colored fluid frequently becomes interposed between the hard corn and the underlying lateral head of the fifth proximal phalanx. When the adventitious bursa becomes infected, infiltration of acute and chronic inflammatory cells such as polymorphonuclear leukocytes, lymphocytes, plasma cells, histiocytes; foci of necrosis and hemorrhage; and reparative fibrosis may be present. Arthritic changes of the

PIP joint are usually accompanied by degeneration of articular cartilage, subchondral osteosclerosis, synovial proliferation, and periarticular soft tissue fibrosis.

Nonsurgical Treatment

A. Shoe modifications: roomy, extra-depth, and space shoes and stretching of the outer border of the toe box over the hard corn of the fifth toe with a shoemaker's swan can provide relief for painful dorsal corn of the fifth toe (Figures 1–7—1–12).

B. Padding of the toe: soft pads applied directly to the painful dorsal corn of the fifth toe can render symptomatic relief (Figure 1–8). Careful shaving of the corn can also be helpful.

C. Commercially available foot aids: corn pads, toe caps, and adhesive-backed foam strips can all be used to relieve pain (Figures 1–16 and 1–18).

Surgical Treatment

A. Excision of the head of the fifth proximal phalanx (Figures 4–4A and B, 4–5).

B. Proximal phalangectomy of the fifth toe (Figures 4–4C and 4–5).

C. Proximal phalangectomy of the fifth toe plus syndactylization of the fourth and fifth toes (Figure 4–4D).

REFERENCES

Corn on the Dorsolateral Aspect of the Fifth Proximal Phalanx

1. Avellan, L., and Johanson, B.: Hyperkeratosis of scars in the weight-bearing areas of the foot. Acta Chir. Scand., *131*:269, 1966.
2. Durlacher, L.: A Treatise on Corns, Bunions, Disease of the Nails and the General Management of the Feet. London, Simkin, Marshall & Co., 1845.
3. Galland, W.I.: An operative treatment for corns. J.A.M.A., *100*:880, 1933.
4. Gibbs, R.C.: Calluses, corns and warts. Am. Fam. Physician, *3*:92, 1971.
5. Lapidus, P.W.: Orthopaedic skin lesions of the soles and toes—calluses, corns, plantar warts, keratomas,

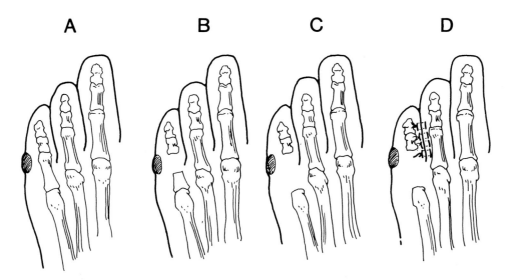

A   **B**   **C**   **D**

Figure 4–4. Surgical procedures for the treatment of painful corn on the dorsolateral aspect of the fifth toe. **A,** hard corn over the dorsolateral aspect of the head of the fifth proximal phalanx. **B,** excision of the head of the fifth proximal phalanx. **C,** proximal phalangectomy of the fifth toe. **D,** proximal phalangectomy of the fifth toe plus syndactylization of the fourth and fifth toes.

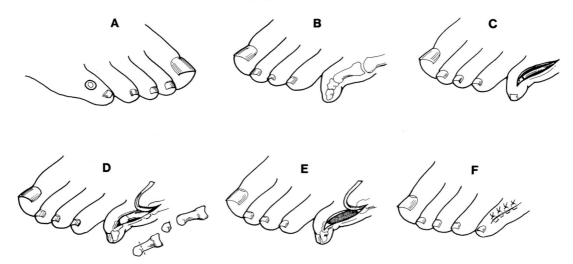

Figure 4-5. Surgical technique for the excision of the head or the entirety of the fifth proximal phalanx. **A** and **B,** lateral views show the hard corn on the dorsolateral aspect of the fifth toe and its relationship to the head of the fifth proximal phalanx. **C,** make a dorsal longitudinal incision from the level of the middle phalanx to the neck of the fifth metatarsal. Cut the extensor digitorum longus tendon near the PIP joint. **D,** cut the collateral ligaments and joint capsule of the PIP joint and free the undersurface of the head and neck of the fifth proximal phalanx from the digital sheath. Amputate the head of the fifth proximal phalanx with a narrow microsaw blade. **E,** proximal phalangectomy can be achieved by cutting the joint capsules, the collateral ligaments, and the tendon of the third plantar interosseous muscle of the M-P and PIP joint of the fifth toe, and by detaching the digital sheath from the undersurface of the fifth proximal phalanx. **F,** suture the cut extensor digitorum longus tendon to its distal stump. Close the skin in a regular manner.

neurovascular growths, onychomas. Clin. Orthop., *45:*87, 1966.
6. McElvenny, R.T.: Corns—their etiology and treatment. Am. J. Surg., *50:*761, 1940.
7. Whitfield, A.: On development of callosities, corns and warts. Br. J. Dermatol., *44:*580, 1932.

OVERLAPPING FIFTH TOE

Incidence

Overlapping fifth toe (also known as varus or overriding fifth toe) is usually a bilateral congenital toe deformity with a strong familial tendency and without any apparent sex predilection. It is often completely asymptomatic during childhood, and only about one half of these patients develop symptoms during adult life. Some patients insist on having their asymptomatic overlapping fifth toes surgically corrected because of their cosmetically unacceptable appearance. The prominent varus and hyperextended position of the overlapping fifth toe subjects the toe to concentrated pressure from the dorsolateral aspect of the shoe, which can produce painful corn on the

dorsal aspect of the PIP joint of the overlapping fifth toe, especially when the shoe has a high heel and a narrow and pointed toe box.

Clinical Symptoms and Signs

The typical deformities consist of overlapping of the fourth toe by the fifth toe, external rotation of the fifth toe along its longitudinal axis with its toenail facing laterally, dorsal subluxation or dislocation of the M-P joint, contracture of the extensor digitorum longus and brevis, painful corn on the dorsolateral aspect of the head of the fifth proximal phalanx, inability to plantar flex the M-P joint of the fifth toe, and tight skin on the dorsal aspect of the fifth toe. When arthritic changes have occurred in the M-P joint, pain, tenderness, and crepitation may be present.

Roentgenographic Manifestations

On the anteroposterior view of the foot, an overlapping fifth toe shows varus deformity and overlapping of the phalanges of the fourth toe and lateral displacement of the nail shadow

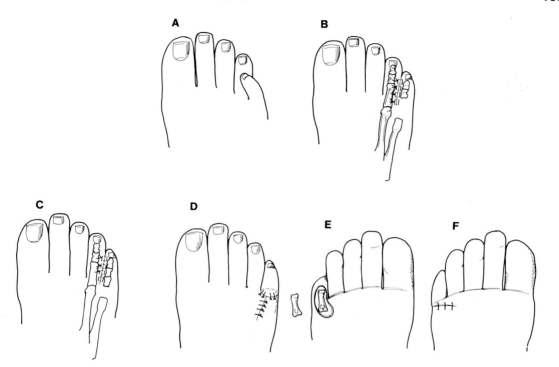

Figure 4–6. Various surgical procedures for the correction of an overlapping fifth toe. **A,** dorsal view of an overlapping fifth toe. **B,** proximal phalangectomy of the fifth toe plus syndactylization of the fourth and fifth toes. **C,** excision of the proximal portion of the fifth proximal phalanx plus syndactylization of the fourth and fifth toes. **D,** release of the tight dorsal capsule, collateral ligaments, and tendons of third plantar interosseous and extensor digitorum longus and brevis muscles, plus a Y-V skin plasty to move the overlapping fifth toe downward and laterally to lie in the plantar aspect of the wound in its corrected position. **E** and **F,** proximal phalangectomy of the fifth toe through an elliptical excision of the plantar skin of the fifth toe. Two halves of the elliptical skin incision are sutured to tighten the plantar skin of the fifth toe so to move the fifth toe laterally and plantarward to its anatomic position.

of the fifth toe due to its external rotation deformity. On the standing lateral radiograph, the fifth toe shows hyperextension and subluxation or frank dislocation of the M-P joint, with the phalanges of the fifth toe situated dorsal to those of the fourth toe. When degenerative arthritis has taken place in the M-P joint, joint narrowing and irregularity, osteophyte formation at the joint margins, and osteosclerosis of subchondral bone may be present.

Pathologic Anatomy

Dorsal subluxation or dislocation of the M-P joint in overlapping fifth toe is accompanied by contracture of the dorsal joint capsule, collateral ligaments, and interosseous and extensor digitorum longus and brevis muscles. Great thickening of the stratum corneum

of the skin, atrophy of the subcutaneous tissue, and the presence of an adventitious bursa are associated with the hard corn over the dorsal aspect of the PIP joint. When arthritic changes have occurred in the M-P joint, degeneration of the articular cartilage, synovial proliferation, and periarticular soft tissue fibrosis may be present.

Nonsurgical Treatment

A. Shoe modifications: wide and comfortable, extra-depth, and space shoes, and stretching of the outer border of the shoe with a shoemaker's swan to accommodate the overlapping fifth toe are helpful in relieving symptomatic overlapping fifth toe (Figures 1–7 and 1–12).

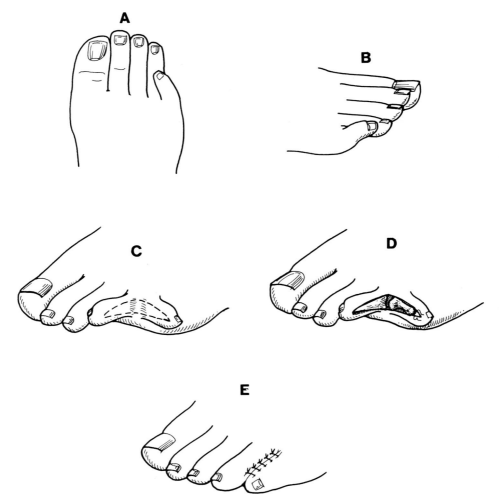

Figure 4–7. Surgical technique to correct an overlapping fifth toe. **A** and **B,** dorsal and lateral views of an overlapping fifth toe. **C,** make a diamond-shaped skin incision in the fourth webspace. Remove the diamond-shaped piece of skin. **D,** perform a proximal phalangectomy of the fifth toe by cutting the collateral ligaments and joint capsules of the M-P and PIP joints and by detaching it from its digital sheath. **E,** close the skin incision by suturing the mirror images of the two halves of the diamond-shaped incision together.

B. Padding of the toe: soft pads applied directly to the dorsal corn of the overlapping fifth toe can provide relief (Figure 1–8).

C. Commercially available foot aids: donut-shaped pads, soft toe caps, and adhesive-backed foam strips can be used to give relief to a painful, overlapping fifth toe (Figures 1–16 and 1–18).

Surgical Treatment

Although many surgical procedures have been described in the treatment of an overlapping fifth toe, only four are described in the subsequent section (Figures 4–6—4–9).

A. Proximal phalangectomy of the fifth toe plus syndactylization of the fourth and fifth toes (Figures 4–6A and B, 4–7). The author's preferred surgical procedure.

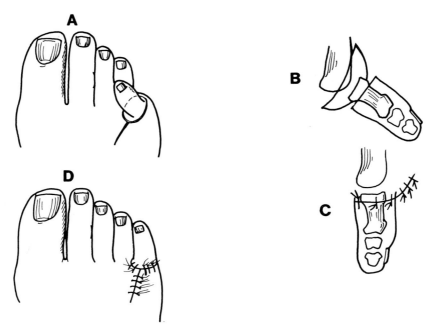

Figure 4–8. A second surgical technique for correcting an overlapping fifth toe. **A,** make a circular skin incision around the base of the fifth toe with two extensions, to the dorsal and plantar aspects of the foot. Release the contracted soft tissue structures on the dorsal aspect of the M-P joint. **B** and **C,** move the fifth toe laterally and plantarward along its plantar incision. **D,** suture the fifth toe in its new anatomic position by closing the entire skin incision.

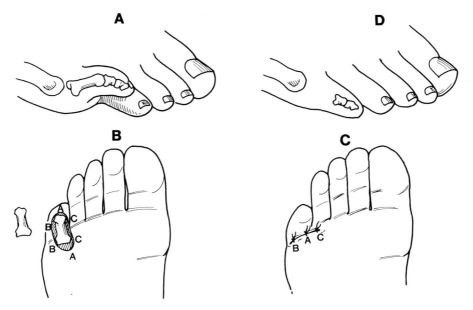

Figure 4–9. A third surgical technique for correcting an overlapping fifth toe. **A,** lateral view shows an overlapping fifth toe. **B,** excise an elliptical piece of skin from the plantar aspect of the fifth toe. Perform a proximal phalangectomy through the same incision by detaching all the soft tissue attachments from the fifth proximal phalanx. **C,** close the two mirror images of the two halves of the elliptical skin incision together to force the fifth toe into a lateral and plantar position to correct its overlapping deformity. **D,** fifth toe is in its anatomic position after its proximal phalangectomy and accurate plication of its plantar skin.

B. Proximal hemiphalangectomy of the fifth proximal phalanx plus syndactylization of the fourth and fifth toes (Figure 4–6C).

C. Release of all the tight dorsal structures plus a Y-V skin plasty to move the overlapping fifth toe downward and laterally to its anatomic position (Figures 4–6D and 4–8).

D. Excision of an elliptical piece of skin from the plantar aspect of the fifth toe plus proximal phalangectomy of the same toe. The two halves of the elliptical skin incision are sutured together to bring the deformed toe plantarward and laterally to its anatomic position (Figures 4–6E, 4–6F, and 4–9).

REFERENCES

Overlapping Fifth Toe

1. Cockin, J.: Butler's operation for an over-riding fifth toe. J. Bone Joint Surg. [Br.], *50:*78, 1968.
2. Colonna, P.C.: Regional Orthopedic Surgery. Philadelphia, W.B. Saunders, 1950, p. 492.
3. Goodwin, F.C., and Swisher, F.M.: The treatment of congenital hyperextension of the fifth toe. J. Bone Joint Surg., *25:*193, 1943.
4. Hulman, S.: Simple operation for the overlapping fifth toe. Nurs. Mirror, *123:*1, 1967.
5. Jahss, M.H.: Diaphysectomy for severe acquired overlapping fifth toe and advanced fixed hammering of the small toes. In Foot Science. J.E. Bateman (ed.). Philadelphia, W.B. Saunders, 1976, pp. 211–221.
6. Janecki, C.J., and Wilde, A.H.: Results of phalangectomy of the fifth toe for hammertoe. The Ruiz-Mora procedure. J. Bone Joint Surg. [Am.], *58:*1005, 1976.
7. Jones, R., and Lovett, R.W.: Orthopaedic Surgery. 2nd Ed. London, Oxford University Press, 1929, p. 666.
8. Kaplan, E.G.: A new approach to the surgical correction of overlapping toes. J. Foot Surg., *3:*24, 1964.
9. Lantzounis, L.A.: Congenital subluxation of the fifth toe and its correction by a periosteo-capsulo-plasty and tendon transplantation. J. Bone Joint Surg. *22:*147, 1940.
10. Lapidus, P.W.: Transplantation of extensor tendon for correction of overlapping fifth toe. J. Bone Joint Surg., *24:*555, 1942.
11. Leonard, M.H., and Rising, E.E.: Syndactylization to maintain correction of overlapping fifth toe. J. Bone Joint Surg., *24:*555, 1942.
12. McFarland, B.: Congenital deformities of the spine and limbs. In Modern Trends in Orthopaedics. H. Platt (ed.). London, Butterworth, 1980, p. 107.
13. Moeller, F.: Surgical Treatment of Digital Deformities. Mount Kisco, NY, Futura Publishing, 1975, pp. 127–131.
14. Morris, E.W., Scullion, J.E., and Mann, T.S.: Varus fifth toe. J. Bone Joint Surg. [Br.], *64:*99, 1982.
15. Rosner, M., Knudsen, H.A., and Sharon, S.M.: Overlapping fifth toe: A new surgical approach. J. Foot Surg., *17:*67, 1978.
16. Ruiz-Mora, J.: Plastic correction of the overriding fifth toe. Orthop. Lett. Vol. 6, 1954.
17. Scrase, W.H.: The treatment of dorsal adduction deformities of the fifth toe. J. Bone Joint Surg. [Br.], *36:*146, 1954.
18. Stamm, T.T.: Minor surgery of the foot—elevated fifth toe. In British Surgical Practice. E.R. Carling and J.P. Ross, (eds.). London, Butterworth, 1948, pp. 161–162.
19. Straub, L.R.: Orthopedic Surgery. In The Specialities in General Practice. R. L. Cecil (ed.). Philadelphia, W.B. Saunders, 1951, p. 60.
20. Tax, H.R.: Podopediatrics. Baltimore, Williams & Wilkins, 1980, p. 188.
21. Weber, R.B.: Surgical criteria for correcting the overlapping fifth toe. J. Foot Surg., *21:*30, 1982.
22. Wilson, J.N.: V-Y correction for varus deformity of the fifth toe. Br. J. Surg., *41:*113, 1953.
23. Young, C.R., and Solomon, M.G.: Surgical management of digiti quinti varus: A case presentation. J. Foot Surg., *17:*87, 1978.

5 SURGERY OF THE METATARSAL REGION

FREIBERG'S DISEASE

Incidence

Freiberg's disease is synonymous with Freiberg's infraction and Köhler's second disease, and was first described by Freiberg in 1914. The condition produces aseptic necrosis of the metatarsal head during a period of rapid growth before the closure of the epiphyseal plate. The disease shows a definite predilection for the second metatarsal head, and adolescent girls about 13 years of age, with a male to female ratio of 1 to 3. It has been postulated that trauma may play a role in the pathogenesis of Freiberg's disease, which is characterized by a disorderliness of endochondral ossification affecting both chondrogenesis and osteogenesis. This articular osteochondrosis produces significant alteration in the shape and form of the joint surfaces, resulting in subsequent symptomatic degenerative arthritis. Although Freiberg's infraction predominantly involves the second metatarsal head, it can affect the third metatarsal head and, rarely, the fourth and fifth metatarsal heads. In addition, Freiberg's disease can occasionally show bilateral involvement or involvement of more than one metatarsal head in the same foot. There are three main types of osteochondrosis:

A. Articular osteochondrosis: affects articular and epiphyseal cartilage and adjacent endochondral ossification. Freiberg's disease and Legg-Calvé-Perthes disease are two typical examples.

B. Nonarticular osteochondrosis: involves the site of tendon insertion. Osgood-Schlatter disease is a good example.

C. Physeal (growth plate) osteochondrosis: affects the growth plate and results in retarded growth and early closure of the growth plate to which tibia vara (or Blount's disease) belongs.

Clinical Symptoms and Signs

Freiberg's disease causes pain, tenderness, and swelling in the affected M-P joint that is aggravated by weight-bearing and movement and is relieved by rest. Examination may reveal crepitation, limited range of joint motion, palpable enlargement of the affected metatarsal head, osteophyte formation at joint margins, and hyperextension and subluxation of the M-P joint.

Roentgenographic Manifestations

The radiologic appearance of Freiberg's disease depends on the stages of the disease:

143

A. Active (early) stage: increased density of the affected metatarsal epiphysis, metaphyseal rarefaction, and widening of the joint space.

B. Latent (late) stage: an irregular and narrow joint space with subchondral osteosclerosis, flattening and enlargement of the metatarsal head, enlargement of the base of the corresponding proximal phalanx, osteophyte formation at joint margins, thickening and hypertrophy of the meta-

tarsal shaft, intra-articular loose bodies, and hyperextension and dorsal subluxation of the M-P joint.

Pathologic Anatomy

The pathology of Freiberg's disease depends largely on its stages. In its early active stage, the synovium and joint capsule are swollen, edematous, and hyperemic, with an excessive amount of joint fluid; this fluid collection produces the radiologic appearance of

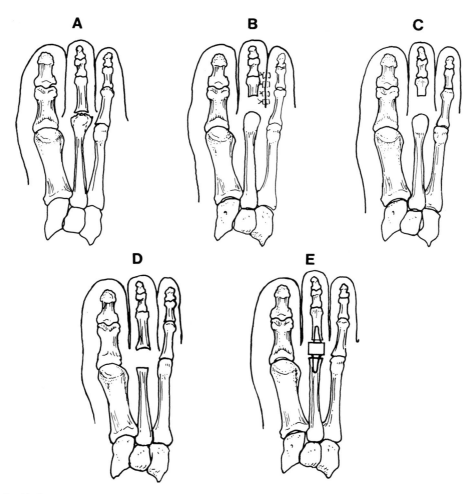

Figure 5–1. Various surgical procedures for the treatment of Freiberg's disease. **A,** anteroposterior view shows irregularity and narrowing of the second M-P joint, enlargement of the second metatarsal head and the corresponding base of the second proximal phalanx, and hypertrophy of the second metatarsal shaft. **B,** reshape the deformed second metatarsal head, excise the base of the second proximal phalanx, and join the second and third toes. **C,** excise the base of the second proximal phalanx. **D,** excise the head and neck of the second metatarsal. **E,** resect the second M-P joint and insert a Silastic prosthesis.

a widening of the joint space. The hyperemia causes dissolution of the metaphyseal bone producing metaphyseal rarefaction. The radiopaque and necrotic metatarsal epiphysis contains many empty lacunae, lacunae with pyknotic nuclei, and necrotic bone marrow. With time, the necrotic epiphysis is invaded by vascular and cellular connective tissue, which resorbs the dead bone and replaces it with immature fibrous bone; this immature bone will be replaced by mature bone with time. When Freiberg's disease has been present for a long time, marked degeneration of the articular cartilage, synovial proliferation, loose body formation, osteophyte formation at joint margins, subchondral osteosclerosis, enlargement of the metatarsal head and shaft, thickening of the M-P joint capsule, and contracture of the collateral ligaments may be present.

Nonsurgical Treatment

A. Shoe modifications: metatarsal pads and bars, low heeled shoes, a rocker-bottom sole, and a soft, total contact insole are useful means to relieve the metatarsalgia associated with Freiberg's disease (Figures 1–4—1–6).

B. Crutches, a walking cast, and marked limitation of activities can provide symptomatic relief during the acute stage of Freiberg's disease.

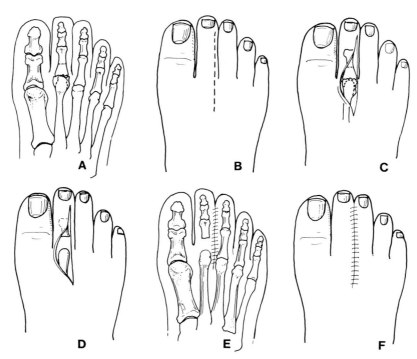

Figure 5–2. Surgical technique in treating Freiberg's disease preferred by author. **A,** anteroposterior view shows the presence of Freiberg's disease in the second metatarsal head. Dotted lines, amount of bone to be resected. **B,** make a longitudinal incision on the dorsolateral aspect of the second toe from the level of the PIP joint to the level of the second metatarsal neck. **C,** expose the second metatarsal head and the base of the second proximal phalanx by detaching the joint capsule and collateral ligaments and then retracting the long and short toe extensors and flexors from them. **D,** trim the osteophytes and round off the second metatarsal head. Resect the proximal portion of the second proximal phalanx. **E** and **F,** join the second and third toes by removing a diamond-shaped piece of skin from the opposing surfaces of the second webspace and then suturing the corresponding sides of the diamond-shaped skin incision.

Surgical Treatment

A. Reshaping of the deformed metatarsal head, excision of the base of proximal phalanx, and syndactylization of the second toe to the third toe: the author's preferred method of treatment because it not only provides relief of pain, but also stabilizes and preserves the length of the second toe (Figures 5–1A and B, 5–2).

B. Excision of the base of the proximal phalanx: creates an unstable second toe that may encourage the development of a hallux valgus deformity (Figure 5–1C).

C. Excision of the affected metatarsal head: encourages proximal migration of the second toe to create a deformed second toe. May also produce a transfer metatarsalgia due to the absence of the weight-bearing function of the second metatarsal head (Figure 5–1D).

D. Insertion of a Silastic prosthesis after proper resection of the diseased M-P joint: breakage of the prosthesis, infection, and inflammation are the possible postoperative complications (Figure 5–1E).

REFERENCES

Freiberg's Disease

1. Bordelon, R.L.: Silicone implant for Freiberg's disease. South. Med. J., *70:*1002, 1977.
2. Braddock, G.T.F.: Experimental epiphyseal injury and Freiberg's disease. J. Bone Joint Surg. [Br.], *41:*154, 1959.
3. Burman, M.S.: Epiphysitis of the proximal or pseudometatarsal epiphyses of the foot. J. Bone Joint Surg., *15:*538, 1933.
4. Campbell, W.C.: Infraction of the head of the second and third metatarsal bones: Report of cases. Am. J. Orthop. Surg., *15:*721, 1917.
5. Freiberg, A.H.: Infraction of the second metatarsal bone—a typical injury. Surg. Gynecol. Obstet., *19:*191, 1914.
6. Freiberg, A.H.: The so-called infraction of the second metatarsal bone. J. Bone Joint Surg., *8:*257, 1926.
7. Hoskinson, J.: Freiberg's disease: A review of the long-term results. Proc. R. Soc. Lond. [Med.], *67:*196, 1974.
8. Kohler, A.: Eine typische Erkrankung des 2 meta-tarsophalangeal Gelenkes. Munch. Med. Wochenschr., *67:*1289, 1920.
9. Painter, C.F.: Infraction of the second metatarsal head. Boston Med. Surg. J., *184:*533, 1921.
10. Siffert, R.S.: Classification of the osteochondroses. Clin. Orthop., *158:*10, 1981.
11. Smillie, I.S.: Freiberg's infraction (Kohler's second disease). J. Bone Joint Surg. [Br.], *37:*580, 1955.
12. Sollitto, R.J.: Silicone implant for Freiberg's disease. South. Med. J., *71:*352, 1978.
13. Swanson, A.B.: Flexible Implant Resection Arthroplasty in the Hand and Extremities. St. Louis, C.V. Mosby, 1973.
14. Wagner, A.: Isolated aseptic necrosis in epiphysis of the first metatarsal bone. Acta Radiol., *11:*80, 1930.

MORTON'S NEUROMA

Incidence

Morton's neuroma, also known as interdigital neuroma, Morton's toe, plantar digital neuroma (neuritis), and Morton's metatarsalgia, was first described in 1876 by Thomas G. Morton, after whom the disease was named. It typically involves the third plantar common digital nerve between the third and fourth metatarsal heads, and less frequently the second and fourth plantar common digital nerves. It is extremely rare that the first plantar common digital nerve is involved. Morton's neuroma is usually unilateral and shows a strong predilection for female patients between 25 and 50 years of age, with a male to female ratio of approximately 1 to 10. It can also have bilateral involvement, however, or more than one neuroma can occur in the same foot. There is little doubt that narrow, pointed, and high-heeled shoes, which concentrate pressure on the forefeet and tightly crowd the toes together, are the main culprits in producing Morton's neuromas. The enlarged neuroma is typically found just proximal to the bifurcation of the plantar common digital nerve into its two plantar proper digital nerves; this is the point at which it goes through the metatarsal (interdigital) canal formed by the two adjacent M-P joint capsules laterally and medially, the deep transverse metatarsal ligament dorsally, and the transverse fibers of the plantar fascia plantarly (Figure 5–3). Several anatomic peculiarities of the third plantar common digital nerve are thought to be re-

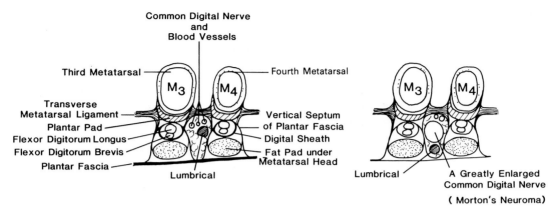

Figure 5–3. Cross-section of the third common digital (metatarsal) canal shows the relative positions of the various bony and soft tissue structures.

sponsible for its frequent involvement by the neuroma formation:

A. This nerve receives its constituent nerve fibers from both the medial and lateral plantar nerves in the third webspace, and has the greatest diameter among all the plantar common digital nerves. Therefore, it is more prone to be compressed in the third metatarsal canal.

B. Because the third plantar common digital nerve is formed by nerve fibers from both the medial and lateral plantar nerves, it is tethered by these two parental nerves. Consequently, it is more prone to sustain microtrauma of daily living.

C. The third metatarsal is bound to the second metatarsal, which is tightly wedged and immobilized in the three cuneiform bones and thus is less movable. In contrast, the fourth and fifth metatarsals articulate with the cuboid bone and are comparatively more movable. The third plantar common digital nerve in the third interdigital space between the third and fourth metatarsals is, therefore, subjected to significantly more shearing forces, which may well contribute

to the development of an interdigital neuroma.

Clinical Symptoms and Signs

Morton's neuroma produces neuralgia that patients describe as a burning, tingling, stabbing, needling, lancing, or electric shock-like pain that may radiate to the affected adjacent toes or sometimes up the leg. The neuralgia typically involves the head and neck region of the third and fourth metatarsals and their corresponding toes, and is aggravated by walking on a hard surface, especially when wearing tight and high-heeled shoes, and is relieved by removal of the shoes, rest, and rubbing the affected toes. The same neuralgic pain can usually be reproduced by applying direct pressure between the metatarsal heads, by transversely compressing the metatarsal heads together, or by pressing the edge of a coin into the affected intermetatarsal space. Localized tenderness in the space btween the two metatarsal heads, rarely a palpable swelling, and occasionally hyperesthesia on opposing surfaces of the involved toes are the other physical findings. The symptoms of Morton's neuroma are usually intermittent in the beginning, and have a tendency to increase in frequency to progress into a chronic condition. Morton's neuroma can even produce paroxysmal and intense pain at night, waking the sufferer from deep sleep. To reconfirm the clinical impression of the presence of a Morton's neuroma, a local anesthetic agent can be injected directly into the affected plantar common digital nerve. If all its symptoms and signs are obliterated by the injection, a positive diagnosis of Morton's neuroma can be established. In addition, motor and sensory nerve conduction tests of Morton's neuromas have shown that digital sensory action potential tends to be absent in the affected toes and can thus be used to confirm the clinical diagnosis of Morton's neuroma, especially in young patients with atypical presentation of pain in their feet.

Roentgenographic Manifestations

Because Morton's neuroma is an enlarged plantar common digital nerve that does not contain any calcification, it is usually not demonstrable by routine roentgenographic examination. New generations of CT scanners, however, with high, soft tissue resolution power may be able to demonstrate the presence or absence of a Morton's neuroma.

Pathologic Anatomy

A. Gross anatomy: Morton's neuroma is a greatly enlarged fusiform swelling of a plantar common digital nerve with marked perineural and intraneural fibrosis.

B. Microscopic anatomy:
  1. Nerve: separation of individual nerve fibers by a proliferating collagenous matrix; absence of proliferation of nerve tissue of the type commonly seen in neuromata; no evidence of Schwann cell proliferation; and marked disruption and drastically decreased number of nerve fibers in severe cases in which nerve bundles appear as interwoven collagenous fibrous tissue, no longer recognizable as nerve tissue, are the possible findings.

  2. Blood vessels: periarterial fibrosis and sclerosis of the blood vessels with narrowing of their lumens, infolding of endothelial lining, irregular disruption of the intimal elastic lamina, and loss of distinction between tunica intima and media are the various microscopic findings.

All of the above pathologic findings seem to support the contention that Morton's neuroma is caused by repeated microtraumas over a long time that cause reparative overgrowth of collagenous connective tissue. This tissue, in turn, disrupts the nerve tissue and causes fibrosis of the walls of blood vessels, disruption of the intimal elastic lamina, and narrowing of the lumens of digital vessels, producing ischemia and further nerve atrophy. These degenerative nerve and blood vessels encased in a dense reactive scar become very sensitive to pressure and consequently produce the excruciating neuritic pain characteristic of Morton's neuroma.

Nonsurgical Treatment

A. Shoe modifications: metatarsal bars and pads; total contact arch support; low-heeled, soft, and thick-soled shoes; and a rocker-bottom sole can provide some degree of pain relief for Morton's neuroma (Figures 1–4—1–6).

B. Padding of the foot: small foam rubber pads applied to the sole of the foot proximal to the two involved metatarsal heads to keep them apart can provide symptomatic relief.

C. Local injection of any anesthetic agent with or without a hydrocortisone preparation: can provide some temporary relief for pain.

Surgical Treatment

Surgical excision of the Morton's neuroma usually produces dramatic symptomatic relief.

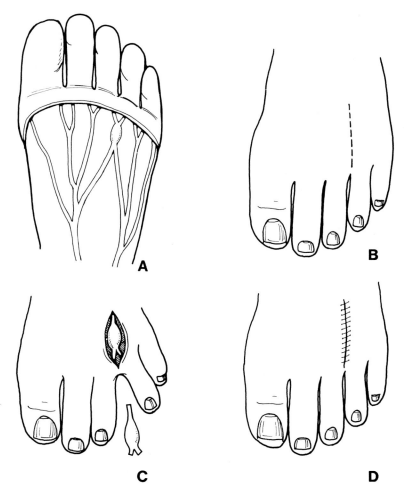

Figure 5–4. Surgical technique for the removal of a Morton's neuroma. **A,** transparent anteroposterior view shows a large Morton's neuroma in the third plantar common digital nerve, which is formed by nerve fibers from both the medial and plantar nerves. **B,** make a longitudinal dorsal skin incision over the third interdigital space. Cut the underlying deep transverse metatarsal ligament to gain access to the neuroma. **C,** by pushing the neuroma upward from the plantar side, remove it by cutting the proximal portion of the plantar common digital nerve at least 1 cm proximal to the neuroma, and by cutting the two proper digital nerves distal to the neuroma. **D,** close the skin in a regular manner.

A longitudinal dorsal skin incision over the involved interdigital cleft can be used to cut the deep transverse metatarsal ligament and to expose the underlying neuroma. Resection of the neuroma should include at least 1 cm of normal nerve proximal to the neuromatous mass to prevent incarceration of the nerve stump in scar tissue forming an amputation neuroma (Figure 5–4).

REFERENCES

Morton's Neuroma

1. Ames, P.A., Lenet, M.D., and Sherman, M.: Joplin's neuroma. J. Am. Podiatry Assoc., *70:*99, 1980.
2. Baker, L.D., and Kuhn, H.H.: Morton's metatarsalgia. South. Med. J., *37:*123, 1944.
3. Berger, M.R.: Morton's neuroma. Orthop. Nurs., *1:*31, 1982.
4. Betts, L.O.: Morton's metatarsalgic neuritis of fourth digital nerve. Med. J. Aust., *1:*514, 1940.

5. Bickel, W.H., and Dockerty, M.B.: Plantar neuromas—Morton's toe. Surg. Gynecol. Obstet., *84:*111, 1947.

6. Bossley, C.J., and Cairney, P.C.: The intermetatarsophalangeal bursitis, significance in Morton's metatarsalgia. J. Bone Joint Surg. [Br.], *62:*184, 1981.

7. Bradford, E.H.: Metatarsal neuralgia, or "Morton's affection of the foot." Boston Med. Surg. J., *125:*52, 1891.

8. Bradley, N., Miller, W.A., and Evans, J.P.: Plantar neuroma: Analysis of results following surgical excision in 145 patients. South. Med. J., *69:*853, 1976.

9. Brahms, M. A.: Common foot problems. J. Bone Joint Surg. [Am.], *49:*1653, 1967.

10. Burke, B.R.: A preliminary report in the use of Silastic nerve caps in conjunction with neuroma surgery. J. Foot Surg., *17:*53, 1978.

11. Cooper, J.W.: Double lesion of the foot, plantar scars associated with interdigital neuroma, report of two cases. J. Bone Joint Surg. [Am.], *45:*657, 1963.

12. Dewberry, J.W., Christian J.D., Jr., and Becton, J.L.: Morton's neuroma. J. Med. Assoc. Ga., *62:*144, 1973.

13. Duncan, T.L., and Wright, A.: Plantar interdigital neuroma. South. Med. J., *51:*49, 1958.

14. Durlacher, L.: A Treatise on Corns, Bunions, The Diseases of Nails and The General Management of The Feet. London, Simpkin, Marshall and Co., 1845, p. 52.

15. Gauthier, G.: Thomas Morton's disease: A nerve entrapment syndrome. A new surgical technique. Clin. Orthop., *142:*90, 1979.

16. Gilmore, W.N.: Morton's metatarsalgia. J. Bone Joint Surg. [Br.], *55:*221, 1973.

17. Graham, W.D., and Johnson, C.R.: Plantar digital neuroma. Lancet, *2:*470, 1957.

18. Haeri, G.B., Fornasier, V.L., and Schatzker, J.: Morton's neuroma—pathogenesis and ultrastructure. Clin. Orthop., *141:*256, 1979.

19. Hauser, E.D.W.: Interdigital neuroma of the foot. Surg. Gynecol. Obstet., *133:*265, 1971.

20. Hoadley, A.E.: Six cases of metatarsalgia. Chicago Med. Rec., *5:*32, 1893.

21. Jones, R.: Plantar neuralgia (metatarsalgia, Morton's painful affection of the foot). Liverpool Med.-Chir. J., *17:*1, 1897.

22. Jones, R., and Tubby, A.H.: Metatarsalgia or Morton's disease. Ann. Surg., *28:*297, 1898.

23. Joplin, R.J.: Surgery of the forefoot in the rheumatoid arthritic patient. Surg. Clin. North Am., *49:*866, 1969.

24. Joplin, R.J.: The proper digital nerve, vatallium stem arthroplasty, and some thoughts about foot surgery in general. Clin. Orthop., *76:*199, 1971.

25. King, L.S.: Pathology of Morton's metatarsalgia. Am. J. Clin. Pathol., *16:*124, 1946.

26. Kite, H.J.: Morton's toe neuroma. South. Med. J., *59:*20, 1966.

27. Lassmann, G., Lassmann, H., and Stockinger, L.: Morton's metatarsalgia. Light and electron microscopic observations and their relation to entrapment neuropathies. Virchows Arch. [Pathol. Anat.], *370:*307, 1976.

28. Litchman, H.M., Silver, C.M., and Simon, S.D.: Morton's metatarsalgia. J. Int. Coll. Surg., *41:*647, 1964.

29. Margo, M.K.: Surgical treatment of conditions of the forepart of the foot. J. Bone Joint Surg. [Am.], *49:*1665, 1967.

30. McElvenny, R.T.: The etiology and surgical treatment of intractable pain about the fourth metatarsophalangeal joint (Morton's), J. Bone Joint Surg., *25:*675, 1943.

31. McKeever, D.C.: Surgical approach for neuroma of plantar digital nerve (Morton's metatarsalgia). J. Bone Joint Surg. [Am.], *34:*490, 1952.

32. Meachim, G., and Abberton, M.J.: Histological findings in Morton's metatarsalgia. J. Pathol., *103:*209, 1971.

33. Merritt, G.N., and Subotnick, S.I.: Medial plantar digital proper nerve syndrome (Joplin's neuroma)—typical presentation. J. Foot Surg., *21:*166, 1982.

34. Milgrim, J.E.: Office methods for relief of the painful foot. J. Bone Joint Surg. [Am.], *46:*1099, 1964.

35. Miller, W.A.: Fasciotomy in the treatment of plantar keratosis and other conditions of the foot. J. Okla. State Med. Assoc., *66:*13, 1973.

36. Miller, W.A.: Plantar neuroma visualization with a laminar spreader. J. Bone Joint Surg. [Am.], *61:*1258, 1979.

37. Morris, M.A.: Morton's metatarsalgia. Clin. Orthop., *127:*203, 1977.

38. Morton, J.G.: A peculiar and painful affection of the fourth metatarsophalangeal articulation. Am. J. Med. Sci., *71:*37, 1876.

39. Morton, T.G.: The application of the x-rays to the diagnosis of Morton's painful affection of the foot, or metatarsalgia. Int. Med. Mag., *5:*322, 1897.

40. Morton, T.S.K.: Metatarsalgia (Morton's painful affection of the foot), with an account of six cases cured by operation. Ann. Surg., *17:*680, 1893.

41. Moshein, J.E., and Portis, R.B.: Plantar incision for plantar neuroma of the foot. J. Bone Joint Surg. [Am.], *45:*657, 1963.

42. Mulder, J.D.: The causative mechanism in Morton's metatarsalgia. J. Bone Joint Surg. [Br.], *33:*94, 1951.

43. Nissen, K.I.: Plantar digital neuritis. J. Bone Joint Surg. [Br.], *30:*84, 1948.

44. Nora, P.F., Nora, E.D., and Ghislandi, E.: Morton's metatarsalgia, a misconception. Ill. Med. J., *127:*155, 1965.

45. Reed, R.J., and Bliss, B.O.: Morton's neuroma. Regressive and productive intermetatarsal elastofibrositis. Arch. Pathol. Lab. Med., *95:*123, 1973.

46. Ringertz, N., and Unander-Scharin, L.: Morton's disease—a clinical and patho-anatomical study. Acta Orthop. Scand., *19:*327, 1950.

47. Rugh, J.T.: A simple method of treatment of common metatarsal disabilities. J. Bone Joint Surg., *16:*151, 1934.

48. Sayle-Creer, W.: A review of Morton's metatarsalgia. J. Bone Joint Surg. [Br.], *43:*603, 1961.

49. Shephard, E.: Intermetatarso-phalangeal bursitis in the causation of Morton's metatarsalgia. J. Bone Joint Surg. [Br.], *57:*115, 1974.

50. Stern, W.F.: Morton's painful disease of the toes. Am. Med., *7:*221, 1904.

51. Thompson, T.C.: Surgical treatment of disorders of the forepart of the foot. J. Bone Joint Surg. [Am.], *46:*1123, 1964.

52. Vainio, K.: Morton's metatarsalgia in rheumatoid arthritis. Clin. Orthop., *142:*85, 1979.

53. Viladot, A.: Metatarsalgia due to biomechanical alterations of the forefoot. Orthop. Clin. North Am., *4*:165, 1973.
54. Whitman, R.: Observations on Morton's painful affection of the fourth metatarso-phalangeal articulation and similar affections of the metatarsal region that may be included with it under the term anterior metatarsalgia. Trans. Am. Orthop. Assoc., *11*:34, 1898.
55. Winkler, H., Feltner, J.B., and Kimmelstiel, P.: Morton metatarsalgia. J. Bone Joint Surg. [Am.], *30*:496, 1948.

TAILOR'S BUNION (BUNIONETTE)

Incidence

Tailor's bunion derives its name from the fact that tailors in the old days used to sit on the floor in a cross-legged fashion, a position that resulted in constant pressure between the unyielding floor and the lateral aspect of the fifth metatarsal head, producing a painful corn over an enlarged fifth metatarsal head with an adventitious bursa between them. Like many other acquired, painful foot conditions, chronic irritation from poorly fitted shoes is the major cause of tailor's bunion; the dorsolateral aspect of the fifth metatarsal head is the lateral limit of the widest portion of the foot and is subjected to maximal pressure from the lateral vamp portion of the shoe. In addition, lateral angulation of the distal portion of the fifth metatarsal, wide splayfoot, and the presence of a symptomatic hallux valgus can all predispose the foot to the development of a tailor's bunion from increased shoe pressure on the dorsolateral aspect of the fifth metatarsal head. Occasionally, a malunited fracture of the fifth metatarsal can cause its distal portion to become laterally angulated, producing a tailor's bunion. Tailor's bunion shows a strong predilection for female patients, and according to personal experience, the male to female ratio of the patients who have undergone surgical excision of tailor's bunion is at least 1 to 10.

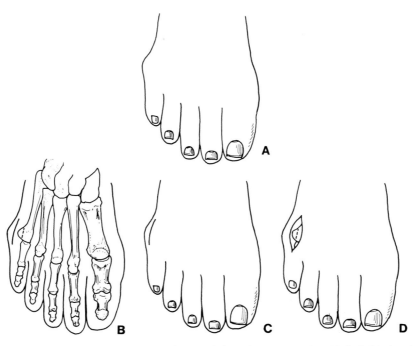

Figure 5–5. Simple excision of the tailor's bunion. **A,** dorsal view shows a prominent tailor's bunion. **B,** tailor's bunion is caused by an enlarged lateral condyle of the fifth metatarsal head. Dotted line, line of resection. **C,** longitudinal dorsal incision is placed directly over the bunion. **D,** expose the lateral aspect of the fifth metatarsal head by detaching the joint capsule and lateral collateral ligament from the lateral aspect of the fifth metatarsal head. Resect the lateral condyle of the fifth metatarsal head with a narrow microsaw blade.

Clinical Symptoms and Signs

A painful corn, swelling, erythema, and tenderness over the dorsolateral aspect of the fifth metatarsal head are common clinical findings. Patients with tailor's bunions often complain of difficulty in finding comfortable shoes to wear. Examination of the shoe frequently reveals a bulge on the lateral border of its vamp corresponding to the exact location occupied by the tailor's bunion inside the shoe. Sometimes a painful plantar callosity under the fifth metatarsal head can also be found. Occasionally, the adventitious bursa over the prominent fifth metatarsal head can become infected and then produce a draining sinus with purulent discharge, which if untreated, may even lead to osteomyelitis of the fifth metatarsal.

Roentgenographic Manifestations

The various abnormal radiographic findings of a tailor's bunion include soft tissue swelling over the lateral aspect of the metatarsal head caused by the presence of a hard corn and its underlying fluid-filled adventitious bursa, which may occasionally become calcified; enlarged lateral condyle of the fifth metatarsal head, and lateral angulation of the distal portion of the fifth metatarsal shaft. In addition, hallux valgus and splayfoot deformity frequently coexist with tailor's bunion.

Pathologic Anatomy

The hard corn over the fifth metatarsal head consists of avascular keratinized tissue that is slightly raised above the surrounding skin surface and is also invaginated beneath the

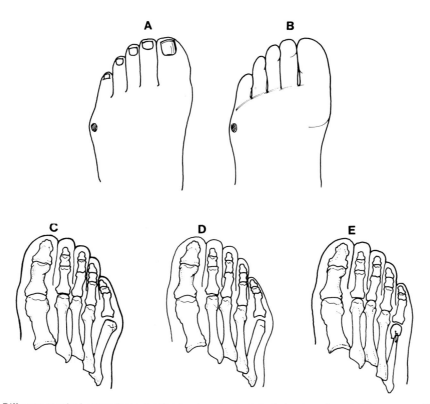

Figure 5–6. Different surgical procedures for the treatment of a tailor's bunion. **A,** painful corn over the dorsolateral aspect of the fifth matatarsal head. **B,** painful plantar callosity under the fifth metatarsal head. **C,** dotted line, line of resection of the tailor's bunion. **D,** tailor's bunion has been removed. **E,** varus osteotomy through the fifth metatarsal neck has been performed to correct a tailor's bunion deformity.

skin surface. The adventitious bursa under the corn is a sac-like structure containing a straw-colored fluid and a rich nerve supply. The surface of the enlarged lateral condyle of the fifth metatarsal head is somewhat irregular and is covered with a thin layer of cartilage.

Nonsurgical Treatment

A. Shoe modifications: comfortable shoes with wide vamps and stretching the outer border of the vamp of shoe with a shoe-maker's swan to accommodate the enlarged fifth metatarsal head can give relief to the painful tailor's bunion (Figures 1–7 and 1–12).

B. Padding of the foot: soft pads applied directly to the tailor's bunion and the callosity under the fifth metatarsal head can provide symptomatic relief (Figure 1–8). In addition, both corns can be pared to minimize their symptoms.

C. Commercially available foot aids: donut-shaped pads and adhesive-backed foam strips can be used to cushion a painful tailor's bunion (Figures 1–16 and 1–18).

Surgical Treatment

Several surgical procedures are available for the treatment of tailor's bunion, depending on whether the tailor's bunion exists alone or is associated with a painful plantar callosity under the fifth metatarsal head.

A. Tailor's bunion without associated plantar callosity under the fifth metatarsal head:
　1. Excision of the lateral condyle of the fifth metatarsal head (Figures 5–5, 5–6A—E, 5–7A1 and 2).
　2. Varus osteotomy of the fifth metatarsal neck (Figures 5–6E, 5–7C1—C3).

B. Tailor's bunion with associated plantar callosity under the fifth metatarsal head:
　1. Excision of the lateral and plantar condyles of the fifth metatarsal head (Figures 5–5, 5–6A—D, 5–7A1—B2).

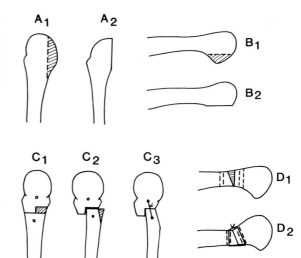

Figure 5–7. Different bone resections for the treatment of tailor's bunion. **A1** and **A2**, excision of the lateral condyle of the fifth metatarsal head. **B1** and **B2**, plantar condylectomy of the fifth metatarsal in the treatment of a painful plantar callosity. **C1** and **C3**, varus osteotomy of the fifth metatarsal neck to eliminate the tailor's bunion. **D1** and **D2**, dorsal angulation osteotomy through the fifth metatarsal neck by removing more bone from the dorsal side than the plantar side. The dorsally angulated fifth metatarsal head is held tightly against the shaft by passing one or two sutures through two drilled holes situated proximal and distal to the osteotomy site and by tying the sutures together.

　2. Varus and dorsal angulation osteotomy of the fifth metatarsal neck (Figures 5–6E and 5–7C1—D2).

REFERENCES

Tailor's Bunion (Bunionette)

1. Addante, J.B., Scardina, R., and Kaufmann, D.: Repair of tailor's bunion by means of fifth metatarsal head resection and insertion of a spherical silicone implant. Arch. Pod. Med. Foot Surg., *4*:450, 1977.
2. Bishop, J., Kahn, III., A., and Turba, J.E.: Surgical correction of the splayfoot: The Giannestras procedure. Clin. Orthop., *146*:234, 1980.
3. Buchbinder, I.J.: Drato procedure for tailor's bunion. J. Foot Surg., *21*:177, 1982.
4. Haber, J.H., and Kraft, J.: Crescentic osteotomy for fifth metatarsal head lesions. J. Foot Surg., *19*:66, 1980.
5. Harris, M.D.: A surgical approach for digiti quinti varus. J. Natl. Assoc. Chirop., *47*:362, 1957.
6. Leach, R.E., and Igou, R.: Metatarsal osteotomy for bunionette deformity. Clin. Orthop., *100*:171, 1974.
7. Lelievre, J.: Exostosis of head of the 5th metatarsal

bone, tailor's bunion. Concourse Med., *78:*4815, 1956.
8. Margo, M.K.: Surgical treatment of conditions of the forepart of the foot. J. Bone Joint Surg. [Am.], *49:*1665, 1967.
9. McKeever, D.C.: Excision of the fifth metatarsal head. Clin. Orthop., *13:*321, 1959.
10. Petrich, R.J., and Dull, D.D.: Interpositional sphere implant in the fifth metatarsophalangeal joint. J. Foot Surg., *20:*93, 1981.
11. Rappaport, M.: Wedge osteotomy for tailor's bunion. *In* Reconstructive Surgery of The Foot and Leg. E.D. McGlamry (ed.). New York, Intercontinental Medical Book Corp., 1974, pp. 127–134.
12. Sponsel, K.H.: Bunionette correction by metatarsal osteotomy: Preliminary report. Orthop. Clin. North Am., *7:*809, 1976.
13. Weisberg, M.H.: Resection of the fifth metatarsal head in lateral segment problems. J. Am. Podiatry Assoc., *57:*374, 1967.

PLANTAR FIBROMATOSIS

Incidence

Plantar fibromatosis is a benign fibroblastic proliferative disorder of the plantar fascia, and seems to be associated with Dupuytren's contracture of the hand, Peyronie's disease of the penis, knuckle pads, keloid formation, fibrous nodules in tendons, alcoholism, epilepsy, trauma, and periarthrosis humeri. Meyerding and co-workers (1948) reviewed 882 cases of Dupuytren's contracture of the hand and found only 24 (2.7%) cases with both hand and foot involvement. Plantar fibromatosis usually shows unilateral and multinodular involvement, some familial tendency, and strong predilection for the anterior one third and medial one half of the plantar fascia, with no apparent sex predilection. It is of interest to note that patients with palmar fibromatosis tend to be older than patients with plantar fibromatosis, which can show bilateral involvement.

Clinical Symptoms and Signs

Plantar fibromatosis is a firm, irregular, and nodular growth in the anterior one third and medial one half of the plantar fascia. It is commonly adherent to the overlying skin, producing wrinkles and indentations of the involved skin. Dorsiflexion of the foot and toes tightens the plantar fascia and makes the nodules of plantar fibromatosis more prominent and palpable. Although plantar fibroma-tosis does cause contracture of the plantar fascia, it usually does not produce contracture of the toes like that seen in the hand due to the insignificant extension of plantar fascia to the phalanges of the foot. In the active or early stage of the disease, the nodules are less well defined, softer, somewhat tender, and slightly painful. In contrast, these same nodules are fairly discrete, hard, and non-tender in the late resting or latent stage, with definite associated fascial contracture and scarring. When these fibrous nodules are of sufficient size, they can cause significant discomfort and disability. Plantar fibromatosis should be carefully differentiated from a wide variety of diseases that can all produce a plantar mass. These entities include leiomyoma, rhabdomyosarcoma, clear cell sarcoma, fibrosarcoma, synovial sarcoma, liposarcoma, lipoma, ganglion, giant cell tumor of the tendon sheath, rheumatoid nodule, granuloma annulare, neurofibroma, neurilemmoma, sporotrichosis, melanoma, and sweat gland carcinoma.

Roentgenographic Manifestations

Plantar fibromatosis usually does not show any radiologic abnormality. A very large nodule of plantar fibromatosis, however, may cast a soft tissue shadow in the longitudinal arch of the foot on an oblique view. The nodular mass can also be visualized by CT scanning.

Pathologic Anatomy

A. Gross anatomy: nodules are usually firm, lobulated, and grayish-white. They not only can adhere to the overlying skin to produce wrinkles and indentations, but also can involve the adjacent muscles, tendons, nerves, and blood vessels.

B. Microscopic anatomy: plantar fibromatosis is composed of fibrous tissue of varying degrees of cellular activity and vascularity, and shows perivascular round cell infiltration. It has a tendency for linear extension along the plantar fascia in the direction of the longitudinal arch of the foot, and for infiltration of the overlying skin. Nodules consist of islands of proliferating fibroblasts in a nodular and muticentric fashion. They can compress the surrounding plantar fascia into a pseudocapsule or blend gradually with the surrounding fascial bundles with their collagen fibers in-

versely proportional to the degrees of cellularity. The histologic findings of plantar fibromatosis depend on the stages of maturation.

1. Active stage: characterized by active fibroblastic proliferation with large and hyperchromatic nuclei and loose fascial

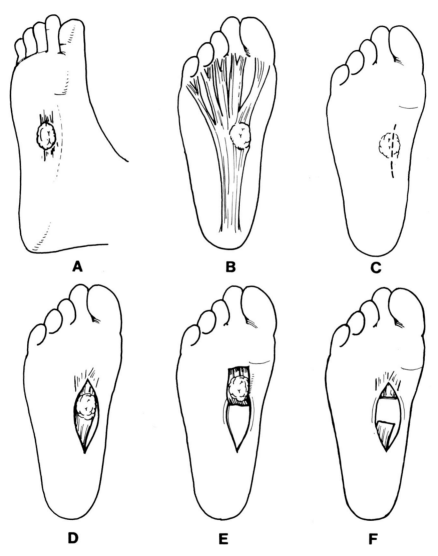

Figure 5–8. Surgical excision of plantar fibromatosis. **A,** transparent view shows a large nodule of plantar fibromatosis involving the medial one half of the plantar fascia. **B,** oblique view shows a bulge in the longitudinal arch of the foot caused by plantar fibromatosis. **C,** longitudinal plantar incision is made along the longitudinal arch of the foot. **D,** nodule of plantar fibromatosis is exposed. **E,** incise the plantar fascia proximal, medial, and lateral to the nodule so it can be lifted out of the wound. **F,** cut the plantar fascia distal to the nodule, to complete the excision. The skin is closed in a regular manner.

strands; higher cellularity, vascularity and perivascular round cell infiltration; a mild degree of atypism; and small number of mitotic figures which may raise the question of the presence of a low-grade fibrosarcoma.

2. Resting (latent) stage: characterized by thick and mature fibrous tissue with little cellular activity and small nuclei and by loss of subcutaneous areolar tissue.

Nonsurgical Treatment

Thick and soft pads can be inserted into shoes to provide a cushion for symptomatic relief of large and tender nodules of plantar fibromatosis (Figure 1–10).

Surgical Treatment

Complete excision of the nodule or nodules of plantar fibromatosis, together with the surrounding plantar fascia, is the treatment of choice when the nodules are large and symptomatic (Figure 5–8).

REFERENCES

Plantar Fibromatosis

1. Allen, P.W.: The fibromatoses: A clinicopathologic classification based on 140 cases. Am. J. Surg. Pathol., *1:*255, 1977.
2. Allen, R.A., Woolner, L.B., and Ghormley, R.K.: Soft tissue tumors of the sole. J. Bone Joint Surg. [Am.], *37:*14, 1955.
3. Aviles, E., Arlen, M., and Miller, T.: Plantar fibromatosis. Surgery, *69:*117, 1971.
4. Cameron, H.: Plantar fibromatosis. Can. Med. Assoc. J., *123:*846, 1980.
5. Clay, R.C.: Dupuytren's contracture: Fibroma of the palmar fascia. Ann. Surg., *120:*224, 1944.
6. Curtin, J.W.: Surgical therapy for Dupuytren's contracture of the foot. Plast. Reconstr. Surg., *30:*568, 1962.
7. Curtin, J.W.: Fibromatosis of the plantar fascia. Surgical technique and design of skin incision. J. Bone Joint Surg. [Am.], *47:*1605, 1965.
8. Dupuytren, G.: De la rétraction des doigts par suite d'une affection de l'aponé vrose palmarie, description de la maladie. Opération chirurgicale qui convient dans de cas. Med. Class., *4:*127, 1939.
9. Gelfarb, M., and Michaelides, P.: Plantar fibromatosis. Arch. Dermatol., *85:*278, 1962.
10. Greenberg, L.: Dupuytren's contracture of palmar and plantar fasciae. J. Bone Joint Surg. *21:*785, 1939.
11. Jaworek, T.E.: A histologic analysis of plantar fibromatosis. J. Foot Surg., *15:*47, 1976.
12. Kanavel, A.B., Koch, S.L., and Mason, M.L.: Dupuytren's contracture; with a description of the palmar fascia, a review of the literature, and a report of twenty-nine surgically treated cases. Surg. Gynecol. Obstet., *48:*145, 1929.
13. Keasby, L.: Juvenile aponeurotic fibroma, a distinctive tumor of the palms and soles of young children. Cancer, *6:*338, 1953.
14. Lund, M.: Dupuytren's contracture of palmar and plantar fasciae. Acta Psychol. (Amst.), *16:*465, 1941.
15. Meyerding, H.W.: Dupuytren's contracture. Arch. Surg., *32:*320, 1936.
16. Meyerding, H.W., and Jackson, A.E.: Epidermoid cyst of the left palm with Dupuytren's contracture of the hands and right foot: Report of case. Surg. Clin. North Am., *28:*1031, 1948.
17. Meyerding, H.W., and Shellito, J.G.: Dupuytren's contracture of the foot. J. Int. Coll. Surg., *11:*596, 1948.
18. Pedersen, H.E., and Day, A.J.: Dupuytren's disease of the foot. J.A.M.A., *154:*33, 1954.
19. Pickren, J.W., Smith, A.G., Stevenson, T.W., and Stout, A. P.: Cancer, *4:*846, 1951.
20. Pojer, J., Radivojevic, M., and Williams, T.F.: Dupuytren's disease: Its association with abnormal liver functions in alcoholism and epilepsy. Arch. Intern. Med., *129:*561, 1972.
21. Powers, H.: Dupuytren's contracture one hundred years after Dupuytren: Its interpretation. J. Nerv. Ment. Dis., *80:*386, 1934.
22. Warthan, T.L., Rudolph, R.I., and Gross, P.R.: Isolated plantar fibromatosis. Arch. Dermatol., *108:*823, 1973.
23. Westerkamp, M.: A case history of recurrent plantar fibromatosis (Dupuytren's contracture). J. Foot Surg., *17:*73, 1978.
24. White, S.W.: Plantar fibromatosis. Arch. Dermatol., *117:*375, 1981.
25. Wiseman, G.G.: Multiple recurring plantar fibromatosis and its surgical excision. J. Foot Surg., *22:*121, 1983.
26. Wright, D.J., and Rennels, D.C.: A study of the elastic properties of plantar fascia. J. Bone Joint Surg. [Am.], *46:*482, 1964.

DORSAL TARSAL AND TARSOMETATARSAL EXOSTOSES

Incidence

Dorsal tarsal and tarsometatarsal exostoses typically involve the medial naviculocuneiform joint and the first metatarsocuneiform joint. They usually affect female patients over 40 years of age and do not seem to be related to any specific trauma. These exostoses tend to be associated with mild cavus feet with tight heel cords and evidence of increased plantar weight-bearing, or with arthritic pronated feet. Dorsal tarsal and tarsometatarsal exostoses are localized osteoarthritic conditions that can be irritated by lacing the shoes tightly or by any other abnormal pressure applied directly or indirectly to the dorsal aspect of the foot.

Clinical Symptoms and Signs

Patients usually complain of pain in their exostoses when wearing snugly fitting shoes or oxford-type shoes with laces. The symptoms are insidious but tend to be slowly progressive until patients seek medical attention for pain relief. Examination often reveals tenderness, redness, and swelling over a palpable bony prominence over either the first tarsometatarsal joint or the medial naviculocuneiform joint. Careful palpation may also reveal some thickening and tenderness of the overlying tibialis anterior tendon sheath.

Roentgenographic Manifestations

The roentgenographic abnormalities associated with dorsal naviculocuneiform and metatarsocuneiform exostoses include narrowing and irregularity of these joints, subchondral osteosclerosis, osteophyte formation at their joint margins, and soft tissue swelling over these dorsal exostoses caused by the adventitious bursae and the heavily keratinized skin over these bony prominences. To identify the exact location of dorsal exostosis, a lead marker, such as the letter O, can be taped directly to the exostosis, and radiographs of the foot are then obtained.

Pathologic Anatomy

Because dorsal exostoses of the tarsal and tarsometatarsal joints are caused by localized

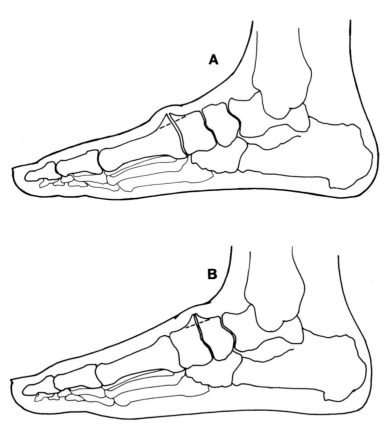

Figure 5–9. Dorsal tarsal and tarsometatarsal exostoses. **A,** dorsal exostosis of the first metatarsocuneiform joint. **B,** dorsal exostosis of the medial cuneiform-navicular joint.

osteoarthritis of these joints, articular cartilage degeneration, chronic synovitis, formation of osteophytes at joint margins, and periarticular soft tissue fibrosis are commonly
present. In addition, the bony exostosis is
covered by a thin layer of hyaline cartilage,
which in turn is covered by a fluid-filled adventitious bursa and thickly keratinized skin.

Nonsurgical Treatment

Any shoes that do not create pressure on
the dorsal exostoses, such as loosely fitting,
slipper- and pump-style shoes, can provide
symptomatic relief. In addition, a soft pad can
be applied directly to the dorsal exostosis or
glued to the undersurface of the tongue of the
shoe to cushion the painful exostoses (Figures 1–8 and 1–11).

Surgical Treatment

When a dorsal tarsal or tarsometatarsal exostosis is symptomatic and fails to respond to
nonsurgical treatment, it can be surgically excised under local anesthesia (Figures 5–9 and
5–10). Care should be taken, however, to
prevent cutting the branches of the dorsal
sensory nerve so to avoid formation of trou-
blesome neuromas. In addition, the dorsal joint
capsule should be closed in a meticulous
manner to avoid formation of a postoperative
dorsal ganglion.

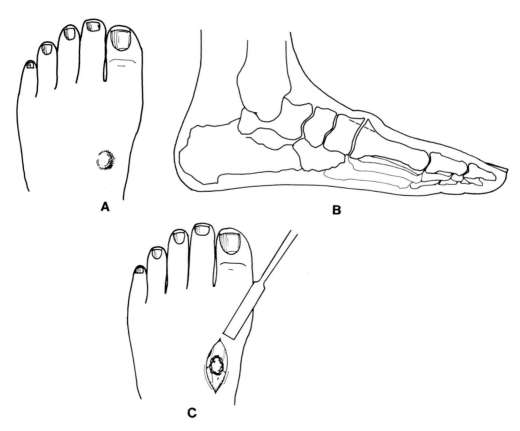

Figure 5–10. Surgical excision of a dorsal exostosis of the first metatarsocuneiform joint. **A,** lateral view shows a
dorsal exostosis of the first metatarsocuneiform joint and its associated soft tissue swelling. **B,** make a longitudinal
dorsal incision directly over the exostosis. Dotted line, line of bone resection. **C,** by carefully retracting the branches
of the dorsal sensory nerve and stripping the joint capsule from the exostosis, the exostosis can be removed with a
small osteotome. Its bony bed is then smoothed with a bone rasp. The joint capsule should be meticulously repaired
to prevent the possibility of subsequent dorsal ganglion formation.

REFERENCES

Dorsal Tarsal and Tarsometatarsal Exostoses

1. DuVries, H.L.: Surgery of The Foot. St. Louis, C.V. Mosby, 1959, pp. 150–151.
2. Giannestras, N.J.: Foot Disorders. 2nd Ed. Philadelphia, Lea & Febiger, 1973, pp. 589–590.
3. Jahss, M.H. (ed.): Disorders of The Foot. Philadelphia, W.B. Saunders, 1982, pp. 722–723.

SURGERY OF THE M-P JOINTS IN RHEUMATOID ARTHRITIS

Incidence

Rheumatoid arthritis affects the forefoot, especially the M-P joints, in at least 90% of its victims, with hallux valgus and hammer toe or clawtoe deformity of the lesser toes being the most common toe deformities. The rheumatoid synovitis of the M-P joints causes joint effusion that distends and stretches the joint capsules and collateral ligaments and produces synovial panus, which erodes the articular cartilage and subchondral bone. This erosion results in a relative lengthening of the joint capsules and collateral ligaments and multiple unstable M-P joints. Spasm and contracture of foot muscles, weight-bearing stress, and the deforming forces of improperly fitted shoes greatly encourage the long toe flexors and extensors to overpower the intrinsic muscles that normally flex the M-P joints and extend the PIP and DIP joints; hyperextension and subluxation or dislocation of the M-P joints and flexion contracture of the PIP and DIP joints results. Similarly, the unstable M-P joint of the great toe favors the overpull of the adductor hallucis over the abductor hallucis to produce a hallux valgus deformity. These typical forefoot deformities of rheumatoid arthritis can also be seen in psoriatic arthritis, systemic lupus erythematosus, and ankylosing spondylitis.

Clinical Symptoms and Signs

Clinical manifestations of rheumatoid arthritis in the M-P joints of the foot depend on the stages of the disease. In the early and acute stage, the M-P joints tend to be warm, swollen, erythematous, tender, and irritable, with synovial thickening and effusion. In the late or chronic stage, hyperextension and subluxation or dislocation of the M-P joints of the lesser toes, depressed metatarsal heads associated with painful plantar callosities and atrophy of the plantar fat pads, painful corns over the dorsal aspect of the PIP joints, end corns at the tips of the lesser toes in association with a fixed flexion contracture of the PIP and DIP joints, metatarsus primus varus, hallux valgus, painful bunion, internal rotation deformity of the great toe associated with a corn under the mediobasal portion of the distal phalanx of the great toe, a planovalgus foot, or even a rocker-bottom flatfoot deformity are the possible clinical findings. Patients with severe rheumatoid foot deformities tend to walk on their heels in an attempt to avoid the pain of putting their forefeet to the ground. They commonly complain of unsteady gait, difficulty in finding suitable shoes to wear, inability to walk any significant distance, and the uncomfortable weight-bearing sensation of "walking on pebbles." Examination of the shoes frequently reveals bulges in the foreparts of the shoes caused by bunions and cocked-up lesser toes. Occasionally, subcutaneous rheumatoid nodules can also be found in the feet of rheumatoid patients; these nodules can cause considerable discomfort when located in the weight-bearing portions of the foot.

Roentgenographic Manifestations

Feet affected by rheumatoid arthritis usually exhibit various degrees of generalized osteoporosis. The great toe frequently shows hallux valgus, metatarsus primus varus, prominent bunion formation, internal rotation deformity along its longitudinal axis with its toenail facing medially, and lateral migration of the sesamoids with subluxation or dislocation of the medial and lateral sesamoidometatarsal joints. The lesser toes commonly show hyperextension and subluxation or dislocation of their M-P joints and hyperflexion of their PIP and DIP joints. Planovalgus deformity of the foot and arthritic changes of the

M-P, metatarsotarsal, intertarsal, subtalar, or ankle joints are frequently present.

Pathologic Anatomy

The joints of the foot affected by rheumatoid arthritis usually show destruction of the articular cartilage by the ingrowth of synovial panus, atrophy and destruction of subchondral bone manifested by a decrease in the thickness and in the number of its bony trabeculae, and proliferation of the synovium with infiltration of many chronic inflammatory cells. The hallux valgus deformity is associated with plantar migration of the abductor hallucis tendon and the medial head of the flexor hallucis brevis, dorsal migration and contracture of the adductor hallucis and lateral head of flexor hallucis brevis, and formation of an adventitious bursa over the dorsomedial aspect of the first metatarsal head. The clawtoe deformity of the lesser toes is accompanied by contracture of the collateral ligaments of the M-P, PIP, and DIP joints; contracture of the dorsal joint capsules of M-P joints and plantar joint capsules of the PIP and DIP joints; contracture of the flexor digitorum longus, extensor digitorum longus and brevis, and interosseous muscles; and hyperkeratotic skin lesions under the metatarsal heads, above the PIP joints and at the tips of the lesser toes.

Nonsurgical Treatment

A. Shoe modifications: wide and comfortable shoes, metatarsal pads and bars, custom-made total contact arch supports, rocker-bottom soles, and stretching of the shoes' uppers to accommodate the bunion and clawtoe deformity can provide some degree of symptomatic relief for painful forefeet in rheumatoid arthritis (Figures 1–4—1–7, 1–12).

B. Padding of the feet and shoes: soft pads of various sizes applied directly to the painful corns and callosities or inserted into the shoes can provide relief (Figures 1–8—1–10).

C. Commercially available foot aids: donut-shaped pads, hallux valgus splints, bunion shields, arch cuffs, hammer toe shields, and toe crests are useful foot appliances for patients with painful forefeet affected by rheumatoid arthritis (Figures 1–16—1–18).

Surgical Treatment

A. Hallux valgus with arthritis of the M-P joint:
   1. Resection of the first M-P joint (Figures 5–11B and 5–12).
   2. Resection of the first metatarsal head (Figure 5–11C).
   3. Resection of the base of the first proximal phalanx (Figure 5–11D).
   4. Fusion of the first M-P joint (Figure 5–11E).
   5. Insertion of a Silastic prosthesis into the first M-P joint (Figure 5–11H).

B. Clawtoe deformity of the lesser toes:
   1. Resection of the four lateral M-P joints (Figures 5–11B and 5–12).
   2. Resection of the four lateral metatarsal heads (Figure 5–11C and H).
   3. Resection of the proximal portions of the four lateral proximal phalanges and the plantar condyles of the four lateral metatarsals, and extensor tenotomies of the four lateral toes (Figure 5–11D–G).

REFERENCES

Surgery of the M-P Joints in Rheumatoid Arthritis

1. Amuso, S.J., et al.: Metatarsal head resection in the treatment of rheumatoid arthritis. Clin. Orthop., *74:*94, 1971.
2. Ananthaknishan, C.V., and Wiedel, J.D.: Forefoot resection in rheumatoid arthritis. A long term follow up. Orthop. Trans., *3:*243, 1978.
3. Barton, N.J.: Arthroplasty of the forefoot in rheumatoid arthritis. J. Bone Joint Surg. [Br.], *55:*126, 1973.
4. Benson, G.M., and Johnson, E.N.: Management of the foot in rheumatoid arthritis. Orthop. Clin. North Am., *2:*733, 1971.
5. Brattstrom, H.: Surgery in metatarsophalangeal joint II–V in rheumatoid arthritis. Acta Orthop. Belg., *58:*107, 1972.

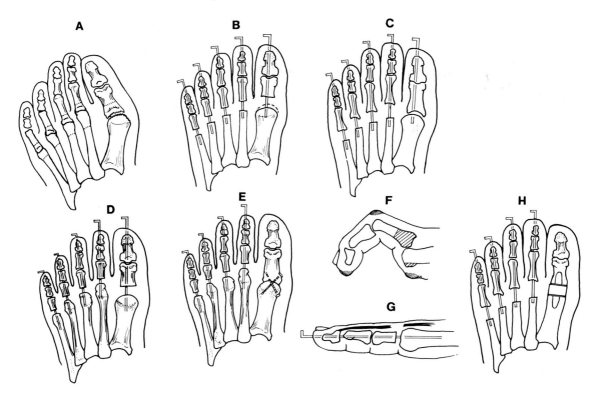

Figure 5–11. Various surgical procedures for the treatment of hallux valgus and multiple clawtoes caused by rheumatoid arthritis. **A,** rhematoid foot shows hallux valgus and arthritis of the first M-P joint, plus dislocation of three middle M-P joints. **B,** resection of the bases of all five proximal phalanges and the heads of all five metatarsals. Each toe is fixed to its corresponding metatarsal with a small smooth K-wire. **C,** resection of the heads of all five metatarsals and alignment of all five toes with their respective metatarsals by using small smooth K-wires. **D,** resection of the bases of all five proximal phalanges, plantar condylectomies, and extensor tenotomies of all four lateral toes. All five toes are fixed to their corresponding metatarsals with small smooth K-wires. **E,** resection of the bases of four lateral proximal phalanges, fusion of the first M-P joint with two mini-screws, plantar condylectomies of all four lateral metatarsal heads, and extensor tenotomies of all four lateral toes. All four lateal toes are aligned to their respective metatarsals with small smooth K-wires. **F,** typical lesser toe affected by rheumatoid arthritis shows dislocation of the M-P joint and flexion contracture of the PIP and DIP joints. Dark elliptical areas, sites of painful corns and callosity; shaded areas, amount of bone to be excised. **G,** same toe as in **F,** after resection of the base of the proximal phalanx and plantar condyle of the metatarsal head; extensor tenotomy; and alignment of the toe with its metatarsal by means of a small smooth K-wire. **H,** resection of the heads of all four lateal metatarsals plus insertion of a Silastic prosthesis into the arthritic first M-P joint. The four lateral toes are fixed to their individual metatarsals with small smooth K-wires.

6. Brattstrom, H., and Brattstrom, M.: Resection of the metatarsophalangeal joint in rheumatoid arthritis. Acta Orthop. Scand., *41:*213, 1970.
7. Calabro, J.J.: A clinical evaluation of the diagnostic features of the feet in rheumatoid arthritis. Arthritis Rheum., *5:*19, 1962.
8. Chand, K.: Rheumatoid arthritis of the foot. Int. Surg., *58:*12, 1973.
9. Clayton, M.L.: Surgery of the forefoot in rheumatoid arthritis. Arthritis Rheum., *2:*84, 1959.
10. Clayton, M.L.: Surgery of forefoot in rheumatoid arthritis. Clin. Orthop., *16:*136, 1960.
11. Clayton, M.L.: Surgery of lower extremity in rheumatoid arthritis. J. Bone Surg. [Am.], *45:*1517, 1963.
12. Dixon, A.S.J.: The rheumatoid foot. *In* Modern Trends in Rheumatology. A.G.S. Hill (ed.). New York, Appleton-Century-Crofts, 1971, pp. 158–173.
13. Dwyer, A.E.: Correction of severe toe deformities. J. Bone Joint Surg. [Br.], *52:*192, 1970.
14. Dwyer, A.E.: The correction of severe toe deformities. J. West. Orthop. Assoc., *7:*19, 1970.
15. Faithful, D.K., and Savill, D.L.: Review of the results of excision of the metatarsal heads in patients with rheumatoid arthritis. Ann. Rheum. Dis., *30:*201, 1971.
16. Fink, F.J., Jr.: Surgery of the foot in rheumatoid arthritis. Semin. Arthritis Rheum., *1:*25, 1971.
17. Flint, M., and Sweetnam, R.: Amputation of all toes: A review of forty-seven amputations. J. Bone Joint Surg. [Br.], *42:*90, 1960.
18. Fowler, A.W.: A method of forefoot reconstruction. J.

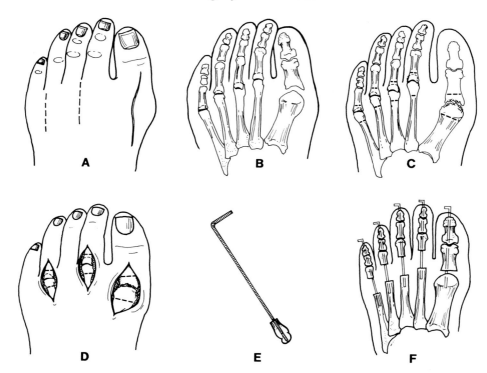

Figure 5–12. Surgical technique for resection of the M-P joints of the foot. **A,** rheumatoid foot with severe hallux valgus and clawtoe deformity. Three longitudinal dorsal skin incisions are shown. **B,** anteroposterior view of the same foot shows hallux valgus and dislocation of three middle M-P joints. **C,** dotted lines, extent of the M-P joint resection. **D,** expose the M-P joints by freeing the attachments of the joint capsules and collateral ligaments from the metatarsal heads and bases of the proximal phalanges. **E,** to facilitate the removal of a metatarsal head that has undergone osteotomy, a Steinmann pin can be inserted into the medullary canal and advanced to the articular surface. By applying steady traction to the pin, the soft tissue attachments to the metatarsal head can be safely and easily detached. **F,** fixation of all five toes to their corresponding metatarsals with small smooth K-wires for 4 weeks maintains the surgical correction and minimizes the chances of osteophyte formation at the ends of the resected metatarsals.

Bone Joint Surg. [Br.], *41:*507, 1959.

19. Funk, F.J., Jr.: Surgery of the foot in rheumatoid arthritis. Semin. Arthritis Rheum., *1:*25, 1971.
20. Gould, N.: Surgery of the forepart of the foot in rheumatoid arthritis. Foot Ankle, *3:*173, 1982.
21. Hoffmann, P.: An operation for severe grades of contracted or clawed toes. Am. J. Orthop. Surg., *9:*441, 1912.
22. Jones, W.N.: Treatment of rheumatoid arthritis of the foot and ankle. *In* Surgery of Rheumatoid Arthritis. R.L. Creuss and N.S. Mitchell (eds.). Philadelphia, J.B. Lippincott, 1971, pp. 87–92.
23. Joplin, R.J.: Surgery of the forefoot in the rheumatoid arthritic foot. Surg. Clin. North Am., *49:*847, 1969.
24. Kates, A., Kessel, L., and Kay, A.: Arthroplasty of the forefoot. J. Bone Joint Surg. [Br.], *49:*552, 1967.
25. Keller, W.L.: Further observations on the surgical treatment of hallux valgus and bunions. N.Y. State J. Med., *95:*696, 1912.
26. Key, J.A.: Surgical revision of arthritic feet. Am. J. Surg., *79:*667, 1950.
27. Kuhas, J.: The foot in chronic arthritis. Clin. Orthop., *16:*141, 1960.

28. Larmon, W.A.: Surgical treatment of deformities of rheumatoid arthritis of the forefoot and toes. Q. Bull. Northwestern Med. School, *25:*39, 1951.
29. Leavitt, D.G.: Surgical treatment of arthritic feet. Northwest Med., *55:*1086, 1956.
30. Lipscomb, P.R.: Surgery for rheumatoid arthritis—timing and technique: Summary. J. Bone Joint Surg. [Am.], *50:*614, 1968.
31. Lipscomb, P.R., Benson, G.M., and Sones, D.A.: Resection of proximal phalanges and metatarsal condyles for deformities of the forefoot due to rheumatoid arthritis. Clin. Orthop., *82:*24, 1972.
32. MacClean, C.R., and Silver, W.A.: Dwyer's operation for the rheumatoid foot. Foot Ankle, *1:*343, 1981.
33. Marmor, L.: Rheumatoid deformity of the foot. Arthritis Rheum., *6:*749, 1963.
34. Marmor, L.: Resection of the forefoot in rheumatoid arthritis. Orthop. Clin. North Am., *108:*223, 1975.
35. McKeever, D.C.: Arthrodesis of the first metatarsophalangeal joint for hallux valgus, hallux rigidus, and metatarsus primus varus. J. Bone Joint Surg. [Am.], *34:*129, 1952.
36. Minaker, K., and Little, H.: Painful feet in rheumatoid

arthritis. Can. Med. Assoc. J., *109:*724, 1973.
37. Newman, R.J., and Fitton, J.M.: Conservation of metatarsal heads in surgery of rheumatoid arthritis of the forefoot. Acta Orthop. Scand., *54:*417, 1983.
38. Preston, R.L.: The Surgical Management of Rheumatoid Arthritis. Philadelphia, W.B. Saunders, 1968.
39. Regnauld, B.: Surgery of the rheumatic forefoot. Acta Orthop. Belg., *35:*557, 1971.
40. Schwartzmann, J.R.: The surgical management of foot deformities in rheumatoid arthritis. Clin. Orthop., *36:*86, 1964.
41. Susman, M.H., and Clayton, M.L.: Surgery of the rheumatoid foot. Ann. Acad. Med. Singapore, *12:*225, 1983.
42. Thomas, W.: Surgery of the foot in rheumatoid arthritis. Orthop. Clin. North Am., *6:*831, 1975.
43. Thompson, T.C.: The management of the painful foot in arthritis. Med. Clin. North Am., *21:*1785, 1937.
44. Tillmann, K.: The rheumatoid foot. Diagnosis, pathogenesis and treatment. Stuttgart, Thieme, 1979.
45. Tillmann, K.: Surgical treatment of the foot in rheumatoid arthritis. Scand. J. Rheum., *9:*257, 1981.
46. Vahvanen, V., Piirainen, H., and Kettunen, P.: Resection arthroplasty of the metatarsophalangeal joints in rheumatoid arthritis. A follow-up study of 100 patients. Scand. J. Rheumatol., *9:*257, 1980.
47. Vanio, K.: Orthopaedic surgery in the treatment of rheumatoid arthritis. Ann. Clin. Res., *7:*216, 1975.
48. Waxman, J.: Joint surgery for rheumatoid arthritis. South. Med. J., *70:*270, 1977.

CLASSIFICATION OF SURGERY OF THE METATARSALS

Although a wide variety of surgical procedures can be performed on the metatarsals, they can be classified into several distinctive groups: Osteotomy—cutting a bone into two halves; ostectomy—removal of a portion of a bone or the whole bone; arthrodesis—fusion of a joint; repair of bony defects; arthroplasty—surgery of a joint with or without insertion of a prosthesis to provide pain relief and/or to improve joint function.

The purpose of this section is to give a bird's eye view on the surgery of all five metatarsals, most of which has been discussed in detail in preceding chapters, and to cover some miscellaneous surgical procedures that are of interest to practicing surgeons.

Osteotomy of the Metatarsals

A. Osteotomy of the first metatarsal: can be performed through the distal portion, midportion, or basal portion, and is most commonly employed in correcting metatarsus primus varus. This osteotomy is frequently performed with removal of plantarly based wedge of bone so to plantar flex this first metatarsal; this restores its normal weight-bearing function, which is often lost when hallux valgus deformity is well established due to the medial and dorsal splaying of the first metatarsal and the subluxation or dislocation of the medial and lateral sesamoidometatarsal joints. When the first intermetatarsal angle is wide and the first metatarsal is short, correction of hallux valgus should take place at the base of the first metatarsal by means of an opening-wedge basal osteotomy so to preserve the length of the first metatarsal and to correct the wide first intermetatarsal angle. There are several surgical techniques for the proximal osteotomy of the first metatarsal:

1. Opening-wedge proximal osteotomy of the first metatarsal by using the excised exostosis (the bunion) from the medial aspect of the first metatarsal head as the wedge-shaped bone graft (Figures 5–13A—E).
2. Opening-wedge proximal osteotomy of the first metatarsal by rotating a bony wedge obtained at the basal portion of the first metatarsal through an arc of 180° (Figures 5–13F and G). This technique is used only when the excised exostosis from the first metatarsal head is not big enough for the bone graft and the first metatarsal is of sufficient length. Similar wedge-shaped bone grafts can be easily obtained from the proximal tibia or the ilium.
3. A crescentic osteotomy of the base of the first metatarsal (see Figure 5–18). In addition, in a low-grade cavus foot in which only the first metatarsal is in a fixed plantar flexion associated with severe metatarsalgia of the first ray, a crescentic or a closing-wedge dorsal angulation osteotomy performed through the proximal portion of the first metatarsal can give significant symptomatic relief to the metatarsalgia. There are

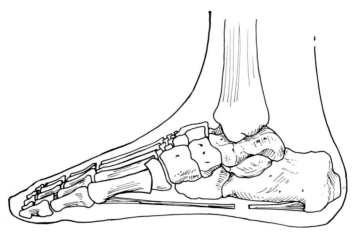

Figure 5–16. A crescentic dorsal angulation osteotomy of all five metatarsals plus release of plantar fascia and the short plantar muscles from the calcaneus for treatment of a cavus foot.

the involved metatarsal.

2. Cavus foot deformity with its apex at the metatarsotarsal joints: can be treated with a straight-line, circular-line, or V-shaped, closing-wedge dorsal angulation osteotomy.

3. A plantarly flexed metatarsal in association with a painful plantar callosity caused by a malunited fracture: can be treated with a dorsal angulation osteotomy.

4. An enlarged lateral condyle of the fifth metatarsal or a laterally angulated fifth metatarsal accompanied by a tailor's bunion and a painful plantar callosity under the fifth metatarsal head: can be treated with a varus and dorsally angulated osteotomy through the fifth metatarsal neck.

5. Resistant varus deformity of the metatarsals in clubfoot: can be treated with a valgus metatarsal osteotomy through their bases.

C. Osteotomy of the first and fifth metatarsals to correct a wide splayfoot can be achieved by a varus osteotomy of the base of the fifth metatarsal and a valgus osteotomy of the base of the first metatarsal to narrow the foot significantly (Figure 5–18).

Osteotomy of the Metatarsals

A. Simple bunionectomy.

B. Exostectomy of the dorsal exostosis of the first metatarsal head.

C. Exostectomy of the dorsal tarsometatarsal exostosis.

D. Resection of the metatarsal head in the treatment of Freiberg's disease.

E. Excision of the lateral condyle of the fifth metatarsal in the treatment of tailor's bunion.

F. Plantar condylectomy of the metatarsal head in the treatment of intractable plantar callosity.

G. Excision of multiple metatarsal heads in the treatment of dislocated M-P joints in rheumatoid arthritis.

H. Excision of the deformed fifth metatarsal head and syndactylization of the fourth and fifth toes in the treatment of a symptomatic dislocated fifth M-P joint caused by excessive resection of the lateral portion

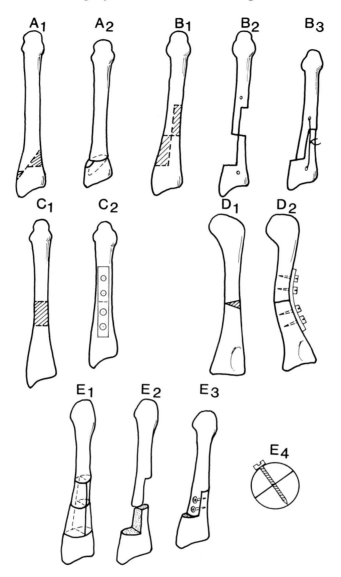

Figure 5–17. Various surgical techniques for shortening metatarsals or for producing dorsally angulated metatarsals in the treatment of intractable metatarsalgia. **A1** and **A2,** telescoping shortening of the metatarsal base. **B1** and **B3,** step-cut shortening of the metatarsal. **C1** and **C2,** segmental shortening of the metatarsal shaft and fixation with a mini-bone plate. **D1** and **D2,** closing-wedge dorsal angulation osteotomy by removal of a dorsally based wedge from the metatarsal shaft and fixation of the osteotomy site with a mini-bone plate. **E1–E4,** oblique step-cut shortening of the metatarsal and fixation with two mini-screws.

of the fifth metatarsal head in treating a tailor's bunion (Figure 5–19).

Arthrodesis of the Metatarsals

A. Arthrodesis of the M-P joint of the great toe: for hallux rigidus, infections, fracture and dislocation of the M-P joint, hallux varus, hallux extensus, and hallux flexus.

B. Arthrodesis of the tarsometatarsal joints: for fracture and dislocation, arthritis, infections, failed fusion, and pes cavus with its

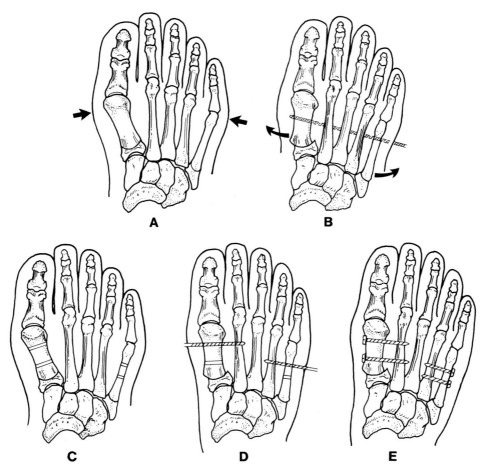

Figure 5–18. Osteotomy of the first and fifth metatarsals to correct a wide splayfoot. **A,** mark the crescentic osteotomy lines on the bases of the first and fifth metatarsals and squeeze the first and fifth metatarsals toward each other. **B,** fix the first and fifth metatarsal necks together with a Steinmann pin before performing the crescentic osteotomy at the first and fifth metatarsal bases. **C,** drill two transverse holes through the shaft portion of the first and fifth metatarsals and mark the crescentic osteotomy lines on their bases. **D,** squeeze the first and fifth metatarsals toward each other. Fix them to the second and fourth metatarsals with two drill bits and then perform the basal osteotomies. **E,** fix the first metatarsal to the second metatarsal and the fifth metatarsal to the fourth metatarsal with the two proximal screws. Withdraw the two drill bits and put in the two distal screws to complete the osteotomies.

apex at the tarsometatarsal joints (Figures 5–20 and 5–21).

Repair of Bony Defects of the Metatarsals

A. Non-unions from fracture and osteotomies (Figures 5–22—5–24).

B. Destruction of the metatarsals by benign bone tumors.

C. Palliative treatment of destruction of the metatarsals by malignant tumors.

Arthroplasty

A. Silastic prosthesis for arthritis of the first M-P joint and treatment of Freiberg's disease.

B. Resection of the base of the first proximal phalanx and/or part of the first metatarsal

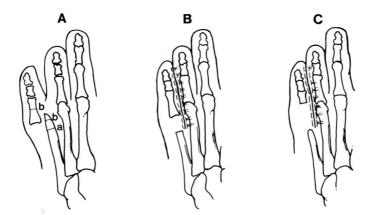

Figure 5–19. Surgical treatment of dislocation of the fifth M-P joint caused by excessive bone resection of a tailor's bunion. **A,** excise the proximal portion of the fifth proximal phalanx and the deformed tip of the fifth metatarsal head, or the whole deformed fifth metatarsal head. **B,** join the fourth and fifth toes after excision of the whole deformed fifth metatarsal head. **C,** join the fourth and fifth toes after excision of the proximal portion of the fifth proximal phalanx and the deformed tip of the fifth metatarsal head.

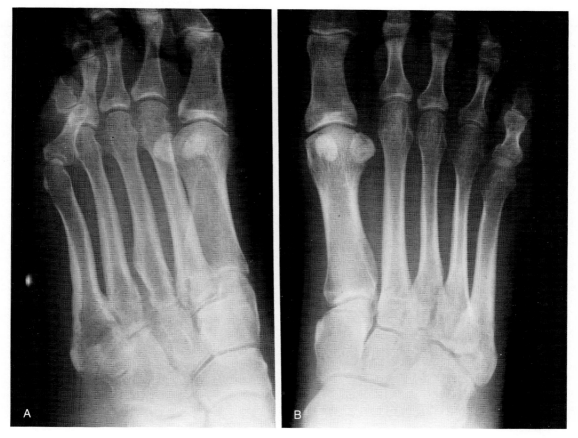

Figure 5–20. A 31-year-old woman who had a failed fusion of her right fifth metatarsocuboid joint as evidenced by the irregular joint space (**A**). **B,** the solid fusion of the fifth metatarsocuboid joint achieved by means of an inlaid iliac bone graft across the arthritic joint.

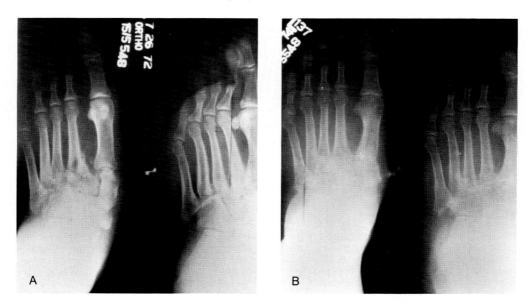

Figure 5–21. **A,** anteroposterior and oblique views. A 35-year-old man sustained a severe fracture and dislocation of his left metatarsotarsal joints in an automobile accident 6 months before being evaluated by the author. Owing to severe rocker-bottom deformity and constant pain of his left foot, he subsequently underwent fusion of all five left tarsometatarsal joints. **B,** anteroposterior and oblique views 2 years later. The tarsometatarsal fusion is still solid and the patient had no left foot symptoms.

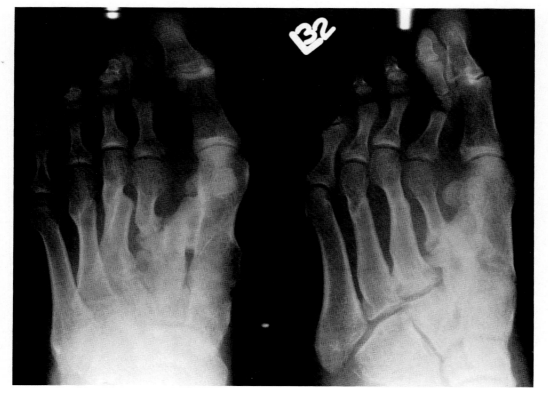

Figure 5–22. A 26-year-old man had a non-union of his left second metatarsal shaft for 6 years. Anteroposterior and oblique views show a solid bony union was achieved by an inlaid iliac bone graft across the non-union site.

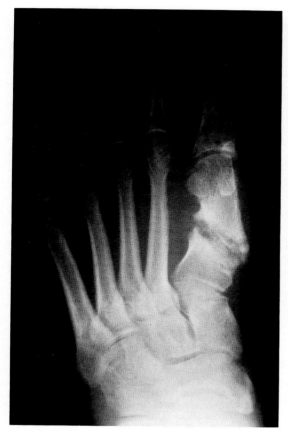

Figure 5-23. A 43-year-old woman underwent an oblique shaft osteotomy of her left first metatarsal for correction of a hallux valgus deformity. A radiolucent line across the osteotomy site in this anteroposterior radiograph is caused by a non-union.

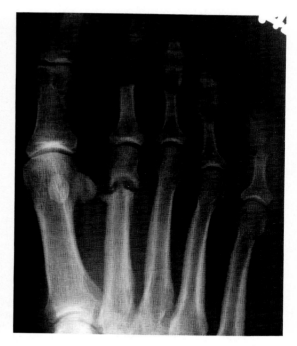

Figure 5-24. A 44-year-old man had an osteotomy of his right second metatarsal neck for treatment of metatarsalgia. An anteroposterior radiograph reveals a bony defect between the head and the shaft of the second metatarsal caused by a well-established non-union, which can be treated by an inlaid bone graft.

head in treating arthritis of the first M-P joint.

C. Resection of the M-P joints or only the metatarsal heads in treating severe arthritis and subluxation and dislocation of the M-P joints caused by rheumatoid arthritis, psoriatic arthritis, and ankylosing spondylitis.

D. Resection of the base of the proximal phalanx of a lesser toe in the treatment of Freiberg's disease and hammer toe.

E. Resection of part or the whole M-P joint of the fifth toe plus syndactylization of the fourth and fifth toes in the treatment of a symptomatic dislocation of the fifth M-P joint caused by excessive resection of the lateral portion of the fifth metatarsal head in the excision of a tailor's bunion.

REFERENCES

Surgery of the Metatarsals

1. Allum, R.L., and Higginson, D.W.: Keller's operation with basal osteotomy of first metatarsal. J.R. Soc. Med., *76:*116, 1983.
2. Amuso, S.J., et al. Metatarsal head resection in the treatment of rheumatoid arthritis. Clin. Orthop., *24:*94, 1971.
3. Artz, T., and Rogers, S.C.: Osteotomy for correction of hallux valgus. Clin. Orthop., *88:*50, 1972.
4. Austin, D.W., and Leventen, F.O.: A new osteotomy for hallux valgus: A horizontally directed "V" displacement osteotomy of the metatarsal head for hallux valgus and primus varus. Clin. Orthop., *157:*25, 1981.
5. Billig, H.E.: Condylectomy for metatarsalgia: Indications and results. J. Int. Coll. Surg., *25:*220, 1956.

6. Bishop, J., Kahn, 3rd. A., and Turba, J.E.: Surgical correction of the splayfoot: The Giannestras procedure. Clin. Orthop., *146:*234, 1980.
7. Bonnel, F., and Barthelemy, M.: Injuries of Lisfranc's joint: Severe sprains, dislocations, fractures. Study of 39 personal cases and biomechanical classification. J. Chir. (Paris), *111:*573, 1976.
8. Bonney, G., and Macnab, I.: Hallux valgus and hallux rigidus: A critical survey of operative results. J. Bone Joint Surg. [Br.], *34:*366, 1952.
9. Bordelon, R.L.: Silicone implant for Freiberg's disease. South. Med. J., *70:*1002, 1977.
10. Bourdillon, J.F.: Metatarsophalangeal fusion for hallux valgus. Can. Med. Assoc. J., *121:*1351, 1979.
11. Cedell, C.A., and Astrom, J.: Proximal metatarsal osteotomy in hallux valgus. Acta Orthop. Scand., *53:*1013, 1982.
12. Clayton, M.L.: Surgery of forefoot in rheumatoid arthritis. Clin. Orthop., *16:*136, 1960.
13. Dewar, F.P., and Rathburn, J.B.: Oblique transposition osteotomy of the first metatarsal for adolescent hallux valgus. J. Bone Joint Surg. [Br.], *35:*663, 1973.
14. Ellis, V.H.: A method of correcting metatarsus primus varus; A preliminary report. J. Bone Joint Surg. [Br.], *33:*415, 1951.
15. Fitzgerald, J.A., and Wilkinson, J.M.: Arthrodesis of the metatarsophalangeal joint of the great toe. Clin. Orthop., *157:*70, 1981.
16. Frieberg, A.H.: Infraction of the second metatarsal bone—a typical injury. Surg. Gynecol. Obstet., *19:*191, 1914.
17. Ganel, A., Chechick, A., and Farine, I.: Chevron osteotomy. Clin. Orthop., *154:*300, 1981.
18. Giannestras, N.J.: Shortening of the metatarsal shaft and the treatment of plantar keratosis and end result studies. J. Bone Joint Surg. [Am.], *40:*61, 1958.
19. Giannestras, N.J.: Plantar keratosis, treatment by metatarsal shortening: Operative technique and end-result study. J. Bone Joint Surg. [Am.], *48:*72, 1966.
20. Giannestras, N.J.: Foot Disorders. 2nd Ed. Philadelphia, Lea & Febiger, 1973, pp. 589–590.
21. Gibbs, R.C., and Boxer, M.C.: Abnormal biomechanics of feet and their cause of hyperkeratoses. J. Am. Acad. Dermatol., *6:*1061, 1982.
22. Golden, G.N.: Hallux valgus, the osteotomy operation. Br. Med. J., *1:*1361, 1961.
23. Groulier, P., and Pinaud, J.C.: Tarso-metatarsal dislocations (10 cases). Rev. Chir. Orthop., *56:*303, 1970.
24. Gudas, C.J.: Compression screw fixation in proximal first metatarsal osteotomies for metatarsus primus varus: Initial observations. J. Foot surg., *18:*10, 1979.
25. Gudmundsson, G., and Robertsson, K.: Silastic arthroplasty of the first metatarso-phalangeal joint. Acta Orthop. Scand., *51:*575, 1980.
26. Haddad, R.J., Jr.: Hallux valgus and metatarsus primus varus treated by bunionectomy and proximal metatarsal osteotomy. South. Med. J., *68:*684, 1975.
27. Harty, M.: Metatarsalgia. Surg. Gynecol. Obstet., *136:*105, 1973.
28. Helal, B.: Metatarsal osteotomy of metatarsalgia. J. Bone Joint Surg. [Br.], *57:*187, 1975.
29. Hoffmann, P.: An operation for severe grade of contracted or clawed toes. Am. J. Orthop. Surg., *9:*441, 1912.
30. Hulbert, K.F.: Compression clamp for arthrodesis of the first metatarsophalangeal joint. Lancet, *1:*597, 1955.
31. Jahss, M.H.: Tarsometatarsal truncated-wedge arthrodesis for pes cavus and equinovarus deformity of the fore part of the foot. J. Bone Joint Surg. [Am.], *62:*713, 1980.
32. Jahss, M.H. (ed.): Disorders of the Foot. Philadelphia, W.B. Saunders, 1982, pp. 722–723.
33. Jeremin, P.J., DeVincentis, A., and Goller, W.: Closing base wedge osteotomy: An evaluation of twenty-four cases. J. Foot Surg., *21:*316, 1982.
34. Lapidus, P.W.: The operative correction of the metatarsus primus varus in hallux valgus. Surg. Gynecol. Obstet., *58:*183, 1934.
35. Leach, R.E., and Igou, R.: Metatarsal osteotomy for bunionette deformity. Clin. Orthop., *100:*171, 1974.
36. Lewis, R.J., and Feffer, H.L.: Modified chevron osteotomy of the first metatarsal. Clin. Orthop., *157:*105, 1981.
37. Lipscomb, P.R.: Arthrodesis of the first metatarsophalangeal joint for severe bunions and hallux rigidus, Clin. Orthop., *142:*48, 1979.
38. Marmor, L.: Resection of the forefoot in rheumatoid arthritis. Orthop. Clin. North Am., *108:*223, 1975.
39. Mayo, C.H.: The surgical treatment of bunion. Ann. Surg., *48:*300, 1908.
40. McDowell, F.: Plantar warts, plantar calluses and such. Plast. Reconstr. Surg., *51:*196, 1973.
41. McElvenney, R.T., and Caldwell, G.D.: A new operation for correction of cavus foot: Fusion of first metatarsocuneiform navicular joints. Clin. Orthop., *11:*85, 1958.
42. McKeever, D.C.: Arthrodesis of the first metatarsophalangeal joint for hallux valgus, hallux rigidus, and metatarsus primus varus. J. Bone Joint Surg. [Am.], *34:*129, 1952.
43. McKeever, D.C.: Excision of the fifth metatarsal head. Clin. Orthop., *13:*321, 1959.
44. Mitchell, C.L., et al. Osteotomy-bunionectomy for hallux valgus. J. Bone Joint Surg. [Am.], *40:*41, 1958.
45. Pelet, D.: Osteotomy and fixation for hallux valgus. Clin. Orthop., *157:*42, 1981.
46. Rogers, J.E., Sharon, S.M., Knudsen, H.A., and Mann, I.: Delayed reduction of a dislocation at Lisfranc's joint: A case report. J. Foot Surg., *16:*162, 1977.
47. Rokkanen, P., et al. Basal osteotomy of the first metatarsal bone in hallux valgus: Experiences with the use of A-O plate. Arch. Orthop. Trauma. Surg., *92:*233, 1978.
48. Samilson, R.L., and Dillin, W.: Cavus, cavovarus, and calcaneocavus. An update. Clin. Orthop., *177:*125, 1983.
49. Simmonds, F.A., and Menelaus, M.B.: Hallux valgus in adolescents. J. Bone Joint Surg. [Br.], *42:*761, 1960.
50. Sollitto, R.J.: SIlicone implant for Freiberg's disease. South. Med. J., *71:*352, 1978.
51. Sponsel, K.H.: Bunionette correction by metatarsal osteotomy: Preliminary report. Orthop. Clin. North Am., *7:*809, 1976.
52. Swanson, B.: Implant arthroplasty for the great toe. Clin. Orthop., *86:*74, 1972.
53. Swanson, A.B.: Flexible Implant Resection Arthroplasty in the Hand and Extremities. St. Louis, C.V. Mosby, 1973.
54. Swanson, A.B., Browne, H.S., and Coleman, J.D.,

The cavus foot concept of production and treatment by metatarsal osteotomy. J. Bone Joint Surg. [Am.], *48:*1019, 1966.

55. Trethowan, J.: Hallux valgus. *In* A System of Surgery. C. C. Choyce (ed). New York, P.B. Hoeber, 1923, p. 1046.

56. Trillat, A., Lerat, J.L., Leclerc, P., and Schuster, P.: Fracture-dislocation of the tarso-metatarsal joint. Classification. Treatment. Apropos of 81 cases. Rev. Chir. Orthop., *62:*685, 1976.

57. Wang, G.J., and Shaffer, L.W.: Osteotomy of the metatarsals for pes cavus. South. Med. J., *70:*77, 1977.

58. Wilson, J.N.: Oblique displacement osteotomy of hallux valgus. J. Bone Joint Surg. [Br.], *45:*552, 1963.

59. Wilson, J.N.: Cone arthrodesis of the first metatarsophalangeal joint. J. Bone Joint Surg. [Br.], *49:*98, 1967.

60. Wolf, M.D.: Metatarsal osteotomy for the relief of painful metatarsal callosities. J. Bone Joint Surg. [Am.], *55:*1760, 1973.

6 SURGERY OF THE TARSAL REGION

CALCANEAL SPUR (PLANTAR FASCIITIS)

Incidence

Calcaneal spur is a bridge of bone that is frequently across the entire width of the anteroinferior edge of the tuberosity of the calcaneus where the plantar fascia, abductor hallucis, flexor digitorum brevis, and abductor digiti quinti attach. It is a wear-and-tear type of osteophyte formation in response to traction forces of the plantar fascia and the intrinsic muscles of the foot, and shows a predilection for overweight middle-aged and older patients. It has been estimated that 15% of adults have calcaneal spurs. Tanz (1963), however, showed that 50% of adults with heel pain had calcaneal spurs of different sizes. This finding suggests that heel spur probably contributes to the plantar heel pain, in spite of the fact that many patients with heel pain do not have heel spurs, and many patients with heel spurs do not have heel pain. It should be noted that os calcis has two bony prominences, the medial and lateral tubercles, on the posterior aspect of its inferior surface that serve as points of origin of plantar fascia and intrinsic muscles of the foot. Beneath these two tubercles is the subcalcaneal bursa, and below the bursa is the thick heel pad. The heel pad consists of strong vertical fibrous septa that run from the thick plantar skin to the periosteum of the inferior surface of the calcaneus and divide the fatty tissue of the heel pad into small and tight compartments (Figure 6–1). A list of the many different causes of heel pain follows.

A. Subcalcaneal bursitis.

B. Plantar fasciitis.

C. Tendonitis of the abductor hallucis, flexor digitorum brevis, and abductor digiti quinti.

D. Periostitis of the calcaneus.

E. Calcaneal spur formation.

F. Subcalcaneal nerve entrapment syndrome.

G. Abnormal foot mechanics, such as a valgus foot, may place abnormal stress on the structures on the medial aspect of the foot to cause medial heel pain.

H. Loss of compressibility of the subcalcaneal fat pad by local fat loss or rupture of fibrous tissue septa.

175

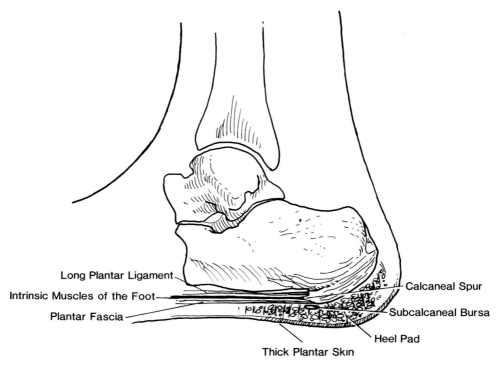

Figure 6–1. Lateral view of the hindfoot shows the relationship of the calcaneal spur with its adjacent soft tissue structures, all of which can produce heel pain.

l. Systemic diseases such as gout, rheumatoid arthritis, ankylosing spondylitis, psoriatic arthritis, Reiter's syndrome, and systemic lupus erythematosus.

The neurogenic cause of heel pain implicates the medial calcaneal nerve, a branch of the posterior tibial nerve, and the nerve to the abductor digiti quinti, a branch of the lateral plantar nerve. Inflammatory reaction due to mechanical stress at the common muscle and fascial origins on the anteroinferior aspect of the calcaneus may irritate the medial calcaneal nerve, which innervates the region of the calcaneal common fascial and muscle origins. The nerve to the abductor digiti quinti runs between the abductor hallucis muscle and the medial one half of the quadratus plantae muscle and crosses the plantar aspect of the foot between the calcaneal spur and the most proximal portion of the long plantar ligament.

It then enters the abductor digiti quinti muscle at its musculotendinous junction, where it is vulnerable to pressure from the calcaneal spur (Figure 6–2).

Clinical Symptoms and Signs

Pain from calcaneal spur is usually located at the medial portion of the heel and is aggravated by prolonged standing and walking. Patients with symptomatic calcaneal spurs frequently complain of significant heel pain on arising in the morning and must limp for some time to let the heel pain subside. This same heel pain tends to recur after periods of sitting, and patients must walk it off or decrease its intensity by walking. Examination usually reveals localized tenderness at the medial tubercle, and occasionally at the lateral tubercle; tenderness can also be present in the proximal portion of the plantar fascia. Passive dorsiflexion of the toes, which increases ten-

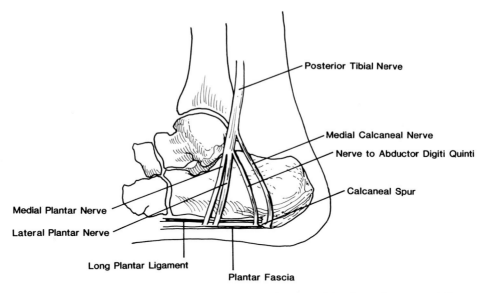

Posterior Tibial Nerve

Medial Calcaneal Nerve

Nerve to Abductor Digiti Quinti

Calcaneal Spur

Medial Plantar Nerve

Lateral Plantar Nerve

Long Plantar Ligament

Plantar Fascia

Figure 6–2. Lateral view of the hindfoot shows the courses of the medial calcaneal nerve and the nerve to the abductor digiti quinti, which can become entrapped to produce neurogenic heel pain.

sion in the plantar fascia and the intrinsic muscles of the foot, may accentuate pain beneath the heel and along the plantar fascia. A large calcaneal spur is usually palpable through the heel pad, and the pain associated with the calcaneal spur is usually nonradiating and ordinarily does not produce paresthesia, which is an important clinical symptom to differentiate a painful calcaneal spur from a tarsal tunnel syndrome.

Roentgenographic Manifestations

The calcaneal spur is best demonstrated by a lateral radiograph of the foot, and almost always points directly forward in the same line of stress as the plantar fascia. On technetium bone scans patients with heel pain show increased uptake of radionuclide at a site corresponding to that of the insertion of the short plantar tendons into the base of the calcaneus; this nuclear medicine study is a useful diagnostic tool in identifying the painful lesion within or around the calcaneus. In the absence of calcaneal fracture, tumors, and infection, sharply increased uptake at the base of the calcaneus usually indicates periostitis associated with plantar fasciitis.

Pathologic Anatomy

The pathologic findings of calcaneodynia (painful heel) naturally depend on its true etiology, which may include plantar fasciitis, tendonitis of short plantar muscles, subcalcaneal bursitis, periostitis of the calcaneus, calcaneal spur formation, subcalcaneal nerve entrapment syndrome, and deterioration of the subcalcaneal heel pad.

Nonsurgical Treatment

The main principle in treating a painful heel is to minimize stress on the painful heel region. There are several useful methods:

A. Soft, custom-made total contact arch supports distribute weight-bearing stress over the entire sole (Figure 1–6).

B. Sponge rubber heels, soft and thick-soled shoes, and ripple-soled shoes to absorb the reaction force from the walking surface (Figures 1–3 and 1–4).

C. A soft heel pad with a depression or a circular cut-out area under the tender spot of the heel (Figure 1–11).

D. A Thomas heel plus a medial heel wedge to invert the heel and to decrease weight-bearing pressure on the medial tubercle of the calcaneus (Figure 1–3).

E. Heel cups reduce the flattening of the heel pad on weight-bearing, allow a more uniform pressure transmission, and tend to shift vertical pressure from the hindfoot to the mid- or forefoot (Figure 1–17).

F. UCBL (University of California Biomechanics Laboratory) Shoe inserts hold the foot in inversion to relieve tension on the plantar fascia by applying forces against the navicular and outer side of the forefoot.

Additional nonsurgical measures in treating a painful heel include weight reduction, anti-inflammatory medications, and injection of a local anesthetic agent and hydrocortisone into the painful heel.

Surgical Treatment

Resection of the calcaneal spur, resection of part of the plantar fascia near its origin, stripping of the soft tissues from the plantar surface of the calcaneus, and excision of the medial inferior tubercle of the calcaneus can be employed when a painful calcaneal spur fails to respond to various methods of nonsurgical treatment (Figure 6–3).

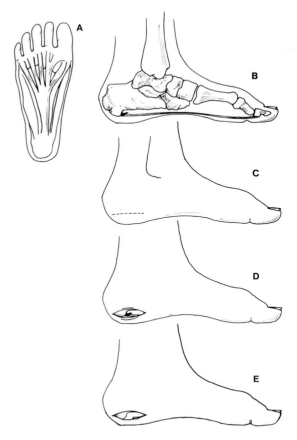

Figure 6–3. Surgical treatment of painful calcaneal spur. **A,** bottom view shows the normal anatomy of plantar fascia. **B,** lateral view shows the relationship of the calcaneal spur with the plantar fascia and short muscles of the foot. **C,** make a short transverse incision on the medial side of the heel at the level of the calcaneal spur. **D,** expose the medial aspect of the calcaneal spur and its associated origins of the plantar fascia and short plantar muscles by carefully protecting and retracting the medial calcaneal nerve. **E,** remove the calcaneal spur and strip the plantar fascia and the short plantar muscles from their origins at the anteroinferior aspect of the calcaneus. Close the incision in a regular manner.

REFERENCES

Calcaneal Spur (Plantar Fasciitis)

1. Ali, E.: Calcaneal spur in Guyana. West Indian Med. J., *29:*125, 1980.
2. Bojsen-Moller, F., and Flagstad, K.E.: Plantar aponeurosis and internal architecture of the ball of the foot. J. Anat., *121:*599, 1976.
3. Bordelon, R.L.: Subcalcaneal pain. A method of evaluation and plan for treatment. Clin. Orthop., *177:*49, 1983.
4. Borovoy, M., and Hertzberg, N.: Pivotal resection of heel spurs in sports medicine: A case study and presentation. J. Foot Surg., *17:*162, 1978.
5. Campbell, J.W., and Inman, V.T.: Treatment of plantar fasciitis and calcaneal spur with the UC-BL shoe insert. Clin. Orthop., *103:*57, 1974.
6. Davies-Colley, N.: Fibroma of plantar fascia. Trans. Pathol. Soc. Lond., *45:*150, 1894.
7. Davis, J.B., and Blair, H.C.: Spurs of the calcaneus in Strumpell-Marie disease. J. Bone Joint Surg. [Am.], *32:*838, 1950.
8. DuVries, H.L.: Heel spur (calcaneal spur). Arch. Surg., *74:*536, 1957.
9. Eggers, G.W.N.: Shoe pad treatment for calcaneal spur. J. Bone Joint Surg. [Am.], *39:*219, 1957.
10. Fairbank, H.A.T.: Dupuytren's contracture of plantar fascia. Proc. R. Soc. Lond. [Med.], *26:*103, 1932.
11. Furey, J.G.: Plantar fasciitis. The painful heel syndrome. J. Bone Joint Surg. [Am.], *57:*672, 1975.

12. Gerster, J.C.: Plantar fasciitis and Achilles tendonitis among 150 cases of seronegative spondarthritis. Rheumatol. Rehabil., *19:*218, 1980.
13. Goetzee, A.E., and Williams, H.O.: Case of Dupuytren's contracture involving hand and foot in child. Br. J. Surg., *42:*417, 1955.
14. Greenberg, L.: Dupuytren's contracture of palmar and plantar fasciae. J. Bone Joint Surg., *21:*785, 1939.
15. Grimes, D.W., and Garner, R.W.: Medial calcaneal neurotomy for painful heel spurs—a preliminary report. Orthop. Rev., *7:*57, 1978.
16. Hassab, H.K., and El-Sherif, A.S.: Drilling of the oscalcis for painful heel with calcaneal spur. Acta Orthop. Scand., *95:*152, 1974.
17. Hicks, J.H.: The mechanics of the foot. II. The plantar aponeurosis and the arch. J. Anat., *88:*25, 1944.
18. Kanavel, A.B., Koch, S.L., and Mason, M.L.: Dupuytren's contracture; with a description of the palmar fascia, a review of the literature, and a report of twenty-nine surgically treated cases. Surg., Gynecol. Obstet., *48:*145, 1929.
19. Katoh, Y., Chao, E.Y., Morrey, B.F., and Laughman, R.K.: Objective technique for evaluating painful heel syndrome and its treatment. Foot Ankle, *3:*227, 1983.
20. Kopel, H.P.: Peripheral Entrapment Neuropathy. New York, Robert E. Krieger, 1976.
21. Lapidus, P.W., and Guidotti, F.P.: Painful heel: Report of 323 patients with 364 painful heels. Clin. Orthop., *39:*178, 1965.
22. Leach, R.E., Diiorio, E., and Harney, R.A.: Pathologic hindfoot conditions in the athlete. Clin. Orthop., *177:*116, 1983.
23. Leach, R.E., Jones, R., and Silva, T.: Rupture of the plantar fascia in athletes. J. Bone Joint Surg. [Am.], *60:*537, 1978.
24. Michele, A.A., and Krueger, F.J.: Plantar heel pain treated by counter sinking osteotomy. Milit. Med., *109:*26, 1950.
25. Myerding, H.W., and Shellito, J.G.: Dupuytren's contracture of the foot. J. Int. Coll. Surg., *11:*595, 1948.
26. Pedersen, H.E., and Day, A.J.: Dupuytren's disease of foot. J.A.M.A., *154:*33, 1954.
27. Przylucki, H., and Jones, C.L.: Entrapment neuropathy of muscle branch of lateral plantar nerve. J. Am. Podiatry Assoc., *7:*119, 1981.
28. Rose, G.K.: The painful heel. Br. Med. J., *2:*831, 1955.
29. Rugh, J.T.: An operation for the correction of plantar and adduction contraction of the foot arch. J. Bone Joint Surg. *6:*664, 1924.
30. Scranton, Jr., P.E., Pedegana, L.R., and Whitesel, J.P.: Gait analysis. Alterations in support phase forces using supportive devices. Am. J. Sports Med., *10:*6, 1982.
31. Sewell, J.R., et al. Quantitative scintigraphy in diagnosis and management of plantar fasciitis (calcaneal periostitis): Concise communication. J. Nucl. Med., *21:*633, 1980.
32. Snook, G.A., and Chrisman, O.D.: The management of subcalcaneal pain. Clin. Orthop., *82:*163, 1972.
33. Steindler, A.: Stripping of calcis. J. Orthop. Surg., *2:*8, 1920.
34. Steindler, A., and Smith, A.R.: Spurs of the os calcis. Surg. Gynecol. Obstet., *66:*663, 1938.
35. Tanz, S.S.: Heel pain. Clin. Orthop., *28:*169, 1963.
36. Taunton, J.E., Clement, D.B., and McNicol, K.: Plantar fasciitis in runners. Can. J. Appl. Sport Sci., *7:*41, 1982.
37. Woolnough, J.: Tennis heel. Med. J. Aust., *2:*857, 1954.

TARSAL COALITION

Incidence

Tarsal coalition is also known as peroneal spastic flatfoot and congenital rigid flatfoot, and is caused by failure of segmentation of the tarsal bones during the embryonic development of the foot. The various forms of tarsal coalition include talocalcaneal, calcaneonavicular, naviculocuneiform, talonavicular, calcaneocuboid, and naviculocuboid coalitions, of which talocalcaneal coalition between the medial articular surfaces of the talus and the sustentaculum tali of the calcaneus, and calcaneonavicular coalition are the most common forms (Figures 6–4A and 6–5). Bone (synostosis), cartilage (synchondrosis), and

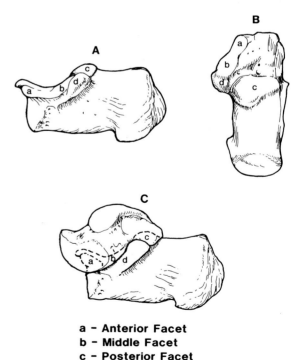

a – Anterior Facet
b – Middle Facet
c – Posterior Facet
d – Sustentaculum Tali

Figure 6–4. The three articular facets of the subtalar joint: anterior, middle, and posterior articular facets.

A	B	C	D	E
Normal Foot	Bony Cuneiform–Navicular Coalition	Bony Naviculocuboid Coalition	Bony Calcaneonavicular Coalition	Fibrocartilaginous Calcaneonavicular Coalition

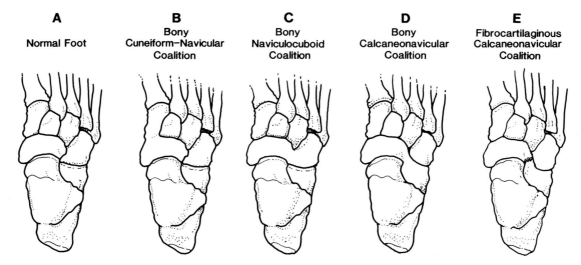

Figure 6–5. Various forms of tarsal coalition.

fibrous tissue (syndesmosis) are the three kinds of tissues found at the sites of tarsal coalitions. It is of interest that Wray and Herndon (1963) reported calcaneonavicular coalition in members of each of three different generations, and Leonard (1974) found a 39% incidence of tarsal coalition in first-degree relatives, as well as an 81% incidence of bilateral involvement of tarsal coalitions of various types. In addition, Kendrick (1972) and Wheeler et al. (1981) described patients with bilateral talocalcaneal and calcaneonavicular coalitions.

Tarsal coalition greatly diminishes or completely eliminates the motion of the involved tarsal joint and disturbs the normal mechanics of the affected foot; secondary foot strain, spasm, and adaptive shortening of the peronei, and degenerative arthritis may result. It should be mentioned that painful peroneal spastic flatfoot can also be produced by trauma, arthritis, neoplasms, and infections of the subtalar joint.

Clinical Symptoms and Signs

Tarsal coalitions are usually asymptomatic during early childhood, but can become symptomatic during late childhood and adolescence when some minor trauma or prolonged and vigorous activities precipitate the onset of foot pain. Such pain is frequently ac-

companied by spasm of the peroneal muscles and rarely of the anterior and posterior tibial muscles. Examination often reveals tenderness over the area of coalition, limitation or absence of subtalar motion, tightness of the peroneal muscles that actively resist active inversion of the heel, and forefoot abduction and pronation. To perform a proper examination of the range of motion of the subtalar joint, the ankle joint should be immobilized in slight dorsiflexion by taking advantage of the peculiar configuration of the superior articular surface of the talus, which is much wider in its anterior than its posterior aspect. In this way, true subtalar motion in inversion and eversion can be adequately evaluated.

Calcaneonavicular coalition can have relatively or significantly restricted subtalar joint motion, and synostosis of the talocalcaneal coalition usually produces complete absence of subtalar motion. Syndesmosis and synchondrosis tend to produce less restriction of the tarsal joint motion than is found with synostosis. When some subtalar joint motion is still present, passive inversion of the heel tends

→

Figure 6–6. A, anteroposterior view of the feet, and lateral (**B**) and anteroposterior (**C**) views of the ankle of a 15-year-old girl show a left bony talonavicular coalition and a ball-and-socket left ankle joint.

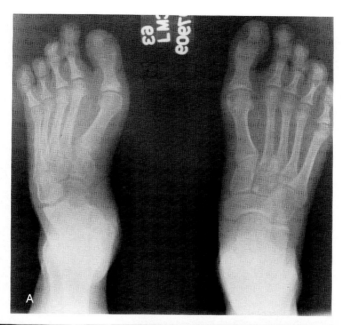

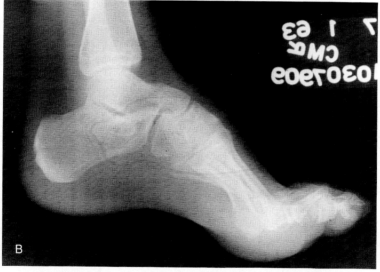

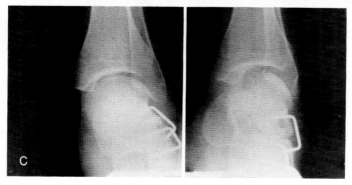

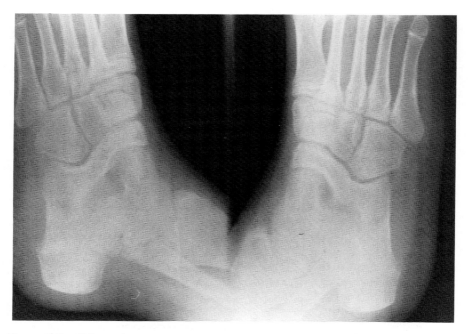

Figure 6–7. Oblique views. A 10-year-old girl with bilateral bony calcaneonavicular coalitions.

to cause the shortened peroneal muscles to contract in a spastic manner to protect the symptomatic subtalar joint. When tarsal coalition is occasionally associated with spasm of the anterior and posterior tibial muscles, a tibial spastic varus foot with tight anterior and posterior tibial muscles and a varus heel can usually be found.

Roentgenographic Manifestations

Although naviculocuneiform, talonavicular, calcaneocuboid, and naviculocuboid coalitions can be seen easily on an anteroposterior radiograph of the foot (Figure 6–6), calcaneonavicular coalition is best demonstrated with an oblique view (Figures 6–7—6–9). The medial and posterior talocalcaneal coalitions are best visualized on an axial (Harris) view (Figures 6–10—6–13), whereas the inconspicuous anterior talocalcaneal coalition can be shown clearly only by regular or computed tomography. The calcaneonavicular coalition is often cartilaginous and is characterized by irregularity, flattening, and osteosclerosis of

the calcaneus and navicular at their junction (Figures 6–8A and 6–9).

When the calcaneonavicular coalition is osseous, the bony trabeculae of the calcaneus and navicular is continuous from one into the other (Figure 6–7). When a bony talocalcaneal coalition is present, axial (Harris) views of the calcaneus show complete obliteration of the medial talocalcaneal joint (Figure 6–10). On the other hand, a cartilaginous or fibrous coalition produces a narrow, irregular, and obliquely oriented medial talocalcaneal joint (Figure 6—11). When regular or computed tomography shows irregularity of the anterior talocalcaneal joint or the undersurface of the talar head, an anterior talocalcaneal coalition is likely to be present. In addition, lateral radiographs of a foot with subtalar coalition are likely to show beaking of the talus secondary to increased stress and motion at the talonavicular joint, rounding of the lateral process of the talus, narrowing of the posterior talocalcaneal space, failure of visualization of the middle talocalcaneal joint, and asymmetry of

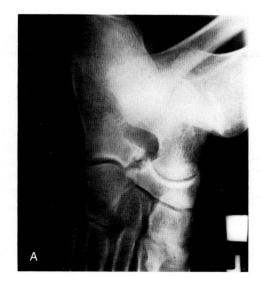

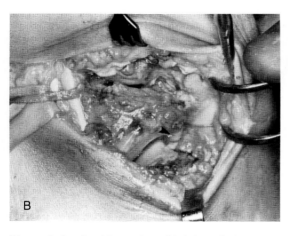

Figure 6–8. **A,** oblique view of left foot; **B,** intraoperative photograph. A 15-year-old boy with a cartilaginous calcaneonavicular coalition (*arrow*), with no detectable arthritis of the midtarsal and subtalar joints, which can be treated with resection of the cartilaginous coalition and insertion of the extensor digitorum brevis muscle into the defect created by the resection.

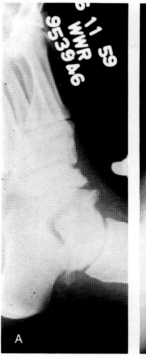
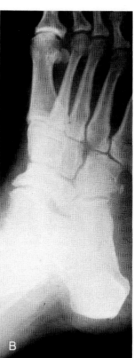

Figure 6–9. Lateral (**A**) and oblique (**B**) views of the right foot. A 29-year-old man with a cartilaginous calcaneonavicular coalition with talar beaking and arthritis of the talonavicular joint, which may eventually require a triple arthrodesis for pain relief.

Pathologic Anatomy

When synostosis is the mode of tarsal coalition, continuity of the bony trabeculae are found at the site of coalition. When synchondrosis has produced the tarsal coalition, hyaline cartilage, fibrocartilage, dense fibrosis, and subchondral osteosclerosis are present. When syndesmosis is responsible, dense collagenous tissue tightly binding the bones involved in tarsal coalition is found during gross and microscopic analysis. In addition, when a tarsal coalition has been present for a long time, arthritic changes such as degeneration of the articular cartilage, synovial proliferation, osteophyte formation at joint margins, and subchondral osteosclerosis are noted in the related tarsal joints due to the presence of excessive motion and stress.

the anterior subtalar joint (Figures 6–14 and 6–15). Furthermore, a secondary ball-and-socket type of joint change (Figures 6–6C and 6–12) may occur in the ankle joint or in the midtarsal joints when subtalar coalition is present.

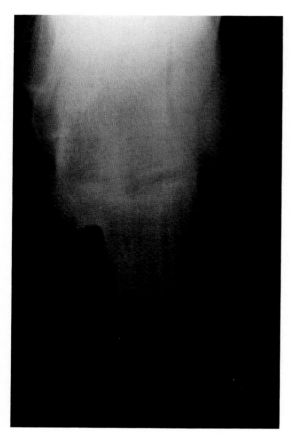

Figure 6–10. A 22-year-old man had a bony talocalcaneal coalition of its middle facet. Axial (Harris) view shows the middle talocalcaneal joint is completely absent.

Nonsurgical Treatment

The aim in the nonsurgical treatment of tarsal coalition is to support and minimize the planovalgus deformity of the foot. Consequently, well-made shoes with a medial heel wedge and Thomas heel, custom-made total contact arch supports, ankle-foot orthoses, and UCBL (University of California Biomechanics Laboratory) shoe inserts can be used to relieve symptoms of painful peroneal spastic flatfoot (Figures 1–3 and 1–6). When foot symptoms are acute a short walking cast with a well-molded arch should be used to speed recovery; the use of oral anti-inflammatory medications may provide further symptomatic relief.

Surgical Treatment

The surgical treatment of tarsal coalition largely depends on the patient's age and the condition of other tarsal joints.

A. In the absence of arthritis of the tarsal joints, calcaneonavicular and naviculocuboid coalitions should be treated with generous resection of the coalition areas (calcaneonavicular and naviculocuboid bars) plus interposition of the proximal portion of the extensor digitorum brevis muscle into the space created by the resection (Figure 6–16).

B. Resection of the medial talocalcaneal coalition is occasionally indicated in an adolescent patient to provide pain relief when the coalition either presses on the medial plantar nerve or causes a mechanical disturbance of the ankle.

C. Symptomatic tarsal coalition in late adolescent and adult patients that fail to respond to various nonsurgical treatments should be treated with triple arthrodesis, especially in those individuals with significant arthritis in other tarsal joints (Figures 6–17—6–19).

REFERENCES

Tarsal Coalition

1. Anderson, R.J.: The presence of an astragaloscaphoid bone in man. J. Anat., *14:*452, 1880.
2. Andreason, E.: Calcaneonavicular coalition. Late results of resection. Acta Orthop. Scand., *39:*424, 1968.
3. Austin, F.H.: Symphalangism and related fusions of tarsal bones. Radiology, *56:*882, 1951.
4. Badgeley, C.E.: Coalition of the calcaneus and the navicular. Arch. Surg., *15:*75, 1927.
5. Bass, S.S.: Naviculo-cuneo-metatarsophalangeal synostoses. Indian J. Surg., *25:*750, 1963.
6. Beckly, D.E., Anderson, P.W., and Pedegana, L.R.: The radiology of the subtalar joint with special reference to talo-calcaneal coalition. Clin. Radiol., *26:*333, 1975.
7. Bentzon, P.G.K.: Bilateral congenital deformity of the astragalocalcaneal joint. Bony coalescence between the os trigonum and the calcaneus. Acta Orthop. Scand., *1:*359, 1930.
8. Bersani, F.A., and Samilson, R.L.: Massive familial tarsal synostosis. J. Bone Joint Surg. [Am.], *39:*1187, 1957.

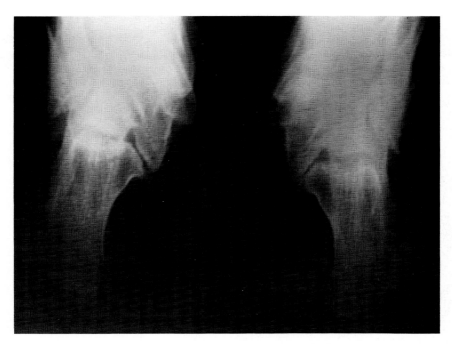

Figure 6–11. An 18-year-old man had bilateral cartilaginous talocalcaneal coalitions. Axial views of both feet reveal obliquity, irregularity, and sclerosis of the middle talocalcaneal articular facets.

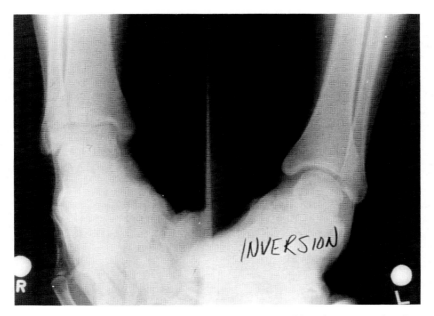

Figure 6–12. A 15-year-old girl had a cartilaginous left talocalcaneal coalition. Anteroposterior views of both ankles show a round top talus in a ball-and-socket ankle joint.

Surgery of the Foot

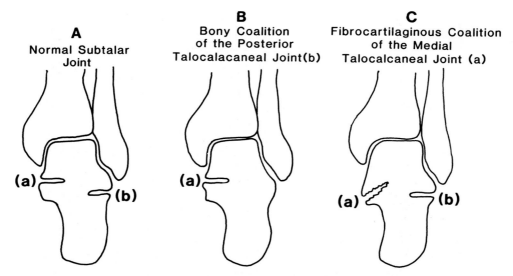

A
Normal Subtalar
Joint

B
Bony Coalition
of the Posterior
Talocalacaneal Joint(b)

C
Fibrocartilaginous Coalition
of the Medial
Talocalcaneal Joint (a)

Figure 6–13. Axial (Harris) view of the calcaneus shows **A** a normal subtalar joint, **B** bony coalition of the posterior talocalcaneal joint, and **C** fibrocartilaginous coalition of the medial talocalcaneal joint.

A Normal Foot

B Talocalcaneal Coalition of its Middle Facet

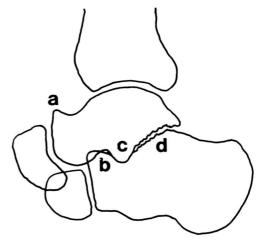

a – Talar Beaking

b – Absence of Visualization of the Middle Subtalar Joint

c – Broadening of the Lateral Process of the Talus

d – Narrowing and Irregularity of the Posterior Subtalar Joint

Figure 6–14. Various radiographic manifestations of talocalcaneal coalition of its middle facet as seen on the lateral view of the ankle.

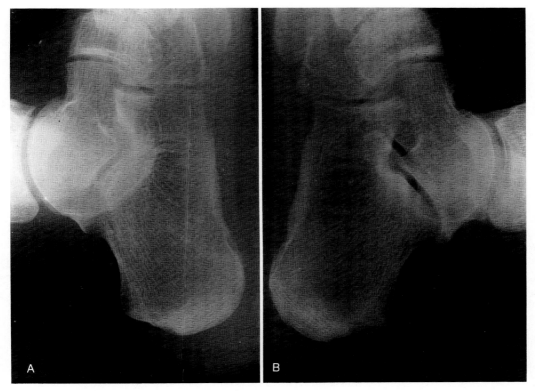

Figure 6–15. Lateral views. Comparison of an abnormal ankle with talocalcaneal coalition of the middle facet (**A**) and a normal foot (**B**) shows absence of visualization of the middle talonavicular joint, broadening of the lateral process of the talus, and slight irregularity and narrowing of the posterior talocalcaneal joint.

9. Blockey, N.J.: Peroneal spastic flatfoot. J. Bone Joint Surg. [Br.], *37:*191, 1955.
10. Boyd, H.B.: Congenital talo-navicular synostosis. J. Bone Joint Surg., *26:*682, 1944.
11. Braddock, G.T.F.: A prolonged follow-up of peroneal spastic flatfoot. J. Bone Joint Surg. [Br.], *43:*734, 1961.
12. Brobeck, O.: Congenital bilateral synostosis of the calcaneus and cuboid and of the triquetral and hamate bones: Report of a case. Acta Orthop. Scand., *26:*217, 1957.
13. Bullitt, J.B.: Variations of the bones of the foot. Fusion of the talus and navicular, bilateral and congenital. Br. J. Radiol., *23:*580, 1950.
14. Challis, J.: Hereditary transmission of talonavicular coalition associated with anomaly of the little finger. J. Bone Joint Surg., [Am.], *52:*1273, 1974.
15. Chambers, C.H.: Congenital anomalies of the tarsal navicular with particular reference to calcaneonavicular coalition. Br. J. Radiol., *23:*580, 1950.
16. Chambers, R.B., Cook, T.M., and Cowell, H.R.: Surgical reconstruction for calcaneonavicular coalition. Evaluation of function and gait. J. Bone Joint Surg. [Am.], *64:*829, 1982.
17. Conway, J.J., and Cowell, H.R.: Tarsal coalition: Clinical significance and roentgenographic demonstration. Radiology, *92:*799, 1969.
18. Coventry, M.B.: Flatfoot, with special consideration of tarsal coalition. Minn. Med., *33:*1091, 1950.
19. Cowell, H.R.: Talocalcaneal coalition and new causes of peroneal spastic flatfoot. Clin. Orthop., *85:*16, 1972.
20. Cowell, H.R.: Diagnosis and management of peroneal spastic flatfoot. Instr. Course Lect., *24:*94, 1975.
21. Cowell, H.R., and Elener, V.: Rigid painful flatfoot secondary to tarsal coalition. Clin. Orthop., *177:*54, 1983.
22. Delsel, J.M., and Grand, N.E.: Cubo-navicular synostosis. A rare tarsal anomaly. J. Bone Joint Surg. [Br.], *41:*149, 1959.
23. Devoldere, J.: A case of familial congenital synostosis in the carpal and tarsal bones. Arch. Chir. Neerl., *12:*185, 1960.
24. Gaynor, S.S.: Congenital astragalocalcaneal fusion. J. Bone Joint Surg., *18:*479, 1936.
25. Glessner, Jr., J.R., and Davis, G.L.: Bilateral calcaneonavicular coalition occurring in twin boys. Clin. Orthop., *47:*173, 1966.
26. Goldner, J.L., and Musgrave, R.: Results of triple arthrodesis for rigid (spastic) flatfeet. South. Med. J., *49:*32, 1956.
27. Gregersen, H.N.: Naviculo-cuneiform coalition. J. Bone Joint Surg. [Am.], *59:*128, 1977.
28. Hark, F.W.: Congenital anomalies of the tarsal bones.

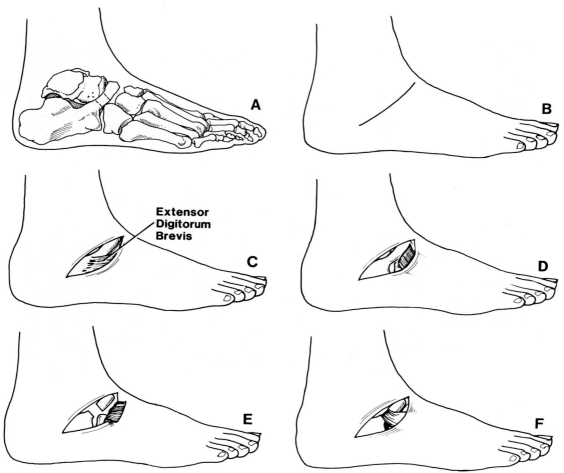

Figure 6–16. Surgical technique for resection of a calcaneonavicular coalition. **A,** lateral view showing a calcaneonavicular coalition. Dotted lines, extent of bone resection. **B,** make an oblique skin incision about 1.5 cm below the tip of the lateral malleolus across the lateral aspect of the calcaneus to the lateral aspect of the tarsal navicular. **C,** strip the origin of the extensor digitorum brevis from the lateral aspect of the calcaneus and retract it forward. **D,** mark the extent of the calcaneonavicular bar to be excised. **E,** remove the calcaneonavicular bar through its entire thickness. **F,** place the origin of the extensor digitorum brevis muscle into the defect created by the resection of the calcaneonavicular bar, and anchor it to either the calcaneus or the navicular before wound closure.

Clin. Orthop., *16:*21, 1960.

29. Harle, T.S., and Stevenson, J.R.: Hereditary symphalangism associated with carpal and tarsal fusion. Radiology, *89:*91, 1967.
30. Harris, R.I.: Rigid valgus foot due to talocalcaneal bridge. J. Bone Joint Surg. [Am.], *37:*169, 1955.
31. Harris, R.I.: Peroneal spastic flatfoot. Instr. Course Lect. *15:* 1958.
32. Harris, R.I.: Retrospect—peroneal spastic flatfoot (rigid valgus foot). J. Bone Joint Surg. [Am.], *47:*1657, 1965.
33. Harris, R.I., and Beath, T.: Etiology of peroneal spastic flatfoot. J. Bone Joint Surg. [Br.], *30:*624, 1948.
34. Heikel, H.V.A.: Coalition calcaneonavicularis and calcaneus secondarius. A clinical and radiographic study of twenty-three patients. Acta Orthop. Scand., *32:*72, 1962.
35. Heiple, K.G., and Lovejoy, C.O.: The antiquity of tarsal coalition. J. Bone Joint Surg. [Am.], *51:*979, 1969.
36. Hodgson, F.G.: Talonavicular synostosis. South. Med. J., *39:*940, 1946.
37. Isherwood, I.: A radiological approach to the subtalar joint. J. Bone Joint Surg. [Br.], *43:*566, 1961.
38. Jack, E.A.: Bone anomalies of the tarsus in relation to peroneal spastic flatfoot. J. Bone Joint Surg. [Br.], *36:*530, 1977.
39. Jayakumar, S., and Cowell, H.R.: Rigid flatfoot. Clin. Orthop., *122:*77, 1977.
40. Kaye, J.J., Ghelman, B., and Schneider, R.: Talo-

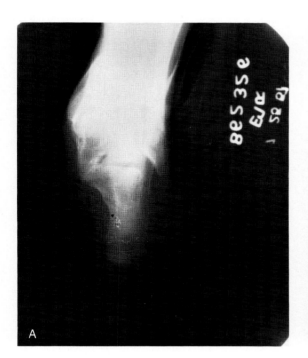

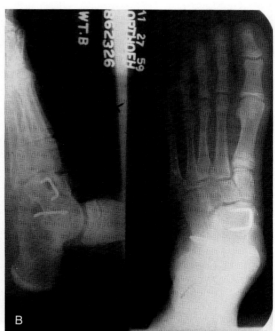

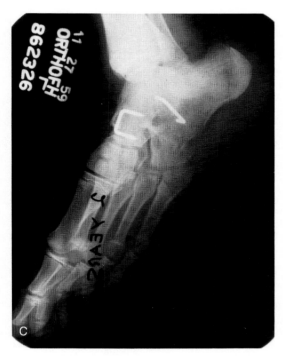

Figure 6–17. **A,** Harris view, **B,** lateral and anteroposterior views, **C,** oblique view. A 13-year-old boy with bilateral symptomatic talocalcaneal coalitions that were not responsive to conservative treatment underwent bilateral triple arthrodesis with good results.

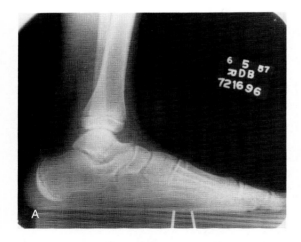

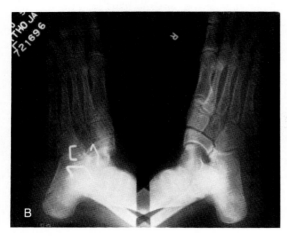

Figure 6–18. A, lateral view; **B,** oblique views. A 13-year-old boy with bilateral symptomatic calcaneonavicular coalitions and talar beaks that failed to respond to conservative treatment had bilateral triple arthrodesis performed on both feet with gratifying results.

calcaneonavicular joint arthrography for sustentacular-talar tarsal coalitions. Radiology, *115:*730, 1975.

41. Kendrick, J.I.: Treatment of calcaneonavicular bar. J.A.M.A., *172:*1242, 1960.
42. Kendrick, J.I.: Tarsal coalitions. Clin. Orthop., *85:*62, 1972.
43. Kyne, P.J., and Mankin, H.J.: Changes in intra-articular pressure with subtalar joint motion with special reference to the etiology of peroneal spastic flatfoot. Bull. Hosp. Joint Dis. Orthop. Inst., *26:*181, 1965.
44. Lapidus, P.W.: Bilateral congenital talonavicular fusion. Report of a case. J. Bone Joint Surg., *20:*775, 1938.
45. Lapidus, P.W.: Spastic flatfoot. J. Bone Joint Surg., *28:*126, 1946.
46. Leonard, M.A.: The inheritance of tarsal coalition and

its relationship to spastic flat foot. J. Bone Joint Surg. [Br.], *56:*520, 1974.
47. Lisoos, I., and Soussi, J.: Tarsal synostosis with partial adactylia. Med. Proc., *11:*224, 1965.
48. Lusby, H.I.J.: Naviculo-cuneiform synostosis. J. Bone Joint Surg. [Br.], *41:*140, 1959.
49. Mahaffey, H.W.: Bilateral congenital calcaneocuboid synostosis. Case report. J. Bone Joint Surg., *27:*164, 1945.
50. Mitchell, G.P., and Gibson, J.M.C.: Excision of calcaneonavicular bar for painful spasmoidic flatfoot. J. Bone Joint Surg. [Br.], *49:*281, 1967.
51. Musgrave, R.E., and Goldner, J.L.: Results of triple arthrodesis for rigid (spastic) flat feet. South. Med. J., *49:*32, 1956.
52. O'Donoghue, D.H., and Sell, L.S.: Congenital talonavicular synostosis. J. Bone Joint Surg., *25:*925, 1943.
53. O'Rahilly, R.: A survey of carpal and tarsal anomalies. J. Bone Joint Surg. [Am.], *35:*626, 1953.
54. Outland, T., and Murphy, I.D.: Relation of tarsal anomalies to spastic and rigid flatfeet. Clin. Orthop., *1:*217, 1953.
55. Outland, T., and Murphy, I.D.: The pathomechanics of peroneal spastic flatfoot. Clin. Orthop., *16:*64, 1960.
56. Pearlman, H.S., Edkin, R.E., and Warren, R.F.: Familial tarsal and carpal synostosis with radial head subluxation. J. Bone Joint Surg. [Am.], *46:*585, 1964.
57. Rankin, E.A., and Baker, G.I.: Rigid flatfoot in the young adult. Clin. Orthop., *104:*244, 1974.
58. Richards, J.F.: Peroneal spastic flatfoot syndrome due to fibrosarcoma. Interclin. Info. Bull., *11:*9, 1971.
59. Rothberg, A.S., Feldman, J.W., and Schuster, O.F.: Congenital fusion of the astragalus and scaphoid: Bilateral, inherited. N.Y. State J. Med., *35:*29, 1935.
60. Sanghi, J.K., and Roby, H.R.: Bilateral peroneal spastic flatfeet associated with congenital fusion of the navicular and talus. A case report. J. Bone Joint Surg. [Am.], *43:*1237, 1961.
61. Schreiber, R.R.: Talonavicular synostosis. J. Bone Joint Surg. [Am.], *45:*170, 1963.
62. Seddon, H.J.: Calcaneo-scaphoid coalition. Proc. R. Soc. Lond. [Med.], *26:*419, 1932.
63. Simmons, E.H.: Tibialis spastic varus foot with tarsal coalition. J. Bone Joint Surg. [Br.], *47:*533, 1965.
64. Slomann, H.C.: On coalition calcaneonavicularis. J. Orthop. Surg., *3:*586, 1921.
65. Slomann, H.C.: On the demonstration and analysis of calcaneo-navicular coalition by roentgen examination. Acta Radiol. [Diagn.] (Stockh.), *5:*304, 1926.
66. Sutro, C.: Anomalous talocalcaneal articulation. Cause for limited subtalar movements. Am. J. Surg., *74:*64, 1947.
67. Swiontkowski, M.F., Scranton, P.E., and Hansen, S.: Tarsal coalitions: Long-term results of surgical treatment. J. Pediatr. Orthop., *3:*287, 1983.
68. Vaughan, W.H., and Segal, G.: Tarsal coalition, with special reference to roentgenographic interpretation. Radiology, *60:*855, 1953.
69. Veneruso, L.C.: Unilateral congenital calcaneocuboid synostosis with complete absence of a metatarsal and the case report. J. Bone Joint Surg., *27:*718, 1945.
70. Wagoner, G.W.: A case of bilateral congenital fusion of the calcanei and cuboids. J. Bone Joint Surg., *10:*220, 1928.

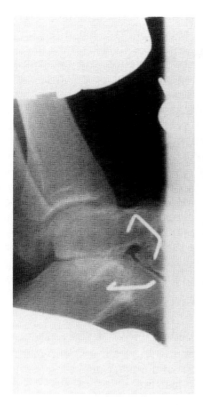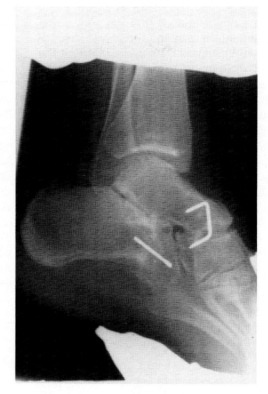

Figure 6–19. A 15-year-old girl with a left bony talonavicular coalition and a ball-and-socket left ankle joint underwent triple arthrodesis (requiring only subtalar and calcaneocuboid fusions) with satisfactory results.

71. Waugh, W.: Partial cubo-navicular coalition as a cause of peroneal spastic flatfeet. J. Bone Joint Surg. [Br.], *39:*520, 1957.
72. Webster, F.S.: Treatment of symptomatic calcaneo-navicular anomalies of the foot. Surg. Gynecol. Obstet., *107:*758, 1958.
73. Webster, F.S., and Roberts, W.M.: Tarsal anomalies and peroneal spastic flatfoot. J.A.M.A., *146:*1099, 1951.
74. Wheeler, R., Guevera, A., and Bleck, E.E.: Tarsal coalitions: Review of the literature and case report of bilateral dual calcaneonavicular and talocalcaneal coalitions. Clin. Orthop., *156:*175, 1981.
75. Wilkinson, R.H.: Tarsal coalition. Postgrad. Med., *47:*69, 1970.
76. Wray, J.B., and Herndon, C.N.: Hereditary transmission of congenital coalition of the calcaneus to the navicular. J. Bone Joint Surg. [Am.], *45:*365, 1963.

TARSAL TUNNEL SYNDROME

Incidence

Tarsal tunnel syndrome is an entrapment neuropathy of the posterior tibial nerve as it goes through the fibroosseous tunnel under the flexor retinaculum (laciniate ligament), which extends from the inferior aspect of the medial malleolus downward and backward to attach to the periosteum over the medial aspect of the calcaneus. The contents of the tarsal tunnel include tendons of the posterior tibialis, flexor digitorum longus, and flexor hallucis longus muscles, and the posterior tibial artery, vein, and nerve. Within the tarsal tunnel or immediately distal to it, the posterior tibial nerve divides into three branches, the calcaneal, lateral, and medial plantar nerves. The calcaneal nerve innervates the skin on the medial aspect of the heel; the medial plantar nerve, the skin and muscles of the medial portion of the sole; and the lateral plantar nerve, the lateral part of the sole and the rest of the plantar muscles. In the tarsal tunnel, the neurovascular bundle is flanked superiorly, anteriorly, and medially by the flexor digitorum longus tendon; and inferiorly, posteriorly, and laterally by the flexor hallucis longus tendon. In addition, fibrous septa from the flexor retinaculum to the periosteum on the medial surface of the calcaneus form individual compartments within the tarsal tunnel. Consequently, the posterior tibial nerve and its branches are relatively fixed in position in the tarsal tunnel and are prone to being compressed. Furthermore, the posterior tibial nerve is richly supplied with arterial blood, making it susceptible to the effects of localized vascular insufficiency, which may produce sensory symptoms.

With an understanding of the anatomy of the tarsal tunnel, it is clear that any disease or condition that reduces the available space of the tarsal tunnel can produce tarsal tunnel syndrome. Fractures or dislocations of the ankle and tarsal bones, tenosynovitis of the tendons in the tarsal tunnel from inflammatory diseases, lipoma, ganglion, osteochondroma

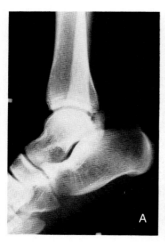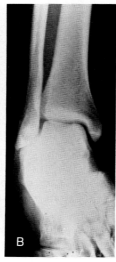

Figure 6–20. Lateral (**A**) and anteroposterior (**B**) views. A 26-year-old man with worsening pain and numbness in the plantar aspect of his left foot for several weeks was found to have an osteochondroma originating in the posteromedial aspect of his left talus and extending directly into the tarsal tunnel. He underwent a decompression of his left tarsal tunnel with removal of the talar osteochondroma through the same incision. His foot symptoms disappeared postoperatively.

(Figure 6–20), post-traumatic fibrosis, neuroma, neurilemmoma, enlarged and tortuous veins, severe planovalgus deformity of the foot, and thrombophlebitis can diminish the tarsal tunnel to cause compression of the posterior tibial nerve. It should be emphasized, however, that in most cases of bona fide tarsal tunnel syndrome, no demonstrable pathologic condition can be found. In addition to the compression of the posterior tibial nerve in the tarsal tunnel, entrapment neuropathy can also occur at the fibrous origin of the abductor hallucis muscle, where the medial and lateral plantar nerves enter the foot. The differential diagnosis of tarsal tunnel syndrome should include interdigital neuroma, sciatic nerve pain, peripheral neuritis, peripheral vascular diseases, and degenerative lumbar disc disease.

Clinical Symptoms and Signs

Patients with tarsal tunnel syndrome often complain of burning pain in the plantar aspect of their feet that is aggravated by prolonged standing and walking and is relieved by rest. They may also experience nocturnal burning pain, which frequently wakes them from a sound sleep; foot massage and hanging the affected feet over the edge of the bed tend to render some symptomatic relief. Occasionally, the foot pain can also radiate proximally along the calf. Physical examination may reveal a positive Tinel sign, tenderness over the course of the posterior tibial nerve under the flexor retinaculum, hypo- or hyperaesthesia in the area innervated by the posterior tibial nerve, muscle weakness and atrophy in advanced cases, diminished two-point discrimination, and occasionally a palpable fusiform swelling of the nerve.

It should be mentioned that a tourniquet test is useful in confirming the clinical diagnosis of tarsal tunnel syndrome. To perform the test, a sphygmomanometer is applied and inflated around the affected leg to produce venous congestion. If the symptoms of tarsal tunnel syndrome are reproduced, the condition can be positively identified. In addition, electromyographic studies frequently show delayed conduction velocity of the posterior tibial nerve at the tarsal tunnel region, and fibrillation and diminished amplitude of action potentials of intrinsic muscles of the foot, which make the diagnosis of tarsal tunnel syndrome a certainty.

Roentgenographic Manifestations

Most feet with tarsal tunnel syndrome show no detectable radiologic abnormalities. If an osteochondroma or a large bony spur is responsible for producing tarsal tunnel syndrome, however, it can easily be seen on routine radiographic analysis.

Pathologic Anatomy

Constriction of the posterior tibial nerve with a proximal fusiform swelling, fibrous band encircling the nerve, intraneural fibrosis, and degenerative changes of nerve fibers, are the common pathologic findings. In addition, tenosynovitis, lipoma, ganglion, osteochondroma, neuroma, and neurilemmoma of the posterior tibial nerve, and, enlarged and tortuous veins are the other possible pathologic

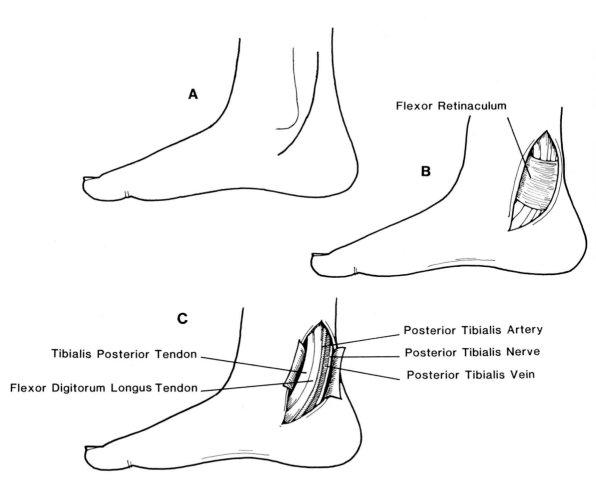

Figure 6–21. Surgical technique for release of tarsal tunnel syndrome. **A,** make a slightly curved skin incision over the tarsal tunnel behind the medial malleolus. **B,** longitudinally transect the entire flexor retinaculum. **C,** perform neurolysis of the posterior tibial nerve from the proximal margin of the tarsal tunnel down to the fibrous origin of the abductor hallucis, where both the medial and lateral plantar nerves enter the foot.

conditions responsible for producing tarsal tunnel syndrome.

Nonsurgical Treatment

The injection of steroids into the tarsal tunnel area may provide some symptomatic relief.

Surgical Treatment

Division of the flexor retinaculum and the small fibrous bands encircling the posterior tibial nerve, and neurolysis of the posterior tibial nerve down to the origin of the abductor hallucis, where the medial and lateral plantar nerves enter the foot through an opening in the fibrous origin of the abductor hallucis muscle by a partial excision of this fibrous tendenous origin, should be performed (Figure 6–21). In addition, tenosynovectomy of the tendons in the tarsal tunnel in rheumatoid arthritis, and excision of lipoma, osteochondroma, neuroma, ganglion, and neurilemmoma in the tarsal tunnel should also be undertaken.

REFERENCES

Tarsal Tunnel Syndrome

1. DiStefano, V., Sack, J.T., Waittaker, R., and Nixon, J.E.: Tarsal-tunnel syndrome. Review of the literature and two case reports. Clin. Orthop., *88:*76, 1972.
2. Edwards, W.G., Lincoln, C.R., Bassett, III, F.H., and Goldner, J.L.: The Tarsal tunnel syndrome. Diagnosis and treatment. J.A.M.A., *207:*716, 1969.
3. Goodgold, J., Kopell, H.P., and Spielholtz, N.J.: The tarsal tunnel syndrome: Objective diagnostic criteria. N. Engl. J. Med., *273:*742, 1965.
4. Haeck, L., and DeConinck, D.: Tarsal tunnel syndrome caused by a talo-calcaneal joint cyst. Case report. Acta Orthop. Belg., *46:*83, 1980.
5. Janecki, C.J., and Dorberg, J.L.: Tarsal-tunnel syndrome caused by neurilemmoma of the medial plantar nerve. J. Bone Joint Surg. [Am.], *59:*127, 1977.
6. Johnson, E.W., and Ortiz, P.R.: Electro-diagnosis of tarsal tunnel syndrome. Arch. Phys. Med. Rehabil., *47:*776, 1966.
7. Keck, C.: The tarsal tunnel syndrome. J. Bone Joint Surg. [Am.], *44:*180, 1962.
8. Kojima, T.: A case of carpal tunnel syndrome associated with tarsal-tunnel syndrome. Tohuku J. Orthop. Traumatol., *7:*214, 1963.
9. Kopell, H.P., and Thompson, W.A.L.: Peripheral entrapment neuropathies. Baltimore, Williams & Wilkins, 1963.
10. Lam, S.J.S.: Tarsal-tunnel syndrome. Lancet, *2:*1354, 1962.
11. Lam, S.J.S.: Tarsal tunnel syndrome. J. Bone Joint Surg. [Br.], *49:*87, 1967.
12. Mann, R.A.: Tarsal tunnel syndrome. Orthop. Clin. North Am., *5:*109, 1974.
13. McGill, D.A.: Tarsal tunnel syndrome. Proc. R. Soc. Lond. [Med.], *57:*1125, 1964.
14. Moloney, S.: Tarsal tunnel syndrome pain abated by operation to relieve pressure. Calif. Med., *101:*378, 1964.
15. Pho, R.W., and Rasjid, C.: A ganglion causing the tarsal tunnel syndrome: Report of a case. Aust. N.Z. Surg., *48:*96, 1978.

ACCESSORY NAVICULAR (PREHALLUX DEFORMITY)

Incidence

Accessory navicular, also known as prehallux, os tibiale externum, and os naviculare secundium, is situated posteriorly and medially behind the scaphoid (navicular) tuberosity. It can exist in three forms:

A. Type 1: a small pea-sized sesamoid embedded in the posterior tibialis tendon, with no direct connection with the tarsal scaphoid.

B. Type 2: a direct connection of the accessory navicular to the tuberosity of the tarsal scaphoid by means of a fibrous or fibrocartilaginous union, with insertion of a portion of the posterior tibialis tendon into the accessory navicular.

C. Type 3: a cornuate scaphoid, probably brought about by fusion of the accessory navicular with the tarsal scaphoid to produce a bony prominence on the medial aspect of the tarsal navicular, to which part or all of the posterior tibialis tendon is inserted.

Normally, one-third of the posterior tibialis tendon inserts into the tuberosity of the navicular, the other two-thirds into the plantar surfaces or the sustentaculum tali, three cuneiforms, the cuboid, and the bases of the second, third, and fourth metatarsals. The extensive insertion of the posterior tibialis tendon acts as a medial sling to support the arch of the foot and to prevent excessive heel valgus. When the accessory navicular receives a major portion of the insertion of the posterior tibialis tendon, the arch-supporting function of the medial sling is lost; the development of a symptomatic flatfoot is then possible. Sullivan and Miller (1979), however, reported a mean calcaneometatarsal angle (a measurement of the longitudinal arch of the foot) of 134.7° in 108 patients without accessory navicular, and a mean calcaneometatarsal angle of 132.6° in 29 patients with accessory navicular, results that suggest the accessory navicular may not be responsible for the development of planovalgus foot deformity. With regard to the prevalence of accessory navicular in the general population, Harris and Beath (1947) and Veitch (1978) reported an incidence of 5%.

Clinical Symptoms and Signs

Clinical symptoms of accessory navicular commonly appear during adolescence or early adulthood. Patients often complain of shoe pressure on the prominent accessory navicular and may have pain in the midfoot from prolonged walking and standing and from wearing narrow shoes. Examination frequently reveals a palpable bony protuberance on the medial aspect of the navicular associated with localized redness, swelling, tenderness, and callus and adventitious bursal formation over the accessory navicular. Swelling and tenderness may also be present in the posterior tibial tendon, which inserts into the accessory navicular, and pain may be produced by inverting the foot against resistance. Planovalgus foot deformity with a fallen longitudinal arch, forefoot pronation and abduction, and heel valgus may also be present.

Roentgenographic Manifestations

Routine radiographs of the foot usually show one of the three forms of accessory navicular, which include a small sesamoid bone embedded in the posterior tibial tendon near its insertion into the navicular, an accessory bone connected with the medial tuberosity of the tarsal navicular with a fibrous or fibrocartilaginous union that is represented radiologically by a smooth radiolucent line, and a horn-like enlargement of the medial navicular tuberosity. When a planovalgus foot deformity is associated with an accessory navicular, medial deviation of the talus with an increased talocalcaneal angle, valgus position of the calcaneus, and a talonavicular sag with loss of the normal height of the longitudinal arch may be present on the foot and ankle films of the involved foot.

Pathologic Anatomy

Microscopic examination of the junction between the navicular tuberosity and the accessory navicular may show organized fibrous tissue, multinucleated giant cells, chondroblasts, chondrocytes, subchondral callus-like reparative tissue, fibrocartilaginous attachment of the accessory navicular to the tarsal navicular, and the presence of inflammatory cells and hemorrhage secondary to direct and repeated trauma to the region. In addition, formation of an adventitious bursa and hyperkeratotic skin over the accessory navicular as well as edematous and inflammatory tissue changes associated with tenosynovitis of the posterior tibial tendon are the other possible pathologic findings.

Nonsurgical Treatment

When an accessory navicular is accompanied by a painful overlying adventitious bursa and a hard callosity, the use of a soft, donut-shaped pad can provide symptomatic relief (Figure 1–8). Accessory navicular associated with symptomatic planovalgus deformity of the foot can be treated with arch supports and shoes with Thomas heels, a medial heel wedge, arch supports, and a stiff shank (Figures 1–3, 1–5, 1–6). When acute symptoms of accessory navicular are present, especially those caused by acute trauma or associated with chronic posterior tibialis tendonitis, a short walking cast with a well-molded longitudinal arch and that holds the heel in a slightly varus position can give significant pain relief.

Warm soaks, gentle massage, rest, crutches, and anti-inflammatory medications are other useful means of nonsurgical treatment.

Surgical Treatment

Surgical treatment of a symptomatic accessory navicular is indicated only when all the

various methods of nonsurgical treatment have failed. The principals of surgical treatment of accessory navicular follow.

A. When an accessory navicular is associated with a painful adventitious bursa and a callosity, but is not associated with a

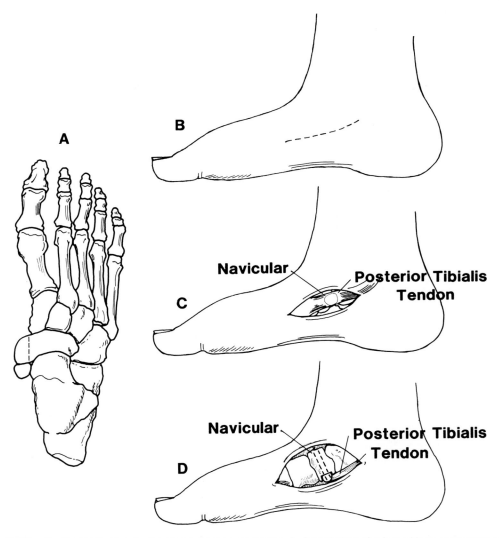

Figure 6–22. Surgical technique for treating accessory navicular. **A,** Dorsal view of a foot with an accessory navicular and a large medial navicular tuberosity. **B,** longitudinal incision directly over the accessory navicular region. **C,** exposure of the accessory navicular and its posterior tibialis tendon. **D,** detachment of the accessory navicular from the medial navicular tuberosity, ostectomy of the enlarged medial navicular tuberosity, and transplantation of the accessory navicular and its posterior tibialis tendon into a hole carved into the undersurface of the navicular. The accessory navicular can then be held tightly to the navicular bone by means of one or two stout sutures that can be passed to the dorsal aspect of the navicular through a drilled hole and tied together.

symptomatic planovalgus foot deformity or a major portion of the insertion of the posterior tibialis tendon, simple excision of the accessory navicular is all that is needed.

B. When an accessory navicular is associated with a symptomatic planovalgus deformity of the foot, receives a major portion of the posterior tibialis tendon insertion, or is in the form of a horn-like enlargement of the medial navicular tuberosity, the excision of which usually results in complete detachment of the navicular insertion of the posterior tibialis tendon, transfer of the posterior tibialis tendon to the under-

surface of the navicular with or without the accessory navicular bone should be performed (Figures 6–22 and 6-23).

REFERENCES

Accessory Navicular (Prehallux Deformity)

1. Basmajian, J.V., and Stecko, G.: The role of muscles in arch support of the foot. J. Bone Joint Surg. [Am.], *45:*1184, 1963.
2. Charter, E.H.: Foot pain and the accessory navicular bone. Ir. J. Med. Sci., *442:*471, 1962.
3. Dwight, T.: Variations of the bone of the hand and foot. Philadelphia, J.B. Lippincott, 1907.
4. Ferguson, Jr., A.B., and Gingrich, R.M.: The normal and the abnormal calcaneal apophysis and tarsal navicular. Clin. Orthop., *10:*87, 1957.
5. Geist, E.S.: The accessory scaphoid bone. J. Bone Joint Surg., *7:*570, 1925.
6. Harris, R.I., and Beath, T.: Army foot survey. National Research Council of Canada, Ottawa, *1:*52, 1947.
7. Jones, R.L.: The human foot. An experimental study of its mechanisms and the role of its muscles and ligaments in the support of the arch. Am. J. Anat., *68:*1, 1941.
8. Leonard, M.H., et al. Lateral transfer of the posterior tibial tendon in certain selected cases of pes plano valgus (Kidner operation). Clin. Orthop., *40:*139, 1965.
9. Kidner, F.C.: The pre-hallux (accessory scaphoid) in its relation to flat foot. J. Bone Joint Surg., *11:*831, 1929.
10. Kidner, F.C.: The prehallux in relation to flat foot. J.A.M.A., *101:*1539, 1933.
11. Monahan, J.J.: The human pre-hallux. Am. J. Med. Sci., *160:*708, 1920.
12. O'Rahilly, R.: A survey of carpal and tarsal anomalies. J. Bone Joint Surg. [Am.], *35:*626, 1953.
13. Ray, S., and Goldberg, V.M.: Surgical treatment of the accessory navicular. Clin. Orthop., *177:*61, 1983.
14. Shands, A.R., and Wentz, I.J.: Congenital anomalies, accessory bones, and osteochondritis in the feet of 850 children. Surg. Clin. North Am., *33:*1643, 1953.
15. Strayhorn, G., and Puhl, J.: The symptomatic accessory navicular bone. J. Fam. Pract., *15:*59, 1982.
16. Sullivan, J.A., and Miller, W.A.: The relationship of the accessory navicular to the development of the flat foot. Clin. Orthop., *144:*233, 1979.
17. Swenson, P.C., and Wilner, D.: Unfused ossification centers associated with pain in the adult. AJR, *61:*341, 1949.
18. Veitch, J.M.: Evaluation of the Kidner procedure in treatment of symptomatic accessory tarsal scaphoid. Clin. Orthop., *131:*210, 1978.
19. Waugh, W.: The ossification and the vascularization of the tarsal navicular and their relation to Kohler's disease. J. Bone Joint Surg. [Br.], *40:*765, 1958.
20. Zadek, I.: The significance of the accessory tarsal scaphoid. J. Bone Joint Surg., *8:*618, 1926.
21. Zadek, I., and Gold, A.M.: The accessory tarsal scaphoid. J. Bone Joint Surg. [Am.], *30:*957, 1948.

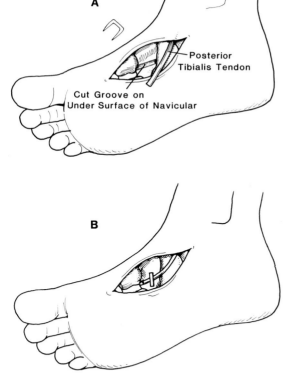

Figure 6–23. An alternative surgical technique for anchoring the posterior tibialis tendon to the undersurface of the navicular. **A,** carve a small groove on the plantar surface of the navicular that is deep enough to receive the detached posterior tibialis tendon. **B,** tightly wedge the posterior tibialis tendon into the groove and hold it in place with a small staple.

PUMP BUMP

Incidence

Pump bump is also known as retrocalcaneal bursitis, Haglund's disease, tendo Achilles bursitis, knobby heel, calcaneus altus, high-prow heel, winter heel, policeman heel, and cucumber heel. It is a bony enlargement on the posterolateral surface of the calcaneus at the insertion of the calcaneal tendon. Pump bump is almost invariably found in women who wear high-heeled shoes with short vamps (pumps) whose closely contoured heel counters press on the posterolateral aspect of the calcaneus, resulting in thickening, enlargement, and inflammation of the tendo Achilles bursa (a subcutaneous bursa superficial to the insertion of Achilles tendon) and the retrocalcaneal bursa (a bursa situated between the posterosuperior border to the calcaneus and the Achilles tendon), and Achilles tendonitis.

There are three anatomic abnormalities that may contribute to the pathogenesis of pump bump: a prominent posterosuperior calcaneal tuberosity, a relatively increased horizontal length of the calcaneus, and a posterior calcaneal step. These abnormalities can cause repeated trauma to the Achilles tendon, producing collagen fiber disruption, decreased tendon vascularity and elasticity, dystrophic calcification, and scar formation, which may eventually lead to rupture of the calcaneal tendon. Pump bump usually shows bilateral involvement with a female to male ratio of approximately 20 to 1. Although pump bump is usually caused by improperly fitting shoes, it is also occasionally found in people who do not wear pumps (or high-heeled shoes) but who have a calcaneus shaped like a hatchet.

Clinical Symptoms and Signs

Although the majority of pump bumps do not produce significant symptoms, patients with symptomatic pump bumps frequently complain of pain in the posterosuperior aspect of the calcaneus when wearing tight and high-heeled shoes. Examination usually reveals swelling, tenderness, redness, and callosity over the posterolateral aspect of the heel at the insertion of the calcaneal tendon (Figure 6–24). When the tendo Achilles bursa has become infected, skin ulceration and the formation of a sinus tract with purulent discharge are likely present. In addition, when Achilles tendonitis is associated with retrocalcaneal bursitis, tenderness and palpable swelling of the Achilles tendon can usually be found.

Roentgenographic Manifestations

The various radiologic abnormalities associated with pump bump are best seen on the lateral radiographs of the foot and ankle; a list follows (Figures 6–25—6–27).

A. A prominent and sharply angled posterior and superior surface of the calcaneus (a hatchet-shaped calcaneus) whose posterior configuration can be measured by means of the so-called Fowler-Phillip angle (an angle formed between the posterosuperior and the plantar surfaces of the calcaneus). According to Fowler and Phillip (1945), this angle ranged from 44 to 62° in normal people, but was greater than 75° in patients with Haglund's disease (pump bump).

B. An oval subcutaneous, soft tissue swelling at the level of the insertion of the Achilles tendon caused by superficial tendo Achilles bursitis.

C. Swelling, loss of sharpness of outline, and calcification of the distal portion of the Achilles tendon caused by Achilles tendonitis. Calcification of the calcaneal tendon is approximately eight times more common in patients with symptomatic heels than in those with normal heels.

D. Obliteration of the sharp interface along the anterior margin of the Achilles tendon (the retrocalcaneal recess) caused by retrocalcaneal bursitis.

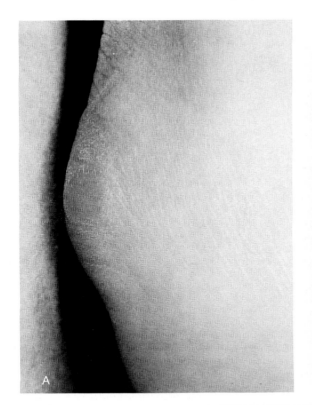

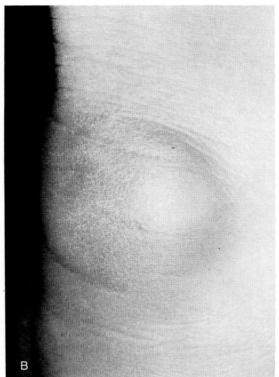

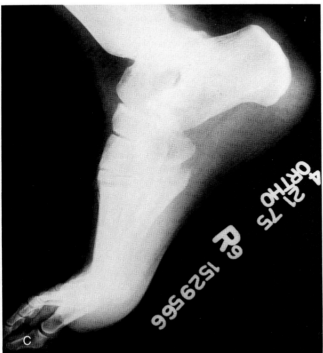

Figure 6—24. A 15-year-old girl with a symptomatic pump bump had an enlargement on the posterosuperior aspect of the right calcaneus (**A** and **B**) associated with redness and hyperkeratotic skin changes. Lateral radiograph (**C**) revealed a prominent posterosuperior angle of the calcaneus.

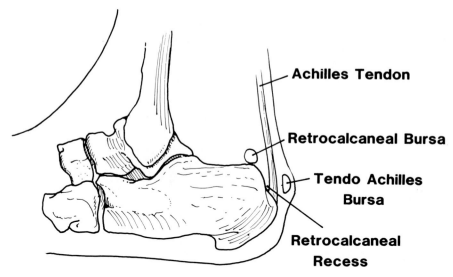

Figure 6–25. Various structures that can be associated with pump bump. Pathologic conditions include tendo Achilles bursitis, Achilles tendonitis, and retrocalcaneal bursitis.

E. A bony step in the middle of the posterior surface of the calcaneus (a posterior calcaneal step).

Pathologic Anatomy

Thickening and swelling of the tendo Achilles bursa, the retrocalcaneal bursa, and the Achilles tendon are accompanied by fibrosis, edema, infiltration of inflammatory cells, dystrophic calcification, and increased intrabursal fluid. Polymorphonuclear leukocytes, tissue necrosis, and bacteria may all be seen when the tendo Achilles bursa becomes infected. Great thickening of the stratum corneum of

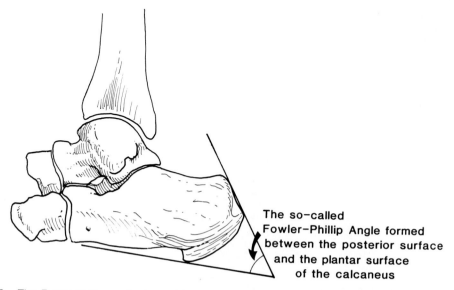

The so-called Fowler–Phillip Angle formed between the posterior surface and the plantar surface of the calcaneus

Figure 6–26. The Fowler-Phillip angle, formed by the posterosuperior and the plantar surfaces of the calcaneus, can be used to measure the degree of prominence of a pump bump.

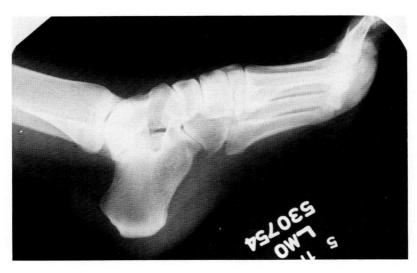

Figure 6–27. Lateral view. A 30-year-old woman with a clinical diagnosis of a pump bump of her left heel had a soft tissue swelling superficial and proximal to the insertion of the calcaneal tendon, indicating the presence of a tendo Achilles bursitis.

the skin is commonly found in the callosity overlying the prominent posterolateral calcaneal tuberosity.

Nonsurgical Treatment

Sandals, open-back shoes, and sling-heel pumps can all be used to eliminate the pressure of the stiff shoe counters on painful pump bumps. In addition, removal of a rectangular portion of the shoe counter over the pump bump area and stiching the margins of the U-shaped cut to prevent separation of the posterior seam can also be employed to relieve painful pump bump (Figure 1–14). Soft U-shaped pads applied directly to the painful pump bump (Figure 1–8) or to the inside of the counter of a shoe directly over the pump bump (Figure 1–11) may provide some symptomatic relief.

Surgical Treatment

A. An ostectomy of the posterosuperior calcaneal prominence to remove enough bone so that the previously palpable calcaneal prominence is no longer present is the surgical treatment of choice. Care should be taken to avoid damage to the attach-ment of the calcaneal tendon. Postoperatively, a walking cast should be used for 4 weeks to protect the weakened calcaneal insertion of the Achilles tendon (Figure 6–28A).

B. A dorsally based, closing-wedge calcaneal osteotomy, can be performed to shorten the horizontal length of the calcaneus and to decrease the Fowler-Phillip angle of the calcaneus at the same time (Figures 6–28B and C).

The surgical technique for removal of a pump bump requires the following steps (Figures 6–29):

A. Make a longitudinal incision parallel and lateral to the Achilles tendon over the pump bump (Figure 6–29A—C).

B. Free the superior and posterior aspect of the calcaneus from the surrounding soft tissues (Figure 6–29D).

C. Remove the posterosuperior calcaneal prominence with a straight osteotome or

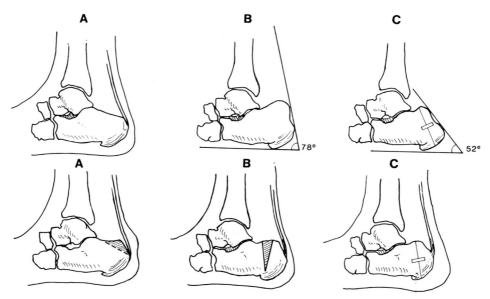

Figure 6–28. Surgical technique for treatment of a pump bump. **A,** osteotomy of the posterosuperior calcaneal prominence. **B** and **C,** performing a dorsally based, closing-wedge calcaneal osteotomy to shorten the horizontal length of the calcaneus and at the same time decrease the Fowler-Phillip angle of the calcaneus.

an oscillating saw (Figure 6–29). Close the skin in a regular manner.

REFERENCES

Pump Bump

1. Berlin, D., Coleman, W., and Nickamin, A.: Surgical approaches to Haglund's disease. J. Foot Surg., *21:*42, 1982.
2. Brahms, M.A.: Common foot problems—heel tuberosities. Heel bursitis. J. Bone Joint Surg. [Am.], *49:*1653, 1967.
3. Cozen, L.: Bursitis of the heel. Am. J. Orthop., *3:*372, 1961.
4. Dickinson, P.H., Coutts, M.B., and Woodward, E.P., and Handler, D.: Tendo Achilles bursitis. J. Bone Joint Surg. [Am.], *48:*77, 1966.
5. DiMonte, P., and Light, H.: Pathomechanics, gait deviations, and treatment of the rheumatoid foot: A clinical report. Phys. Ther., *62:*1148, 1982.
6. Hagergren, C., and Lindholm, A.: Vascular distribution in the Achilles tendon: An angiographic and microangiographic study. Acta Chir. Scand., *116:*491, 1958–1959.
7. Fiamengo, S.A., et al. Posterior heel pain associated with a calcaneal step and Achilles tendon calcification. Clin. Orthop., *167:*203, 1982.
8. Fischer, E.: Soft tissue diagnosis on the extremities using soft tissue radiography. Part II. Diseases of Achilles tendon and the surrounding tissues. Radiologe, *14:*457, 1974.
9. Fowler, A., and Phillip, J.F.: Abnormality of the calcaneus as a cause of painful heel: Its diagnosis and operative treatment. Br. J. Surg., *32:*494, 1945.
10. Fuglsang, F., and Torup, D.: Bursitis retrocalcanearis. Acta, Orthop. Scand., *30:*315, 1961.
11. Gerster, J.C., Langier, R., and Boivin, G.: Achilles tendonitis associated with chondrocalcinosis. J. Rheumatol., *7:*82, 1980.
12. Gerster, J.C., Vischer, T.L., Bennani, A., and Fallet, G.H.: The painful heel. Comparative study in rheumatoid arthritis, ankylosing spondylitis, Reiter's syndrome, and generalized osteoarthrosis. Ann. Rheum. Dis., *36:*343, 1977.
13. Haglund, P.: Beitrag zur klinikder Achillessehne. Aschr. Orthop. Chir., *49:*49, 1928.
14. Keck, S.W., and Kelly, P.J.: Bursitis of the posterior part of the heel. Evaluation of surgical treatment of eighteen patients. J. Bone Joint Surg. [Am.], *47:*267, 1965.
15. Lotker, P.A.: Ossification of the Achilles tendon. J. Bone Joint Surg. [Am.], *52:*157, 1970.
16. Miller, B.F., and Buhr, A.J.: Pump bumps or knobby heels. NZ Med. Bull., *48:*191, 1969.
17. Nielson, A.L.: Diagnosis and therapeutic point in retrocalcaneal bursitis. J.A.M.A., *77:*463, 1921.
18. Nisbet, N.W.: Tendo-Achilles Bursitis ("winter heel"). Br. Med. J., *2:*1394, 1954.
19. Pavlov, H., et al. The Haglund syndrome: Initial and differential diagnosis. Radiology, *144:*83, 1982.
20. Resnick, D., et al. Calcaneal abnormalities in articular disorders. Rheumatoid arthritis, ankylosing spondylitis, psoriatic arthritis, and Reiter syndrome. Radiology, *125:*355, 1977.
21. Roaas, A., and Nilsson, S.: Disorders of the Achilles tendon in athletics. Tidsskr. Nor. Laegeforen., *96:*1606, 1976.

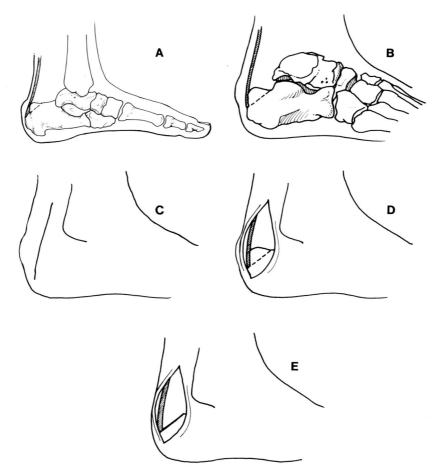

Figure 6–29. Surgical technique for removal of a pump bump. **A** and **B,** medial and lateral views show a prominent posterosuperior angle of the calcaneus. **C,** make a skin incision parallel and lateral to the Achilles tendon over the pump bump. **D,** isolate the prominent posterosuperior calcaneal tuberosity and mark the amount of bone to be removed. **E,** by carefully protecting the Achilles tendon, remove the prominent posterosuperior portion of the calcaneus with either a straight osteotome or an air-driven oscillatory saw. Close the skin in a regular manner.

22. Ruch, J.A.: Haglund's disease. J. Am. Podiatry Assoc., *64:*1000, 1974.
23. Sndenaa, K.: Achillobursitis. A 10-year material with operative treatment. Tidsskr. Nor. Laegeforen., *98:*955, 1978.
24. Steffensen, J.C.A., and Evensen, A.: Bursitis retrocalcanea Achilli. Acta Orthop. Scand., *27:*229, 1958.
25. Zadek, I.: An operation for the cure of Achillo-bursitis. Am. J. Surg., *43:*542, 1939.

CALCANEAL TENDON (TENDO ACHILLES) LENGTHENING

The calcaneal tendon is the conjoined tendon of the gastrocnemius and soleus muscles, and is the biggest and strongest tendon in the human body. To gain a good understanding of the pathologic conditions affecting the calcaneal tendon, a thorough knowledge of the normal anatomy of the gastrocnemius and soleus muscles is of vital importance.

GASTROCNEMIUS MUSCLE (Figure 6–30).

ORIGIN. Its medial head originates from a depression at the proximal and posterior part of the medial femoral condyle and the adjacent part of the femur. Its lateral head is from the posterior aspect and the side of the lateral femoral condyle and the posterior sur-

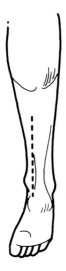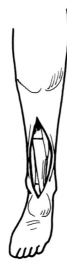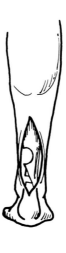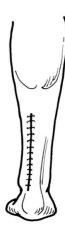

Figure 6–38. Sliding lengthening of the calcaneal tendon is achieved by cutting different fibers of the same Achilles tendon at the proximal and distal partial tenotomy sites so that tendon continuity is maintained at the lengthened position.

Surg. [Am.], *58:*497, 1976.

5. Cameron, H.U.: Symmetrical muscle contractures in tumorous sarcoidosis: Report of a case. Clin. Orthop., *155:*108, 1981.

6. Campos Da Paz, Jr., A., and De Souza, V.: Talipes equinovarus: Pathomechanical basis of treatment. Orthop. Clin. North Am., *9:*171, 1978.

7. Campos Da Paz, Jr., A., De Souza, V., and Conceicao de Souza, D.: Cogenital convex pes valgus. Orthop. Clin. North Am., *9:*207, 1978.

8. Clark, M.W., D'Ambrosia, R.D., and Ferguson, A.B.: Congenital vertical talus: Treatment by open reduction and navicular excision. J. Bone Joint Surg. [Am.], *59:*816, 1977.

9. Conrad, J.A., and Frost, H.M.: Evaluation of subcutaneous heel-cord lengthening. Clin. Orthop., *64:*121, 1969.

10. Cozen, L.: Effect of lengthening the Achilles tendon on the strength of gastrocnemius-soleus musculature. Clin. Orthop., *49:*179, 1966.

11. Craig, J.J., and Van Vuren, J.: The importance of gastrocnemius recession in the correction of equinus deformity in cerebral palsy. J. Bone Joint Surg. [Br.], *58:*84, 1976.

12. Cumminus, E.J., et al. The structure of the calcaneal tendon of Achilles in relation to orthopaedic surgery with additional observation on the plantaris muscle. Surg. Gynecol. Obstet., *83:*107, 1946.

13. Dillin, W., and Samilson, R.L.: Calcaneus deformity in cerebral palsy. Foot Ankle, *4:*167, 1983.

14. Frost, H.M.: Subcutaneous tendo Achilles lengthening. Am. J. Orthop., *256:*257, 1963.

15. Garland, D.E., Lucie, R.S., and Waters, R.L.: Current uses of phenol nerve block for adult acquired spasticity. Clin. Orthop., *165:*217, 1982.

16. Goldwyn, R.M.: Z-plasty skin closure after lengthening of Achilles tendon. Plast. Reconstr. Surg., *52:*431, 1973.

17. Grabe, R.P., and Thompson, P.: Lengthening of the Achilles tendon in cerebral palsies. Basic principles and follow-up study. S. Afr. Med. J., *56:*993, 1979.

18. Green, N.E., Griffin, P.P., and Shiavi, R.: Split posterior tibial tendon transfer in spastic cerebral palsy. J. Bone Joint Surg. [Am.], *65:*748, 1983.

19. Hatt, R.N., and Lamphier, T.A.: Triple hemisection: A simplified procedure for lengthening of Achilles tendon. N. Engl. J. Med., *236:*166, 1947.

20. Hoffer, M.M., and Brink, J.: Orthopedic management of acquired cerebrospasticity in childhood. Clin. Orthop., *110:*244, 1975.

21. Hoover, G.H., and Frost, H.M.: Dynamic correction of spastic rocker bottom foot. Peroneal to anterior tibial tendon transfer and heel-cord lengthening. Clin. Orthop., *65:*175, 1969.

22. Martin, L.W., and Kosloske, A.M.: Heel cord shortening with ganglioneuroblastoma. Am. J. Dis. Child., *129:*254, 1975.

23. McCauley, Jr., J.C.: Operative treatment of clubfeet. N.Y. State J. Med., *47:*255, 1947.

24. McCauley, Jr., J.C.: Clubfoot. History of the development and concepts of pathogenesis and treatment. Clin. Orthop., *44:*51, 1966.

25. Melkonian, G.J., Cristofaro, R.L., Perry, J., and Hsu, J.D.: Dynamic gait electromyography study in Duchenne muscular dystrophy (DMD) patients. Foot Ankle, *1:*78, 1980.

26. Ozonoff, M.B.: Orthopedic procedures in neuromuscular diseases. Radiol. Clin. North Am., *13:*139, 1975.

27. Perry, J., et al. Gait analysis of the triceps surae in cerebral palsy. A preoperative and postoperative clinical and electromyographic study. J. Bone Joint Surg. [Am.], *56:*511, 1974.

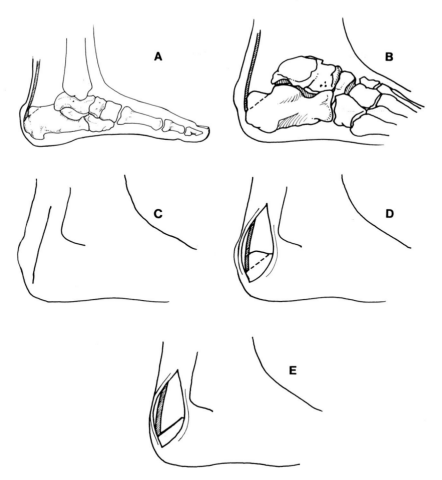

Figure 6–29. Surgical technique for removal of a pump bump. **A** and **B,** medial and lateral views show a prominent posterosuperior angle of the calcaneus. **C,** make a skin incision parallel and lateral to the Achilles tendon over the pump bump. **D,** isolate the prominent posterosuperior calcaneal tuberosity and mark the amount of bone to be removed. **E,** by carefully protecting the Achilles tendon, remove the prominent posterosuperior portion of the calcaneus with either a straight osteotome or an air-driven oscillatory saw. Close the skin in a regular manner.

22. Ruch, J.A.: Haglund's disease. J. Am. Podiatry Assoc., *64:*1000, 1974.
23. Sndenaa, K.: Achillobursitis. A 10-year material with operative treatment. Tidsskr. Nor. Laegeforen., *98:*955, 1978.
24. Steffensen, J.C.A., and Evensen, A.: Bursitis retrocalcanea Achilli. Acta Orthop. Scand., *27:*229, 1958.
25. Zadek, I.: An operation for the cure of Achillo-bursitis. Am. J. Surg., *43:*542, 1939.

CALCANEAL TENDON (TENDO ACHILLES) LENGTHENING

The calcaneal tendon is the conjoined tendon of the gastrocnemius and soleus muscles, and is the biggest and strongest tendon in the human body. To gain a good understanding of the pathologic conditions affecting the calcaneal tendon, a thorough knowledge of the normal anatomy of the gastrocnemius and soleus muscles is of vital importance.

GASTROCNEMIUS MUSCLE (Figure 6–30).

ORIGIN. Its medial head originates from a depression at the proximal and posterior part of the medial femoral condyle and the adjacent part of the femur. Its lateral head is from the posterior aspect and the side of the lateral femoral condyle and the posterior sur-

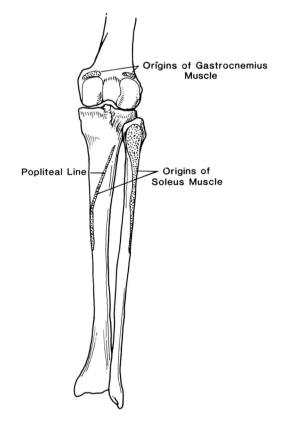

Origins of Gastrocnemius Muscle

Popliteal Line

Origins of Soleus Muscle

Figure 6–30. Origins of the gastrocnemius and soleus muscles.

face of the femur immediately proximal to the lateral femoral condyle.

INSERTION. The middle part of the posterior surface of the calcaneus by means of a conjoined tendon, the calcaneal tendon (tendo Achilles or tendo calcaneus).

ACTION. Plantar flexion and supination of the foot and flexion of the knee joint.

INNERVATION. Branches of the tibial nerve with their origins in the first and second sacral nerves.

SOLEUS MUSCLE (Figure 6–30).

ORIGIN. Posterior surface of the head and the proximal one third of the posterior surface of the body of the fibula, the popliteal line and the middle one third of the medial border of the tibia, and the tendinous arch formed between the tibial and fibular origins of the mus-

cle under which the popliteal vessels and posterior tibial nerve proceed into the lower leg.

INSERTION. Middle part of the posterior surface of the calcaneus through a conjoined tendon, the tendo Achilles.

ACTION. Plantar flexion and supination of the foot.

INNERVATION. Branches of the tibial nerve with their origins in the first and second sacral nerves.

Because the gastrocnemius and soleus muscles insert into the calcaneus through the calcaneal tendon and frequently act as a single muscle, they are commonly referred to as the triceps surae muscle. Owing to the fact that the gastrocnemius muscle spans both the knee and ankle joints, and the soleus muscle traverses only the ankle joint, if the ankle joint cannot be dorsiflexed with the knee in both flexion and extension, the whole triceps surae is contracted and the Achilles tendon should be lengthened. If equinus deformity of the foot is present when the knee is in extension and disappears when the knee is in flexion, however, the deformity is caused by a tight gastrocnemius muscle, and lengthening of this muscle alone should be performed (Figures 6–31).

Although lengthening of the gastrocnemius can be performed at its femoral origins or near its distal insertion into the tendon of soleus to form the Achilles tendon, distal release is usually preferred because it does not alter the shape of the calf, it is simpler to perform, and it is not liable to produce back knee deformity (genu recurvatum). Proximal recession of the gastrocnemius muscle is also contraindicated when the hamstring muscles must be lengthened at a later date, or when on weight-bearing, the knee goes into hyperextension on heel strike.

It should be noted that the position of the foot in the dorsal-plantar plane depends on the balance between the dorsiflexors of the foot, which include the tibialis anterior, extensor hallucis longus, extensor digitorum longus, and peroneus tertius muscles, and the plantar flexors of the foot, which include the

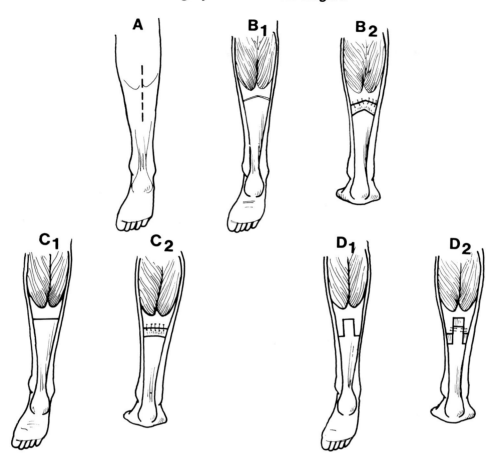

Figure 6–31. Various surgical techniques for performing distal lengthening of the gastrocnemius muscle. **A,** make a posterior longitudinal midline incision in the calf region. **B1** and **B2,** inverted V-shaped lengthening. **C1** and **C2,** transverse lengthening. **D1** and **D2,** tongue-and-groove lengthening.

gastrocnemius, soleus, posterior tibialis, flexor digitorum longus, flexor hallucis longus, peroneus longus, peroneus brevis, and plantaris muscles (Figure 6–32). Whenever the dorsiflexors are overpowered by the plantar flexors of the foot, the foot goes into an equinus position, which if allowed to be present for a significant period will lead to contracture of the triceps surae muscle and eventually the posterior subtalar and ankle joint capsules and ligaments. In addition, because the power of the triceps surae is greater than the combined power of all the dorsiflexors of the foot, whenever the triceps surae is in an advantageous equinus position, it will easily over-come the pull of the dorsiflexors to produce a fixed equinus deformity of the foot. Consequently, many conditions and diseases are capable of producing contracture of the triceps surae muscle that requires lengthening of its tendon.

A. Upper motor neuron diseases, such as stroke, cerebral palsy, myelodysplasia, brain tumors, encephalitis, meningitis, cerebral vascular malformation, and spinal cord tumors.

B. Lower motor neuron diseases, such as

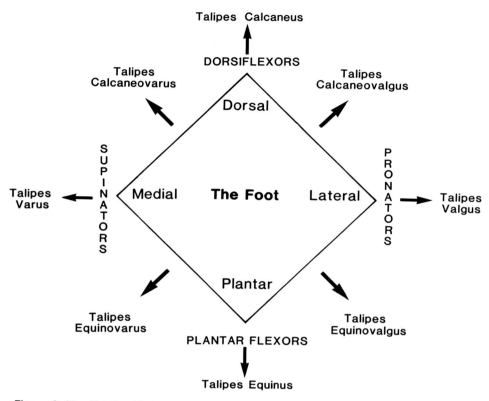

Figure 6–32. Relationship between the various muscle imbalances and the foot deformities.

poliomyelitis, peripheral neuropathies, and injury of the peripheral nerves.

C. Crush injury, fractures, dislocations, and malunited fractures of the lower extremities.

D. Prolonged traction or bed rest with the foot in an equinus position.

E. Prolonged cast immobilization with the foot in an equinus position.

F. Congenital anomalies of the lower extremities, such as arthrogryposis multiplex congenita, congenital short tendo Achilles, talipes equinovarus, pes planovalgus, congenital absence of the fibula, and congenital vertical talus.

G. Amputation through the tarsometatarsal and intertarsal joints.

H. Different muscular dystrophies and myopathies.

I. Pseudarthrosis of the tibia secondary to neurofibromatosis.

J. Leprosy.

K. En block resection of malignant soft tissue tumors of the anterior tibial compartment.

L. Improper transfer of the anterior tibial muscles to other parts of the foot or lower leg.

M. Surgical limb lengthening.

N. Rheumatoid arthritis.

O. Tumorous sarcoidosis.

P. Volkmann's ischemic contracture of the lower extremity.

Q. Postsurgical complication of tibial osteotomy.

R. Constricting bands of the lower leg (Streeter's dysplasia).

S. Burns.

Several surgical techniques are available for lengthening the calcaneal tendon.

A. Closed subcutaneous Achilles tendon lengthening: produces virtually invisible scars and minimal chances of postoperative wound infection, but requires precise placement of the sharp tenotomy knife blade to avoid damage to the nearby important neurovascular structures (Figure 6–33).

B. Z-plasty lengthening of the tendo Achilles: probably the most commonly used method. Technique should include a proximal and lateral cut and a distal and medial cut to help correct a varus heel, and a proximal

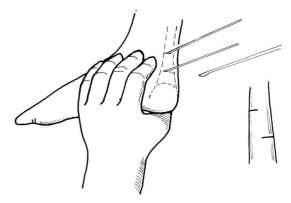

Figure 6–33. Closed subcutaneous Achilles tendon lengthening can be performed by partially cutting the Achilles tendon at two different levels from opposite directions. The foot is then forcefully dorsiflexed to allow the cut portions of the Achilles tendon to slide past each other to achieve the desired degree of calcaneal tendon lengthening.

and medial cut and a distal and lateral cut to help correct a heel valgus (Figures 6–34).

C. Multiple-level Achilles tendon lengthening: takes advantage of the fact that the fibers of the calcaneal tendon are arranged in a longitudinally spiral fashion in that the

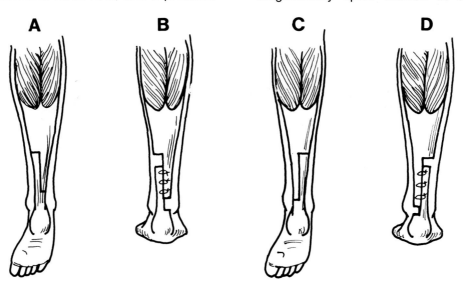

Figure 6–34. Z-plasty lengthening of the Achilles tendon. **A** and **B,** promixal and lateral cut coupled with a distal and medial cut can help the dynamic correction of a varus heel. **C** and **D,** proximal and medial cut coupled with a distal and lateral cut can help the dynamic correction of a valgus heel.

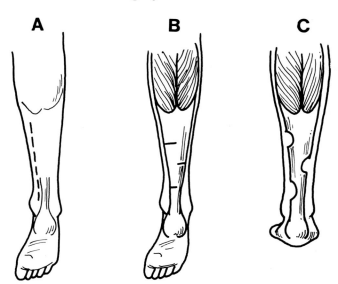

Figure 6–35. Spiral arrangement of the fibers in the Achilles tendon allows the intact and cut fibers to slide past each other and maintain continuity, in spite of the fact that several partial transverse cuts have been made at different levels of the Achilles tendon.

multiple-level partial transverse cuts allow the intact and transected fibers to slide past each other to gain extra tendon length (Figures 6–35).

D. Coronal lengthening of the tendo calcaneus: allows rapid healing of the length-

ened tendon due to the large area of contact of raw tendon surfaces. This technique should be used when the heel is in a neutral position (Figures 6–36A and 6–37).

E. Sliding lengthening of the calcaneal tendon: takes advantage of the longitudinally

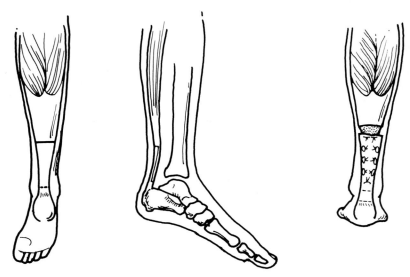

Figure 6–36. Coronal lengthening of the Achilles tendon allows rapid healing but does not help the dynamic correction of heel varus or valgus.

spiral arrangement of the fibers of the calcaneal tendon to achieve tendon lengthening without producing complete tendon
disruption (Figure 6–38).

F. Lengthening of the tendo Achilles in combination with posterior capsulotomy of the
ankle and subtalar joints: should be performed when the foot still cannot be dorsiflexed after tendo Achilles lengthening
(Figure 6–39).

REFERENCES

Calcaneal Tendon Lengthening

1. Baker, L.D.: A rational approach to surgical needs of
   the cerebral palsy patient. J. Bone Joint Surg. [Am.],
   38:313, 1956.
2. Banks, H.H.: The management of spastic deformities
   of the foot and ankle. Clin. Orthop., *122*:70, 1977.
3. Banks, H., and Green. W.: The correction of equinus
   deformity in cerebral palsy. J. Bone Joint Surg. [Am.],
   40:1359, 1958.
4. Bisla, R.S., Louis, H.J., and Albano, P.: Transfer of
   tibialis posterior tendon in cerebral palsy. J. Bone Joint

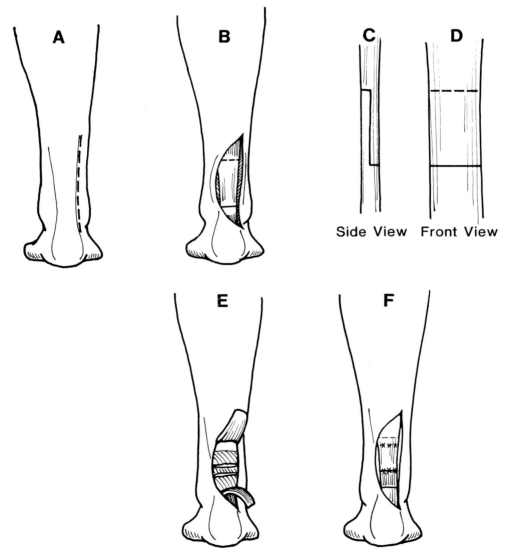

Side View   Front View

Figure 6–37. A–F Coronal lengthening of the tendo Achilles. When the posterior ankle and subtalar joints are contracted, their capsulotomies should be performed in addition to the tendo Achilles lengthening.

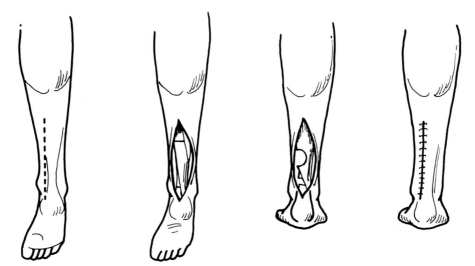

Figure 6–38. Sliding lengthening of the calcaneal tendon is achieved by cutting different fibers of the same Achilles tendon at the proximal and distal partial tenotomy sites so that tendon continuity is maintained at the lengthened position.

Surg. [Am.], *58:*497, 1976.

5. Cameron, H.U.: Symmetrical muscle contractures in tumorous sarcoidosis: Report of a case. Clin. Orthop., *155:*108, 1981.

6. Campos Da Paz, Jr., A., and De Souza, V.: Talipes equinovarus: Pathomechanical basis of treatment. Orthop. Clin. North Am., *9:*171, 1978.

7. Campos Da Paz, Jr., A., De Souza, V., and Conceicao de Souza, D.: Cogenital convex pes valgus. Orthop. Clin. North Am., *9:*207, 1978.

8. Clark, M.W., D'Ambrosia, R.D., and Ferguson, A.B.: Congenital vertical talus: Treatment by open reduction and navicular excision. J. Bone Joint Surg. [Am.], *59:*816, 1977.

9. Conrad, J.A., and Frost, H.M.: Evaluation of subcutaneous heel-cord lengthening. Clin. Orthop., *64:*121, 1969.

10. Cozen, L.: Effect of lengthening the Achilles tendon on the strength of gastrocnemius-soleus musculature. Clin. Orthop., *49:*179, 1966.

11. Craig, J.J., and Van Vuren, J.: The importance of gastrocnemius recession in the correction of equinus deformity in cerebral palsy. J. Bone Joint Surg. [Br.], *58:*84, 1976.

12. Cumminus, E.J., et al. The structure of the calcaneal tendon of Achilles in relation to orthopaedic surgery with additional observation on the plantaris muscle. Surg. Gynecol. Obstet., *83:*107, 1946.

13. Dillin, W., and Samilson, R.L.: Calcaneus deformity in cerebral palsy. Foot Ankle, *4:*167, 1983.

14. Frost, H.M.: Subcutaneous tendo Achilles lengthening. Am. J. Orthop., *256:*257, 1963.

15. Garland, D.E., Lucie, R.S., and Waters, R.L.: Current uses of phenol nerve block for adult acquired spasticity. Clin. Orthop., *165:*217, 1982.

16. Goldwyn, R.M.: Z-plasty skin closure after length-

ening of Achilles tendon. Plast. Reconstr. Surg., *52:*431, 1973.

17. Grabe, R.P., and Thompson, P.: Lengthening of the Achilles tendon in cerebral palsies. Basic principles and follow-up study. S. Afr. Med. J., *56:*993, 1979.

18. Green, N.E., Griffin, P.P., and Shiavi, R.: Split posterior tibial tendon transfer in spastic cerebral palsy. J. Bone Joint Surg. [Am.], *65:*748, 1983.

19. Hatt, R.N., and Lamphier, T.A.: Triple hemisection: A simplified procedure for lengthening of Achilles tendon. N. Engl. J. Med., *236:*166, 1947.

20. Hoffer, M.M., and Brink, J.: Orthopedic management of acquired cerebrospasticity in childhood. Clin. Orthop., *110:*244, 1975.

21. Hoover, G.H., and Frost, H.M.: Dynamic correction of spastic rocker bottom foot. Peroneal to anterior tibial tendon transfer and heel-cord lengthening. Clin. Orthop., *65:*175, 1969.

22. Martin, L.W., and Kosloske, A.M.: Heel cord shortening with ganglioneuroblastoma. Am. J. Dis. Child., *129:*254, 1975.

23. McCauley, Jr., J.C.: Operative treatment of clubfeet. N.Y. State J. Med., *47:*255, 1947.

24. McCauley, Jr., J.C.: Clubfoot. History of the development and concepts of pathogenesis and treatment. Clin. Orthop., *44:*51, 1966.

25. Melkonian, G.J., Cristofaro, R.L., Perry, J., and Hsu, J.D.: Dynamic gait electromyography study in Duchenne muscular dystrophy (DMD) patients. Foot Ankle, *1:*78, 1980.

26. Ozonoff, M.B.: Orthopedic procedures in neuromuscular diseases. Radiol. Clin. North Am., *13:*139, 1975.

27. Perry, J., et al. Gait analysis of the triceps surae in cerebral palsy. A preoperative and postoperative clinical and electromyographic study. J. Bone Joint Surg. [Am.], *56:*511, 1974.

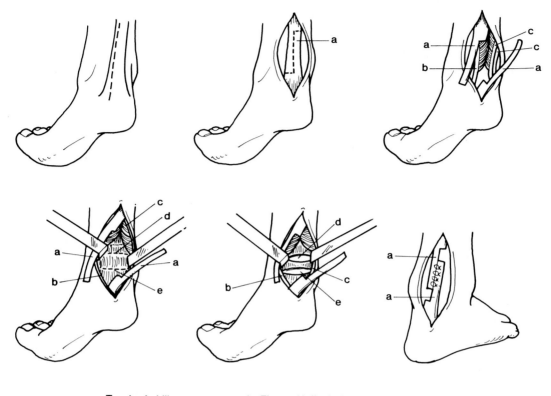

a- Tendo Achilles   b-Flexor Hallucis Longus

c- Peroneal Tendons   d-Posterior Aspect of Ankle Joint

e- Posterior Aspect of Subtalar Joint

Figure 6–39. Capsulotomy of the posterior ankle and subtalar joints should be performed if they are contracted to allow dorsiflexion of the ankle after Achilles tendon lengthening.

28. Pollock, G.A.: Lengthening of the gastrocnemius tendons in cases of spastic equinus deformity. J. Bone Joint Surg. [Br.], *35:*148, 1953.
29. Price, R.I., and Ecker, M.L.: Z-plasty skin closure after lengthening the Achilles tendon. Case report. Plast. Reconstr. Surg., *52:*309, 1973.
30. Schneider, M., and Balon, K.: Deformity of the foot following anterior transfer of the posterior tibial tendon and lengthening of the Achilles tendon for spastic equinovarus. Clin. Orthop., *125:*113, 1977.
31. Schrodt, M.J., et al. Tibial lengthening. A review of 20 cases. Clin. Orthop., *80:*139, 1971.
32. Sgarlato, T.E., Morgan, J., Shane, H.S., and Frenkenberg, A.: Tendo Achilles lengthening and its effect on foot disorders. J. Am. Podiatry Assoc., *65:*849, 1975.
33. Sharma, S.V.: A modified method of Achilles tendon lengthening. Int. Surg., *63:*35, 1978.
34. Silfverskiöld, N.: Reduction of the uncrossed two-joint muscles of the leg to one joint muscles in spastic conditions. Acta Chir. Scand., *56:*315, 1923–1924.
35. Silver, C.M., and Simon, S.D.: Gastrocnemius-muscle recession (Silfverskiöld operation) for spastic equinus deformity in cerebral palsy. J. Bone Joint Surg. [Am.], *41:*1021, 1959.
36. Strayer, Jr., L.J.: Gastrocnemius recession. Five year report of cases. J. Bone Joint Surg. [Am.], *40:*1019, 1958.
37. Strayer, Jr., L.M., Recession of the gastrocnemius, an operation to relieve spastic contracture of the calf muscles. J. Bone Joint Surg. [Am.], *32:*671, 1950.
38. Tardieu, G., Tardieu, C., Colbeau-Justin, P., and Lespargot, A.: Muscle hypoextensibility in children with cerebral palsy. II. Therapeutic implications. Arch. Phys. Med. Rehabil., *63:*103, 1982.
39. Tracy, H.W.: Operative treatment of the plantar-flexed inverted foot in adult hemiplegia. J. Bone Joint Surg. [Am.], *58:*1142, 1976.
40. Truscelli, D., Lespargot, A., and Tardieu, G.: Variation on the long-term results of elongation of the tendo Achilles in children with cerebral palsy. J. Bone Joint Surg. [Br.], *61:*466, 1979.

41. Turco, V.J.: Surgical correction of resistant clubfoot. J. Bone Joint Surg. [Am.], *53:*477, 1971.
42. Vulpius, O., and Stoffel, A.: Orthopäedische Operationslehre. 2nd Ed. Stuttgart, Ferdinand Enke, 1920.
43. White, J.W.: Torsion of Achilles tendon: Its surgical significance. Arch. Surg., *46:*784, 1943.
44. Willert, H.G., Horrig, C., Ewald, W., and Scharrer, I.: Orthopaedic surgery in hemophilic patients. Arch. Orthop. Trauma Surg., *101:*121, 1983.
45. Wittenberg, M.: The criteria for gastrocnemius vs. tendo Achilles surgery. J. Foot Surg., *14:*54, 1975.
46. Zimmermann, R., Ehlers, G., and Ehlers, W.: Congenital factor VII deficiency. A report of four new cases. Blut, *38:*119, 1979.

CALCANEAL OSTEOTOMY

The calcaneus is the only bone of the hindfoot that is in contact with the ground through its thick and strong heel pad; it bears approximately 50% of the body weight of a barefoot person in a standing position. The talus transmits part of the body weight through the subtalar joint to the heel region, and both the talus and calcaneus transmit the remainder of the body weight to the forefoot through the talonavicular joint and calcaneocuboid joint, respectively. In a normal foot, the configurations of foot bones and their joints, joint capsules, and ligaments provide the static structural support for the foot, and all the extrinsic and intrinsic muscles of the foot render dynamic support for the foot. When the calcaneus is significantly deviated from its normal anatomic position, the weight-bearing forces in the ankle, subtalar, intertarsal, tarsometatarsal, M-P, or interphalangeal joints are inevitably altered. Such alteration can be significantly increased in key areas such as the ankle, subtalar, talonavicular, and calcaneocuboid joints, resulting in premature deterioration.

Calcaneal osteotomy can be used to change the weight-bearing alignment of the hindfoot, decreasing stress on the ankle, subtalar, and intertarsal joints. Although subtalar fusion can also correct the abnormal alignment of the calcaneus, the loss of subtalar joint motion tends to put more stress on the ankle and intertarsal joints, and may produce early onset of arthritis in these areas. In addition, calcaneal osteotomy is a simpler and safer surgical procedure with less postoperative com-

plications, shorter hospitalization, and little growth disturbance as compared with subtalar fusion, provided, of course, that no arthritic changes have taken place in the subtalar joint. In practice, calcaneal osteotomy is frequently combined with other surgical procedures of the foot, such as calcaneal tendon lengthening, release of plantar fascia and intrinsic muscles in the plantar aspect of the foot, tendon transfers, osteotomy of the tarsals or metatarsals, and fusion of the tarsal or metatarsotarsal joints.

From an anatomic point of view, any diseases or conditions that cause imbalance between the dorsiflexors and plantar flexors and the supinators and pronators of the foot can produce various foot deformities (Figure 6–40). A list of the four major muscle groups of the foot follows.

A. Dorsiflexors: tibialis anterior, extensor hallucis longus, extensor digitorum longus, and peroneus tertius.

B. Plantar flexors: gastrocnemius, soleus, posterior tibialis, flexor digitorum longus, flexor hallucis longus, peroneus longus, peroneus brevis, and plantaris.

C. Supinators: tibialis anterior, extensor hallucis longus, flexor hallucis longus, flexor digitorum longus, and tibialis posterior.

D. Pronators: peroneus longus, peroneus brevis, peroneus tertius, and extensor digitorum longus.

Neurologic diseases, trauma, complications of surgical procedures of the lower extremities, congenital anomalies and diseases, foot amputations, diseases of the muscles, infections, bone and soft tissue tumors, vascular diseases, inflammatory diseases, and metabolic diseases can all produce muscle imbalance among the various muscle groups of the foot that can easily lead to various foot deformities. A list of the different calcaneal osteotomies that can be used to treat the various kinds of muscle imbalance and the associated foot deformities follows.

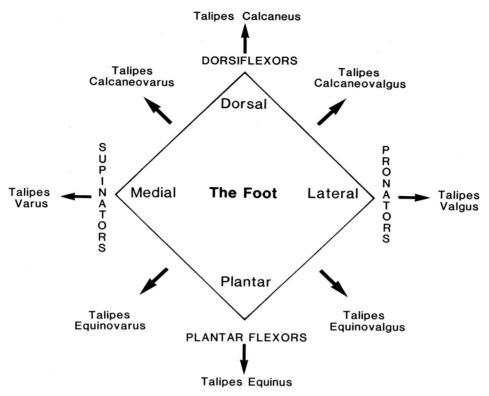

Figure 6–40. Relationship between foot deformities and the various muscle imbalances among the dorsiflexors, plantar flexors, supinators, and pronators of the foot.

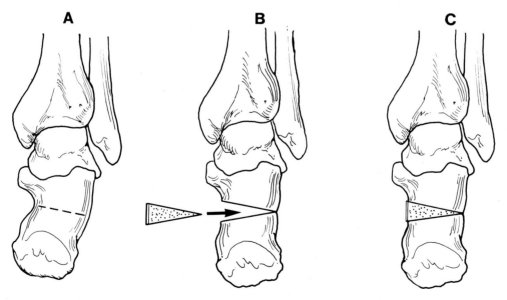

Figure 6–41. An opening-wedge calcaneal osteotomy for correction of varus deformity of the calcaneus. **A,** perform an oblique or horizontal osteotomy through the body of the calcaneus. **B,** open the medial aspect of the osteotomy site, with the lateral calcaneal surface used as a hinge. **C,** insert a wedge-shaped autogenous bone graft into the osteotomy site to maintain the correction.

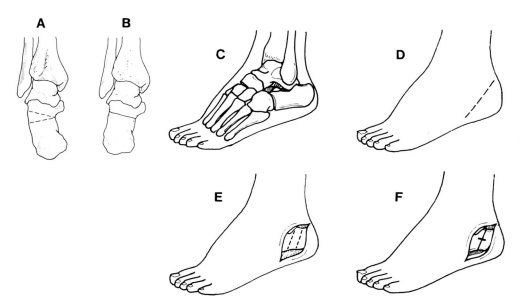

Figure 6–42. Laterally based, closing-wedge calcaneal osteotomy for correction of a varus deformity of the calcaneus. **A,** dotted lines, amount of calcaneal bone to be removed. **B,** calcaneus is in a neutral position after its valgus osteotomy. **C,** lateral view. **D,** make an oblique incision over the lateral aspect of the calcaneus. **E,** remove a laterally based bone wedge from the calcaneus. **F,** bring the two raw bone surfaces into intimate contact and hold them together with a bone staple.

A. Talipes varus: overpowering of the pronators by the supinators of the foot may necessitate a valgus calcaneal osteotomy (Figures 6–41 and 6–42).

B. Talipes valgus: overpowering of the supinators by the pronators of the foot may require a varus calcaneal osteotomy (Figures 6–43, 6–44C and D).

C. Talipes equinus: overpowering of the dorsiflexors by the plantar flexors may need a calcaneus calcaneal osteotomy (Figure 6–45).

D. Talipes calcaneus: overpowering of the plantar flexors by the dorsiflexors of the foot may necessitate the use of an equinus calcaneal osteotomy (Figure 6—44).

E. Talipes equinovarus: overpowering of the dorsiflexors by the plantar flexors, and the pronators by the supinators of the foot may require a valgus and calcaneus calcaneal osteotomy (Figures 6–41, 6–42, 6–45).

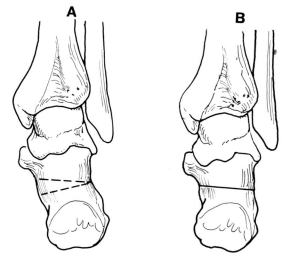

Figure 6–43. A closing-wedge calcaneal osteotomy for correction of valgus deformity of the calcaneus. **A,** remove a medially based wedge of bone from the calcaneus with an osteotome or an oscillating bone saw. **B,** bring the raw and flat bone surfaces into intimate contact and hold them together with a staple. The same valgus deformity of the calcaneus can also be corrected by performing a laterally based, opening-wedge calcaneal osteotomy with insertion of a wedge-shaped autogenous bone graft into the osteotomy site, which is particularly indicated when the calcaneus is relatively small.

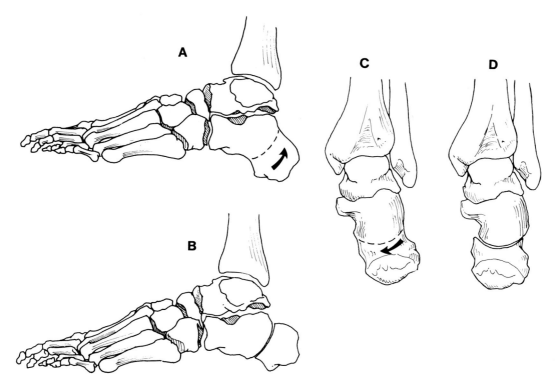

Figure 6–44. A crescentic calcaneal osteotomy for correction of the calcaneus or of valgus deformity of the calcaneus. **A,** make a crescent-shaped osteotomy through the body of the calcaneus. **B,** rotate the basal portion of the calcaneus upward along the crescentic osteotomy line to correct the deformity of the calcaneus. **C,** make a crescent-shaped osteotomy through the body of the calcaneus in a lateral to medial direction. **D,** rotate the inferior portion of the calcaneus medially along the crescentic osteotomy line to correct the valgus deformity of the calcaneus.

F. Talipes equinovalgus: overpowering of the dorsiflexors by the plantar flexors, and the supinators by the pronators of the foot may demand a varus and calcaneus calcaneal osteotomy (Figures 6–43 and 6–45).

G. Talipes calcaneovarus: overpowering of the plantar flexors by the dorsiflexors, and the pronators by the supinators of the foot may necessitate a valgus and equinus calcaneal osteotomy (Figures 6–41, 6–42, 6–44A and B).

H. Talipes calcaneovalgus: overpowering of the plantar flexors by the dorsiflexors, and the supinators by the pronators of the foot may require a varus and equinus calcaneal osteotomy (Figures 6–43 and 6–44).

When arthritic changes of the subtalar joint are associated with varus, valgus, equinus, or calcaneal deformities of the heel, more bone should be simultaneously removed from the lateral, medial, anterior, or posterior aspect of the subtalar joint, respectively, during subtalar fusion to correct the hindfoot deformity.

From a technical point of view, calcaneal osteotomy can be performed in at least three different ways with specific indications for each.

A. An opening-wedge calcaneal osteotomy with an autogenous bone graft: tends to lengthen the calcaneus and correct the calcaneal deformity at the same time. This procedure should be used on a small or underdeveloped calcaneus, or when the foot to be repaired is smaller than its opposite member.

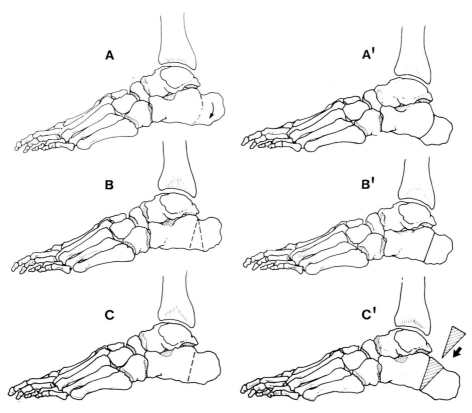

Figure 6–45. Various calcaneal osteotomies for correction of equinus deformity of the calcaneus. **A,** make a crescentic osteotomy through the body of the calcaneus. **A',** rotate the inferior portion of the calcaneus downward along the crescentic osteotomy line to correct its equinus deformity. **B,** remove an inferiorly based bone wedge from the calcaneus. **B',** bring the raw bone surfaces of the calcaneus into intimate contact and hold them together with a bone staple. **C,** perform an opening-wedge osteotomy through the body of the calcaneus. **C',** open the osteotomy site and insert a wedge-shaped autogenous bone graft to displace the basal portion of the calcaneus in a more plantar direction.

B. A closing-wedge calcaneal osteotomy: used when the calcaneus is well developed, the foot is of good size, or the calcaneus must be shortened.

C. A crescentic calcaneal osteotomy: can simultaneously correct calcaneal deformity in two planes, such as surgical correction of equinovalgus, equinovarus, calcaneovalgus, and calcaneovarus hindfoot deformities.

REFERENCES

Calcaneal Osteotomy

1. Baker, L.D., and Hill, L.M.: Foot alignment in the cerebral palsy patient. J. Bone and Joint Surg. [Am.], *46:*1, 1964.

2. Barenfeld, P.A., Weseley, M.S., and Munters, M.: Dwyer calcaneal osteotomy. Clin. Orthop., *53:*147, 1967.
3. Dekel, S., and Weissman, S.L.: Ostectomy of the calcaneus and concomitant plantar stripping in children with talipes cavo-varus. J. Bone Joint Surg. [Br.], *55:*802, 1973.
4. Dwyer, F.C.: Osteotomy of the calcaneus for pes cavus. J. Bone Joint Surg. [Br.], *41:*80, 1959.
5. Dwyer, F.C.: The treatment of relapsed clubfoot by the insertion of a wedge into the calcaneus. J. Bone Joint Surg. [Br.], *45:*67, 1963.
6. Dwyer, F.C.: The present status of the problem of pes cavus. Clin. Orthop., *106:*254, 1975.
7. Evans, D.: Calcaneo-valgus deformity. J. Bone Joint Surg. [Br.], *57:*270, 1975.
8. Fisher, R.L., and Shaffer, S. R.: An evaluation of calcaneal osteotomy in congenital clubfoot and other disorders. Clin. Orthop., *70:*141, 1970.
9. Handelsman, J.E., Youngleson, J., and Malkin, C.: A modified approach to the Dwyer os calcis osteotomy in clubfoot. S. Afr. Med. J., *39:*989, 1965.
10. Kleiger, B., and Mankin, H.J.: A roentgenographic

study of the development of the calcaneus by means of the posterior tangential view. J. Bone Joint Surg. [Am.], *43:*961, 1961.

11. Liscomb, P.R.: Osteotomy of calcaneus, triple arthrodesis, and tendon transfer for severe paralytic calcaneocavus deformity. J. Bone Joint Surg. [Am.], *51:*548, 1969.

12. Lord, J.P.: Corrections of extreme flatfoot. Value of osteotomy of os calcis and inward displacement of posterior fragment (Gleich operation). J.A.M.A., *81:*1502, 1923.

13. Mitchell, G.P.: Posterior displacement osteotomy of the calcaneus. J. Bone Joint Surg. [Br.], *59:*233, 1977.

14. Samilson, R.L.: Crescentic osteotomy of the os calcis for calcaneocavus feet. *In* Foot Science. J.E. Bateman (ed.). Philadelphia, W.B. Saunders, 1976, pp. 18–25.

15. Sedgwick, J.: Dwyer osteotomy of the calcaneus. J. Bone Joint Surg. [Br.], *54:*381, 1972.

16. Silver, C.M., et al. Calcaneal osteotomy for valgus and varus deformities of the foot in cerebral palsy. J. Bone Joint Surg. [Am.], *49:*232, 1967.

17. Weseley, M.S., and Barenfeld, P.A.: Calcaneal osteotomy for the treatment of cavus deformity. Bull. Hosp. Jt. Dis., Orthop. Inst., *31:*93, 1970.

18. Weseley, M.S., and Barenfeld, P.A.: Mechanism of the Dwyer calcaneal osteotomy. Clin. Orthop., *70:*137, 1970.

SUBTALAR ARTHRODESIS

The subtalar joint is also known as the talocalcaneal, calcaneoastragaloid, or subastragaloid joint. This articulation is between the calcaneus and the talus and can be divided into the anterior and posterior parts. The anterior part of the subtalar joint forms part of the talocalcaneonavicular joint and includes anterior and medial articular facets of the calcaneus, which articulate with the undersurface of the head of the talus. The posterior part is formed by the posterior articular facets of the calcaneus and the talus, and is separated from the anterior part of the subtalar joint by a wide and strong interosseous talocalcaneal ligament. A subtalar joint capsule connects the calcaneus and talus together and is strengthened on all four sides by the anterior, posterior, medial, and lateral talocalcaneal ligaments. The peculiar configuration of the subtalar joint allows minimal extension, flexion, and rotation, but does provide a certain amount of inversion and eversion (side to side motion). This motion tends to smooth the rough axes of ambulation of the pelvis, hips, knees, and ankles by providing a subtle shift of weight-bearing points on the feet to achieve a smooth plantigrade support during walking or running, particularly on uneven terrain.

When the subtalar joint is damaged, pain in the anterolateral aspect of the hindfoot is usually present, especially on weight-bearing. With the patient in a sitting position with the affected foot dangling free, inspection of a foot with significant subtalar joint disease frequently reveals a slightly dorsiflexed and valgus position with visible peroneal tendons behind the lateral malleolus. Palpation almost invariably reveals localized tenderness at the sinus tarsi. In addition, subtalar motion is painful and limited, and any attempt to invert the heel is resisted by the peroneal muscles, which tend to stand out prominently due to their adaptive shortening. Lateral radiographs of the foot may show a talar beak due to increased stress in the talonavicular joint, and the subtalar joint is likely to show irregularity, narrowing, and osteosclerosis.

The nonsurgical treatments of a painful subtalar joint include inversion-eversion splint, ankle-foot orthosis, and an ankle arthrodesis brace. Painful subtalar joints that do not respond to nonsurgical treatments may benefit from a subtalar arthrodesis. It should be emphasized, however, that subtalar fusion is only effective in relieving pain of a purely subtalar origin. When arthritis is also present in the calcaneocuboid and talonavicular joints, triple arthrodesis instead of subtalar fusion should be employed. A list of the conditions and diseases that may necessitate subtalar arthrodesis follows.

A. Fracture of the talus.

B. Fracture of the calcaneus.

C. Dislocation of the subtalar joint with articular damage.

D. Rheumatoid subtalar arthritis.

E. Gouty subtalar arthritis.

F. Benign bone tumors of the talus or calcaneus with destruction of the subtalar joint.

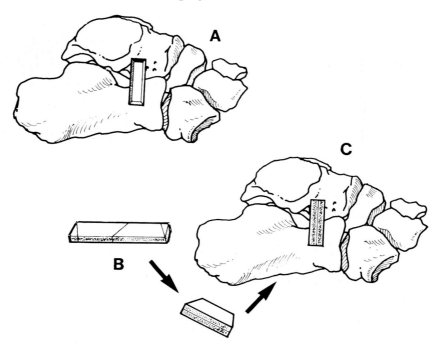

Figure 6–46. Extra-articular (Grice) subtalar arthrodesis. **A,** cut a rectangular slot in the region of the sinus tarsi into the neck of the talus and the anterolateral aspect of the calcaneus. **B,** obtain a tibial graft large enough to make two identical trapezoid grafts, which should be squeezed together with their raw bone surfaces in intimate contact to form a composite bone graft. **C,** composite bone graft is tightly wedged into the rectangular slot with its longest side going in first. The whole graft is gently tapped until it is even with the lateral surfaces of the talus and the calcaneus.

G. Tuberculous subtalar arthritis.

H. Fungal subtalar arthritis.

I. Pyogenic infection of the subtalar joint.

J. Pes planovalgus, equinovalgus, calcaneo-valgus, and so forth. Due to neurologic, neuromuscular, and myodystrophic diseases, or any other congenital anomalies.

K. Painful non-union of a previous subtalar arthrodesis.

L. Arthrodesis of the subtalar joint in a mal-position.

M. Vertical talus.

From the above mentioned surgical indications for subtalar arthrodesis, it should be apparent that the main aims of subtalar arthrodesis include relief of subtalar pain, balance and stabilization of the subtalar joint, correction of subtalar deformities, and arrest of subtalar infections or neoplastic processes. Subtalar arthrodesis is frequently combined with other surgical procedures of the foot such as Achilles tendon lengthening, release of the plantar fascia and short plantar muscles, different tendon transfers, tarsal or metatarsal osteotomies or fusions, and correction of toe deformities. It should be noted that subtalar fusion is relatively contraindicated under the following circumstances:

A. Advanced age.

B. Normal subtalar joint.

C. Deformity of the subtalar joint without pain.

D. Insensitive foot.

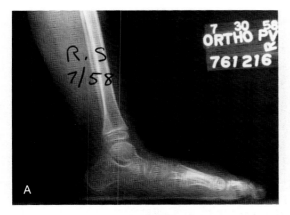
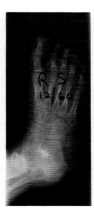
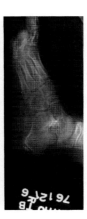

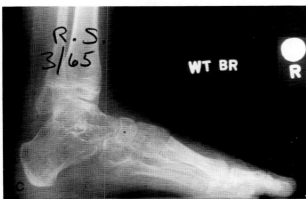

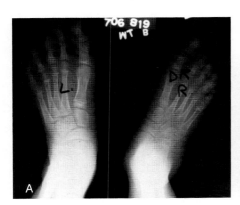

Figure 6–47. A 7-year-old boy with severe pla-novalgus deformity of his right foot caused by po-liomyelitis underwent an extra-articular subtalar ar-throdesis (**A,** lateral view). Follow-up radiographs taken 2 years and 5 months (**B,** lateral, oblique and anteroposterior views) and 6 years and 8 months (**C,** lateral view) later show that the arch of the right foot is well maintained and there is no evidence of significant growth retardation of the right talus and calcaneus.

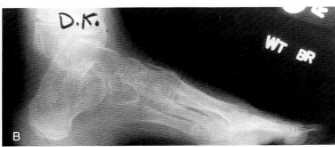

Figure 6–48. An 8-year-old boy who had marked calcaneovalgus deformity of his right foot caused by poliomyelitis underwent an extra-articular subtalar arthrodesis (**A,** anteroposterior view). A follow-up examination 4 years later (**B,** lateral view) showed absence of significant heel valgus, although the calcaneus remained in a calcaneal position.

E. Meningomyelocele.

F. Presence of pathologic processes of the ankle or midtarsal.

G. Vascular insufficiency.

H. Severe diabetes mellitus with peripheral neuropathy.

I. Presence of local or systemic infections.

J. Poor local soft tissues.

From a surgical point of view, there are three types of subtalar arthrodesis:

A. Extra-articular subtalar arthrodesis: popularized by Grice (1952) and tends to produce less growth disturbance of the foot.

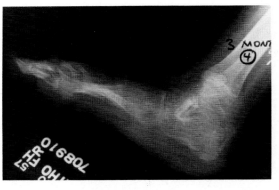

Figure 6–49. Follow-up lateral radiograph of an 8-year-old girl with rocker-bottom flatfoot caused by myelodysplasia shows solid fusion of the extra-articular subtalar arthrodesis and a reasonably good longitudinal arch of her right foot.

It is therefore useful in treating deformities in immature feet (Figures 6–46—6–50).

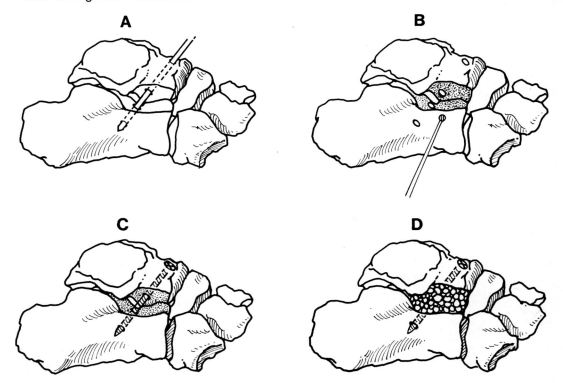

Figure 6–50. An alternative surgical technique for performing an extra-articular subtalar arthrodesis. **A,** run a drill bit from the head of the talus obliquely across the sinus tarsi into the distal portion of the calcaneus to emerge from the lateral aspect of the calcaneus. **B,** thoroughly roughen the bone surfaces of the entire sinus tarsi with an air-driven burr down to bleeding bone surfaces. **C,** transfix the subtalar joint by inserting a bone screw of appropriate length through the drilled hole. **D,** tightly pack the entire sinus tarsi with small iliac bone chips.

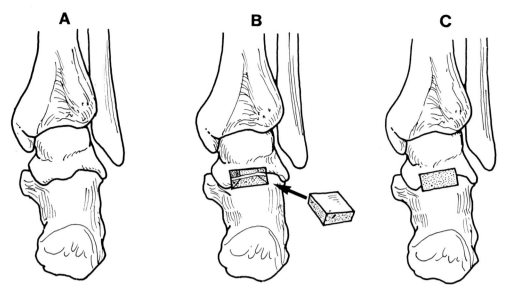

Figure 6–51. Posterior subtalar fusion. **A,** posterior view of the subtalar joint. **B,** cut a slot through the entire depth of the posterior articular facet of the subtalar joint. **C,** tightly insert an autogenous bone graft into the prepared bone slot.

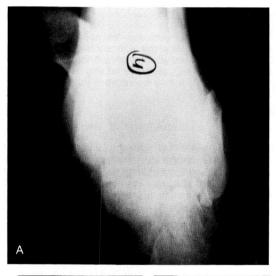

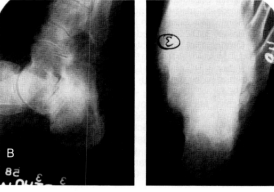

Figure 6–52. **A,** axial view of a right calcaneus. A 44-year-old man sustained a severely comminuted and transarticular fracture of his right calcaneus in a fall. Several fracture lines involve both the middle and posterior calcaneal articular facets. Because of persistent foot pain, he eventually underwent a posterior subtalar fusion of his right foot. **B,** lateral and axial views fo the hindfoot 2 years and 6 months later. A solid subtalar fusion is shown. The patient no longer had subtalar symptoms.

cular arthrodesis of the subtalar joint. Clin. Orthop., *61:*223, 1968.

36. Kleiger, B., and Ahmed, M.: Injuries of the talus and its joints. Clin. Orthop., *121:*243, 1976.

37. Lahdenranta, U., and Pylkkanen, P.: Subtalar extra-articular fusion in the treatment of valgus and varus deformities in children. A review of 162 operations in 136 patients. Acta Orthop. Scand., *43:*438, 1972.

38. Leavitt, D.G.: Subastragaloid arthrodesis for the os calcis type of flat foot. Am. J. Surg., *59:*501, 1943.

39. Mortens, J., Moller, H., and Salmonsen, L.: Early stabilizing operations for spastic talipes equino-valgus by Grice's extra-articular osteoplastic subtalar arthrodesis. Acta Orthop. Scand., *32:*485, 1965.

40. Noble, J., and McQuillan, W.M.: Early posterior subtalar fusion in the treatment of fractures of the os calcis. J. Bone Joint Surg. [Br.], *61:*90, 1979.

41. Paluska, D.J., and Blount, W.P.: Ankle valgus after the Grice subtalar stabilization: The late evaluation of a personal series with a modified technic. Clin. Orthop., *59:*137, 1959.

42. Pantazopoulos, T.: Extra-articular arthrodeses of the subtalar joint for correction of paralytic flat feet in children. J. Bone Joint Surg. [Br.], *43:*398, 1961.

43. Pennal, G.F., and Yadav, M.P.: Operative treatment of comminuted fractures of the os calcis. Orthop. Clin. North Am., *4:*197, 1973.

44. Pforringer, W., Matzen, K., and Hinterberger, J.: Electronic studies of gait disturbances. A new method of gait examination in patients with arthrodesis of the ankle and/or subtalar joint. Arch. Orthop. Trauma. Surg., *96:*115, 1980.

45. Pipino, F., and Mori, F.: The resection-arthrodesis operation on the mediotarsal and subastragalic joints. Chir. Organi. Mov., *62:*123, 1975.

46. Pollock, J.H., and Carrell, B.: Subtalar extra-articular arthrodesis in the treatment of paralytic valgus deformities: A review of 112 procedures in 100 patients. J. Bone Joint Surg. [Am.], *46:*533, 1964.

47. Ross, P.M., and Lyne, E.D.: The Grice procedure: Indications and evaluation of long-term results. Clin. Orthop., *153:*194, 1980.

48. Rugtveit, A.: Extra-articular subtalar arthrodesis, according to Green-Grice in flatfoot. Acta Orthop. Scand., *34:*367, 1964.

49. Schneider, F.R.: Subtalar extra-articular arthrodesis; 6 year follow-up post polio paralytic foot. J. Bone Joint Surg. [Am.], *45:*653, 1963.

50. Schwartz, R.P.: Arthrodesis of subtalus and midtarsal joints of the foot: Historical review, pre-operative determinations and operative procedure. Surgery, *20:*619, 1946.

51. Seymour, N., and Evans, D.K.: A modification of the Grice subtalar arthrodesis. J. Bone Joint Surg. [Br.], *50:*372, 1968.

52. Schneider, D.A., and Smith, C.F.: Medial subtalar stabilization with posterior medial release in the treatment of varus feet: A preliminary report. Orthop. Clin. North Am., *7:*949, 1976.

53. Smith, J.B., and Westin, G.W.: Subtalar extra-articular arthrodesis. J. Bone Joint Surg. [Am.], *50:*1027, 1968.

54. Staples, S.: Posterior arthrodesis of the ankle and subtalar joints. J. Bone Joint Surg. [Am.], *38:*50, 1956.

55. Thomas, F.B.: Arthrodesis of the subtalar joint. J. Bone Joint Surg. [Br.], *49:*93, 1967.

56. Tohen, A., Carmona, J., Chow, L., and Rosas, J.: Extra-articular subtalar arthrodesis. A review of 286 operations. J. Bone Joint Surg. [Br.], *51:*45, 1969.

57. Ward, F.G.: Grice's operation. J. Bone Joint Surg. [Br.], *51:*190, 1969.,

58. Westin, G.W., and Hall, C.B.: Subtalar extra-articular arthrodesis. J. Bone Joint Surg. [Am.], *39:*501, 1957.

59. Willard, D.P.: Subastragalar arthrodesis in lateral deformities of paralytic feet. Am. J. Orthop. Surg., *14:*323, 1916.

60. Wilson, Jr., F.C., Fay, G.F., Lamotte, P., and Williams, J.C.: Triple arthrodesis: a study of the factors affecting fusion after three hundred and one procedures. J. Bone Joint Surg. [Am.], *47:*340, 1965.

61. Wilson, P.D.: Treatment of fractures of os calcis by arthrodesis of the subastragalar joint. J.A.M.A., *80:*1676, 1927.

62. Zachariae, L.: Experience with the Grice operation for the paralytic foot after poliomyelitis. J. Bone Joint Surg. [Br.], *43:*853, 1961.

TRIPLE ARTHRODESIS

Triple arthrodesis fuses the talonavicular, calcaneocuboid, and talocalcaneal joints, which normally form a biomechanical linkage between the tibia and the foot. Body weight is usually transmitted to the first, second, and third rays of the forefoot through the talonavicular joint, and to the fourth and fifth rays through the calcaneocuboid joint. Biomechanically, the axes of rotation of the midtarsal joints and the subtalar joint cross at the center of motion of the talonavicular joint, making this point common to both motions. The talonavicular joint is of the ball-and-socket type and forms the highest point on the medial side of the longitudinal arch. Similarly, the calcaneocuboid joint, a trochlear joint, forms the highest point on the lateral side of the longitudinal arch. These two midtarsal (talonavicular and calcaneocuboid) joints permit limited dorsiflexion and plantar flexion and minimal rotation of the forefoot on the hindfoot. In contrast, the subtalar joint allows minimal extension, flexion, and rotation, but does provide a certain amount of inversion and eversion (side-to-side motion).

Although the range of motions of the midtarsal and subtalar joints are relatively small, they are important in providing constant fine adjustments to help the feet achieve smooth plantigrade support during walking or running,

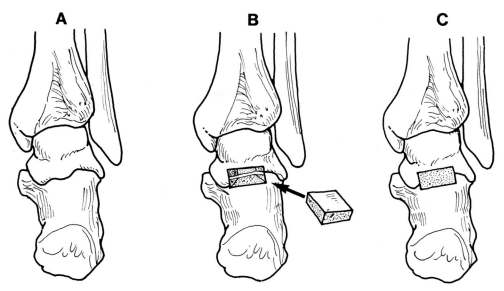

A **B** **C**

Figure 6–51. Posterior subtalar fusion. **A,** posterior view of the subtalar joint. **B,** cut a slot through the entire depth of the posterior articular facet of the subtalar joint. **C,** tightly insert an autogenous bone graft into the prepared bone slot.

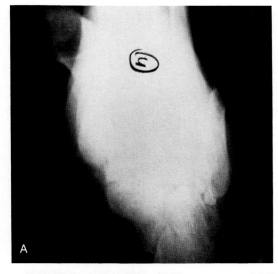

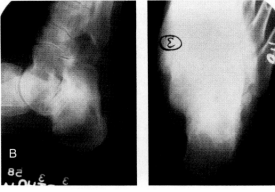

Figure 6–52. A, axial view of a right calcaneus. A 44-year-old man sustained a severely comminuted and transarticular fracture of his right calcaneus in a fall. Several fracture lines involve both the middle and posterior calcaneal articular facets. Because of persistent foot pain, he eventually underwent a posterior subtalar fusion of his right foot. **B,** lateral and axial views fo the hindfoot 2 years and 6 months later. A solid subtalar fusion is shown. The patient no longer had subtalar symptoms.

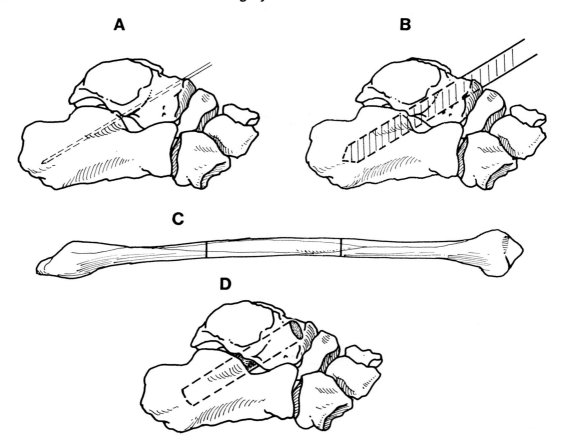

Figure 6–53. Subtalar fusion with a fibular graft. **A,** drive a K-wire or a small drill bit from the center of the head of the talus across the subtalar joint into the central portion of the calcaneus; correct placement of this guide wire is confirmed radiographically. **B,** by using drill bits of increasing diameters, the drilled hole is gradually enlarged until it can accommodate a fibular graft. **C,** measure the depth of the drilled hole and obtain a segment of the fibula of equal length from its middle portion. **D,** drive the fibular graft into the drilled hole to transfix the subtalar joint.

B. Intra-articular subtalar arthrodesis: usually involves the fusion of the posterior talocalcaneal joint, which contains the largest portion of the articular surface of the subtalar joint. A solid bony union is therefore easier to achieve (Figures 6–51—6–53).

C. A combined extra-articular and intra-articular subtalar arthrodesis: the author's preferred method of performing a subtalar arthrodesis, because it can achieve the highest degree of bony union. Its main drawback is that it requires a longer intra-operative time and a significant amount of autogenous bone from the anterior iliac crest (Figures 6–54—6–57).

REFERENCES

Subtalar Arthrodesis

1. Alban, S.L., Alban, H., and Fixler, R.H.: Subtalar arthrodesis utilizing autogenous calcaneal grafts. J. Bone Joint Surg. [Am.], *57:*133, 1975.
2. Baker, L.D., and Dodelin, C.D.: Extra-articular arthrodesis of the subtalar joint (Grice procedure). J.A.M.A., *168:*1005, 1958.
3. Baker, L.D., and Hill, L.M.: Foot alignment in the cerebral palsy patient. J. Bone Joint Surg. [Am.], *46:*1, 1964.
4. Banks, H.H.: The foot and ankle in cerebral palsy. Clin. Dev. Med., *52/53:*195, 1975.
5. Bratberg, J.J., and Scheer, G.E.: Extra-articular arthrodesis of the subtalar joint: A clinical study and review. Clin. Orthop., *126:*220, 1977.
6. Broms, J.D.: Sub-talar extra-articular arthrodesis—follow-up study. Clin. Orthop., *42:*139, 1965.
7. Brown, A.: A simple method of fusion of the subtalar

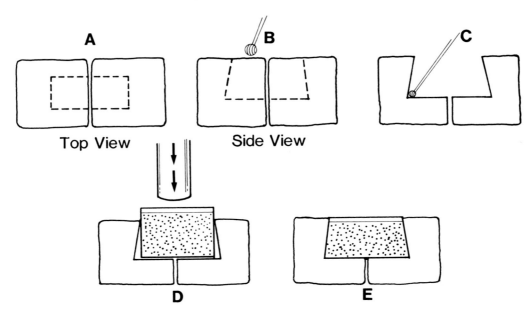

Figure 6–54. Surgical technique for performing an inlaid bone graft. **A,** mark the fusional area. **B,** perform a rough carving of the fusional site with a large burr. **C,** complete the carving with a small burr and make the bottom of the slot slightly larger than its surface portion. **D,** insert a bone graft having the same dimensions as those of the surface portion, but with greater thickness. Drive the graft into the slot until its surface is flush with the surrounding bones. **E,** as the bone graft is deformed by the driving tamp, its bottom portion is forced to spread and locks the bone graft in the fusional site.

joint in children. J. Bone Joint Surg. [Br.], *50:*369, 1968.

8. Burghele, N., and Serban, N.: Reappraisal of the treatment of fractures of the calcaneus involving the subtalar joint. Ital. J. Orthop. Traumatol., *2:*273, 1976.

9. Coleman, S.S., Martin, A.F., and Jarrett, J.: Congenital vertical talus: Pathomechanics and treatment. J. Bone Joint Surg. [Am.], *48:*1442, 1966.

10. Coleman, S.S., Stelling, III, F.H., and Jarrett, J.: Pathomechanics and treatment of congenital vertical talus. Clin. Orthop., *70:*62, 1970.

11. Dennyson, W.G., and Fulford, G.E.: Subtalar arthrodesis by cancellous grafts and metallic internal fixation. J. Bone Joint Surg. [Br.], *58:*507, 1976.

12. Dick, I.L.: Primary fusion of the posterior subtalar joint in the treatment of fractures of the calcaneum. J. Bone Joint Surg. [Br.], *35:*375, 1953.

13. Engstrom, A., Erikson, V., and Hjelmstedt, A.: The results of extra-articular subtalar arthrodesis according to the Green-Grice method in cerebral palsy. Acta Orthop. Scand., *45:*945, 1974.

14. Friedman, M.S.: Subtalar bone block for pes planovalgus. J. Bone Joint Surg. [Am.], *47:*1087, 1965.

15. Gallie, W.E.: Sub-astragalar arthrodesis in fractures of the os calcis. J. Bone Joint Surg., *25:*731, 1943.

16. Gresham, J.L.: Correction of flat feet in children. Grice-Green subastragalar arthrodesis. South. Med. J., *61:*177, 1968.

17. Grice, D.S.: An extra-articular arthrodesis of the subastragalar joint for correction of paralytic flat feet in children. J. Bone Joint Surg. [Am.], *34:*927, 1952.

18. Grice, D.S.: Further experience with extra-articular arthrodesis of the subtalar joint. J. Bone Joint Surg. [Am.], *36:*246, 1955.

19. Grice, D.S.: The role of subtalar fusion in the treatment of valgus deformities of the feet. Instr. Course Lect., *16:*127, 1959.

20. Griffin, W.C.: Grice operation. J. Bone Joint Surg. [Br.], *46:*156, 1964.

21. Gross, R.H.: A clinical study of the Batchelor subtalar arthrodesis. J. Bone Joint Surg. [Am.], *58:*343, 1976.

22. Guttmann, G.: Modification of the Grice-Green subtalar arthrodesis in children. J. Pediatr. Orthop., *1:*219, 1981.

23. Hall, M.C.: Complications at the ankle and the midtarsal joints following subtalar arthrodesis by the Gallie method: A case report. Clin. Orthop., *28:*207, 1963.

24. Hall, M.C., and Pennal, G.F.: Primary subtalar arthrodesis in the treatment of severe fractures of the calcaneum. J. Bone Joint Surg. [Br.], *42:*336, 1960.

25. Harris, R.I.: Fractures of the os calcis: Treatment by early subtalar arthrodesis. Clin. Orthop., *30:*100, 1963.

26. Herold, H.Z.: Extra-articular subtalar arthrodesis of Grice. J. Bone Joint Surg. [Br.] *47:*199, 1965.

27. Howorth, M.B.: Triple subtalar arthrodesis. Clin. Orthop., *99:*175, 1974.

28. Hsu, L.C.S., Obrien, J.P., Yau, A.C., and Hodgson, A.R.: Batchelor's extra-articular subtalar arthrodesis. J. Bone Joint Surg. [Am.], *58:*243, 1976.

29. Hsu, L.C.S., Yau, A.C., Obrien, J.P., and Hodgson, A.R.: Valgus deformity of the ankle resulting from fi-

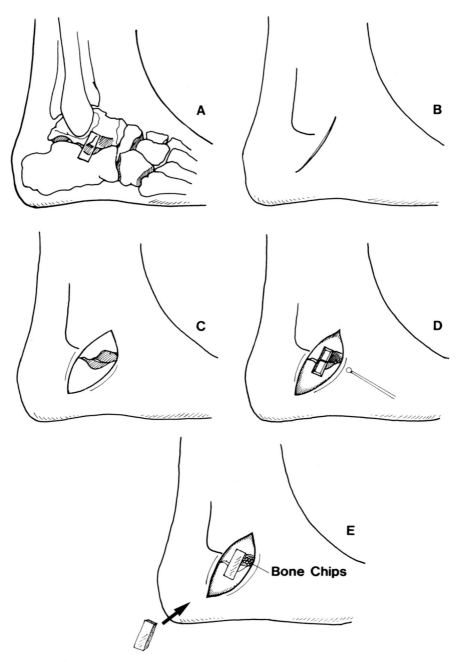

Figure 6–55. Author's preferred surgical technique for performing a subtalar fusion. **A,** lateral view of the hindfoot shows the correct location of placement of an inlaid bone graft. **B,** make an oblique skin incision across the sinus tarsi. **C,** expose the entire sinus tarsi and the anterior portion of the posterior articular facet of the subtalar joint. **D,** thoroughly roughen the sinus tarsi down to bleeding bones with a burr. Carve a slot across the posterior articular facet of the subtalar joint with different burrs (also see Figure 6–56A). **E,** tightly pack the partially decorticated sinus tarsi with iliac bone chips and insert an iliac bone graft of appropriate size into the prepared bone slot (also see Figure 6–56B).

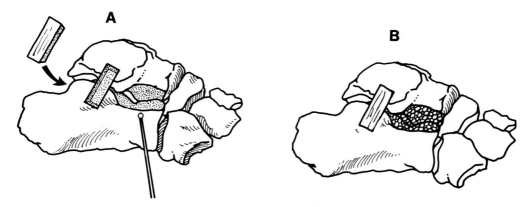

Figure 6–56. A and **B,** See legend to Figure 6–58.

bular resection for a graft in subtalar fusion in children. J. Bone Joint Surg. [Am.], *54:*585, 1972.

30. Hunt, J.C., and Brooks, A.L.: Subtalar extra-articular arthrodesis for correction of paralytic valgus deformity of the foot: Evaluation of forty-four procedures with particular reference to associated tendon transference. J. Bone Joint Surg. [Am.], *47:*1310, 1965.
31. Isherwood, I.: A radiological approach to the subtalar joint. J. Bone Joint Surg. [Br.], *43:*566, 1961.
32. Jackson, C.T., and Weighill, F.J.: A combined per-

oneal tendon transfer and subtalar fusion using excised fibular bone. Br. J. Clin. Pract., *27:*329, 1973.
33. Johansson, J.E., Harrison, J., and Greenwood, F.A.: Subtalar arthrodesis for adult traumatic arthritis. Foot Ankle, *2:*294, 1982.
34. Kalamchi, A., and Evans, J.G.: Posterior subtalar fusion. A preliminary report on a modified Gallie's procedure. J. Bone Joint Surg. [Br.], *59:*287, 1977.
35. Keats, S., and Kouten, J.: Early surgical correction of the planovalgus foot in cerebral palsy. Extra-arti-

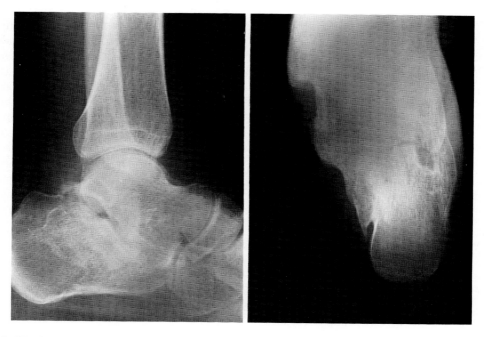

Figure 6–57.   Lateral and axial views. A 40-year-old man had a comminuted transarticular fracture of his right calcaneus in an automobile accident, which caused persistent pain of his right subtalar joint. Eventually, he had to undergo a subtalar fusion of his right foot, performed by means of the combined intra-articular and extra-articular subtalar arthrodesis technique.

cular arthrodesis of the subtalar joint. Clin. Orthop., *61:*223, 1968.

36. Kleiger, B., and Ahmed, M.: Injuries of the talus and its joints. Clin. Orthop., *121:*243, 1976.
37. Lahdenranta, U., and Pylkkanen, P.: Subtalar extra-articular fusion in the treatment of valgus and varus deformities in children. A review of 162 operations in 136 patients. Acta Orthop. Scand., *43:*438, 1972.
38. Leavitt, D.G.: Subastragaloid arthrodesis for the os calcis type of flat foot. Am. J. Surg., *59:*501, 1943.
39. Mortens, J., Moller, H., and Salmonsen, L.: Early stabilizing operations for spastic talipes equino-valgus by Grice's extra-articular osteoplastic subtalar arthrodesis. Acta Orthop. Scand., *32:*485, 1965.
40. Noble, J., and McQuillan, W.M.: Early posterior subtalar fusion in the treatment of fractures of the os calcis. J. Bone Joint Surg. [Br.], *61:*90, 1979.
41. Paluska, D.J., and Blount, W.P.: Ankle valgus after the Grice subtalar stabilization: The late evaluation of a personal series with a modified technic. Clin. Orthop., *59:*137, 1959.
42. Pantazopoulos, T.: Extra-articular arthrodeses of the subtalar joint for correction of paralytic flat feet in children. J. Bone Joint Surg. [Br.], *43:*398, 1961.
43. Pennal, G.F., and Yadav, M.P.: Operative treatment of comminuted fractures of the os calcis. Orthop. Clin. North Am., *4:*197, 1973.
44. Pforringer, W., Matzen, K., and Hinterberger, J.: Electronic studies of gait disturbances. A new method of gait examination in patients with arthrodesis of the ankle and/or subtalar joint. Arch. Orthop. Trauma. Surg., *96:*115, 1980.
45. Pipino, F., and Mori, F.: The resection-arthrodesis operation on the mediotarsal and subastragalic joints. Chir. Organi. Mov., *62:*123, 1975.
46. Pollock, J.H., and Carrell, B.: Subtalar extra-articular arthrodesis in the treatment of paralytic valgus deformities: A review of 112 procedures in 100 patients. J. Bone Joint Surg. [Am.], *46:*533, 1964.
47. Ross, P.M., and Lyne, E.D.: The Grice procedure: Indications and evaluation of long-term results. Clin. Orthop., *153:*194, 1980.
48. Rugtveit, A.: Extra-articular subtalar arthrodesis, according to Green-Grice in flatfoot. Acta Orthop. Scand., *34:*367, 1964.
49. Schneider, F.R.: Subtalar extra-articular arthrodesis; 6 year follow-up post polio paralytic foot. J. Bone Joint Surg. [Am.], *45:*653, 1963.
50. Schwartz, R.P.: Arthrodesis of subtalus and midtarsal joints of the foot: Historical review, pre-operative determinations and operative procedure. Surgery, *20:*619, 1946.
51. Seymour, N., and Evans, D.K.: A modification of the Grice subtalar arthrodesis. J. Bone Joint Surg. [Br.], *50:*372, 1968.
52. Schneider, D.A., and Smith, C.F.: Medial subtalar stabilization with posterior medial release in the treatment of varus feet: A preliminary report. Orthop. Clin. North Am., *7:*949, 1976.
53. Smith, J.B., and Westin, G.W.: Subtalar extra-articular arthrodesis. J. Bone Joint Surg. [Am.], *50:*1027, 1968.
54. Staples, S.: Posterior arthrodesis of the ankle and subtalar joints. J. Bone Joint Surg. [Am.], *38:*50, 1956.
55. Thomas, F.B.: Arthrodesis of the subtalar joint. J. Bone Joint Surg. [Br.], *49:*93, 1967.
56. Tohen, A., Carmona, J., Chow, L., and Rosas, J.: Extra-articular subtalar arthrodesis. A review of 286 operations. J. Bone Joint Surg. [Br.], *51:*45, 1969.
57. Ward, F.G.: Grice's operation. J. Bone Joint Surg. [Br.], *51:*190, 1969.,
58. Westin, G.W., and Hall, C.B.: Subtalar extra-articular arthrodesis. J. Bone Joint Surg. [Am.], *39:*501, 1957.
59. Willard, D.P.: Subastragalar arthrodesis in lateral deformities of paralytic feet. Am. J. Orthop. Surg., *14:*323, 1916.
60. Wilson, Jr., F.C., Fay, G.F., Lamotte, P., and Williams, J.C.: Triple arthrodesis: a study of the factors affecting fusion after three hundred and one procedures. J. Bone Joint Surg. [Am.], *47:*340, 1965.
61. Wilson, P.D.: Treatment of fractures of os calcis by arthrodesis of the subastragalar joint. J.A.M.A., *80:*1676, 1927.
62. Zachariae, L.: Experience with the Grice operation for the paralytic foot after poliomyelitis. J. Bone Joint Surg. [Br.], *43:*853, 1961.

TRIPLE ARTHRODESIS

Triple arthrodesis fuses the talonavicular, calcaneocuboid, and talocalcaneal joints, which normally form a biomechanical linkage between the tibia and the foot. Body weight is usually transmitted to the first, second, and third rays of the forefoot through the talonavicular joint, and to the fourth and fifth rays through the calcaneocuboid joint. Biomechanically, the axes of rotation of the midtarsal joints and the subtalar joint cross at the center of motion of the talonavicular joint, making this point common to both motions. The talonavicular joint is of the ball-and-socket type and forms the highest point on the medial side of the longitudinal arch. Similarly, the calcaneocuboid joint, a trochlear joint, forms the highest point on the lateral side of the longitudinal arch. These two midtarsal (talonavicular and calcaneocuboid) joints permit limited dorsiflexion and plantar flexion and minimal rotation of the forefoot on the hindfoot. In contrast, the subtalar joint allows minimal extension, flexion, and rotation, but does provide a certain amount of inversion and eversion (side-to-side motion).

Although the range of motions of the midtarsal and subtalar joints are relatively small, they are important in providing constant fine adjustments to help the feet achieve smooth plantigrade support during walking or running, particularly on uneven ground. Triple arthrodesis does stabilize the hindfoot and midtarsal region, but will create more stress on the ankle joint. Consequently, ankle stability is a prerequisite for triple arthrodesis. The stability of the ankle joint can be determined by means of stress views with the ankle in eversion and abduction, and in inversion and adduction. In addition, triple arthrodesis should be performed on skeletally mature feet, should remove most bone from the calcaneus and a minimal amount of bone from the talus, and should achieve a 5 to 10° valgus position of the heel. Like many other arthrodeses, the main purposes of a triple arthrodesis are: to correct deformity, to provide stability, to relieve pain, to improve function, and to arrest pathologic processes (e.g., infections and benign bone tumors).

There are many diseases capable of producing deformities or destruction of the foot that may require triple arthrodesis:

A. Neurologic diseases.
   1. Poliomyelitis.
   2. Spinal cord tumors.
   3. Brain tumors and malformations.
   4. Friedreich's ataxia.
   5. Charcot-Marie-Tooth dis
   6. Cerebral palsy.
   7. Diastematomyelia.
   8. Meningomyelocele.
   9. Multiple sclerosis.
  10. Spina bifida.
  11. Syringomyelia.
  12. Hemiplegia.
  13. Trauma or degenerative diseases of the peripheral nerves.
  14. Congenital or postnatal encephalopathy.

B. Myogenic diseases.

C. Congenital diseases.
   1. Talipes equinovarus.
   2. Arthrogryposis multiplex congenita.
   3. Congenital vertical talus (congenital rocker-bottom flatfoot or congenital convex pes valgus).
   4. Tarsal coalitions (congenital rigid flatfoot or peroneal spastic flatfoot).

D. Fractures and dislocations of the calcaneus, the talus, the subtalar joint, and the midtarsal joints.

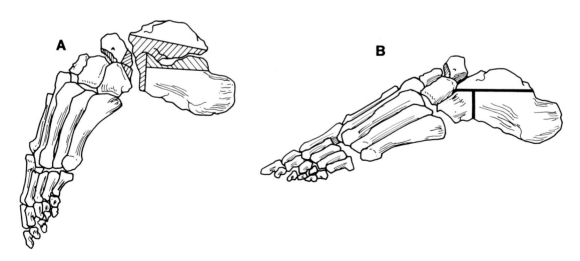

Figure 6–58. Lambrinudi's triple arthrodesis for severe talipes equinus. **A,** shaded areas, amount of bone that should be excised from the subtalar and midtarsal joints to bring the foot up to the desired degree of dorsiflexion. **B,** completed Lambrinudi's triple arthrodesis yields a neutral foot with the anterior portion of the talus in intimate contact with the inferior aspect of the navicular.

E. Various kinds of arthritis.
  1. Rheumatoid.
  2. Gouty.
  3. Tuberculous.
  4. Pyogenic.
  5. Fungal.
  6. Traumatic and degenerative.

F. Bone tumors.

It should be noted that it is for the Lambrinudi dropfoot triple arthrodesis that the plantar-flexed position of the talus is used to bring the foot up to the desired degree of dorsiflexion by excising an anteriorly based wedge from the subtalar joint. Its success largely depends on the strength of the dorsal ligaments of the ankle joint (Figures 6–58). The indications for Lambrinudi arthrodesis include: dropfoot (pes equinus), pes equinovarus, pes equinovalgus, and pes cavus.

The contraindications for Lambrinudi arthrodesis include:

A. Ankle instability.

B. Marked knee instability.

C. Patients under 11 years of age who tend to have a greater risk of avascular necrosis of the talus.

D. Painful ankle arthritis.

E. An unbalanced dropfoot. A pantalar arthrodesis is the procedure of choice.

The complications of Lambrinudi arthrodesis include:

A. Pseudarthrosis of the talonavicular joint due to inadequate contact between the talar beak and the navicular base.

B. Ankle instability may result from the smaller posterior part of the talus, which tends to fit loosely between the malleoli.

C. Avascular necrosis of the talus.

D. Residual varus or valgus foot deformity secondary to muscle imbalance.

In performing a triple arthrodesis, when the cuneiform wedge resected from the midtarsal (talonavicular and calcaneocuboid) joints is wide superiorly and laterally and narrow medially and inferiorly, it can correct adduction, supination, and cavus deformity of the foot (a cavovarus foot). In contrast, when the same cuneiform wedge is wide medially and inferiorly and narrow laterally and superiorly, it can be used to correct the abduction and pronation deformity of a planovalgus foot. In addition, a wide lateral and narrow medial wedge resected from the subtalar joint can be used to correct varus deformity of the heel; a wide anterior and narrow posterior wedge can correct equinus deformity of the heel. Likewise, a wide medial and narrow lateral wedge resected from the subtalar joint will correct a valgus deformity of the heel, and a wide pos-

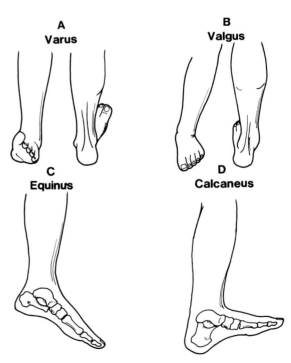

Figure 6–59. Various deformities of the foot. **A,** varus deformity; **B,** valgus deformity; **C,** equinus deformity; **D,** calcaneal deformity.

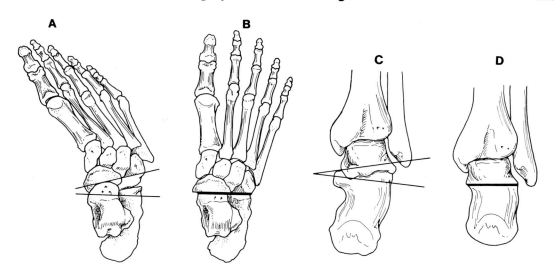

Figure 6–60. Triple arthrodesis in persistent or untreated talipes equinovarus (clubfoot). **A,** resect a bone wedge from the midtarsal joints that is wide laterally and narrow medially. **B,** align the forefoot with the hindfoot in a neutral position. **C,** resect a bone wedge from the subtalar joint that is wide laterally and narrow medially. **D,** align the calcaneus with the ankle joint in its normal neutral position.

terior and narrow anterior wedge will correct a calcaneal deformity of the heel (Figures 6–59—6–63). It should be emphasized that during the performance of triple arthrodesis, it is wise to remove too little bone rather than

too much bone and then to adjust the opposing raw bone surfaces as needed.

The three resected joints in a triple arthrodesis can be held together with small K-wires, and radiographs should be taken to check the

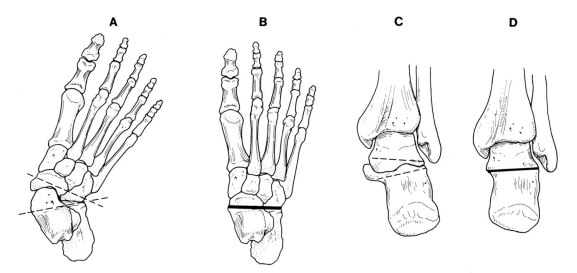

Figure 6–61. Triple arthrodesis in severe talipes planovalgus. **A,** resect a bone wedge from the midtarsal joints that is wide medially and narrow laterally. **B,** align the forefoot with the hindfoot in a neutral position. **C,** resect a bone wedge from the subtalar joint that is wide medially and narrow laterally. **D,** align the calcaneus with the ankle joint in its normal neutral position.

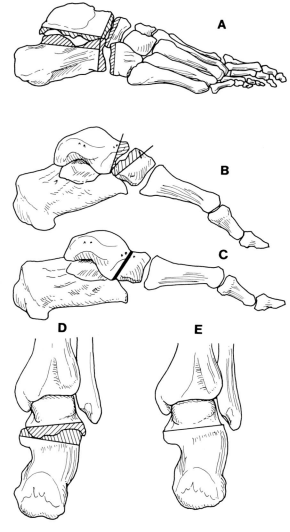

Figure 6–62. Triple arthrodesis in talipes cavovarus with its apex at the midtarsal joints. **A,** shaded areas, amount of bone to be removed from the midtarsal and subtalar joints. **B,** resect a bone wedge from the midtarsal joints that is wide superiorly and narrow inferiorly. **C,** bring the midtarsal bone surfaces altered at osteotomy into intimate contact to restore the normal longitudinal and transverse arches of the foot. **D,** resect a bone wedge from the subtalar joint that is wide laterally and narrow medially. **E,** align the calcaneus with the ankle joint in its normal neutral position.

correction of foot deformity and the closeness of the opposing raw bone surfaces at all three fusional sites. If everything is satisfactory, three staples can be used to secure the three fu-

sional sites, and fine cancellous bone chips can be forced into the small crevices at all three fusional sites to improve the chances of achieving an early bony union. When there is minimal malalignment in the talonavicular, calcaneocuboid, and talocalcaneal joints, except for arthritis, three corticocancellous iliac bone blocks can be inlaid across the talocalcaneal, talonavicular, and calcaneocuboid joints (Figures 6–64—6–66). The advantages of using inlaid iliac bone grafts in triple arthrodesis include its simpler technique, less postoperative bleeding and edema, less pseudarthrosis, no shortening, minimal chances of developing postoperative avascular necrosis, and no lowering of the foot.

Every effort should be made to minimize the chances of developing recurrent deformities and postoperative complications, a list of which follows.

A. Inadequate immobilization to permit bone fusion to take place.

B. Malalignment of the foot with the ankle.

C. Loss of position during cast change.

D. Pseudarthrosis, especially the talonavicular joint.

E. Muscle imbalance.

F. Operation on an immature foot resulting in a growth disturbance of the foot.

G. Inadequate or excessive joint resection to produce over or under correction.

H. Avascular necrosis of the talus due to excessive bone resection from its undersurface.

I. Skin slough.

J. Instability of the ankle joint.

K. Postoperative infections.

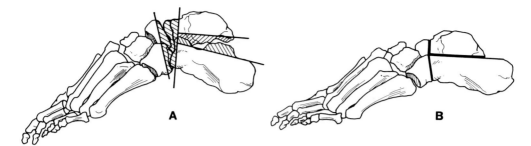

Figure 6–63. Triple arthrodesis in talipes calcaneocavus. **A,** resect a bone wedge from the midtarsal joints that is wide superiorly and narrow inferiorly, and another bone wedge from the subtalar joint that is wide posteriorly and narrow anteriorly. **B,** align the forefoot with the hindfoot and the calcaneus with the ankle joint in their normal neutral positions.

L. Surgically induced neurovascular compromise of the foot.

To gain a better understanding of the relationship between the various foot deformities and the various bone wedge resections in triple arthrodesis, the following list is provided (Figure 6–67):

A. Talipse varus: heel in inversion and forefoot in inversion and adduction requiring removal of a wedge from the midtarsal joints with its wider base located laterally, and removal of another wedge from the

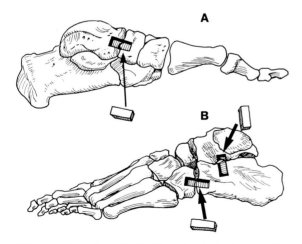

Figure 6–64. Bone block triple arthrodesis. **A,** cut a slot across the talonavicular joint and sink an iliac bone block into it. **B,** cut two additional slots across the calcaneocuboid and talocalcaneal joints, and sink an iliac bone block into each.

subtalar joint with its wider base located laterally.

B. Talipes valgus: heel in eversion and forefoot in eversion and abduction requiring removal of a wedge from the midtarsal joints with its wider base located medially, and removal of another wedge from the subtalar joint with its wider base located medially.

C. Talipes equinus: foot in plantar flexion with the heel higher than the toes requiring removal of a wedge from the subtalar joint with its wider base located anteriorly.

D. Talipes calcaneus: foot in dorsiflexion with the heel lower than the toes requiring removal of a wedge from the subtalar joint with its wider base located posteriorly.

E. Talipes equinovarus: heel in inversion and dorsiflexion and the forefoot in inversion and adduction requiring removal of a wedge from the midtarsal joints with its wider base located laterally, and removal of another wedge from the subtalar joint with its wider base located laterally and anteriorly.

F. Talipes equinovalgus: heel in eversion and dorsiflexion and the forefoot in eversion and abduction requiring removal of a wedge from the midtarsal joints with its wider base located medially, and removal of another

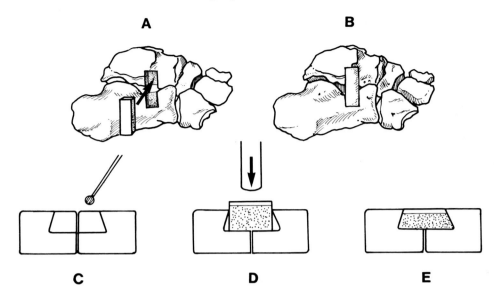

Figure 6-65. Surgical technique for performing an arthrodesis with an inlaid bone graft. **A,** cut a slot across the lateral aspect of the subtalar joint and obtain an autogenous bone graft to fill the slot. **B,** tightly insert the bone graft into the slot. **C,** remove bone from the fusional site with burrs and purposely undercut the slot. **D,** drive a bone graft into the slot with a bone tamp so that the bone graft will broaden at its base, locking itself into the slot. **E,** finished fusional site with the bone graft completely filling the slot.

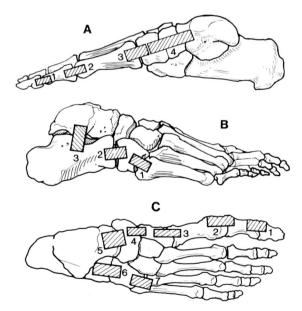

Figure 6-66. Wide applications of the inlaid bone graft arthrodesis technique. **A,** 1: interphalangeal joint; 2: M-P joint; 3: tarsometatarsal joint; 4: talonaviculocuneiform joint. **B,** 1: metatarsocuboid joint; 2: calcaneocuboid joint; 3: talocalcaneal joint. **C,** 1: interphalangeal joint; 2: M-P joint; 3: metatarsocuneiform joint; 4: naviculocuneiform joint; 5: talonavicular joint; 6: calcaneocuboid joint; 7: metatarsocuboid joints.

wedge from the subtalar joint with its wider base located medially and anteriorly.

G. Talipes calcaneovarus: heel in inversion and plantar flexion and the forefoot in inversion and adduction requiring removal of a wedge from the midtarsal joints with its wider base located laterally, and removal of another wedge from the subtalar joint with its wider base located laterally and posteriorly.

H. Talipes calcaneovalgus: heel in eversion and plantar flexion and the forefoot in eversion and abduction requiring removal of a wedge from the midtarsal joints with its wider base located medially, and removal of another wedge from the subtalar joint with its wider base located medially and posteriorly.

The author's preferred surgical technique for performing a triple arthrodesis requires the following steps (Figure 6-68):

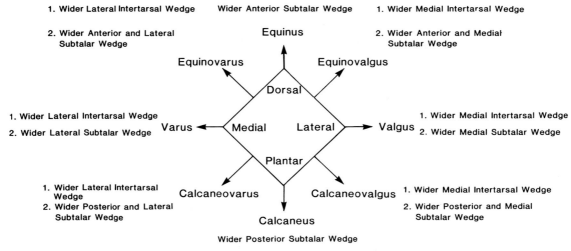

1. Wider Lateral Intertarsal Wedge   Wider Anterior Subtalar Wedge   1. Wider Medial Intertarsal Wedge

2. Wider Anterior and Lateral Subtalar Wedge   Equinus   2. Wider Anterior and Medial Subtalar Wedge

Equinovarus   Equinovalgus

Dorsal

1. Wider Lateral Intertarsal Wedge   Varus ← Medial   Lateral → Valgus   1. Wider Medial Intertarsal Wedge

2. Wider Lateral Subtalar Wedge   2. Wider Medial Subtalar Wedge

Plantar

1. Wider Lateral Intertarsal Wedge   Calcaneovarus   Calcaneovalgus   1. Wider Medial Intertarsal Wedge

2. Wider Posterior and Lateral Subtalar Wedge   2. Wider Posterior and Medial Subtalar Wedge

Calcaneus

Wider Posterior Subtalar Wedge

Figure 6–67. Relationship between bone wedge resection in triple arthrodesis and the various foot deformities.

A. Make an oblique skin incision from a point about 1.3 cm below the tip of the lateral malleolus and carry it upward and distally across the sinus tarsi to the lateral aspect of the tarsal navicular (Figure 6–68B).

B. By stripping the extensor digitorum brevis muscle from its calcaneal origin and retracting it forward, expose and denude the sinus tarsi, the calcaneocuboid and talonavicular joints, and the anterior aspect of the posterior articular facet of the subtalar joint (Figure 6–68C).

C. Cut a slot through the posterior articular facet of the subtalar joint and tightly insert an iliac graft into it. Fill the sinus tarsi with iliac bone chips, and staple the denuded calcaneocuboid joint together with a bone staple (Figure 6–68D).

D. Make a second incision on the dorsomedial aspect of the foot from the level of the head of the talus to the first cuneiform bone (Figure 6–68F).

E. Remove the articular cartilage from the medial aspect of the talonavicular joint (Figure 6–68G).

F. Hold the denuded talonavicular joint together with a bone staple (Figure 6–68H).

G. Fill all the small crevices of the talonavicular, calcaneocuboid, and talocalcaneal joints with small cancellous iliac bone chips before closure of the incisions (Figure 6–68I).

When a significant amount of bone must be resected from the subtalar and midtarsal joints, the staples are inserted at the same time after all the foot deformities have been corrected by bone wedge resections from the subtalar and midtarsal joints.

REFERENCES

Triple Arthrodesis

1. Adelaar, R.S., Dannelly, E.A., and Meunier, P.A.: A long term study of triple arthrodesis in children. Orthop. Clin. North Am., *7*:895, 1976.
2. Benyi, P.: A modified Lambrinudi operation for drop foot. J. Bone Joint Surg. [Br.], *42*:333, 1960.
3. Bernau, A.: Long term results following Lambrinudi arthrodesis. J. Bone Joint Surg. [Am.], *59*:473, 1977.
4. Canale, S.T., and Kelly, Jr., F.B.: Fractures of the neck of the talus. Long-term evaluation of seventy-one cases. J. Bone Joint Surg. [Am.], *60*:143, 1978.
5. Cowell, H.R., and Elener, V.: Rigid painful flatfoot secondary to tarsal coalition. Clin. Orthop., *177*:54, 1983.

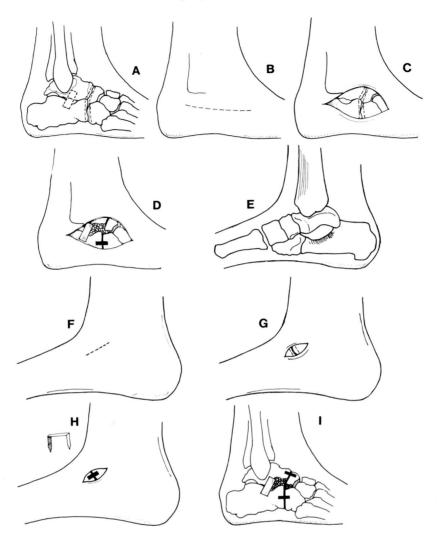

Figure 6–68. Author's preferred method of performing a triple arthrodesis. **A,** lateral view of the hindfoot. Dotted line, amount of bone to be removed. **B,** lateral skin incision. **C,** exposure of the sinus tarsi and the midtarsal and subtalar joints. **D,** fusion of the calcaneocuboid and subtalar joints with staples and bone grafts. **E,** medial view of the hindfoot. **F,** medial skin incision. **G,** removal of cartilage from the medial aspect of the talonavicular joint. **H,** fusion of the talonavicular joint with a bone staple. **I,** completed triple arthrodesis.

6. Davis, R.J., and Millis, M.B.: Ankle arthrodesis in the management of traumatic ankle arthrodesis: A long term retrospective study. J. Trauma, *20:*674, 1980.
7. DeKelver, L., Fabry, G., and Mulier, J.C.: Triple arthrodesis and Lambrinudi arthrodesis: Literature review and follow-up study. Arch. Orthop. Trauma Surg., *96:*23, 1980.
8. Drummond, D.S., and Cruess, R.L.: The management of the foot and ankle in arthrogryposis multiplex congenita. J. Bone Joint Surg. [Br.], *60:*96, 1978.
9. Duncan, J.W., and Lovell, W.W.: Hoke triple arthrodesis. J. Bone Joint Surg. [Am.], *60:*795, 1978.
10. El Ghawabi, M.H.: Centripetal compression triple arthrodesis. Acta Orthop. Scand., *49:*306, 1978.
11. Fusfield, F.D., and Burney, D.W.: Bone plug technique for triple arthrodesis. Am. J. Orthop., *3:215;* 1961.
12. Ghali, N.N., Smith, R.B., Clayden, A.D., and Silk, F.F.: The results of pantalar reduction in the management of congenital talipes equinovarus. J. Bone Joint Surg. [Br.], *65:*1, 1983.
13. Goldner, J.L., and Musgrave, R.: Results of triple arthrodesis for rigid (spastic) flat feet. South. Med. J., *49:*32, 1956.

14. Guidal, P., and Sodermann, T.: Results of 256 triarticular arthrodeses of the foot in sequelae of infantile paralysis. Acta Orthop. Scand., *1:*13, 1930.
15. Gupta, S.P., Mayanger, J.C., and Gagrani, M.R.: The place of Lambrinudi triple arthrodesis in the management of paralytic feet. Indian J. Orthop., *14:*20, 1980.
16. Harold, H.Z., and Torok, G.: Surgical correction of neglected clubfoot in the older children and adult. J. Bone Joint Surg. [Am.], *55:*1385, 1973.
17. Hart, V.L.: Lambrinudi operation for drop foot. J. Bone Joint Surg., *22:*937, 1940.
18. Hersh, A., and Fuchs, L.A.: treatment of the uncorrected clubfoot by triple arthrodesis. Orthop. Clin. North Am., *4:*103, 1973.
19. Hill, N.A., Wilson, J.J., and Cheeres, F.: Triple arthrodesis in the young children. Clin. Orthop., *70:*186, 1970.
20. Hoke, M.: An operation for stabilizing paralytic feet. Am. J. Orthop. Surg., *3:*494, 1921.
21. Howorth, M.B.: Triple arthrodesis. J. Bone Joint Surg. [Br.], *55:*439, 1973.
22. Kaplan, E.G., and Kaplan, G.S.: Triple arthrodesis. J. Foot Surg., *15:*93, 1976.
23. Kilfoyle, R.M., and Byrne, D.P.A.: Nonexcision triple arthrodesis of the foot. Orthop. Clin. North Am., *7:*841, 1976.
24. Kivilaakso, R., and Salenius, P.: Triple arthrodesis of the tarsus as a treatment for posttraumatic conditions. Acta Orthop. Scand., *37:*328, 1966.
25. Krause, M., and Siegel, A.: Experiences with triple arthrodesis in severe paralysis of the foot. Zentralbl. Chir., *45:*227, 1970.
26. Krigsten, E.J., and Janes, J.M.: A method of triple arthrodesis using autogenous tibial bone grafts. Mayo Clin. Proc., *43:*205, 1968.
27. Lambrinudi, C.: A new operation on drop foot. Br., J. Surg., *15:*193, 1927.
28. Lipscomb, P.R.: Osteotomy of the calcaneus, triple arthrodesis and tendon transfer for severe paralytic calcaneocavus deformity. J. Bone Joint Surg. [Am.], *51:*548, 1969.
29. Main, B.J., and Jowett, R.L.: Injuries of the midtarsal joint. J. Bone Joint Surg. [Br.], *57:*89, 1975.
30. McCall, R.E., Mondo, P.J., and Jones, R.E.: Bone block method of triple arthrodesis. Orthopedics, *6:*50, 1983.
31. McCauley, J.: Triple arthrodesis for congenital talipes equinovarus deformities. Clin. Orthop., *34:*25, 1964.
32. McKenzie, J.: Lambrinudi arthrodesis. J. Bone Joint Surg. [Br.], *41:*738, 1959.
33. Meznik, F.: On arthrodesis of the lower tarsal joint according to Lambrinudi. Z. Orthop., *103:*533, 1967.
34. Monson, R., and Gibson, D.A.: Long-term follow-up of triple arthrodesis. Can. J. Surg., *21:*249, 1978.
35. Monteleone, V., and Riccio, V.: The residual function of the foot after double and triple arthrodesis operations. Orizz. Ortop. Odie Riabil., *11:*535, 1966.
36. Nelson, C.L., and Janecki, C.J.: Surgical management of the rheumatoid foot. Clin. Rheum. Dis., *4:*461, 1978.
37. Patterson, R.L.: Various factors involved in triple arthrodesis. Clin. Orthop., *85:*59, 1972.
38. Ryerson, E.W.: Arthrodesing operation on the feet. J. Bone Joint Surg., *5:*453, 1923.
39. Samilson, R.L.: Calcaneocavus feet. A plan of management in children. Orthop. Rev., *10:*121, 1981.
40. Samilson, R.L., and Dillin, W.: Cavus, cavovarus and calcaneocavus. An update. Clin. Orthop., *177:*125, 1983.
41. Seitz, D.G., and Carpenter, E.B.: Triple arthrodesis in children: A ten year review. South. Med. J., *67:*1420, 1974.
42. Sennara, H.: Triple arthrodesis: A modified new technique. Clin. Orthop., *83:*237, 1972.
43. Siffert, R.J., Forster, R.I., and Nachamie, B.: "Beak" triple arthrodesis for correction of severe cavus deformity. Clin. Orthop., *45:*101, 1966.
44. Smith, A.D.: Stabilization of the feet in poliomyelitis. Clin. Orthop., *34:*14, 1964.
45. Southwell, R.B., and Sherman, F.C.: Triple arthrodesis: A long-term study with force plate analysis. Foot Ankle, *2:*15, 1981.
46. Stein, H., Simkin, A., and Joseph, K.: Foot-ground pressure distribution following triple arthrodesis. Arch. Orthop. trauma. Surg., *98:*263, 1981.
47. Thompson, K.R.: Treatment of comminuted fractures of the calcaneus by triple arthrodesis. Orthop. Clin. North Am., *4:*189, 1973.
48. Thompson, K.R., and Friesen, C.M.: treatment of comminuted fractures of the calcaneus by primary triple arthrodesis. J. Bone Joint Surg. [Am.], *41:*1423, 1959.
49. Williams, P.F., and Menelaus, M.B.: Triple arthrodesis by inlay grafting—a method suitable for the undeformed or valgus foot. J. Bone Joint Surg. [Br.], *59:*333, 1977.
50. Wilson, F., Gardner, F., and Lanotte, P.: Triple arthrodesis: A study of the factors affecting fusions after 301 procedures. J. Bone Joint Surg. [Am.], *47:*340, 1965.

7 AMPUTATIONS

An amputation can be performed through a joint or joints (disarticulation), or through a bone or bones, and is usually the last resort in treating a variety of diseases. A list of the various indications for foot amputations follows.

A. Ischemia: arterial thrombosis and laceration, peripheral vascular diseases, diabetic arteriosclerosis, and others.

B. Trauma.
   1. Severe compound fractures and dislocations and crush injury.
   2. Thermal burns.
   3. Cold injury (frost bite).
   4. Electrical burns.
   5. Chemical burns.
   6. Accidental injection of a foreign substance into the foot under high pressure.

C. Malignant bone and soft tissue tumors.

D. Benign bone and soft tissue tumors that have produced grotesque deformities of the foot (e.g., Ollier's disease, Maffucci's disease, and neurofibromatosis).

E. Infections: severe bacterial, fungal, and parasitic infections of bones and soft tissues of the foot may require different amputations to control the infections or to eliminate severe foot deformities.

F. Severe congenital anomalies: marked leg length discrepancy, pseudarthrosis, and severe limb and foot deformities.

G. A completely useless lower extremity may require amputation to eliminate dead weight and hindrance of function.

H. Large trophic ulcers in an anesthetic foot.

The general principles of foot amputations are as follows:

A. Use of a clean operative field.

B. Amputation through the level of good function.

C. Preservation of as much length as possible.

D. Use of skin flaps with good blood supply and normal sensation.

E. Employment of myodesis (fixation of muscle to bone or over the end of bone to fix it to opposing muscle or muscles) to achieve a better control of the amputation stump.

F. High severance of the nerve to minimize the chances of forming a symptomatic neuroma.

G. Double ligation of major blood vessels to prevent postoperative bleeding.

H. Making all bone ends as smooth as possible to avoid future pressure problems.

I. Preservation of the heel pad whenever possible.

Although surgical techniques for amputation through every level of the foot have been described, only the amputation levels that have stood the test of time are discussed in this chapter.

BOYD AMPUTATION

This procedure was first described by Boyd in 1939, and is principally used in ankle amputation in children. The surgical indications for a Boyd amputation include:

A. Severe foot deformities that require the use of expensive and cosmetically unacceptable shoes.

B. Severe leg length discrepancy.

C. Absence or deficiency of the fibula accompanied by severe foot deformity.

D. Congenital femoral deficiency with a markedly shortened extremity.

E. Severe osteomyelitis of the forefoot.

F. Ollier's and Maffucci's diseases with multiple phalangeal and metatarsal involvements.

G. Grotesque deformity of the foot caused by neurofibromatosis.

H. Congenital deficiency of the tibia with severe foot deformity.

I. Severe burns of the forefoot.

J. Severe crush injury of the forefoot.

K. Mutilation of the forefoot by a lawn mower.

L. Gangrene of the forefoot.

Although the Boyd amputation shares many common surgical indications with the Syme's amputation, it does have its advantages and disadvantages when compared with the Syme's procedure. The main advantages include preservation of leg length by saving the calcaneus, and no risk of heel pad injury, which may occur with the Syme's amputation when the heel pad must be completely detached from the calcaneus. The disadvantages include the need to achieve a solid bony calcaneotibial fusion, which requires precise placement of the calcaneus under the tibia and resection of the anterior aspect of the calcaneus, plus intramedullary threaded pin fixation or interosseous screw fixation with their possible postoperative complications.

The surgical technique for the Boyd amputation consists of the following steps (Figure 7–1):

A. Start the skin incision slightly anterior to the tip of the lateral malleolus, carry it across the dorsal aspect of the foot at the level of the naviculocuneiform joints to a point slightly anterior to the tip of the medial malleolus, and then curve it inferiorly and distally across the sole of the foot at the level of the tarsometatarsal joints to complete the whole skin incision (Figure 7–1A).

B. Cut the anterior tibialis, extensor hallucis longus, extensor digitorum longus, and peroneus tertius tendons; doubly ligate the dorsalis pedis artery and vein at the level of skin incision; but cut the superficial and deep peroneal nerves as proximal to the skin incision as possible (Figure 7–1B).

C. Transversely cut the heel pad, plantar aponeurosis, abductor hallucis, flexor digitorum brevis, abductor digiti quinti, quadratus plantae, flexor digitorum longus, flexor hallucis longus, tibialis posterior, peroneus

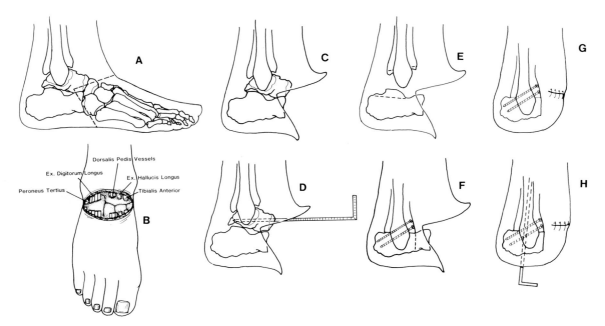

Figure 7–1. Surgical technique for Boyd amputation. **A,** skin incision. **B,** cutting of dorsal tendons and neurovascular structures. **C,** intertarsal disarticulation. **D,** insertion of a Steinmann pin into the talus. **E,** removal of the talus and the tibial and calcaneal articular surfaces. **F,** fixation of the calcaneotibial fusional site with two screws. **G,** removal of the protruding anterior portion of the calcaneus and closure of the skin flaps. **H,** an alternative method of fixing the calcaneotibial fusional site with a large Steinmann pin in a skeletally immature foot.

longus, peroneus brevis, long and short plantar ligaments, plantar calcaneonavicular ligament (spring ligament), dorsal calcaneocuboid and talonavicular ligaments, and the joint capsules of the calcaneocuboid and talonavicular joints; doubly ligate the posterior tibial artery and vein; but cut the posterior tibial nerve at a higher level to complete the disarticulation at the intertarsal joint level (Figure 7–1C).

D. Insert a Steinmann pin into the talus (Figure 7–1D).

E. By manipulating the talus with the Steinmann pin, perform a talectomy by cutting the medial and lateral collateral ligaments of the ankle, the interosseous talocalcaneal ligament, and the ankle and subtalar joint capsules. Remove the articular cartilage from the tibia and the calcaneus by making two cuts parallel to the ground through the subchondral bone of the tibia and the calcaneus with an air-driven oscillating saw (Figure 7–1E).

F. Bring the raw and flat tibial and calcaneal bone surfaces into intimate contact and fix them together with two bone screws of the foot, which is skeletally mature or near skeletal maturity (Figure 7–1F).

G. Trim the protruding anterior aspect of the calcaneus with an air-powered oscillating saw and close the skin flaps in a regular manner (Figure 7–1G).

H. In a skeletally immature foot, the calcaneotibial fusional site can be temporarily held together with a large threaded Steinmann pin, which can be removed 4 to 6 weeks later, before a cast is applied (Figure 7–1H).

REFERENCES

Boyd Amputation

1. Achterman, C., and Kalamchi, A.: Congenital deficiency of fibula. J. Bone Joint Surg. [Br.], *61:*133, 1979.
2. Blum, C.E., and Kalamchi, A.: Boyd amputations in children. Clin. Orthop., *165:*138, 1982.
3. Boyd, H.B.: Amputation of the foot with calcaneotibial arthrodesis. J. Bone Joint Surg., *21:*997, 1939.
4. Edvardsen, P.: Resection osteosynthesis and Boyd amputation for congenital pseudarthrosis of the tibia. J. Bone Joint Surg. [Br.], *55:*179, 1973.
5. Eilert, R.E., and Jayakumar, S.S.: Boyd and Syme ankle amputations in children. J. Bone Joint Surg. [Am.], *58:*1138, 1976.
6. Farmer, A.W., and Laurin, C.A.: Congenital absence of the fibula. J. Bone Joint Surg. [Am.], *42:*1, 1960.
7. Kruger, L.M., and Talbor, R.D.: Amputation and prosthesis as definitive treatment in congenital absence of the fibula. J. Bone Joint Surg. [Am.], *42:*625, 1961.
8. McCollough, N.C., Matthews, J.G., Taut, A., and Caldwell, C.P.: Early opinion concerning the importance of bony fixation of the heel pad to the tibia in the juvenile amputee. N.Y.U. Interclin. Bull., *3:*1, 1964.
9. Tooms, R.E.: Amputations. *In* Campbell's Operative Orthopaedics. 6th Ed. A.S. Edmonson and A.H. Crenshaw (eds.). St. Louis, C.V. Mosby, 1980, p. 833.
10. Williams, M.: Treatment of childhood disability. *In* Orthopaedic Surgery in Infancy and Childhood. A.B. Ferguson (ed.). Baltimore, Williams & Wilkins, 1975, p. 47.

SYME'S AMPUTATION

Syme's amputation is an excellent method of performing an ankle disarticulation, and was first described by James Syme in 1843. Preservation of the thick and strong heel pad virtually eliminates the problem of skin breakdown at the stump end, which is a common problem in below-knee and above-knee amputations. Patients with Syme's amputation can ambulate at home without crutches or prosthesis, especially the ones with bilateral Syme's amputations. Modern surgical techniques and prosthetic designs have enabled patients with Syme's amputations to wear comfortable and cosmetically acceptable prostheses.

Syme's amputation is used in the treatment of a variety of diseases and conditions; a list of the surgical indications follows (Figures 7–2—7–7).

A. Severe crush injury of the forefoot.

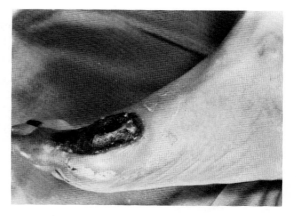

Figure 7–2. A 58-year-old man with a long history of diabetes mellitus developed gangrene of the distal portion of the dorsomedial aspect of his right foot. A Syme's amputation was eventually required.

B. Severe open fractures of the tarsus or ankle that are not suitable for more distal amputations.

C. Failure of a transmetatarsal amputation because of prosthetic fitting difficulty or indolent healing problem.

D. Severe bone and soft tissue infection and gangrene of the forefoot.

E. Leprosy and other neurotrophic diseases of the foot caused by tabes dorsalis, syringomyelia, diabetes, and meningomyelocele.

F. Intractable ulceration of the forefoot from irreparable injury to the sciatic nerve and its major branches.

G. Severe congenital deformities of the foot that make plantigrade weight-bearing and proper fitting of shoes difficult.

H. Deficiency or absence of the tibia or the fibula accompanied by marked deformity of the foot.

I. Benign soft tissue and bone tumors (e.g., Ollier's disease, Maffucci's disease, and neurofibromatosis) that have produced

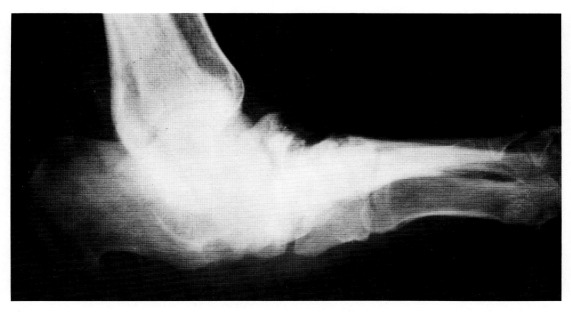

Figure 7–3. A 56-year-old man with diabetic peripheral neuropathy and neurotrophic arthropathy of his left foot developed a large plantar ulcer. Various nonsurgical treatments failed and a Syme's amputation was performed.

grotesque deformities of the foot, making proper shoe fitting difficult.

J. Congenital pseudarthrosis of the tibia.

K. Extensive necrosis of the forefoot due to thermal, electrical, and chemical burns and to frost bite.

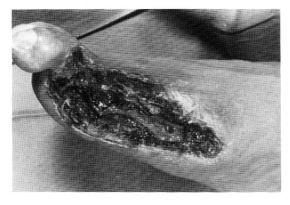

Figure 7–4. A 59-year-old man with arteriosclerosis obliterans developed gangrene of the distal portion of the medial aspect of his right foot. A Syme's amputation was required to salvage the foot.

L. Gangrene of the forefoot caused by diabetes or other peripheral vascular diseases.

M. Palliative treatment for large metastatic tumors of the foot.

In carrying out a Syme's amputation, several important points of the surgical technique should be borne in mind:

A. Ligation of the posterior tibial artery below its bifurcation to achieve maximal preservation of the blood supply to the skin flap.

B. Careful subperiosteal stripping of the thick heel fat pad from the calcaneus to avoid damage to the heel fat pad.

C. Cutting the tibia parallel to the ground immediately above its articular surface, and careful trimming and rounding off of the peripheral portion of the tibia and fibula to facilitate subsequent fitting of the cosmetically acceptable prosthesis.

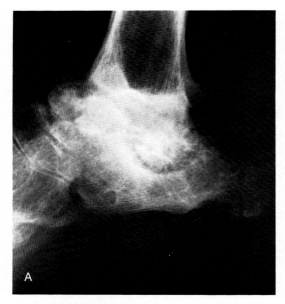

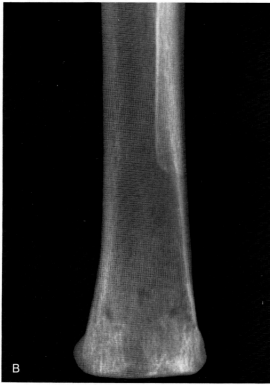

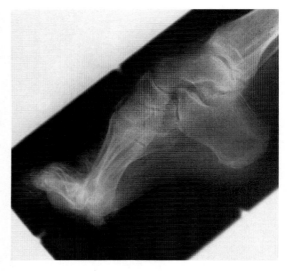

Figure 7–6. A 63-year-old man with a severe clawfoot and 6-inch leg length discrepancy caused by childhood poliomyelitis developed severe metatarsalgia and peripheral vascular disease. A Syme's amputation yielded gratifying results: the patient no longer had metatarsalgia or had to wear the heavy and unsightly shoe.

D. Anchoring the fascia of the heel pad to the stump end through drilled holes in the anterior aspect of the tibia and fibula.

The surgical technique for Syme's amputation includes the following steps (Figure 7–8):

A. Start the skin incision from the tip of the lateral malleolus and carry it across the dorsal aspect of the foot at the level of the talonavicular joint to the tip of the medial malleolus, where the incision is curved inferiorly across the sole of the foot at the level of the distal portion of the calcaneus to complete the whole skin incision (Figure 7–8A).

B. Cut the anterior tibialis, extensor hallucis longus, extensor digitorum longus, and peroneus tertius tendons; doubly ligate the dorsalis pedis artery and vein at the level of the skin incision; but sever the superficial and deep peroneal nerves as proximal to the skin incision as possible (Figure 7–8B).

Figure 7–5. A 47-year-old woman sustained a severe crush injury to her right ankle region (**A** and **B**). Initial treatment with a plantar arthrodesis yielded unsatisfactory results, and a Syme's amputation was eventually required for pain relief.

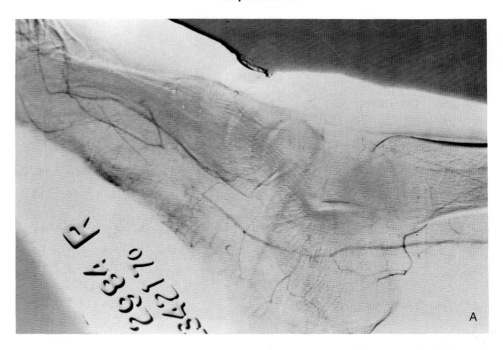

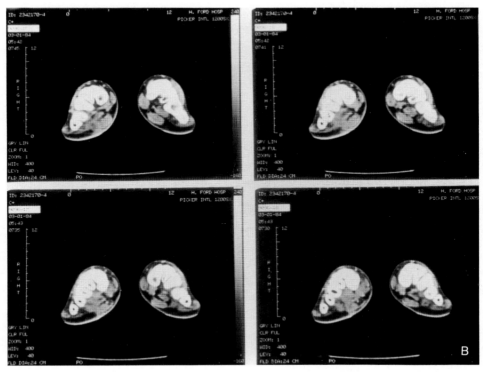

Figure 7–7. A 23-year-old woman had a clear cell sarcoma in her right foot. **A,** arteriography showed increased vascularity and neovascularization of the tumor in the plantar aspect. **B,** CT scan of both feet shows distortion of the normal anatomy of the plantar soft tissue structures of the right foot caused by the presence of the sarcoma.

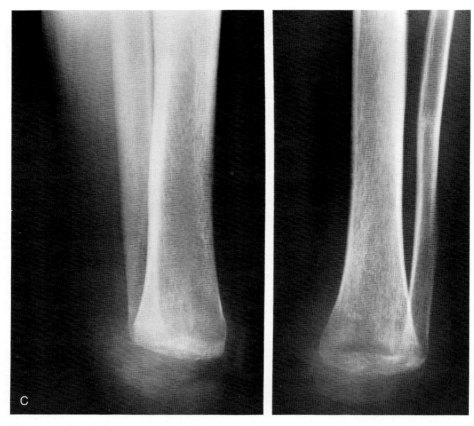

Figure 7–7. Continued. C, Anteroposterior and lateral ankle radiographs show complete absence of the right foot after Syme's amputation. Careful gross and microscopic examination of the margins of the amputated foot showed complete absence of tumor cells.

C. Perform an intertarsal amputation by transversely cutting the heel pad, plantar aponeurosis, abductor hallucis, flexor digitorum brevis, abductor digiti quinti, quadratus plantae, flexor digitorum longus, flexor hallucis longus, tibialis posterior, peroneus longus, peroneus brevis, long and short plantar ligaments, plantar calcaneonavicular ligaments (spring ligament), dorsal calcaneocuboid and talonavicular ligaments, and the joint capsules of the calcaneocuboid and talonavicular joints. Doubly ligate the posterior tibial artery and vein, and cut the posterior tibial nerve at a higher level than the incision site (Figure 7–8C).

D. Insert a Steinmann pin from the head of the talus across the subtalar joint into the calcaneus. Remove the medial and lateral malleoli at the level of the ankle joint to facilitate the posterior dissection (Figure 7–8D).

E. By manipulating the Steinmann pin, remove the talus and the calcaneus as a unit by carefully detaching the calcaneal tendon and the entire heel pad from the calcaneus (Figure 7–8E).

F. Carefully round off the tibial and fibular bone ends and then drill several holes through the anterior aspect of the tibia and fibula (Figure 7–8F).

G. Pass stout sutures through the plantar fascia and the drilled holes in the tibia and fibula (Figure 7–8G).

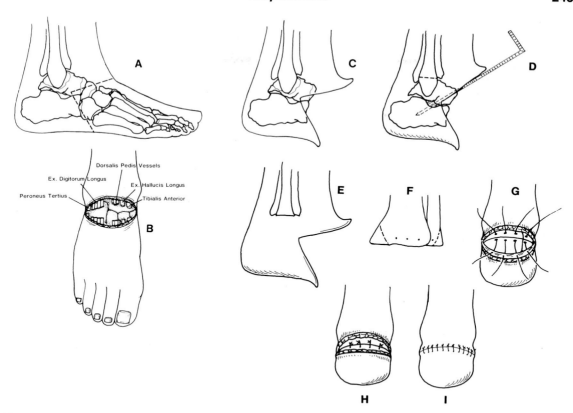

Figure 7–8. Surgical technique for Syme's amputation. **A,** skin incision. **B,** cut the dorsal tendons and neurovascular structures. **C,** intertarsal disarticulation. **D,** insert a Steinmann pin into both the talus and the calcaneus, and remove the medial and lateral malleoli. **E,** remove the talus and the calcaneus as a unit. **F,** round off the bony amputation stump and drill holes through the anterior aspect of the tibia and fibula. **G,** put sutures through the plantar fascia and the drilled holes in the tibia and the fibula. **H,** anchor the heel pad to the end of the amputation stump. **I,** close the skin flaps.

H. Anchor the heel pad to the anterior margin of the tibia and fibula by tying the sutures tightly together (Figure 7–8H).

I. Close the skin flaps in a regular manner (Figure 7–8I).

REFERENCES

Syme Amputation

1. Alldredge, R.H., and Thompson, T.C.: The technique of Syme amputation. J. Bone Joint Surg., 28:415, 1946.
2. Baker, G.C.W., and Stableforth, P.G.: Syme's amputation. A review of 67 cases. J. Bone Joint Surg. [Br.], 51:482, 1969.
3. Burgess, E.M.: Sites of amputation election according to modern practice. Clin. Orthop., 37:17, 1964.
4. Catterall, R.C.F.: Syme's amputation by Joseph Lister after sixty-six years. J. Bone Joint Surg. [Br.], 49:144, 1967.
5. Chen, K.T., McGann, P.D., and Flam, M.S.: Ewing's sarcoma of the phalangeal bone. J. Surg. Oncol., 22:92, 1983.
6. Dale, G.M.: Syme's amputation for gangrene from peripheral vascular disease. Artif. Limbs, 6:44, 1961.
7. Davidson, W.H., and Bohne, W.H.O.: The Syme amputation in children. J. Bone Joint Surg. [Am.], 57:905, 1975.
8. Eilert, R.E., and Jayakumar, S.S.: Boyd and Syme ankle amputations in children. J. Bone Joint Surg. [Am.], 58:1138, 1976.
9. Ghandur-Mnaymneh, L., and Mnaymneh, W.: Solitary bony metastasis to the foot with long survival following amputation. Clin. Orthop., 166:117, 1982.
10. Haig, G.: Syme's amputation. Injury, 4:164, 1972.
11. Harding, H.E.: Knee disarticulation and Syme's amputation. Ann. R. Coll. Surg. Engl., 40:235, 1967.
12. Harris, R.I.: Syme's amputation: The technical details essential for success. J. Bone Joint Surg. [Br.], 38:614, 1956.

13. Harris, R.I.: The history and development of Syme's amputation. Artif. Limbs, *6:*4, 1961.
14. Hinterbuchner, C., Sakuma, J., and Saturen, P.: Syme's amputation and prosthetic rehabilitation in focal scleroderma. Arch. Phys. Med. Rehabil., *53:*78, 1972.
15. Hornby, R., and Harris, W.R.: Syme's amputation. Follow-up study of weight bearing in sixty-eight patients. J. Bone Joint Surg. [Am.], *57:*346, 1975.
16. Jacobsen, S.T., Crawford, A.H., Millar, E.A., and Steel, H.H.: The Syme amputation in patients with congenital pseudarthrosis of the tibia. J. Bone Joint Surg. [Am.], *65:*533, 1983.
17. Lindquist, C., and Riska, E.B.: Chopart, Pirogoff and Syme amputations. A survey of twenty-one cases. Acta Orthop. Scand., *37:*110, 1966.
18. Marx, H.W.: An innovation in Syme's prosthetics. Prosthet. Orthot. Int., *23:*131, 1969.
19. Mazet, R.: Syme's amputation: A follow-up study of fifty-one adults and thirty-two children. J. Bone Joint Surg. [Am.], *50:*1549, 1968.
20. McCarthy, R.E.: Amputation for congenital pseudarthrosis of the tibia. Indications and techniques. Clin. Orthop., *166:*58, 1982.
21. Mercer, W.: Syme's amputation. J. Bone Joint Surg. [Br.], *36:*611, 1956.
22. Millard, I.L.: Amputations at the ankle. J. Arkansas Med. Soc., *80:*108, 1983.
23. Murdoch, G.: Syme's amputation. J. R. Coll. Surg. Edinb., *21:*15, 1976.
24. Ratliff, A.H.: Syme's amputation: Result after forty-four years. Report of a case. J. Bone Joint Surg. [Br.], *49:*142, 1967.
25. Rentoul, W.W.: Syme's amputation. J. Bone Joint Surg. [Br.], *36:*672, 1954.
26. Romano, R.L., Zettl, J.H., and Burgess, E.M.: The Syme's amputation: A new prosthetic approach. Interclin. Info. Bull., *11:*1, 1972.
27. Rosenman, L.D.: Syme amputation for ischemic disease in the foot. Am. J. Surg., *118:*194, 1969.
28. Rubin, G.: Prosthetic fitting problem of the quasi-Syme amputation. Clin. Orthop., *160:*233, 1981.
29. Sarmiento, A.: A modified surgical-prosthetic approach to the Syme's amputation: A follow-up report. Clin. Orthop., *85:*11, 1972.
30. Sarmiento, A., Gilmer, Jr., R.E., and Finnieston, A.: A new surgical-prosthetic approach to the Syme's amputation: A preliminary report. Artif. Limbs, *10:*52, 1966.
31. Shelswell, J.H.: Syme's amputation. Lancet, *2:*1296, 1954.
32. Sinclair, W.F.: Below the knee and Syme's amputation prostheses. Orthop. Clin. North Am., *3:*349, 1972.
33. Spittler, A.W., Brennan, J.J., and Payne, J.W.: Syme amputation performed in two stages. J. Bone Joint Surg. [Am.], *36:*37, 1954.
34. Srinivasan, H.: Syme's amputation in insensitive feet. J. Bone Joint Surg. [Am.], *55:*558, 1973.
35. Syme, J.: Amputation at the ankle joint. Mon. J. Med. Sci., *3:*93, 1843.
36. Thompson, R.G.: Amputation in the lower extremity. J. Bone Joint Surg. [Am.], *45:*1723, 1963.
37. Wagner, Jr., F.W.: Amputations of the foot and ankle. Current status. Clin. Orthop., *122:*62, 1977.
38. Warner, R., Daniel, R., and Leswing, A.L.: Another new prosthetic approach for the Syme's amputation. Interclin. Info. Bull., *12:*7, 1972.
39. Warren, R., Thayer, T.R., Schenbach, H., and Kendall, L.G.: The Syme amputation in peripheral arterial disease. A report of 6 cases. Surgery, *37:*156, 1955.
40. Westin, G.W., Sakai, D.N., and Wood, W.L.: Congenital longitudinal deficiency of the fibula. Follow-up of treatment by Syme amputation. J. Bone Joint Surg. [Am.], *58:*492, 1976.
41. Wilson, Jr., A.B.: Prostheses for Syme's amputation. Artif. Limbs, *6:*52, 1961.
42. Wood, W.L., Zlotsky, N., and Westin, G.W.: Congenital absence of the fibula. Treatment by Syme amputation—indication and techniques. J. Bone Joint Surg. [Am.], *47:*1159, 1965.

TRANSMETATARSAL AMPUTATION

Transmetatarsal amputation, when properly indicated, is an excellent level for amputation, because the amputees have absence of leg length discrepancy, no need for a prosthesis, wide base of support for good balance, and good heel pad and plantar pad of the foot for weight-bearing. The disability of amputation is directly proportional to the level of amputation in such a manner that the more proximal the level, the greater the disability. Transmetatarsal amputation, however, does deprive the foot of the push-off function of the toes, causing the amputee to walk with a flat-footed gait and to run with a significant limp. The surgical indications for transmetatarsal amputation include (Figures 7–9—7–14):

A. Diabetic or arteriosclerotic gangrene of the toes and a small area of the forefoot.

B. Malignant soft tissue or bone tumors of the toes.

C. Severe lawn mower injury to the dorsal or plantar aspect of the forefoot.

D. Trophic ulcer of the forefoot associated with neurologic diseases.

E. Thermal, chemical, electric, or cold injury of the toes.

F. Severe crush injury of multiple toes.

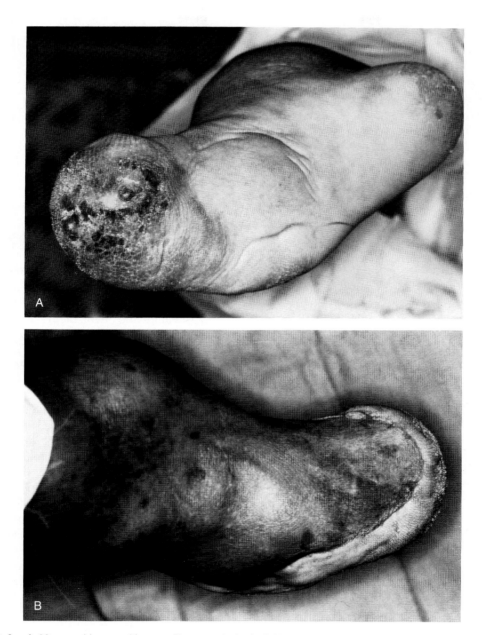

Figure 7–9. A 29-year-old man with neurofibromatosis had all his right toes amputated during childhood because of grotesque toe deformities (**A** and **B**). He was seen by the author because of a persistent ulcer at the tip of the amputation stump, and difficulty and high expense in obtaining a size 19 shoe.

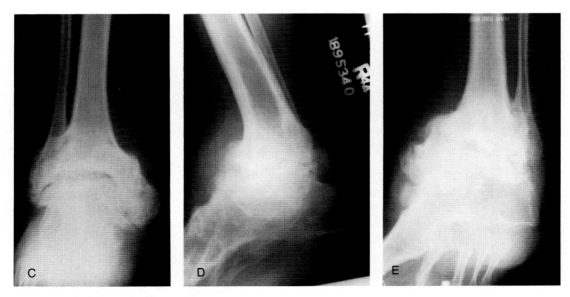

Figure 7–9. Continued. Anteroposterior (**C**), lateral (**D**), and oblique (**E**) views of the right ankle show severe arthritic changes with marked osteophyte formation.

G. Severe congenital or acquired deformities of the toes.

H. Shotgun wound of the toes and forefoot.

A standard transmetatarsal amputation requires the following steps (Figure 7–15):

A. Make a skin incision transversely across the dorsal aspect of the foot at the level of transmetatarsal amputation (Figure 7–15A).

B. Extend the two ends of the dorsal incision distally and plantarly across the plantar aspect of the foot at the level of the M-P joints to complete the whole skin incision (Figure 7–15B).

C. Through the dorsal incision, cut the extensor hallucis longus, extensor digitorum brevis, and extensor digitorum longus tendons and ligate the dorsal metatarsal blood vessels at the level of the skin incision. Then, cut the branches of the superficial and deep peroneal nerves as proximal to the dorsal skin incision site as possible (Figure 7–15C).

D. Through the plantar incision, cut the plantar fascia, abductor hallucis, flexor digitorum brevis, abductor digiti quinti, flexor hallucis longus, flexor digitorum longus, lumbricals, adductor hallucis, flexor hallucis brevis, and flexor digiti quinti; ligate the plantar digital vessels and cut the plantar digital nerves as proximal to the plantar skin incision as possible; and complete the transmetatarsal amputation by cutting all five metatarsals with a microsaw and cutting the plantar and dorsal interosseous muscles with a scalpel (Figure 7–15D).

E. After carefully smoothing the amputated metatarsal ends with a bone rasp, approximate the dorsal and plantar skin flaps (Figure 7–15E).

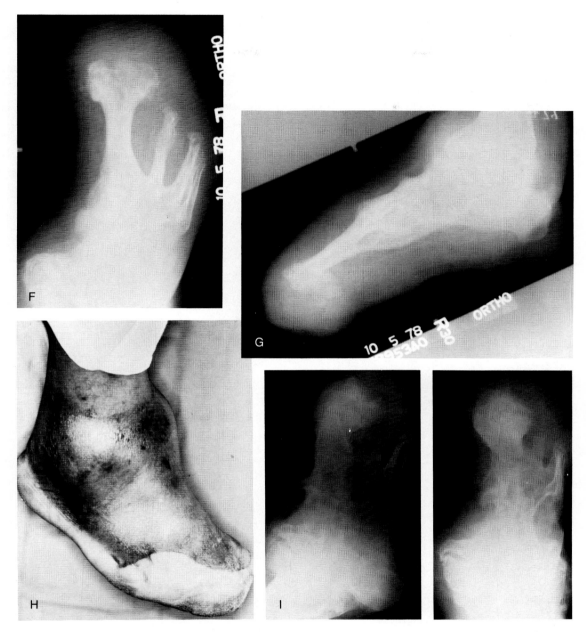

Figure 7–9. Continued. Anteroposterior (**F**) and lateral (**G**) views of the right foot show a mushroom-shaped enlargement of the first metatarsal head, which measures 6.5 cm in diameter, and absence of all five toes. The patient subsequently had a transmetatarsal amputation of his right foot, which eliminated the foot ulcer and reduced his shoe size from 19 to 13. The same patient was again seen by the author 3 years and 8 months later because of enlargement of his right foot, which required the use of a size 16 shoe (**H**). Follow-up anteroposterior and oblique (**I**) right foot radiographs taken 3 years and 8 months later show regrowth of the bulbous first metatarsal head. Because there was no new ulceration and the foot was only minimally symptomatic, no further surgery was recommended.

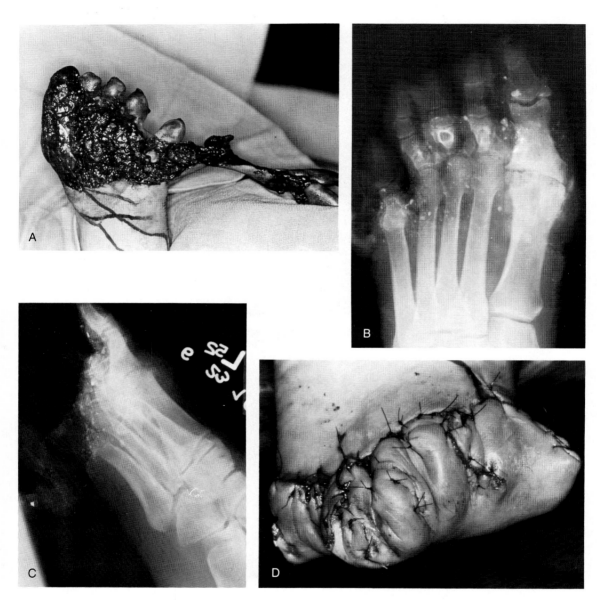

Figure 7–10. A 59-year-old factory worker sustained this severe avulsion of skin and soft tissues from the plantar aspect of his left forefoot (**A**) when the blade of a fork-lift truck went through his safety shoe and nailed his left foot to a brick wall. Anteroposterior (**B**) and lateral (**C**) views of the left foot show multiple fractures of the phalanges and the plantar condyles of the metatarsals, and numerous small pieces of foreign bodies in the open wound. **D,** after initial irrigation and debridement, the wound was closed 1 week later by filleting all the toes plus a transmetatarsal amputation.

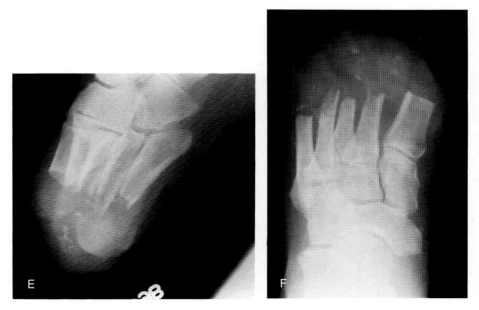

Figure 7–10. Continued. Anteroposterior (**E**) and oblique (**F**) radiographs after the complete closure of the wound show the transmetatarsal amputation. There are still small pieces of bone chips imbedded in the soft tissues distal to the partially amputated metatarsals.

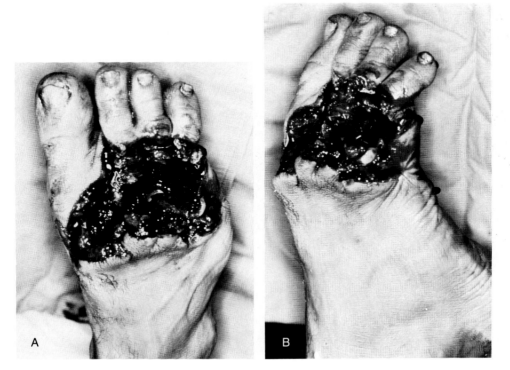

Figure 7–11. **A** and **B,** a 33-year-old man sustained a severe lawn mower injury to his right forefoot, which lacerated multiple toe extensors and flexors and neurovascular structures, and produced multiple distal metatarsal fractures. A transmetatarsal amputation of his right foot was required.

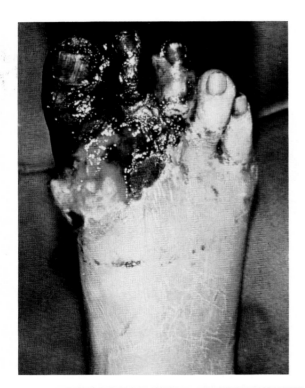

Figure 7–12. A 47-year-old factory worker's right foot was crushed by several tons of steel and developed dry gangrene of the medial three toes and their bases. A transmetatarsal amputation was required to salvage the foot.

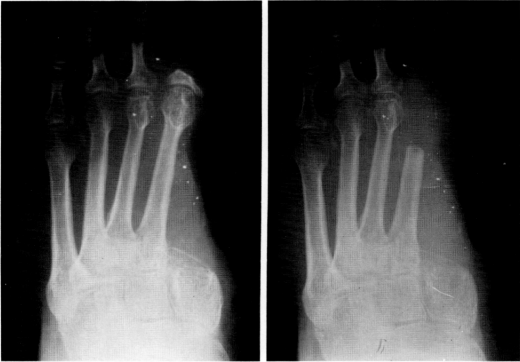

Figure 7–13. A 32-year-old man accidentally shot his left foot with a shotgun at close range. The injury resulted in transmetatarsal amputation of the first and second rays and extensive scar formation around the medial aspect of his left foot, which made proper shoe fitting difficult.

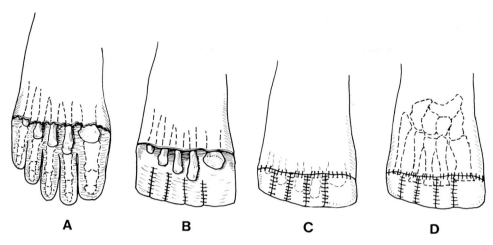

Figure 7–14. Filleting of the toes to cover full thickness skin loss plus deep soft tissue injuries of the dorsal or plantar aspect of the distal portion of the forefoot. **A,** severe soft tissue loss from the dorsal or plantar aspect of the distal portion of the forefoot. **B,** fillet all toes by removing all the phalanges, toenails, and tendons, preserve all the available neurovascular structures, and suture the adjacent sides of the toe skin flaps together. **C,** suture the end of the joined toe skin flaps to the proximal wound margins to achieve complete closure of the open wound. **D,** for more extensive loss of skin from either the dorsal or plantar aspect of the forefoot, transmetatarsal amputation can be combined with filleting of the toes to achieve complete closure of the wound.

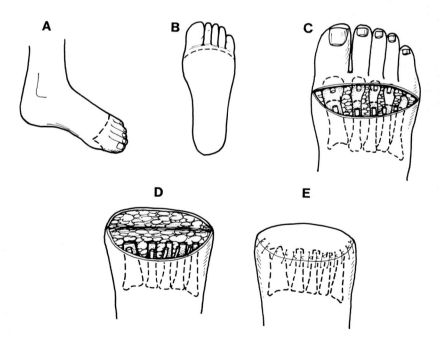

Figure 7–15. Surgical technique for a transmetatarsal amputation. **A,** dorsal skin incision. **B,** plantar skin incision. **C,** cut the dorsal tendons and the neurovascular structures. **D,** cut the plantar tendons, muscles, neurovascular structures, and all five metatarsals to complete the amputation. **E,** approximate the dorsal and plantar skin flaps.

REFERENCES

Transmetatarsal Amputation

1. Bradham, G.B., Lee, W.H., and Stallworth, J.M.: Transmetatarsal amputation. Angiology, *11:*495, 1960.
2. Dvir, E., and Kaufmann-Friedman, K.: Bilateral plantar neurotrophic ulcers treated by transmetatarsal amputation and filleting. Ann. Plast. Surg., *8:*250, 1982.
3. Effeney, D.J., Lim, R.C., and Schecter, W.P.: Transmetatarsal amputation. Arch. Surg., *112:*1366, 1977.
4. Furste, W., and Herrmann, L.G.: Value of transmetatarsal amputations in the management of gangrene of toes. Arch. Surg., *57:*497, 1948.
5. Haimovici, H.: Criteria for and results of transmetatarsal amputation for ischemic gangrene. Arch. Surg., *70:*45, 1955.
6. McKittrick, L.S., McKittrick, J.B., and Risley, T.S.: Transmetatarsal amputations for infection of gangrene in patients with diabetes mellitus. Ann. Surg., *130:*826, 1949.
7. Menacker, L.W., and Litman, M.: Transmetatarsal amputation: A literature review and case presentation. J. Am. Podiatry Assoc., *71:*302, 1981.
8. Pedersen, H.E., and Day, A.J.: The transmetatarsal amputation in peripheral vascular disease. J. Bone Joint Surg. [Am.], *36:*1190, 1954.
9. Rosendahl, S.: Transmetatarsal amputation in diabetic gangrene. Acta Orthop. Scand., *43:*78, 1972.
10. Schwindt, C.D., Lulloff, R.S., and Rogers, S.C.: Transmetatarsal amputations. Orthop. Clin. North Am., *4:*31, 1973.
11. Warren, R., Crawford, E.S., Hardy, I.B., and McKittrick, J.B.: The transmetatarsal amputation in arterial deficiency of the lower extremity. Surgery, *31:*132, 1952.
12. Wheelock, Jr., F.C.: Transmetatarsal amputations and arterial surgery in diabetic patients. N. Engl. J. Med., *264:*316, 1961.
13. Wheelock, Jr., F.C., McKittrick, J.B., and Root, H.F.: Evaluation of the transmetatarsal amputation in patients with diabetes mellitus. Surgery, *41:*184, 1957.

TOE AMPUTATION

The loss of one or more of the three lateral toes produces minimal disability or disturbance in stance and gait. Amputation of the great toe, however, will produce a limp during rapid walking and running due to loss of push-off by the great toe. Amputation of the second toe predisposes the great toe to develop hallux valgus deformity. Toe amputation can be performed through its DIP, PIP, or M-P joint, or through its proximal phalanx. Partial amputation of the toe through its DIP joint is a common surgical procedure and may be indicated under the following circumstances: mallet toe, clawtoe, hammer toe, curly toe, osteomyelitis of the distal phalanx, large epidermoid inclusion cyst of the distal phalanx, glomus tumor of the distal phalanx, and crush injury of the tip of a toe.

Amputation through the PIP joint or the proximal phalanx of a toe is unusual, but amputation through the M-P joint of a toe (a complete toe amputation) is a common surgical procedure and is indicated under the following circumstances (Figures 7–16—7–19).

A. Malignant soft tissue tumors confined to the tip of a toe, or malignant bone tumors of the distal phalanx with no proximal extension.

B. Diabetic or arteriosclerotic dry gangrene of a toe.

C. Traumatic amputation or necrosis of a toe due to crush or lawn mower injury.

D. A severe overlapping toe (usually the second toe) in an elderly patient that prevents the patient from wearing shoes comfortably.

E. Transfer of a toe to the hand to replace a lost or nonfunctional digit.

F. Ainhum.

G. Severe thermal, electric, chemical, and cold injury of toes.

H. Leprosy.

I. Tuberculous, pyogenic, and fungal infections of the toes.

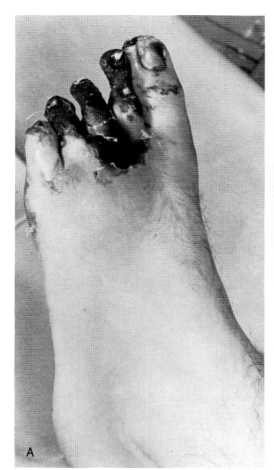
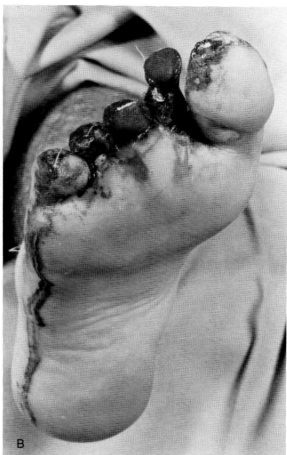

A

B

Figure 7–16. **A** and **B,** a 24-year-old man sustained a severe crushing injury to the three middle toes when an engine block was accidentally dropped on his left foot. Gangrene of the three middle toes resulted and the digits were subsequently amputated.

J. Congenital or acquired grotesque deformity of a toe.

The surgical technique for distal phalangectomy requires the following steps (Figure 7–20):

A. Make a skin incision completely around the nail and nail bed. Remove the nail and nail bed together (Figure 7–20A).

B. Separate the tip of the distal phalanx from the digital pulp and carry the dissection proximally to free the whole distal phalanx from the insertions of the extensor digitorum longus and flexor digitorum longus, and the collateral ligaments and joint capsule of the DIP joint (Figure 7–20B).

C. Approximate the skin flap to the proximal margin of the skin incision to close the wound (Figure 7–20C).

The surgical techniques for M-P and PIP disarticulations follows (Figure 7–21):

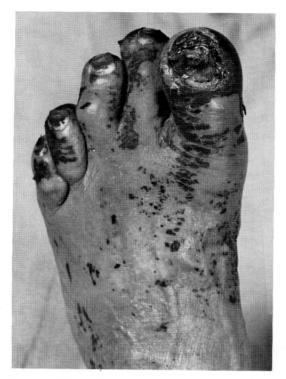

Figure 7–17. A 39-year-old man sustained a thermal burn injury to his great toe when molten iron was accidentally poured on his left foot. Necrosis of the dorsal aspect of the distal portion of the left great toe resulted, which subsequently required a partial amputation of the left great toe.

A. Two racquet-shaped skin incisions are made around the proximal portions of the great toe and second toe (Figure 7–21A—C).

B. The M-P disarticulation of the great and second toe is completed by cutting the extensor hallucis longus, extensor digitorum longus, extensor digitorum brevis, flexor hallucis longus, flexor digitorum longus, flexor digitorum brevis, abductor hallucis, adductor hallucis, flexor hallucis brevis, dorsal and plantar interossei, and lumbrical muscles; ligating the digital vessels to the great and second toes; cutting the digital nerves of the great toe and second toes as proximal to the skin incisions as pos-

sible; and cutting the collateral ligaments and joint capsules of the M-P joints of the great and second toes. The skin is then closed (Figure 7–21D).

C. A racquet-shaped skin incision is made at the level of the midportion of the middle phalanx of a lesser toe (Figure 7–21E).

D. A PIP disarticulation is completed by cutting the extensor digitorum longus, flexor digitorum brevis, collateral ligaments, and joint capsule of the PIP joint; ligating the digital vessels; and cutting the digital nerves as high above the incision as possible. The skin is then closed (Figure 7–21F).

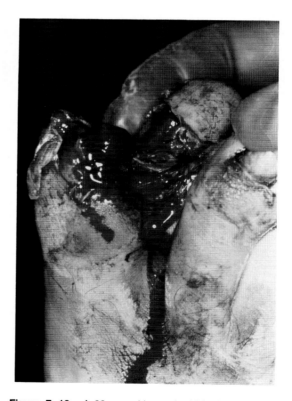

Figure 7–18. A 22-year-old man had his right great toe almost completely amputated by a rotary lawn mower. In spite of an attempt to save the toe, it turned gangrenous and had to be amputated at a more proximal level in order to close the skin.

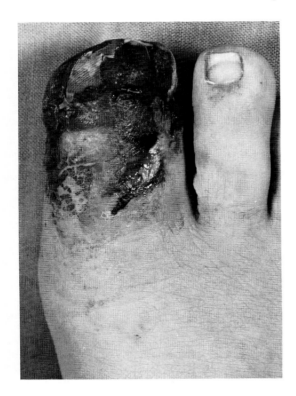

Figure 7–19. A 52-year-old man sustained a crush injury to his right great toe. The toe became gangrenous and a partial amputation was required to salvage the toe.

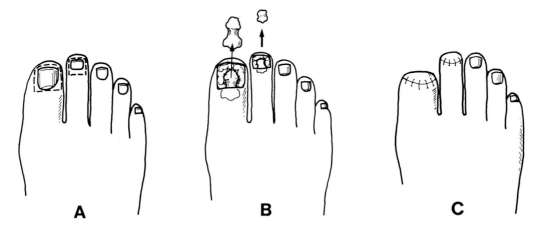

Figure 7–20. Surgical technique for distal phalangectomy of the great and lesser toes. **A,** skin incisions around the nails and nailbeds of the great and second toes. **B,** distal phalangectomies of the great and second toes. **C,** skin closure of the great and second toes.

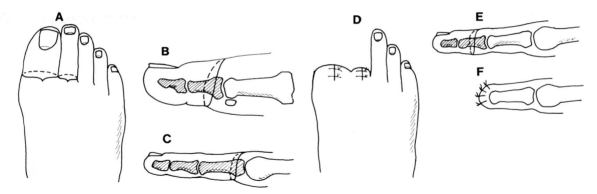

Figure 7–21. Surgical techniques for disarticulation of the PIP and M-P joints of the great and lesser toes. **A,** dorsal view of the skin incisions for disarticulation of the M-P joints of the great and second toes. **B** and **C,** lateral view of the skin incisions for disarticulation of the M-P joints of the great and second toes. **D,** completed disarticulation of the M-P joints. **E,** lateral view of the skin incision for disarticulation of the PIP joint of a lesser toe. **F,** completed disarticulation of the PIP joint of a lesser toe.

REFERENCES

Toe Amputation

1. Attiyeh, F.F., Shah, J., Booher, R.J., and Knapper, W.H.: Subungual squamous cell carcinoma. J.A.M.A., *241:*262, 1979.
2. Baddeley, R.M., and Fulford, J.C.: A trial of conservative amputations for lesions of the feet in diabetes mellitus. Br. J. Surg., *52:*38, 1965.
3. Buncke, H.J.: Toe digital transfer. Clin. Plast. Surg., *3:*49, 1976.
4. Dasgupta, T., and Brasfield, R.: Subungual melanoma. Ann. Surg., *161:*545, 1965.
5. DiGiovanni, J.E., and Fallat, L.M.: Ainhum. Report of a case. J. Am. Podiatry Assoc., *67:*401, 1977.
6. Finseth, F., and Buncke, H.J.: Thumb and digit reconstruction: Toe-to-hand microvascular composite tissue transplantation. Int. Surg., *66:*13, 1981.
7. Flint, M., and Sweetname, R.: Amputations of all toes: A review of forty-seven amputations. J. Bone Joint Surg., [Br.], *42:*90, 1960.
8. Foucher, G., Merle, M., Maneaud, M., and Michon, J.: Microsurgical free partial toe transfer in hand reconstruction: A report of 12 cases. Plast. Reconstr. Surg., *65:*616, 1980.
9. Glubo, S.M., Lenet, M., and Sherman, M.: Lawn-mower foot: The surgical reconstruction of the traumatically injured forefoot. J. Foot Surg., *16:*78, 1977.
10. Hibi, N., et al. Toe-to-hand transfer—our method an indication. Tokushima J. Exp. Med., *27:*69, 1980.
11. Hill, J.A., Victor, T.A., Dawson, W.J., and Milgram, J.W.: Myxoma of the toe: A case report. J. Bone Joint Surg. [Am.], *60:*128, 1978.
12. Hulme, J.R., and Askew, A.R.: Rotary lawn mower injuries. Injury, *5:*217, 1974.
13. Kritter, A.E.: A technique for salvage of the infected diabetic gangrenous foot. Orthop. Clin. North Am., *4:*21, 1973.
14. Leonard, A.G., and Colville, J.: Reconstruction of the thumb by microvascular transfer of the great toe. A case report. Ulster Med. J., *48:*142, 1979.
15. Leppard, B., Sanderson, K.V., and Behan, F.: Subungual malignant melanoma: Difficulty in diagnosis. Br. Med. J., *1:*310, 1924.
16. Letts, R.M., and Mardirosian, A.: Lawn mower injury in children. Can. Med. Assoc. J., *116:*1151, 1977.
17. Leung, P.C.: Transplantation of the second toe to the hand. A preliminary report of sixteen cases. J. Bone Joint Surg. [Am.], *62:*990, 1980.
18. Leung, P.C.: Prolonged refrigeration in toe-to-hand transfer—case report. J. Hand Surg., *6:*152, 1981.
19. Leung, P.C.: Problems in toe-to-hand transfer. Ann. Acad. Med. Singapore, *12:*377, 1983.
20. Leung, P.C.: Thumb reconstruction using second-toe transfer. Hand, *15:*15, 1983.
21. Lichtman, D.M., Ahbel, D.E., Murphy, R.B., and Buncke, Jr., H.J.: Neurovascular double toe transfer for opposable digits—case report and rationale for treatment. J. Hand Surg., *7:*279, 1982.
22. Lithner, F., and Tornblom, N.: Gangrene localized to the feet in diabetic patients. Acta Med. Scand., *218:*75, 1984.
23. Little, J.M., Stephen, M.S., and Zylstra, P.L.: Amputation of the toes for vascular disease: Fate of the affected leg. Lancet, *2:*1318, 1976.
24. London, P.S.: Amputations of the Fingers and Toes. *In* Operative Surgery. 2nd Ed. C. Rob and R. Smith (eds.) London, Butterworth and Co., 1969.
25. Obrien, B., Brennen, M.D., and MacLeod, A.M.: Microvascular free toe transfer. Clin. Plast. Surg., *5:*223, 1978.
26. Obrien, B., et al. Microvascular second toe transfer for digital reconstruction. J. Hand Surg., *3:*235, 1978.
27. Ohmori, K., and Harii, K.: Transplantation of a toe to an amputated finger. Hand, *7:*134, 1975.
28. Ohtsuka, H., Torigai, K., and Shidya, N.: Two toe-to-finger transplants in one hand. Plast. Reconstr. Surg., *60:*561, 1977.

29. Onizuka, T., Noda, H., and Sumiya, N.: Repair of the amputated great toe. J. Trauma, *16:*836, 1976.
30. Pack, G.T., and Adair, F.E.: Subungual melanoma. The differential diagnosis of tumors of the nail bed. *In* Tumors of the Hands and Feet. G.T. Pack (ed.). St. Louis, C.V. Mosby, 1939.
31. Pack, G.T., and Oropeza, R.: Subungual melanoma. Surg. Gynecol. Obstet., *124:*571, 1967.
32. Papachristou, D.N., and Fortner, J.G.: Melanoma arising under the nail. J. Surg. Oncol., *21:*219, 1982.
33. Poppen, N.K., Mann, R.A., Okonski, M., and Buncke, H.J.: Amputation of the great toe. Foot Ankle, *1:*333, 1981.
34. Potempa, R.L., and Lichty, T.: Hallux amputation: A case report. J. Foot Surg., *18:*40, 1979.
36. Rushforth, G.F.: Two cases of subungual malignant melanoma. Br. J. Surg., *58:*451, 1971.
37. Schajowicz, F., Aiello, C.L., and Slullitel, I.: Cystic and pseudocystic lesions of the terminal phalanx with special reference to epidermoid cysts. Clin. Orthop., *68:*84, 1970.
38. Shuman, C.R.: Foot disorders in diabetics, source of serious morbidity. Postgrad. Med., *74:*109, 1983.
39. Shuttleworth, R.D.: Amputation of gangrenous toes— effect of sepsis, blood supply and debridement on healing rates. S. Afr. Med. J., *63:*973, 1983.
40. Sizer, J.W., and Wheelock, F.C.: Digital amputations in diabetic patients. Surgery, *72:*980, 1972.
41. Solonen, K.A., Vastamaki, M., Telaranta, T., and Vilkki, S.: Toe to hand transfer. Ann. Chir. Gynaecol., *71:*28, 1982.
42. Tamai, S., Hori, Y., Tatsumi, Y., and Okuda, H.: Hallux-to-thumb transfer with microsurgical technique: A case report in a 45-year-old woman. J. Hand Surg., *2:*152, 1977.
43. Thompson, R.G., and Harper, I.A.: Lawn mower injuries. Br. Med. J., *3:*687, 1974.
44. Tsai, T.M.: 2nd and 3rd toe transplantation to a transmetacarpal amputated hand. Ann. Acad. Med. Singapore, *8:*413, 1979.
45. Walden, R., Adar, R., and Moies, M.: Gangrene of toes with normal peripheral pulses. Ann. Surg., *185:*269, 1977.
46. Wang, W.: Keys to successful second toe-to-hand transfer: A review of 30 cases. J. Hand Surg., *8:*902, 1983.
47. Werber, K.D., Biemer, E., and Glas, K.: Replantation of the hallux by microsurgical techniques. Arch. Orthop. Trauma Surg., *100:*127, 1982.
48. White, A.A., III, and Feagin, J.A.: The management of foot in leprosy. Clin. Orthop., *85:*115, 1972.
49. Zhong, W.C., Meyer, V.E., and Beasley, R.W.: The versatile second toe microvascular transfer. Orthop. Clin. North Am., *12:*827, 1981.

8 TRAUMA OF THE FOOT

The tremendous functional demands on the human foot in daily living subject it to a wide spectrum of acute and chronic injuries. The function of the bones, joints, joint capsules, and ligaments of the foot is to provide static support; dynamic support is furnished by the various intrinsic and extrinsic foot muscles. As biologic structural materials, the behavior of these bones, joints, ligaments, muscles, and tendons of the foot is governed by the law of physics in terms of stress and strain. The magnitude of this strain is usually far below the limits of elasticity of the foot, thus enabling the foot to return to its normal shape and configuration when the stress is removed. When the amount of acute or chronic stress exerted on the foot exceeds its limits of elasticity, permanent deformity is produced and is clinically manifested by bone fractures, ligament rupture, joint dislocations, and partial or complete rupture of tendons and muscle.

INJURIES OF TENDONS OF THE FOOT

A tendon is a strong collagenous cord that extends from a muscle to a bone or several bones. There are two general types of muscle in the foot, the intrinsic and extrinsic muscles. The intrinsic muscles, which are relatively small and weak, originate in the foot and insert into the different bones of the foot. In contrast, the extrinsic muscles which are larger and stronger, originate outside the foot and

insert into the various foot bones. A list of the intrinsic and extrinsic foot muscles and their respective functions follows.

A. Dorsiflexors of the foot: tibialis anterior, extensor hallucis longus, extensor digitorum longus, and peroneus tertius.

B. Plantar flexors of the foot: gastrocnemius, soleus, posterior tibialis, flexor hallucis longus, flexor digitorum longus, peroneus longus, peroneus brevis, and plantaris.

C. Supinators of the foot: tibialis anterior, tibialis posterior, extensor hallucis longus, flexor hallucis longus, and flexor digitorum longus.

D. Pronators of the foot: peroneus longus, peroneus brevis, peroneus tertius, and extensor digitorum longus.

E. Dorsiflexors of the toes: extensor digitorum longus, extensor hallucis longus, extensor digitorum brevis, and lumbricals and interossei (PIP and DIP joints only).

F. Plantar flexors of the toes: flexor hallucis longus, flexor digitorum longus, quadratus plantae, flexor digitorum brevis, flexor hallucis brevis, flexor digiti minimi brevi, and lumbricals and interossei (M-P joints only).

G. Adductors and abductors of the toes: abductor hallucis, adductor hallucis, abductor digiti minimi, and interossei.

The various injuries of the tendon are usually caused by direct trauma or chronic overuse. Because a tendon is surrounded by tenosynovium and paratenosynovial soft tissue, affections of the tendon can therefore include paratenosynovitis (irritating lesions about the tendon sheath), tenosynovitis (inflammation of a tendon sheath), and tendinitis (inflammation of the tendon itself). These lesions are frequently manifested clinically by swelling, tenderness, pain on passive stretching and active motion, crepitation, and restricted range of excursion of the affected tendon. When acute trauma or degenerative and attritional changes cause a major tendon of the foot to rupture, the patient frequently seeks immediate medical attention because of noticeable functional loss.

Rupture of the Achilles Tendon

The Achilles tendon, the largest and strongest tendon in the human body, is also the one in the foot most frequently ruptured, especially in athletes. Achilles tendinitis, direct injection of cortisone preparations into the Achilles tendon, (Figure 8–1), and previous rupture of the Achilles tendon with or without surgical repair all predispose the tendon to traumatic rupture. The rupture usually takes place near its musculotendinous junction in young people or near its insertion into the calcaneus in middle-aged and older individuals. Patients often experience a snapping or tearing sensation accompanied by pain and

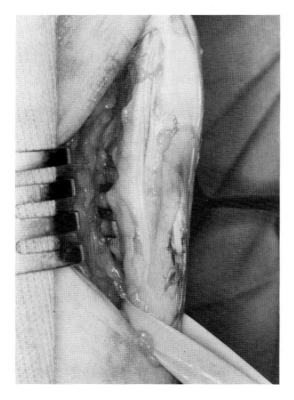

Figure 8–1. A 36-year-old woman with chronic Achilles tendinitis had numerous steroid injections into her Achilles tendon, resulting in partial rupture.

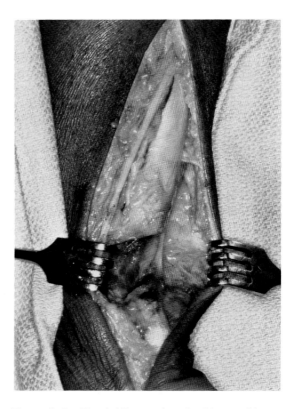

Figure 8–2. The Achilles tendon of a 29-year-old man was completely lacerated by a piece of broken glass. Two smooth, lacerated tendon ends resulted, making surgical repair easy by simply approximating the lacerated tendon ends.

swelling in the posterior aspect of the ankle and weakness of the affected foot. Physical examination often reveals tenderness, ecchymosis, a palpable defect, drastically weakened plantar flexion of the foot, and a positive Thompson's test, which can be performed by gently squeezing the calf muscle to produce plantar flexion of the foot, action that is absent when the tendo Achilles is completely ruptured.

The nonsurgical treatment of a ruptured Achilles tendon consists of immobilization of the ankle joint in a plantar-flexed position in a cast for about 8 weeks to approximate the ruptured tendon ends and to allow scarring to bridge the gap. After the removal of the cast, a lift should be placed under the heel of the affected leg and gentle stretching exercises should be started to bring the foot back gradually into its normal position. The operative treatment of a ruptured Achilles tendon consists of precise approximation of the ruptured tendon ends with sutures (Figure 8–2), and

its postoperative treatment is identical to that of nonoperative treatment. The drawbacks of surgical treatment include the risks of anesthesia, infection, large scar formation, higher medical cost, and skin slough at the incision site. As a rule, however, surgical repair tends to produce less re-rupture and better function and should be reserved for healthy and active individuals with a ruptured calcaneal tendon.

When a completely ruptured Achilles tendon is not treated, the ruptured tendon ends may become widely separated and triceps surae function is completely lost. With time, myostatic contracture of the triceps surae keeps the ruptured tendon ends widely and permanently separated. To repair an old and neglected ruptured Achilles tendon, the gap between the ruptured tendon ends can be bridged by transfer of the peroneal brevis tendon to the calcaneus, plus reinforcement of the transfer with a piece of fascia lata, or by turning down a strip of the tendon from the remaining calcaneal tendon to pass through

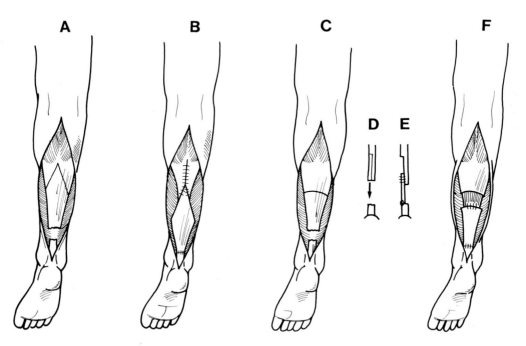

Figure 8–3. Surgical techniques for repairing an old and widely separated Achilles tendon rupture. **A,** widely separated and ruptured tendon ends and an inverted V-shaped tendon incision. **B,** V-Y tendon sliding operation has been performed and the tendon gap has been bridged and repaired. **C–F,** an alternative method of bridging the tendon gap by performing a split-thickness coronal tendon sliding operation.

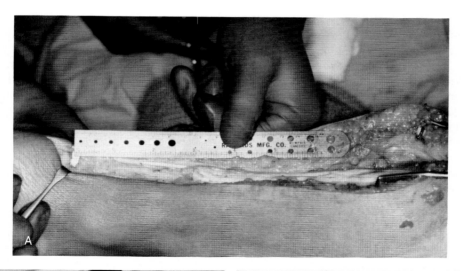

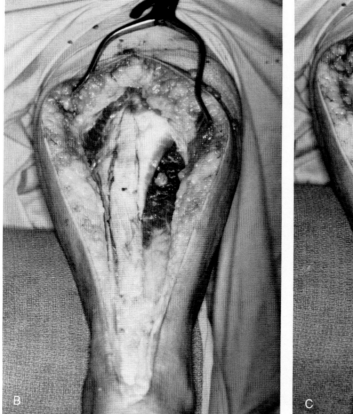

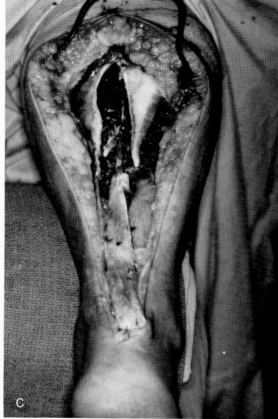

Figure 8–4.   A 28-year-old woman neglected a complete rupture of her right Achilles tendon for 6 months. **A,** a 7.6-cm gap between the ruptured tendon ends. **B,** an inverted V-shaped tendon incision has been marked on the proximal portion of the Achilles tendon in preparation for the full-thickness V-Y tendon sliding operation. **C,** inverted V-shaped tendon incision has been completed and the distal end of this free tendon graft has been sutured to the distal end of the ruptured Achilles tendon.

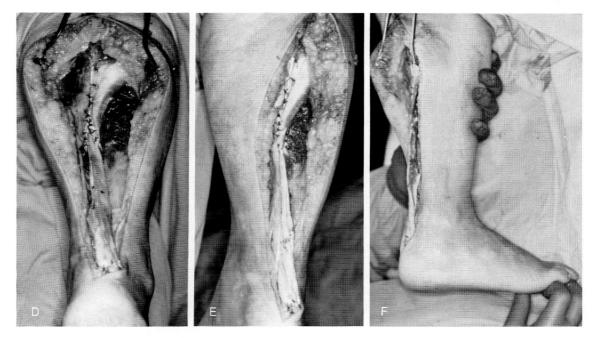

Figure 8–4. Continued. D, full-thickness V-Y tendon sliding operation has been completed and the triceps surae muscle is again continuous. **E,** plantaris tendon has been used to strengthen the Achilles tendon repair by suturing it to the entire length of the repair. **F,** with the knee joint in full extension, the ankle joint can be passively dorsiflexed to the neutral position after the tendon repair, demonstrating that the posterior ankle and subtalar joints are not significantly contracted and subsequently require no surgical release.

the distal stump to bridge the gap. The author prefers either a full-thickness V-Y sliding or a split-thickness coronal tendon sliding of the proximal tendon end to bridge the gap (Figures 8–3 and 8–4).

Rupture of the Posterior Tibial Tendon

The posterior tibial tendon is probably the second most commonly ruptured tendon in the foot, and its rupture most often affects female patients over 40 years of age. Patients with spontaneous rupture of this tendon may not seek medical attention right away due to only moderate loss of foot function. In addition, if they do seek medical attention, many examining physicians may misdiagnose their condition as medial ankle sprain or tendon strain in spite of the fact that these patients commonly give a history of an insidious and gradual development of a painful flatfoot deformity. For those physicians familiar with the symptoms and signs of a ruptured posterior

tibial tendon, however, the diagnosis can be unequivocally established by a careful physical examination of the affected foot.

The clinical signs of a ruptured posterior tibial tendon include swelling and tenderness over the course of the tendon, planovalgus deformity of the foot on weight-bearing, inability to invert the foot from a neutral or plantar-flexed position, absence of a cord-like structure behind the medial malleolus on plantar flexion and inversion of the foot, inability to perform the single-heel rise test, which normally requires strong contraction of the intact posterior tibial tendon to bring the hindfoot into a locked varus position, and the presence of the so-called "too many toes signs" when viewing both feet from a posterior direction due to forefoot abduction in a severely pronated foot. When compared with radiographs of the normal opposite foot, those of a foot with a ruptured posterior tibial tendon tend to show medial and inferior rotation of the talar head and neck from the calcaneus, lateral deviation of the forefoot, increased talocalcaneal angle on both the anteroposterior and lateral views, and subluxation of the talonavicular articulation due to medial deviation of the head of the talus (Figures 8–5 and 8–6).

When the ruptured posterior tibial tendon is diagnosed early, end-to-end repair or reattachment of its end to its normal insertion site may be feasible. When the tendon rupture has been present for a significant period, end-to-end repair is usually no longer possible due to myostatic contracture of the affected posterior tibial muscle or degeneration of the ruptured tendon ends. Under this circumstance, the flexor digitorum longus tendon can be used to bridge the gap by dividing it at an appropriate level, suturing both the proximal and distal ends of the ruptured posterior tibial tendon to the flexor digitorum longus tendon under proper tension, and suturing the distal end of the surgically severed flexor digitorum longus tendon to the neighboring flexor hallucis longus tendon (Figure 8–7).

Dislocation and Rupture of the Peroneal Tendons

Acute trauma is usually the cause of dislocation of the peroneal tendons; congenital shallow groove or absence of the groove be-

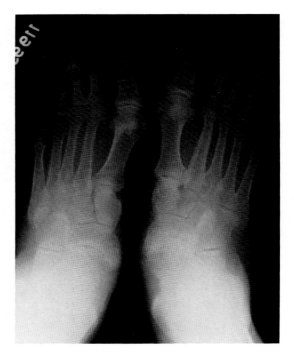

Figure 8–5. A 53-year-old man had a 6-month history of medical foot pain and development of a progressive planovalgus deformity of the right foot caused by spontaneous rupture of the posterior tibial tendon. Note the abduction deformity of the right forefoot and the medial subluxation of the head of right talus from the talonavicular joint.

hind the lateral malleolus may also dispose the peroneal tendons to dislocation. The

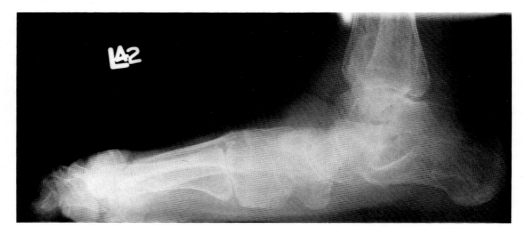

Figure 8–6. A 76-year-old woman had a spontaneous rupture of her left posterior tibial tendon. Over the next 10 years, her foot gradually developed severe planovalgus deformity to the point that she had a rocker-bottom flatfoot on the left with marked heel valgus. Note the plantar-flexed position of the talus and the absence of the longitudinal arch.

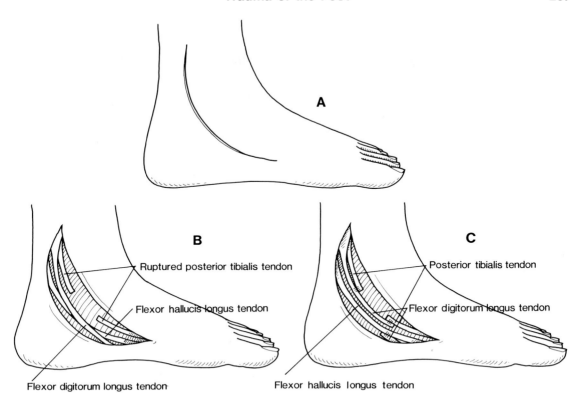

A

B

Ruptured posterior tibialis tendon

Flexor hallucis longus tendon

Flexor digitorum longus tendon

C

Posterior tibialis tendon

Flexor digitorum longus tendon

Flexor hallucis longus tendon

Figure 8–7. Surgical technique for repairing an old and widely separated posterior tibial tendon rupture. **A,** a curved incision behind the medial malleolus along the course of the posterior tibial tendon. **B,** a wide gap between the ruptured tendon ends of the posterior tibial tendon. **C,** proximal end of the surgically severed flexor digitorum longus tendon has been sutured to both ends of the ruptured posterior tibial tendon, and the distal end of the severed flexor digitorum longus tendon has been sutured to the intact flexor hallucis longus tendon to maintain motor function.

mechanism of injury is a combination of forceful contraction of the peroneal muscles and dorsiflexion and eversion of the ankle joint. When a skier's ski accidentally digs into the snow, it forces the ankle joint into acute dorsiflexion. The skier may then experience a tearing or snapping sensation in the lateral ankle region, which is soon followed by pain, tenderness, and swelling in the posterior aspect of the lateral malleolus caused by a detachment of the superior peroneal retinaculum from the lateral surface of the lateral malleolus with its periosteum, or avulsion of a fragment of bone from the lateral margin of the lateral malleolus with the superior peroneal retinaculum still attached to the avulsed bone fragment.

Dislocation of the peroneal tendons is frequently misdiagnosed as a sprain of the lateral aspect of the ankle. By carefully manipulating and examining the injured ankle, however, the peroneal tendons may be found lying obliquely across the lateral surface of the lateral malleolus; the dislocated peroneal tendons can be reduced by plantar flexing the foot, pushing the dislocated tendons downward and backward. In chronic cases, the patients can even voluntarily dislocate their peroneal tendons by dorsiflexing and everting the foot while forcefully contracting the peroneal muscles.

In treating acute dislocation of the peroneal tendons, the author prefers to reattach the detached superior peroneal retinaculum to its original anatomic site surgically. In chronic cases, a strip of the Achilles tendon can be

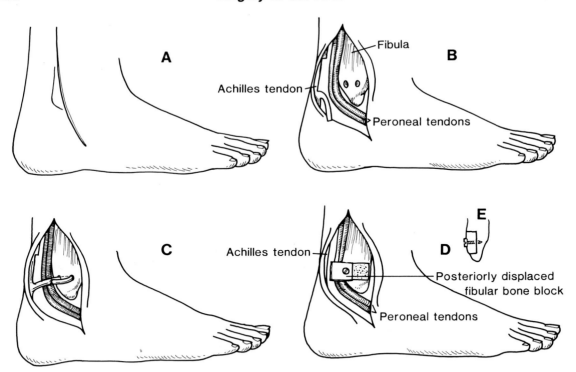

Figure 8–8. Surgical techniques to correct a recurrent anterior dislocation of the peroneal tendons. **A,** a slightly curved incision over the lateral malleolus. **B,** a transverse hole has been drilled through the distal portion of the lateral malleolus and a strip of the Achilles tendon has been prepared. **C,** the Achilles tendon strip has been passed through the drilled hole and its distal end has been sutured to its proximal portion. **D** and **E,** the sliding bone block technique to deepen the groove behind the lateral malleolus and fixation of the bone block with a bone screw.

used to hold the peroneal tendons in place by passing it through a hole drilled transversely in the fibula and then suturing its end tightly to its proximal portion, or by sliding a bone block backward and holding the bone block in place with a bone screw to hold the peroneal tendons in the groove behind the lateral malleolus (Figures 8–8 and 8–9).

Tenosynovitis of the peroneal tendons can be caused by compression of these two tendons between a widened calcaneal body, produced by a calcaneal fracture, and the fibula. The bony encroachment of the peroneal tendons can be clearly demonstrated with a peroneal tendon synoviagram. Pain and impairment of the normal function of the peroneal tendons may require surgical decompression, which is accomplished by either excising the tip of the fibula or resecting the

lateral prominence of the calcaneus to free the peroneal tendons that may be buried in bony callus, held by bony fragment, or fibrosed by scar tissue.

Traumatic rupture of the peroneal tendons is rare. Evans (1966) reported rupture of the peroneal longus tendon from an inversion injury of the foot that occurred playing football. When the peroneal tendons do rupture, however, the tear usually occurs just proximal to the superior peroneal retinaculm. Examination often reveals tenderness, swelling, and ecchymosis along the course of the ruptured portion of the peroneal tendons; weakness of active foot eversion is also a common finding. A defect may also be felt at the site of the peroneal tendon rupture.

The treatment of choice for ruptured peroneal tendons is primary surgical repair plus

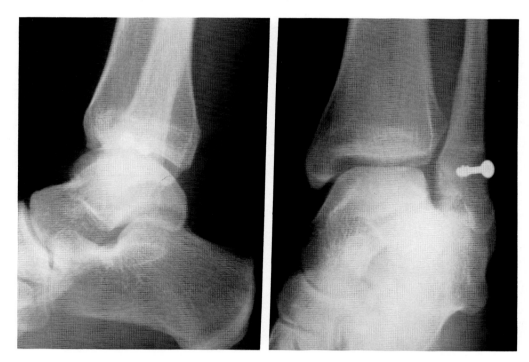

Figure 8–9. An 18-year-old woman sustained a dislocation of her left peroneal tendons in a tennis match and was treated with Ace bandage. With time, the patient could voluntarily dislocate her left peroneal tendons by dorsiflexing and everting her foot while forcefully contracting her peroneal tendons. The recurrent peroneal tendon dislocation was completely cured by sliding a fibular bone block backward to hold the peroneal tendon in the groove behind the lateral malleolus (lateral and mortise views).

cast immobilization for a few weeks for the ruptured tendons to heal. In cases of a neglected rupture, however, a sizable gap may be present between the ruptured tendon ends, making an end-to-end surgical approximation an impossible task. Under this circumstance, if only one of the peroneal tendons is ruptured, its ruptured ends can be sutured directly to the adjacent intact peroneal tendon (Figure 8–10 A–D). If both peroneal tendons are torn, the gap can be bridged with a free sliding peroneus longus tendon graft, the distal end of which should be sutured to the ruptured distal ends of the peroneus longus and brevis tendons, and its proximal end to the proximal end of the ruptured peroneus brevis tendon. In addition, the free peroneus longus muscle should be sutured directly to its adjacent peroneus brevis muscle (Figure 8–10 E and F).

Rupture of the Extensor Hallucis Longus Tendon

The extensor hallucis longus tendon is frequently severed by dropping a sharp object, such as a knife or a broken glass, on the dorsal aspect of the foot, although attritional rupture from constant irritation by a tarsometatarsal exostosis and spontaneous rupture of the same tendon can also occur. The inability to extend the great toe past a neutral position, a palpable defect at the tendon rupture site, and absence of the cord-like structure on the dorsal aspect of the great toe and first metatarsal when the extensor hallucis longus muscle is actively contracting make the diagnosis of a ruptured extensor hallucis longus tendon an easy matter.

The treatment of choice consists of primary surgical repair of the ruptured tendon plus cast

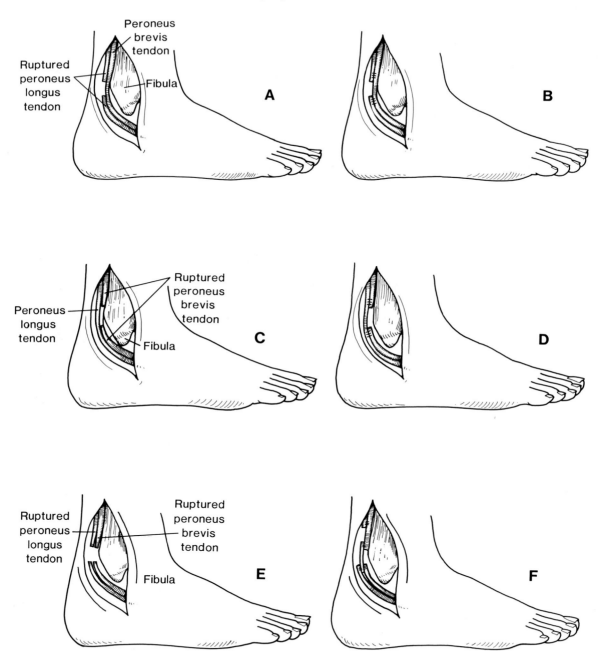

Figure 8–10. Surgical techniques for repairing an old and widely separated single peroneal tendon rupture (**A–D**) and old rupture of both the peroneus longus and brevis tendons (**E** and **F**). **A,** ruptured peroneus longus tendon with a wide gap between the ruptured tendon ends. **B,** ruptured ends of the peroneus longus tendon have been sutured to its adjacent, intact peroneus brevis tendon. **C,** ruptured peroneus brevis tendon with a wide gap between the ruptured tendon ends. **D,** ruptured ends of the peroneus brevis tendon have been sutured to its adjacent, intact peroneus longus tendon. **E,** a wide gap between the ruptured tendon ends of both the peroneus longus and brevis tendons. **F,** a segment of the peroneus longus tendon has been cut, moved distally, and sutured to the distal ends of the ruptured peroneus longus and brevis tendon. The proximal end of the peroneus tendon graft has been sutured to the proximal end of the peroneus brevis tendon, and the peroneus longus muscle to the peroneus brevis muscle.

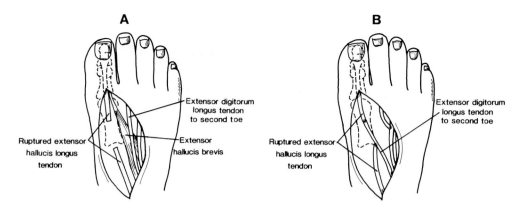

Figure 8–11. Surgical technique for repairing an old ruptured extensor hallucis longus tendon with a large gap between its ruptured tendon ends. **A,** ruptured extensor hallucis longus tendon with a large gap between its ruptured tendon ends. **B,** ruptured ends of the extensor hallucis longus tendon have been sutured to the surgically severed extensor digitorum longus tendon to the second toe, and the severed distal end of the extensor digitorum longus tendon to the second toe has been sutured to the intact extensor digitorum longus tendon to the third toe to provide motor power.

immobilization for a few weeks to allow the repaired tendon to heal. In cases of neglected rupture, a large gap usually exists between the ruptured tendon ends. The extensor digitorum longus tendon to the second toe can then be used to attach to the distal end of the ruptured extensor hallucis longus tendon. In addition, the proximal end of the ruptured extensor hallucis longus can be sutured to the proximal portion of the extensor digitorum longus tendon to the second toe, the severed distal end of which should be sutured to the adjacent extensor digitorum longus tendon to the third toe to preserve its motor function (Figure 8–11 and 8–12).

Rupture of the Anterior Tibial Tendon

The anterior tibial tendon, the largest and strongest tendon in the anterior aspect of the ankle, is rarely ruptured. When rupture does occur, it usually takes place immediately proximal to its insertion and tends to affect patients over 45 years of age, especially in patients in their seventh decade of life. With its slight early disability, weeks or months may pass before the diagnosis of a ruptured anterior tibial tendon is established. Careful examination reveals weakness of dorsiflexion of the ankle, swelling and tenderness about the

dorsum of the ankle and foot, a mild degree of foot drop, a palpable lump in the course of the anterior tibial tendon at the ankle level, a palpable gap near the insertion of the anterior tibial tendon, eversion of the foot on active dorsiflexion of the foot, and the absence of the prominent cord-like structure in the anteromedial aspect of the ankle when the anterior tibialis muscle is actively contracting.

When a fresh rupture of the anterior tibial tendon is diagnosed early, direct surgical repair can usually be accomplished. If the diagnosis is delayed, however, and the anterior tibialis muscle has become contracted, the gap can still be bridged by transferring the extensor hallucis longus tendon to the insertion of the anterior tibial tendon through a drilled hole, and by suturing the end of the extensor hallucis longus tendon to the distal stump of the ruptured anterior tibialis tendon, and the proximal end of the anterior tibial tendon to the more proximal portion of the extensor hallucis longus tendon. In addition, the extensor digitorum longus tendon to the second toe can be sutured to the severed distal end of the extensor hallucis longus to provide motor power for dorsiflexion of the great toe, and the severed distal end of the extensor digitorum longus tendon to the second toe can

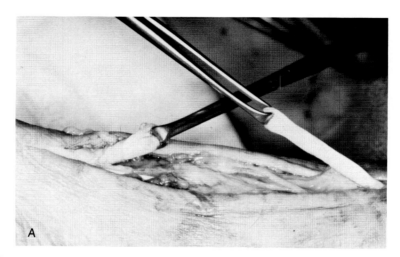

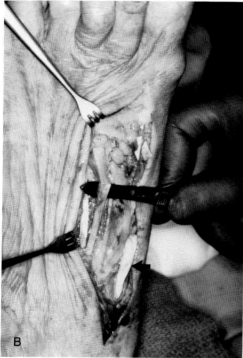
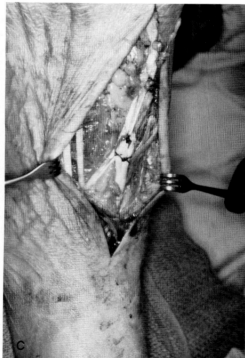

Figure 8–12. A 57-year-old woman developed a spontaneous rupture of her left extensor hallucis longus tendon (**A**). The two ruptured tendon ends could not be repaired in an end-to-end fashion due to myostatic contracture. **B,** the extensor digitorum longus to the second toe has been identified and isolated in preparation for subsequent transfer. Note the ruptured extensor hallucis longus tendon on the right. **C,** the two ruptured ends of the extensor hallucis longus tendon have been sutured to the extensor digitorum longus tendon to the second toe. The severed distal end of the extensor digitorum longus tendon to the second toe can be sutured to the adjacent extensor digitorum longus tendon to the third toe to preserve motor power.

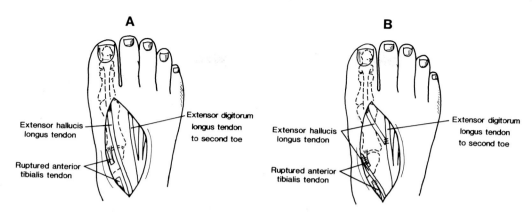

Figure 8–13. Surgical technique for repairing an old ruptured anterior tibial tendon with a wide gap between its ruptured tendon ends. **A,** ruptured anterior tibial tendon with its two ends widely separated. **B,** the two ends of the ruptured anterior tibial tendon are sutured to the surgically severed extensor hallucis longus tendon, and the distal end of the severed extensor hallucis longus tendon to the intact extensor digitorum longus tendon to the second toe so to provide the great toe with new motor power.

be sutured to the same tendon to the third toe to provide active extensor power (Figure 8–13).

Rupture of the Flexor Hallucis Longus Tendon

Laceration of the flexor hallucis longus tendon is usually caused by stepping on a sharp object, such as broken glass, while running or walking barefoot. In addition, depending on the site and depth of the laceration, digital nerves to the toes, medial and lateral plantar nerves, and the flexor hallucis brevis can also be lacerated. Acute rupture has been known to occur in diving accidents, motor cycle accidents, and classic ballet dancing, etc. (Krackow 1980; Sammarco and Miller 1979; and Frenette and Jackson 1977). Physical examination usually reveals absence of flexion of the interphalangeal joint of the great toe when the flexor hallucis longus tendon is lacerated, and inability to flex both the M-P and interphalangeal joints when both the flexor hallucis longus and brevis tendons have been severed. Furthermore, sensory deficit to one or more toes may also be noted when the medial and lateral plantar nerves or their branches have been cut.

Treatment includes thorough debridement and irrigation of the wound plus meticulous surgical repair of the lacerated tendons and nerves. If severe injury to the flexor hallucis brevis tendon has occurred, however, and the proximal end of the flexor hallucis longus tendon cannot be found, suturing the flexor hallucis brevis tendon to the proximal end of the severed distal segment of the flexor hallucis longus tendon should be performed to prevent hyperextension deformity of the great toe. It is of interest to note that Frenette and Jackson (1977) reported that four athletically inclined young people sustained complete laceration of their flexor hallucis longus tendons that were not repaired, and they showed no disability at all. Partial rupture of the flexor hallucis longus tendon, however, can produce a trigger great toe that often requires surgical division of the digital tendon sheath of the great toe to give more room for the scarred flexor hallucis longus tendon to slide forward and backward.

REFERENCES

Achilles Tendon

1. Bosworth, D.M.: Repair of defects in the tendo achilles. J. Bone Joint Surg. [Am.], *38:*111, 1956.
2. Bugg, Jr., E.I., and Boyd, B.M.: Repair of negelected rupture or laceration of the Achilles tendon. Clin Orthop., *56:*73, 1968.

3. Hooker, C.H.: Rupture of tendon Achilles. J. Bone Joint Surg. [Br.], *45:*360, 1963.
4. Inglis, A.E., Scott, W.N., Sculco, T.P., and Patterson, A.H.: Ruptures of tendo Achilles: An objective assessment of surgical and nonsurgical treatment. J. Bone Joint Surg. [Am.], *58:*990, 1976.
5. Lea, R.B., and Smith, L.: Non-surgical treatment of tendo Achilles rupture. J. Bone Joint Surg. [Am.], *54:*1398, 1972.
6. Lindholm, A.: A new method of operation in subcutaneous rupture of the Achilles tendon. Acta Chir. Scand., *117:*261, 1959.
7. Lynn, T.A.: Repair of the torn Achilles tendon, using the plantaris tendon as the reinforcing membrane. J. Bone Joint Surg. [Am.], *48:*268, 1966.
8. Ma, G.W.C., and Griffith, T.G.: Percutaneous repair of acute closed rupture of Achilles tendon—a new technique. Clin. Orthop., *128:*248, 1977.
9. Newmark, H., et al: A new finding in radiographic diagnosis of Achilles tendon rupture. Skeletal Radiol., *8:*223, 1982.
10. Schedl, R., and Fasol, P.: Achilles tendon repair with plantaris tendon compared with repair using polyglycol threads. J. Trauma, *19:*189, 1979.
11. Stein, S.R., and Leukens, Jr., C.A.: Closed treatment of Achilles tendon ruptures. Orthop. Clin. North Am., *7:*241, 1976.
12. Teuffer, A.P.: Traumatic rupture of the Achilles tendon: Reconstruction by transplant and graft using the lateral peroneus brevis. Orthop. Clin. North Am., *5:*89, 1974.
13. Thompson, T.C.: A test for rupture of the tendo Achilles. Acta Orthop. Scand., *32:*461, 1962.
14. White, R.K., and Kraynick, B.M.: Surgical uses of the peroneus brevis tendon. Surg. Gynecol. Obstet., *108:*117, 1959.

Posterior Tibial Tendon

1. Anzel, S.H., Covey, K.W., Weiner, A.D., and Lipscomb, P.R.: Disruption of muscles and tendons. An analysis of 1014 cases. Surgery, *45:*406, 1959.
2. Burman, M.: Stenosing tenovaginitis of the foot and ankle. Arch. Surg., *67:*686, 1953.
3. Cozen, L.: Posterior tibial tenosynovitis secondary to foot strain. Clin. Orthop., *42:*101, 1965.
4. Fowler, A.W.: Tibialis posterior syndrome. J. Bone Joint Surg. [Br.], *37:*520, 1955.
5. Fredenburg, M., Tilley, G., and Yagoobian, E.M.: Spontaneous rupture of the posterior tibial tendon secondary to chronic nonspecific tenosynovitis. J. Foot Surg., *22:*198, 1983.
6. Ghormley, R.K., and Spear, I.M.: Anomalies of the posterior tibial tendon. Arch. Surg., *66:*512, 1953.
7. Goldner, J.L., Keats, P.K., Bassett, F.H., and Clippinger, F.W.: Progressive talipes equinovalgus due to trauma or degeneration of the posterior tibial tendon and medial plantar ligaments. Orthop. Clin. North Am., *5:*39, 1974.
8. Griffiths, J.C.: Tendon injuries around the ankle. J. Bone Joint Surg. [Br.], *47:*686, 1965.
9. Henceroth, II, W.D., and Deyerly, W.M.: The acquired unilateral flat foot in adult: Some causative factors. Foot Ankle, *2:*304, 1982.
10. Jahss, M.H.: Spontaneous rupture of the tibialis posterior tendon: Clinical findings, tenographic studies and a new technique of repair. Foot Ankle, *2:*350, 1982.
11. Johnson, K.A.: Tibialis posterior tendon rupture. Clin. Orthop., *177:*140, 1983.
12. Kettelkamp, D.B., and Alexander, H.H.: Spontaneous rupture of the posterior tibial tendon. J. Bone Joint Surg. [Am.], *51:*759, 1969.
13. Key, J.A.: Partial rupture of the tendon of the posterior tibial muscle. J. Bone Joint Surg. [Am.], *35:*1006, 1953.
14. Kulowski, J.: Tenovaginitis (tenosynovitis): General discussion and report of one case involving posterior tibial tendon. J. Mo. Med. Assoc., *33:*135, 1936.
15. Langenskiold, A.: Chronic nonspecific tenosynovitis of the tibialis posterior tendon. Acta Orthop. Scand., *38:*301, 1967.
16. Lapidus, P.W., and Seidenstein, H.: Chronic nonspecific tenosynovitis with effusion about the ankle. J. Bone Joint Surg. [Am.], *32:*175, 1950.
17. Lewis, O.J.: The tibialis posterior tendon in the primate foot. J. Anat., *98:*209, 1964.
18. Lipscomb, P.R.: Nonsuppurative tenosynovitis and paratendinitis. Instr. Course Lect., *7:*254, 1950.
19. Lipsman, S., Frankel, J.P., and Count, G.W.: Spontaneous rupture of the tibialis posterior tendon. A case report and review of the literature. J. Am. Podiatry Assoc., *70:*34, 1980.
20. Mann, R.A., and Specht, L.H.: Posterior tibial tendon ruptures—analysis of eight cases. Foot Ankle, *2:*350, 1982.
21. Scheller, A.D., Kasser, J.R., and Quigley, T.B.: Tendon injuries about the ankle. Orthrop. Clin. North Am., *11:*801, 1980.
22. Trevino, S., Gould, N., and Korson, R.: Surgical treatment of stenosing tenosynovitis at the ankle. Foot Ankle, *2:*37, 1981.
23. Williams, R.: Chronic nonspecific tenovaginitis of the tibialis posterior. J. Bone Joint Surg. [Br.], *45:*542, 1963.

Peroneal Tendons

1. Abraham, E., and Stirnaman, J.E.: Neglected rupture of the peroneal tendons causing recurrent sprains of the ankle. Case report. J. Bone Joint Surg. [Am.], *61:*1247, 1979.
2. Alm, A., Lamke, L.O., and Liljedahl, S.O.: Surgical treatment of dislocation of the peroneal tendon. Injury. *7:*14, 1975.
3. Burman, M.: Stenosing tenovaginitis of the foot and ankle. Studies with special reference to the stenosing tenosynovitis of the peroneal tendons. Arch. Surg., *67:*686, 1963.
4. De Yerle, W.M.: Long term follow-up of fractures of the os calcis: Diagnostic peroneal synoviagram. Orthrop. Clin. North Am., *4:*213, 1971.
5. Eckert, W.R., and Davis, Jr., E.A.: Acute rupture of peroneal retinaculum. J. Bone Joint Surg. [Am.], *58:*670, 1976.
6. Evans, J.D.: Subcutaneous rupture of the tendon of peroneus longus. Report of a case. J. Bone Joint Surg. [Br.], *48:*507, 1966.
7. Isbister, J.F.S.C.: Calcaneo-fibular abutment follow-

ing crush fracture of the calcaneus. J. Bone Joint Surg. [Br.], *56:*274, 1974.

8. Jackson, M.A., and Gudas, C.J.: Peroneus longus tendonitis: A possible biomechanical etiology. J. Foot Surg., *21:*344, 1982.
9. Jones, E.: Operative treatment of chronic dislocation of peroneal tendon. J. Bone Joint Surg. [Br.], *14:*574, 1932.
10. Kashiwagi, D.: Diagnosis and treatment of fractures of the os calcis. Spectator correspondence club letter, 1965.
11. Kelly, R.E.: An operation for the chronic dislocation of the peroneal tendon. Br. J. Surg., *7:*502, 1920.
12. Munk, R.L., and Davis, P.H.: Longitudinal rupture of the peroneal brevis tendon. J. Trauma, *16:*803, 1976.
13. Murr, S.: Dislocation of the peroneal tendons with marginal fracture of the lateral malleolus. J. Bone Joint Surg. [Br.], *43:*563, 1961.
14. Purnell, M.L., Drummond, D.S., Engber, W.D., and Breed, A.L.: Congenital dislocation of the peroneal tendons in the calcaneovalgus foot. J. Bone Joint Surg. [Br.], *65:*316, 1983.
15. Samiento, A., and Wolf, M.: Subluxation of peroneal tendons: Case treated by rerouting tendons under calcaneofibular ligament. J. Bone Joint Surg. [Am.], *57:*115, 1975.
16. Stover, C.N., and Bryan, D.R.: Traumatic dislocation of the peroneal tendons. Am. J. Surg., *103:*108, 1962.
17. VanMoppes, F.I., and Van Den Hoogenband, C.R.: The significance of the peroneus tendon sheath in ankle arthrography. ROFO, *132:*573, 1980.

Extensor Hallucis Longus Tendon

1. Jahss, M.H. (ed.): Disorders of the Foot. Philadelphia, W.B. Saunders, 1982, p. 864.
2. Griffiths, J.C.: Tendon injuries around the ankle. J. Bone Joint Surg. [Br.], *47:*686, 1965.

Anterior Tibial Tendon

1. Burman, M.S.: Subcutaneous rupture of the tendon of the tibialis anticus. Ann. Surg., *100:*368, 1934.
2. Dooley, B.J., Kudelka, P., and Menelaus, M.B.: Subcutaneous rupture of the tendon of tibialis anterior. J. Bone Joint Surg. [Br.], *62:*471, 1980.
3. Griffiths, J.C.: Tendon injury around the ankle. J. Bone Joint Surg. [Br.], *47:*686, 1965.
4. Lapidus, P.W.: Indirect subcutaneous rupture of the anterior tibial tendon. Report of two cases. Bull. Hosp. J. Dis., Orthop. Inst., *2:*119, 1941.
5. Mensor, M.C., and Ordway, G.L.: Traumatic subcutaneous rupture of the tibialis anterior tendon. J. Bone Joint Surg. [Am.], *35:*675, 1953.
6. Moskowitz, E.: Rupture of the tibialis anterior tendon simulating peroneal nerve palsy. Arch. Phys. Med. Rehabil.. *52:*431. 1971.
7. Richter, R., and Schlitt, R.: Die subkutane ruptur der sehne des musculus tibialis anterior. Z. Orthop., *113:*271, 1975.
8. Moberg, E.: Subcutaneous rupture of the tendon of the tibialis muscle. Acta Chir. Scand., *95:*455, 1947.

Flexor Hallucis Longus Tendon

1. Frenette, J.P., and Jackson, D.W.: Lacerations of the flexor hallucis longus in the young athlete. J. Bone Joint Surg. [Am.], *59:*673, 1977.
2. Gould, N.: Stenosing tenosynovitis of the flexor hallucis longus tendon at the great toe. Foot Ankle, *2:*46, 1981.
3. Hamilton, W.G.: Stenosing tenosynovitis of the flexor hallucis longus tendon and posterior impingement upon the os trigonum in ballet dancers. Foot Ankle, *3:*74, 1982.
4. Krackow, K.A.: Acute, traumatic rupture of a flexor hallucis longus tendon: A case report. Clin. Orthop., *150:*261, 1980.
5. Neely, M.G.: Trigger toes. Report of a case. J. Bone Joint Surg. [Br.], *45:*379, 1963.
6. Sammarco, G.J., and Miller, E.H.: Partial rupture of the flexor hallucis longus tendon in classical ballet dancers. J. Bone Joint Surg. [Am.], *61:*149, 1979.

FRACTURES AND DISLOCATIONS OF THE FOOT

Fractures and Dislocations of the Toes

FRACTURES OF THE GREAT TOE

INCIDENCE. The proximal and distal phalanges of the great toe are larger than the corresponding phalanges of the lesser toes and thus have to bear more body weight and receive more traumatic forces of daily living. In addition, their prominent anatomic site on the leading anteromedial aspect of the foot exposes them to all types of trauma, which may explain why the hallux phalanges sustain more fractures than the phalanges of the four lateral lesser toes.

There are two main mechanisms that produce the majority of fractures of the great toe. In a stubbing injury, the force is applied to the tip of the great toe and is transmitted along its longitudinal axis to produce different displaced and undisplaced fractures of the phalanges (Figure 8–14) as well as dislocation of the interphalangeal and M-P joints of the great toe. Stubbing injury often produces only closed fractures or dislocations and an insignificant degree of bony comminution, all of which are caused by indirect forces. In a crush injury, the force is usually applied directly to the dorsal aspect of the great toe with such a magnitude that bony comminution (particularly the distal phalanx of the great toe), severe soft

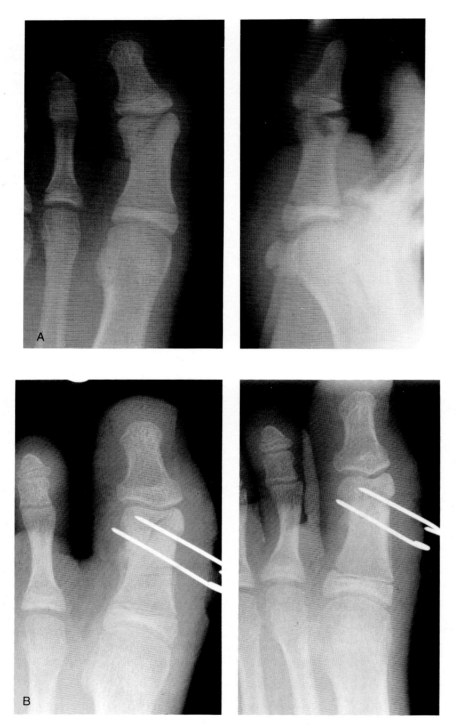

Figure 8–14. A 12-year-old girl in whom anteroposterior and oblique (**A**) radiographs show a displaced transarticular fracture of the distal portion of the proximal phalanx of the left great toe. **B,** Anteroposterior and oblique views show an anatomic reduction of the phalangeal transarticular fracture of the great toe with two small K-wires.

tissue damages that may eventually produce gangrene of the great toe, compound fractures, and minimal to moderate fracture fragment displacement are the likely outcome (Figures 8–15—8–23). Occasionally, avulsion fractures of the proximal and distal phalanges of the great toe can be produced by the tendons and ligaments that are attached to them (Figures 8–24 and 8–25).

CLINICAL SYMPTOMS AND SIGNS. These include pain, tenderness, swelling, ecchymosis, deformity, subungual hematoma, crepitation, and skin laceration.

ROENTGENOGRAPHIC MANIFESTATIONS. Anteroposterior, lateral, and oblique radiographs of the foot usually identify the site and nature of the fracture. A good lateral view of the great toe can be obtained by placing a small dental film between the great and second toes to get an isolated view of the great toe and to show the exact extent of dorsal or plantar angulation of the fracture site.

TREATMENT. When a fresh, tense, and painful subungual hematoma is present, sig-

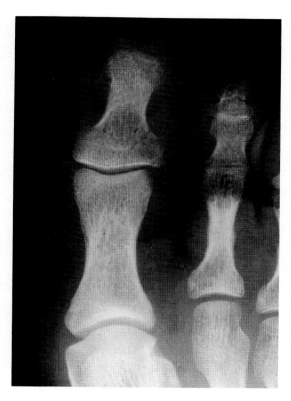

Figure 8–16. Anteroposterior view of the great and second toes shows a nondisplaced fracture of the lateral base of the distal phalanx of the great toe, and a transverse fracture of the distal phalanx of the second toe caused by a crush injury.

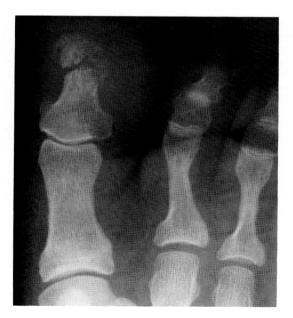

Figure 8–15. A 53-year-old woman dropped a portable computer on her right great toe, which produced a slightly comminuted fracture of the distal portion of the distal phalanx of the great toe. Note the marked soft tissue swelling around the fracture site.

nificant pain relief can be obtained by boring a small hole through the nail with the heated end of a straightened paper clip. When the fracture is extra-articular and stable and shows minimal or no displacement, a piece of felt or some lamb's wool can be placed in the first web space, the great toe can be bound to the second toe with adhesive tape, and a shoe with its toe cap removed and a metatarsal bar on its outer sole or a postoperative wooden-soled shoe can be used to allow early, full weight-bearing. The toe taping should be continued for about 3 weeks to allow fracture callus to form at the fracture site. The patient can then resume wearing comfortable regular shoes.

If the fracture is angulated, closed reduction should first be attempted by applying lon-

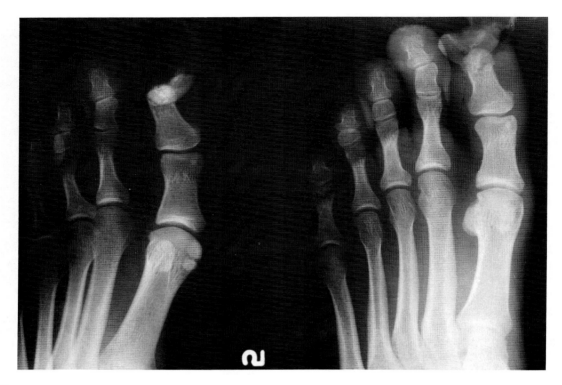

Figure 8–17. A 26-year-old man sustained a compound fracture of the distal portion of the distal phalanx of his left great toe when he accidentally slid his foot under a rotary lawn mower. Oblique and anteroposterior radiographs demonstrate the resulting partial amputation of the distal portion of the great toe.

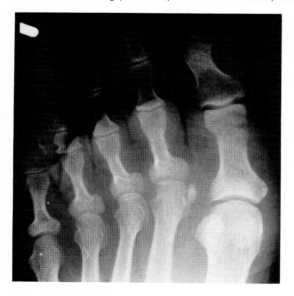

Figure 8–18. A 50-year-old woman dropped a metal block on the dorsal aspect of her left great toe. Anteroposterior radiograph shows a nondisplaced fracture of the neck of the first proximal phalanx.

gitudinal traction by means of Chinese finger traps, and the reduced great toe fracture can then be immobilized and protected by a short walking cast with a big toe spica. If the fracture is unstable, stability can be provided by an intramedullary K-wire, which is driven from the proximal end of the distal fracture fragment to emerge through the tip of the great toe. The fracture is then accurately reduced before driving the K-wire into the proximal fracture fragment in a retrograde manner. The pin should stay in the fractured phalanx for 3 weeks, after which a hard-soled shoe with a metatarsal bar on the outer sole can be worn until the toe is completely asymptomatic.

When a displaced fracture involves an articular surface, closed reduction should be attempted. If the reduction is satisfactory, a short walking cast with a big toe spica can be used to protect the reduced toe fracture. If adequate reduction cannot be achieved by closed

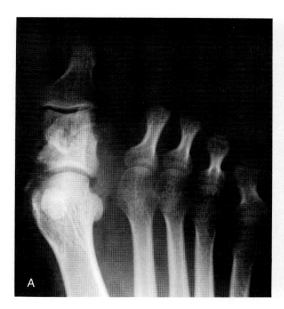 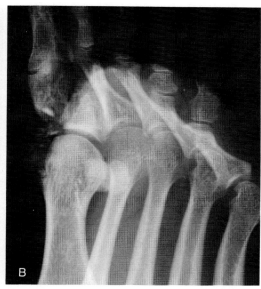

Figure 8–19. A 23-year-old man sustained an open and comminuted fracture of his right great toe when his foot accidentally slid under a lawn mower. On anteroposterior and oblique views, note the extremely comminuted fracture of the first proximal phalanx.

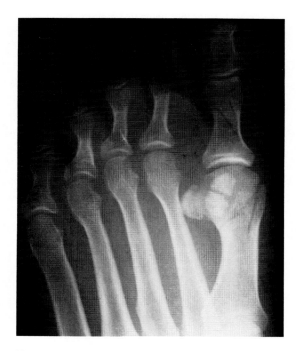

Figure 8–20. Oblique radiograph of the forefoot shows a slightly comminuted fracture of the proximal phalanx of the great toe and the first metatarsal head caused by a crush injury.

means, however, an open reduction through either a midlateral or midmedial skin incision should be performed, and the fracture should be anatomically reduced before fixing it with either a small K-wire or a mini-bone screw (Figure 8–26). It should be mentioned that although it is easy to remove a K-wire, a K-wire can cause skin irritation, necrosis, and pin tract infection. In contrast, a mini-bone screw usually does not cause any skin problem, but it is harder to remove because its head is usually flush with the bone and may not need removal at all.

A small transarticular fracture sometimes fails to heal and produces a painful subcutaneous mass and crepitation on joint motion. Under this circumstance, surgical excision of this non-united and displaced bony fragment and repair of the detached joint capsule and collateral ligament under proper tension should be performed. Compound fractures of the great toe should be irrigated with copious amounts of sterile normal saline solution and meticulously debrided. In addition, prophylactic antibiotic therapy and a tetanus shot should also

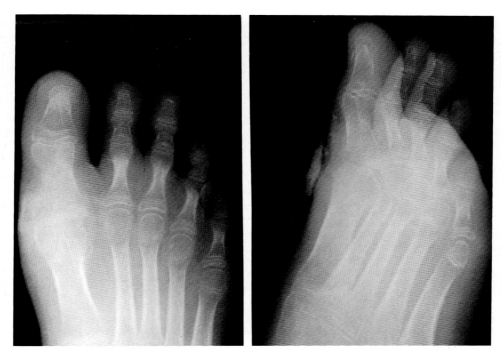

Figure 8–21. An 11-year-old girl sustained a compound fracture of her right great toe, which resulted in the development of a septic arthritis of the M-P joint of that toe. Anteroposterior and oblique radiographs show destruction of the medial portion of the epiphysis of the right first proximal phalanx.

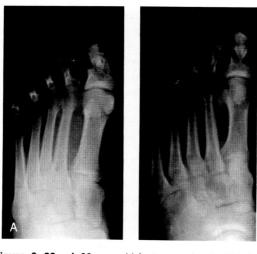

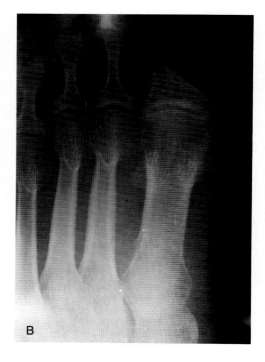

Figure 8–22. A 60-year-old factory worker had his left great and second toes crushed by a 225-kg steel block. **A,** anteroposterior and oblique views show comminuted fractures of the proximal and distal phalanges of the great toe and the head of the second proximal phalanx. **B,** anteroposterior radiograph shows absence of the distal phalanx and the distal portion of the proximal phalanx caused by surgical removal of the gangrenous distal portion of the left great toe.

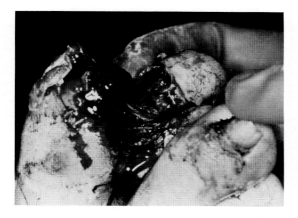

Figure 8–23. A 22-year-old man had his right great toe almost completely amputated by a rotary lawn mower.

direct stubbing injuries account for the majority of the fractures of the lesser toes. Because the proximal phalanges of the lesser toes have basically the same diameter but are at least twice as long as their corresponding middle and distal phalanges, they tend to receive more traumatic forces and are more prone to sustain fractures. Among the proximal phalanges of the four lesser toes, the fifth is most commonly fractured. This fracture is also known as the "night walker's fracture," which is often caused by walking barefoot in the dark and inadvertently striking the fifth toe against a piece of furniture (Figure 8–27). A crush injury is usually produced by a heavy falling object and tends to produce a comminuted fracture or a compound fracture (Figures 8–28—8–31). In contrast, a stubbing injury tends to produce a single oblique fracture of the proximal phalanx with various degrees of displacement (Figure 8–32).

CLINICAL SYMPTOMS AND SIGNS. These include pain on active or passive motion, swelling, gross deformity, ecchymosis, subungual hematoma, nail avulsion, and skin laceration. Severe crush injury frequently results in gangrenous changes of the toes that require toe amputation (Figure 8–33).

be given to minimize the chances of wound infection. When a displaced transarticular fracture is neglected or is improperly treated, traumatic arthritis may develop with time and may eventually require arthrodesis for symptomatic relief.

FRACTURES OF THE LESSER TOES

INCIDENCE. Like the phalangeal fractures of the great toe, direct crushing and in-

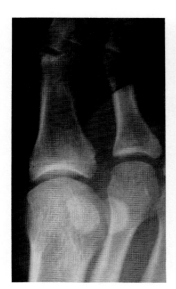
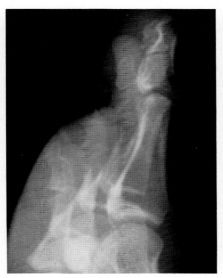
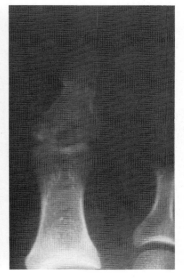

Figure 8–24. A 28-year-old woman fell down a flight of stairs and injured her right great toe. Anteroposterior, lateral, and oblique views show an avulsion fracture of the mid-dorsal aspect of the base of the distal phalanx of the great toe caused by a violent contraction of the extensor hallucis longus muscle.

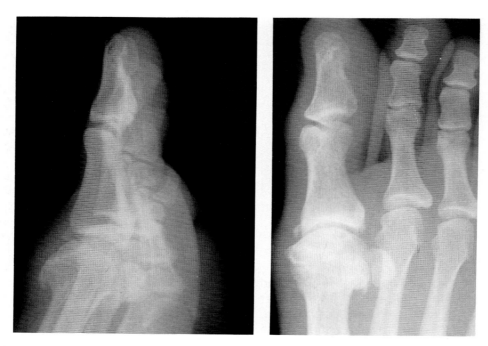

Figure 8–25. A 42-year-old man sustained an abduction injury of his right great toe. Lateral and oblique films reveal a small avulsion fracture of the medial base of the first proximal phalanx.

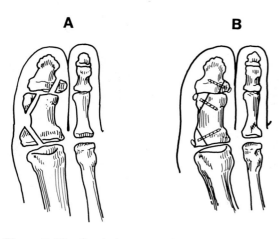

Figure 8–26. Surgical treatment for displaced transarticular fractures of the phalanges of the great toe. **A,** displaced fractures of the bases of the proximal and distal phalanges and the head of the proximal phalanx of the great toe. **B,** reduction of all three phalangeal fractures plus internal fixation with small bone screws.

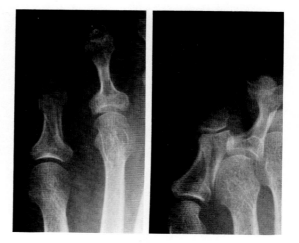

Figure 8–27. Anteroposterior and oblique views of the fourth and fifth toes show an oblique fracture of the fifth proximal phalanx, which is the most common form of the lesser toe fractures.

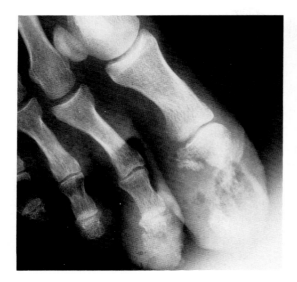

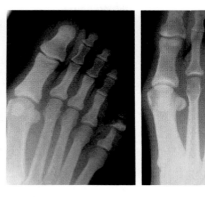

Figure 8–30. A 36-year-old man sustained a severe crush injury to his right small toe, which produced a compound fracture of both the proximal and middle phalanges and severe soft tissue injury (oblique and anteroposterior views). A partial amputation of the fifth toe was required to close the wound.

Figure 8–28. A 68-year-old automobile mechanic had his right great and second toes crushed by an engine block. Oblique view reveals a severely comminuted fracture of the distal phalanges of the great and second toes. Note the presence of air bubbles in the soft tissue of the two injured toes, indicating the presence of a compound fracture.

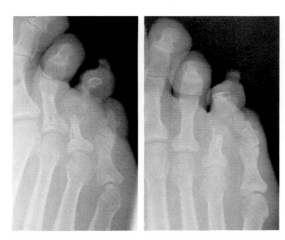

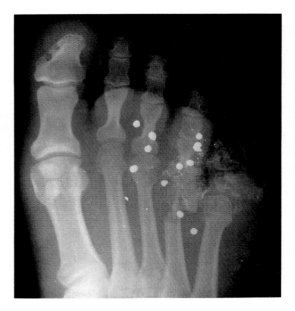

Figure 8–29. A 34-year-old man injured his right foot with a rotary lawn mower. Oblique and anteroposterior radiographs show deformity of the fourth toe and comminuted fractures of the proximal and middle phalanges of the same toe. Amputation of the right fourth toe was eventually required to close the wound.

Figure 8–31. A 45-year-old man was shot with a shotgun in his right foot at close range. Disintegration of the fifth proximal phalanx and fractures of the middle phalanx of the fifth toe, the fourth metatarsal head, and the fourth proximal phalanx are evident on anteroposterior radiograph. The fifth toe was amputated at its M-P level due to severe soft tissue destruction.

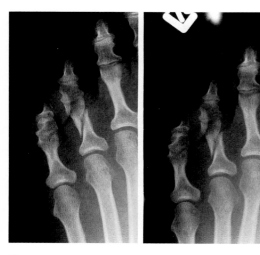

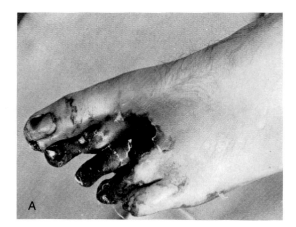

Figure 8–32. A 43-year-old woman struck her left fourth toe against the leg of a dining room table. Anteroposterior and oblique views reveal an oblique fracture through the diaphyseal portion of the fourth proximal phalanx, which can be treated by taping it to adjacent toes.

ROENTGENOGRAPHIC MANIFESTATIONS. Anteroposterior, lateral, and oblique views of the injured toe, with the four uninjured toes held in acute plantar flexion, show the site and extent of the fracture and the degree of comminution and angulation of the fracture site.

TREATMENT. All angulated fractures should be reduced by applying longitudinal traction to the injured toe; the reduced fracture can be stabilized by taping it to its adjacent toe or toes. A postoperative shoe or a shoe with its toe box removed and a metatarsal bar placed on its sole behind the metatarsal heads will allow full weight-bearing. Unstable fractures and fractures with recurrent deformities, however, can be stabilized by means of a small longitudinal K-wire. The pain associated with the fracture usually goes away in about 3 weeks when the fracture site is stabilized by fracture callus; non-union of phalangeal fractures rarely occurs. Compound fractures should be treated with appropriate irrigation, debridement, and antibiotics as for any other open fractures.

DISLOCATIONS OF THE GREAT TOE

INCIDENCE. Dislocations of the interphalangeal and M-P joints are fairly uncom-

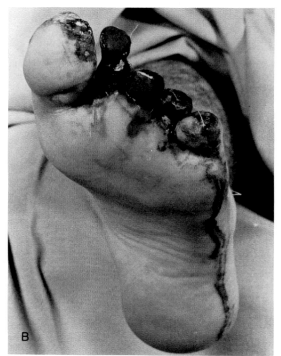

Figure 8–33. A 24-year-old man sustained a severe crush injury to the three middle toes of his left foot (**A** and **B**). Gangrene developed in all three toes and amputation of these digits was required.

mon events and are usually caused by high-energy injuries, such as automobile and motorcycle accidents and striking the great toe against a fixed object while running or jumping down from a height. The traumatic force is usually applied to the tip of the great toe and the force is transmitted along its longitudinal axis to the interphalangeal and M-P joints. The joints are forced into hyperextension, which tears the plantar capsules and causes the distal phalanx to become dislocated to the dorsal aspect of the proximal phalanx, and the proximal phalanx to the dorsal aspect of the first metatarsal head with the collateral ligaments of the interphalangeal and M-P joints remaining basically intact but under tension. Phalangeal and sesamoidal fractures can also accompany the interphalangeal and M-P dislocations, and injuries to other parts of the body may occur. After M-P joint dislocation, further hyperextension can rupture the intersesamoid ligament, can cause the fracture of one of the sesamoids, and may produce interposition of the plantar joint capsule or a fractured bone fragment from the sesamoids into the M-P joint. A complex dorsal dislocation of the M-P joint of the great toe may result, which cannot be reduced by closed means.

CLINICAL SYMPTOMS AND SIGNS. In a dorsally dislocated M-P joint of the great toe, in addition to the pain and swelling, cocked-up deformity of the toe with its interphalangeal joint in flexion, tense dorsal skin, inability to move the M-P joint of the great toe, a prominent and palpable base of the proximal phalanx on the top of the first metatarsal head, and a prominent first metatarsal head under the plantar aspect of the foot are common physical findings. Similarly, in a dorsal interphalangeal joint dislocation, shortening of the great toe, a prominent and palpable base of the distal phalanx on the dorsal aspect of the head of the proximal phalanx, tense dorsal skin, inability to move the interphalangeal joint, and a prominent head of the proximal phalanx under the plantar aspect of the great toe are typically found.

ROENTGENOGRAPHIC MANIFESTATIONS. In a dorsal interphalangeal joint dislocation of the great toe, anteroposterior and oblique views of the foot show that the head of the proximal phalanx is overlapped by the base of the distal phalanx. The lateral view shows that the base of the distal phalanx is sitting on top of the head of the proximal phalanx (Figure 8–34). In addition, fractures of

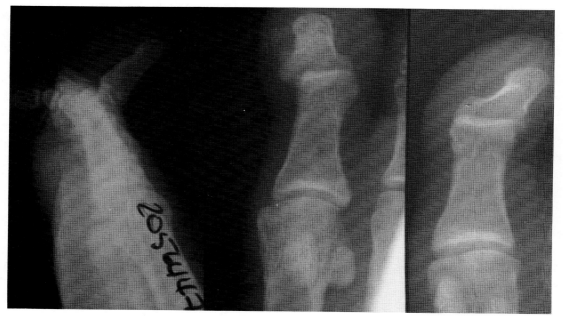

Figure 8–34. A 17-year-old youth injured his right great toe in a motorcycle accident. Lateral anteroposterior, and oblique views, show a dorsal dislocation of the interphalangeal joint of the great toe.

the head of the proximal phalanx and the base of the distal phalanx may also be present. Similarly, in a dorsal dislocation of the M-P joint of the great toe, the anteroposterior and oblique views show overlapping of the first metatarsal head by the base of the first proximal phalanx to produce a double density (Figure 8–35A), the lateral view shows that

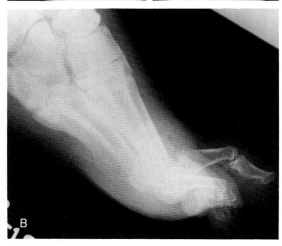

Figure 8–35. Anteroposterior radiographs (**A**) show that the base of the proximal phalanx of the great toe is overlapped by the first metatarsal head caused by a dorsal dislocation of the M-P joint of the great toe. **B,** lateral view clearly shows dorsal dislocation of the M-P joint of the great toe in association with an open wound, as evidenced by air shadows in the soft tissues.

the base of the proximal phalanx is riding on top of the first metatarsal head with the interphalangeal joint in a flexed position (Figure 8–35B). Fractures of the base of the proximal phalanx, the first metatarsal head, and the sesamoids may accompany dorsal dislocation of the M-P joint.

TREATMENT. Closed reduction of the interphalangeal or M-P joint dislocation of the great toe should be performed as soon as possible to minimize the chances of developing necrosis of the dorsal skin. To reduce an interphalangeal dislocation, longitudinal traction should be applied to the distal portion of the great toe, pushing the base of the distal phalanx in a plantar and distal direction, and the head of the proximal phalanx in a dorsal and proximal direction. After confirming the reduction radiographically, if the interphalangeal joint is stable, the great toe can be taped to the second toe for about 3 weeks, which is time for the torn capsular structures to heal. If the joint is unstable after closed reduction, a longitudinal K-wire can be used to stabilize the joint for about 3 weeks (Figure 8–36).

When an interphalangeal joint dislocation is associated with a displaced fracture of the base of the distal phalanx of the head or the head of the proximal phalanx, anatomic reduction can be achieved surgically, and fixation of the fracture site with a small K-wire or a mini-bone screw should also be employed. Occasionally, a dorsal dislocation of the interphalangeal joint of the great toe is accompanied by a herniation of the head of the first proximal phalanx through the plantar joint capsule of the interphalangeal joint, which produces an irreducible dislocation that requires open reduction (Figure 8–37).

Similarly, closed reduction of a dorsally dislocated M-P joint of the great toe usually requires first hyperextending the proximal phalanx on the metatarsal head first, and then applying downward pressure to the dorsal aspect of the base of the proximal phalanx to bring the proximal phalanx into its anatomic alignment with the first metatarsal. A short walking cast with a big toe spica or a toe plate should be used to maintain the reduction for about 3 weeks to allow the torn capsular structures to heal. If the M-P joint is unstable after closed reduction, a small K-wire may be inserted longitudinally through the phalanges into the first metatarsal, and a wooden-soled postoperative shoe can be used to allow early weight-bearing. When a displaced fracture or an intra-articular loose bony fragment is associated with the M-P joint dislocation, the

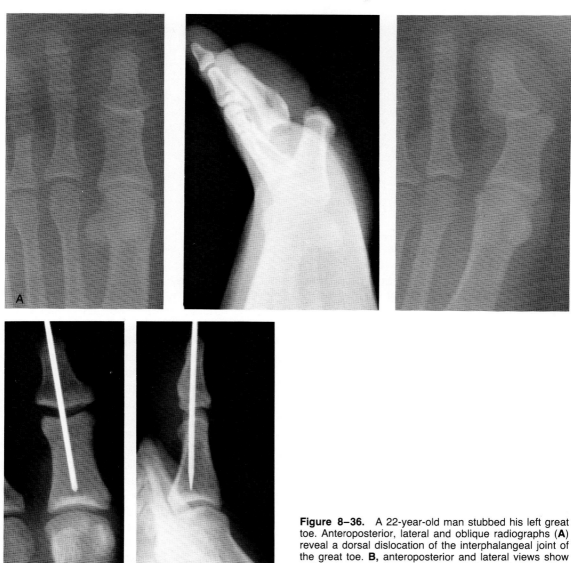

Figure 8–36. A 22-year-old man stubbed his left great toe. Anteroposterior, lateral and oblique radiographs (**A**) reveal a dorsal dislocation of the interphalangeal joint of the great toe. **B,** anteroposterior and lateral views show satisfactory reduction of the interphalangeal dislocation. Instability of that joint reduction required temporary fixation with a small longitudinal K-wire.

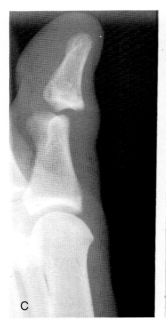
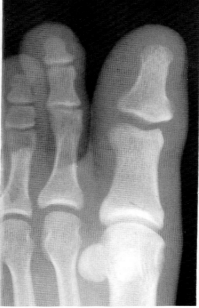
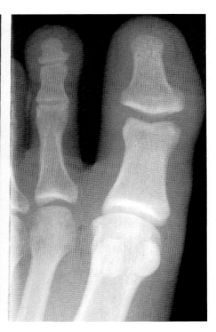

C

Figure 8–36. Continued. C, anteroposterior, oblique, and lateral views 3 months after surgery show satisfactory alignment of the interphalangeal joint of the great toe. The patient had full use of the great toe.

fracture can be anatomically reduced and stabilized with a small K-wire or a mini-bone screw; the loose body can be excised by arthrotomy.

Occasionally, a dorsal dislocation of the M-P joint is irreducible by closed means. The first metatarsal head is tightly held by the interposition of the plantar capsule between the base of the proximal phalanx and the first metatarsal head; medial collateral ligament, abductor hallucis tendon, and medial head of the flexor hallucis brevis medially; lateral collateral ligament, adductor hallucis tendon, and lateral head of the flexor hallucis brevis laterally; the two sesamoids and their intersesamoid ligament dorsally; and the plantar aponeurosis plantarly; all of which tighten around the first metatarsal neck like a noose, making closed reduction impossible (Figure 8–38A). If the intersesamoid ligament is ruptured or one or both of the sesamoids are fractured, however, the strangulating hold of the sesamoids and their associated tendons, muscles, and ligaments is broken and reduction of the M-P joint dislocation can then be

accomplished by closed means (Figure 8–38B).

Open reduction of an irreducible dislocation of the M-P joint of the great toe can be achieved by employing either a transverse plantar incision directly over the prominent metatarsal mead or a medial midline incision through which the incarcerated plantar joint capsule of the M-P joint can be carefully freed. The M-P joint dislocation can then be reduced. After reduction, a short walking cast with a big toe spica or a toe plate should be applied for 3 weeks to allow the ruptured capsular structures to heal. Symptomatic traumatic osteoarthritis may develop from a few months to a few years after dislocations with or without fractures of the interphalangeal and M-P joints of the great toe to the extent that they may require arthrodesis for symptomatic relief.

DISLOCATIONS OF THE LESSER TOES

INCIDENCE. When compared with the dorsal dislocation of the M-P joint of the lesser toes, dislocation of their DIP or PIP joints are

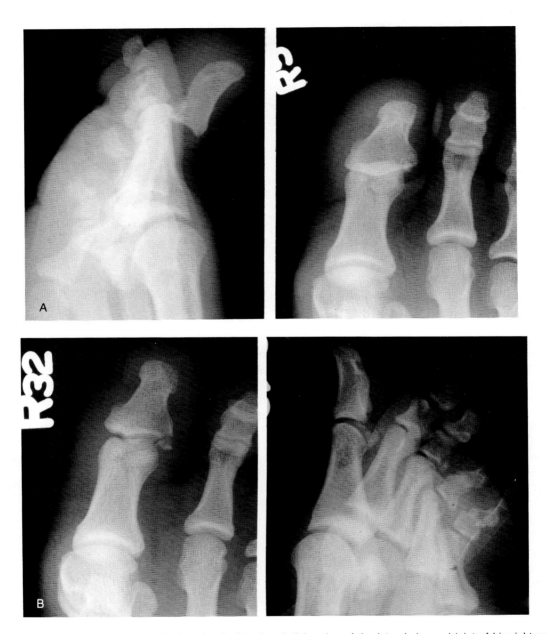

Figure 8–37. A 21-year-old man had an irreducible dorsal dislocation of the interphalangeal joint of his right great toe due to herniation of the head of the proximal phalanx through the plantar fibrocartilaginous plate of the joint. **A,** lateral and anteroposterior radiographs reveal overlapping of the articular surfaces of the interphalangeal joint (anteroposterior view) and riding of the plantar base of the distal phalanx on the head of the proximal phalanx (lateral view) caused by a dorsal dislocation of the interphalangeal joint of the great toe. **B,** anteroposterior and lateral views after open reduction show satisfactory alignment of the interphalangeal joint of the right great toe and a chip fracture of the lateral base of the distal phalanx.

A   B

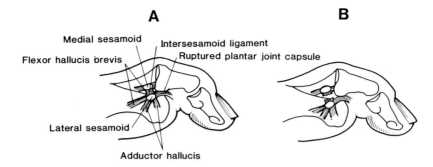

Medial sesamoid   Intersesamoid ligament
Flexor hallucis brevis   Ruptured plantar joint capsule

Lateral sesamoid

Adductor hallucis

Figure 8–38. Irreducible dorsal dislocation of the M-P joint of the great toe. **A,** interposition of the plantar joint capsule between the base of the proximal phalanx and the head of the first metatarsal and the strangulating hold of the first metatarsal neck by both heads of the flexor hallucis brevis, intersesamoid ligament, medial and lateral sesamoids, and abductor and adductor hallucis, all of which work together against a successful closed reduction. **B,** when the intersesamoid ligament is ruptured or one of the two sesamoids sustains a longitudinal fracture, the strangulation hold by the sesamoid complex is released and the reduction can be achieved by closed means.

relatively uncommon. These phalanges are small and are protected by relatively large and strong collateral ligaments and extensor and flexor tendons. Dorsal dislocation of the M-P, PIP, and DIP joints of the three middle toes are usually caused by a longitudinally directed hyperextension force that first tears their plantar capsules and then produces a dorsal dislocation (Figures 8–39 and 8–40). Lateral

dislocation of the M-P joint of the fifth toe is typically caused by forceful abduction, such as catching the fifth toe on a fixed object while walking or running barefoot. This same abduction force can also produce a lateral dislocation of the PIP joint of the fifth toe. It should be noted that automobile accidents are responsible for quite a number of lesser toe dislocations. In addition, the various dislocations of the PIP, DIP and M-P joints of the lesser toes can sometimes be associated with frac-

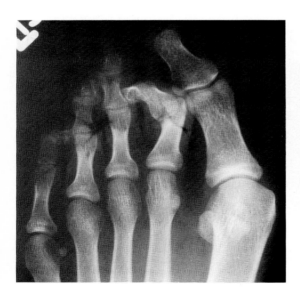

Figure 8–39. Anteroposterior view of the left foot shows a dorsolateral dislocation of the PIP joint of the second toe. Note the overlapping of the base of the middle phalanx and the head of the proximal phalanx.

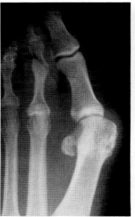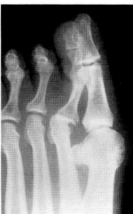

Figure 8–40. A 54-year-old woman stubbed her right second toe and sustained a dorsal dislocation of her second M-P joint. Oblique and anteroposterior views reveal overlapping of the base of the second proximal phalanx and the second metatarsal head.

tures of their corresponding phalanges or metatarsal heads.

CLINICAL SYMPTOMS AND SIGNS. A dislocated lesser toe is usually painful, tender, swollen, and deformed, with tense skin over its dorsal aspect and loss of the normal motion of its DIP, PIP, and M-P joints. The base of the dorsally dislocated phalanx is usually prominent and palpable on the dorsal side of the head of the more proximal phalanx or metatarsal. The metatarsal is also quite prominent on the plantar side, and the whole affected toe appears to be shortened. In a long neglected dorsal dislocation of the M-P joint of any one of the three middle lesser toes, a fixed hammer toe usually develops with its PIP joint in flexion and its proximal phalanx in hyperextension and dorsal dislocation.

In a lateral dislocation of the M-P joint of the fifth toe, the base of the fifth proximal phalanx becomes prominent and palpable on the lateral side of the fifth metatarsal head, with apparent shortening of the fifth toe. Likewise, in a lateral dislocation of the PIP joint of the fifth toe, the base of the middle phalanx becomes prominent and palpable on the lateral aspect of the head of the fifth proximal phalanx instead of in line with the fifth proximal phalanx. The fifth toe is laterally deviated from the fourth toe when its PIP or M-P joint is dislocated laterally.

ROENTGENOGRAPHIC MANIFESTATIONS. Anteroposterior and oblique views of a dorsally dislocated lesser toe usually show overlapping of the head of the more proximal phalanx or metatarsal by the base of the more distal phalanx. Some lateral displacement of these dorsally dislocated phalanges can also be present. Lateral views show that the base of the dislocated phalanx is sitting on top of the head of the more proximal phalanx or the corresponding metatarsal head. Dislocation of the M-P joints can also be associated with comminuted fractures of their respective metatarsal heads and fractures of the necks of the corresponding metatarsals (Figures 8–41—8–43). In addition, lateral dislocation of the PIP and M-P joints of the fifth toe is shown on anteroposterior radiographs with the base of the dislocated phalanx situated at the lateral side of the head of the fifth proximal phalanx and the fifth metatarsal head, respectively.

TREATMENT. Most DIP, PIP, and M-P joint dislocations can be reduced by applying manual traction and manipulation to the affected toes. After reduction, the affected toe should be immobilized by taping it to its adjacent toe or toes for 2 to 3 weeks to allow the torn capsular structure to heal. Occasionally, an irreducible dorsal dislocation of the M-P joint of a lesser toe can be caused by entrapment of the plantar capsule and the deep transverse metatarsal ligament between the base of the proximal phalanx and the dorsal aspect of the metatarsal head, and by the strangulation hold of the flexor digitorum longus and brevis tendons laterally, and the lumbrical tendon medially. This complex dislocation can be reduced by dividing the fibrocartilaginous plate and the deep transverse metatarsal ligament through a dorsal incision.

Another rare cause of an irreducible M-P dislocation is the so-called linked-toe dislocation of the metatarsal bone, in which an

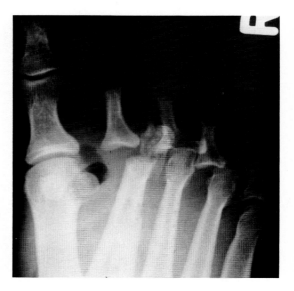

Figure 8–41. Anteroposterior view shows dislocation of the second, third, and fourth M-P joints in association with a comminuted fracture of the second metatarsal head, a fracture of the lateral base of the third proximal phalanx, and a fracture of the shaft of second metatarsal.

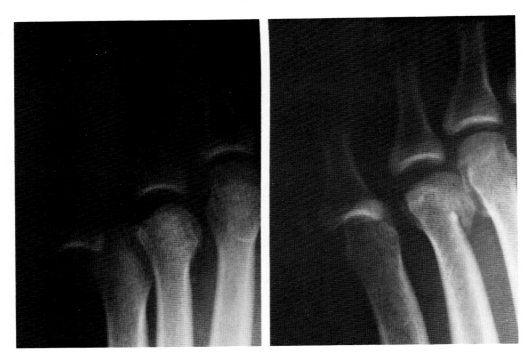

Figure 8–42. Anteroposterior and oblique radiographs of the lateral aspect of the forefoot show complete dislocation of the fifth M-P joint and a fracture of the head of the fourth metatarsal.

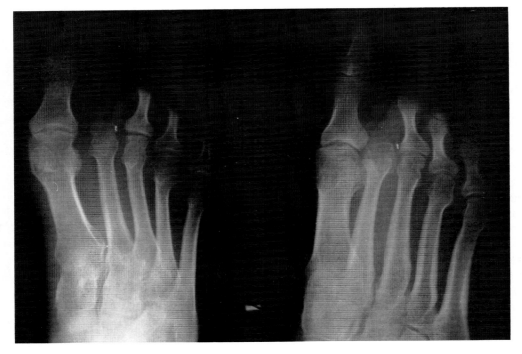

Figure 8–43. A 42-year-old man had his right second toe completely amputated when a sharp metal object was accidentally dropped on this digit. Anteroposterior and oblique radiographs show complete absence of the phalanges of the second toe, and a small metallic particle on the lateral aspect of the second metatarsal head.

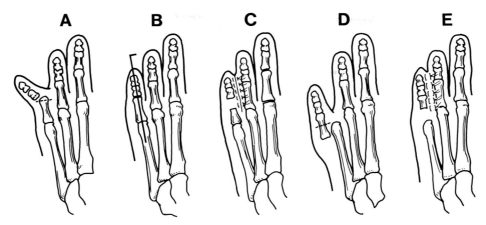

Figure 8–44. Surgical techniques for treating a chronically dislocated PIP and M-P joints of the fifth toe. **A,** a dislocated PIP joint of the fifth toe. Dotted lines, amount of the PIP joint to be resected before a PIP fusion can be performed. **B,** a PIP fusion has been performed and is held in place with a longitudinal, intramedullary K-wire. **C,** head of the fifth proximal phalanx has been excised and the fifth toe is joined to the fourth toe. **D,** dislocated M-P joint of the fifth toe. Dotted line, level of the proximal hemiphalangectomy of the fifth proximal phalanx. **E,** proximal one-half of the fifth proximal phalanx has been removed and the fifth toe is joined to the fourth toe.

isolated dorsal tarsometatarsal dislocation is associated with dislocation of the medially adjacent M-P joint. Because the interosseous muscle originates in the dislocated metatarsal and inserts on the medially adjacent proximal phalanx, the proximal displacement of the dislocated metatarsal carries the interosseous muscle and the medially adjacent proximal phalanx proximally, making closed reduction of the dislocated M-P joint difficult. Once the dislocated metatarsal is reduced, tension is released from the tendon of the interosseous muscle, and the M-P joint dislocation can be easily reduced.

When an M-P joint dislocation is associated with a comminuted fracture of the articular surface of the corresponding metatarsal head, an arthrotomy may be needed to remove all loose articular fragments. The reduced M-P joint can then be stabilized with a longitudinal K-wire through all three phalanges and the metatarsal. Similarly, the occurrence of an M-P joint dislocation and a plantarly angulated metatarsal fracture in the same toe is best treated with a longitudinal K-wire to reduce the M-P joint dislocation and the plantar angulation of the fractured metatarsal, as well as to avoid the future development of painful plantar callosity under the prominent metatarsal head.

When a dorsal M-P joint dislocation is not treated, a fixed hammer toe deformity will develop, with a painful corn on the dorsal aspect of the PIP joint and a symptomatic callosity under the respective metatarsal head. Open reduction of this dislocated M-P joint and fusion of the PIP joint by generous resection of the PIP joint should be followed by insertion of a small K-wire through all three phalanges and the metatarsal to hold the PIP fusion and the reduced M-P joint in place. The surgical treatment for an old dislocation or recurrent dislocation of the PIP joint of the fifth toe includes fusion of the PIP joint or distal hemiphalangectomy of the fifth proximal phalanx plus syndactylization of the fourth and fifth toe (Figure 8–44A—C). Similarly, a long-neglected dislocation of the M-P joint of the fifth toe can be treated with proximal hemiphalangectomy of the fifth proximal phalanx plus syndactylization of the fourth and fifth toe (Figure 8–44D and E).

REFERENCES

Fractures and Dislocations of the Toes

1. Bowers, Jr., K.D., and Martin, R.B.: Turf-toe: A shoe-surface related football injury. Med. Sci. Sports Exerc., *8*:81, 1976.
2. Cobey, J.C.: Treatment of undisplaced toe fractures

with a metatarsal bar made from tongue blades. Clin. Orthop., *103:*56, 1974.

3. Coker, T.P., Arnold, J.A., and Weber, D.L.: Traumatic lesions of the metatarsophalangeal joint of the great toe in athletes. J. Arkansas Med. Soc., *74:*309, 1978.

4. DeLuca, F.N., and Kenmore, P.I.: Bilateral dorsal dislocations of the metatarsophalangeal joints of the great toe with loose body in one of the metatarsophalangeal joints. J. Trauma, *15:*737, 1975.

5. Giannikas, A.C., et al. Dorsal dislocation of the first metatarso-phalangeal joint. Report of four cases. J. Bone Joint Surg. [Br.], *57:*384, 1975.

6. Jahss, M.H.: Unusual diagnostic problems of the foot. Clin. Orthop., *85:*42, 1972.

7. Jahss, M.H.: Traumatic dislocations of the first metatarsophalangeal joint. Foot Ankle, *1:*15, 1980.

8. Jahss, M.H.: Stubbing injuries to the hallux. Foot Ankle. *1:*327, 1981.

9. Jahss, M.H.: Chronic and recurrent dislocations of the fifth toe. Foot Ankle, *1:*275, 1981.

10. Konkel, K.F., and Muehlstein, J.H.: Unusual fracture-dislocation of the great toe: Case report. J. Trauma, *15:*733, 1975.

11. McKinley, L.M., and Davis, G.L.: Locked dislocation of the great toe. J. La. State Med. Soc., *127:*389, 1975.

12. Mullis, D.L., and Miller, W.E.: A disabling sports injury of the great toe. Foot Ankle, *1:*22, 1980.

13. Murphy, J.L.: Isolated dorsal dislocation of the second metatarsophalangeal joint. Foot Ankle, *1:*30, 1980.

14. Nelson, T.L., and Uggen, W.: Irreducible dorsal dislocation of the interphalangeal joint of the great toe. Clin. Orthop., *157:*110, 1981.

15. Pinckney, L.E., Currarino, G., and Kennedy, L.A.: The stubbed great toe: A cause of accult compound fracture and infection. Radiology, *138:*375, 1981.

16. Rao, J.P., and Banzon, M.T.: Irreducible dislocation of the metatarsophalangeal joints of the foot. Clin. Orthop. *145:*224, 1979.

17. Salamon, P.B., Gelberman, R.H., and Huffer, J.M.: Dorsal dislocation of the metatarsophalangeal joint of the great toe. A case report. J. Bone Joint Surg. [Am.], *56:*1073, 1974.

18. Sammarco, G.J., and Miller, E.H.: Forefoot conditions in dancers. Foot Ankle, *3:*93, 1982.

19. Yu, E.C., and Garfin, S.R.: Closed dorsal dislocation of the metatarsophalangeal joint of the great toe. A surgical approach and case report. Clin. Orthop., *185:*237, 1984.

Fractures of the Sesamoids of the Great Toe

INCIDENCE.   The medial and lateral sesamoids are two small, roundish bones that are imbedded in the medial and lateral tendons of the flexor hallucis brevis muscle, and articulate with the plantar articular condyles of the first metatarsal head. Fractures of the sesamoids are uncommon and usually result from direct trauma to the foot that results in crushing of the sesamoids between the first metatarsal head and the ground. The medial sesamoid is fractured more frequently than the lateral sesamoid due to its greater weight-bearing function. Jumping down from a height and landing directly on the ball of the foot, long-distance running, ballet dancing, and dorsal dislocation of the M-P joint of the great toe can cause fractures of these two sesamoids. Although rare, spontaneous fracture of the sesamoid can also occur.

CLINICAL SYMPTOMS AND SIGNS.   Pain, swelling, and localized tenderness may be present on the plantar aspect of the foot directly under the fractured sesamoid. Dorsiflexion of the M-P joint of the great toe puts stress on the fractured sesamoid and greatly aggravates the pain. The patient usually walks with a limp and tends to walk on the outer border of the foot to avoid putting painful stress on the fractured sesamoid.

ROENTGENOGRAPHIC MANIFESTATIONS.   A transverse fracture of a sesamoid can usually be seen on anteroposterior, lateral, and oblique radiographs of the foot, but a longitudinal fracture of the same sesamoid can only be seen on the anteroposterior, oblique, and particularly the tangential (sesamoid or axial) views of the foot. Some soft tissue swelling may be present on the plantar aspect of the foot in the region of the sesamoids on a lateral view. In addition, the irregular fracture line, wide separation between the major bone fragments, comminution, fragments of unequal sizes, soft tissue swelling, fracture callus, and normal sesamoid size are the important radiographic features that differentiate a fractured sesamoid from a bipartite or multipartite sesamoid (Figures 8–45 and 8–46).

TREATMENT.   An undisplaced or minimally displaced fracture of a sesamoid can be treated with a short walking cast and a big toe spica with the first M-P joint in slightly plantar flexion for 5 to 6 weeks. A stiff-soled shoe fitted with a metatarsal bar or pad can then be used until the fractured sesamoid is no longer symptomatic.

Widely separated, comminuted, and painful

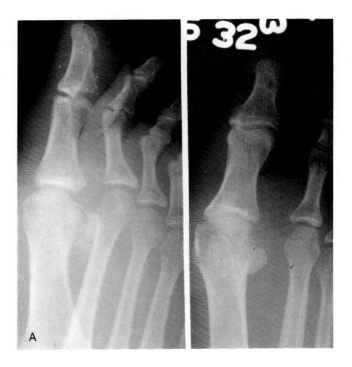

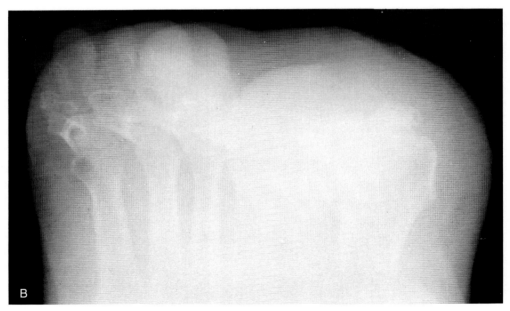

Figure 8–45. A 22-year-old man experienced pain in the medial aspect of the ball of his right foot after jumping down from a height of 4.5 m. Oblique and anteroposterior radiographs (**A**) show a comminuted fracture of the medial sesamoid. **B,** axial view shows a fragmented distal portion of the fractured medial sesamoid.

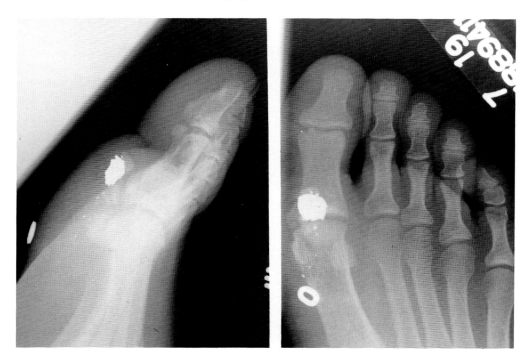

Figure 8-46. A 27-year-old man was shot with a hand gun in his right foot. Lateral and anteroposterior views reveal a comminuted fracture of the medial sesamoid. The lead marker indicates the point of entry of the bullet.

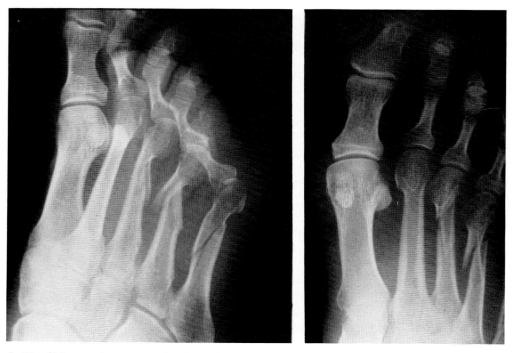

Figure 8–47. Oblique and anteroposterior views show spiral fractures of the third, fourth, and fifth metatarsals caused by a severe twisting injury of the forefoot.

and malunited fractures of the sesamoids are best treated by sesamoidectomy. The medial sesamoid can be excised by making a mid-medial incision through which the medial border of the medial sesamoid can be firmly grasped with a small towel clip. The entire sesamoid can then be shelled out by cutting the intersesamoid ligament and its attachments to the medial head of the flexor hallucis brevis tendon. Alternatively, the lateral sesamoid can be excised through a longitudinal plantar skin incision placed between the first and second metatarsal heads. Care should be taken to avoid injury to the neurovascular bundle that is in the immediate vicinity of the incision.

REFERENCES

Fractures of the Sesamoids of the Great Toe

1. Barnett, J.C., Crespo, A., and Daniels, V.C.: Intra-articular accessory sesamoid dislocation of the great toe. Report of case. J. Fla. Med. Assoc., *66:*613, 1979.
2. Bizarro, A.H.: On the traumatology of the sesamoid structures. Ann. Surg., *74:*783, 1921.
3. Brown, T.I.S.: Avulsion fracture of the fibular sesamoid in association with dorsal dislocation of the metatarsophalangeal joint of the hallux: Report of a case and review of the literature. Clin. Orthop., *149:*229, 1980.
4. Freiberg, A.H.: Injuries to the sesamoid bones of the great toe. J. Orthop. Surg., *2:*453, 1920.
5. Hobart, M.: Fracture of sesamoid bones of the foot. J. Bone Joint Surg., *11:*298, 1931.
6. Inge, G.A.L., and Ferguson, A.B.: Surgery of the sesamoid bones of the great toe. Arch. Surg., *27:*466, 1933.
7. Kliman, M.E., Gross, A.E., Pritzker, K.P., and Greyson, N.D.: Osteochondritis of hallux sesamoid bones. Foot Ankle, *3:*220, 1983.
8. Lapidus, P.W.: A definite fracture of tibial sesamoid of the big toe. Radiology, *36:*235, 1941.
9. Orr, T.G.: Fracture of the great toe sesamoid bones. Ann. Surg., *48:*609, 1918.
10. Parra, G.: Stress fractures of the sesamoids of the foot. Clin. Orthop., *18:*281, 1960.
11. Powers, J.H.: Traumatic and development abnormalities of sesamoid bones of the great toe. Am. J. Surg., *23:*315, 1934.
12. Scranton, Jr., P.E.: Pathologic anatomic variations in the sesamoids. Foot Ankle, *1:*321, 1981.
13. Speed, K.: Injuries of the great toe sesamoids. Ann. Surg., *60:*478, 1913.
14. Van Hal, M.E., Keene, J.S., Lange, T.A., and Clancy, Jr., W.G.: Stress fractures of the great toe sesamoids. Am. J. Sports Med., *10:*122, 1982.
15. Zinman, H., Keret, D., and Reis, N.D.: Fracture of the medial sesamoid bone of the hallux. J. Trauma, *21:*581, 1981.

Fractures of the Metatarsals

INCIDENCE. Metatarsal fractures are common injuries and can be caused by a crush injury from a heavy object that falls on the dorsum of the foot, stubbing injury, avulsion injury caused by forceful muscle pull, or a twisting injury (Figures 8–47—8–50). These fractures can involve the heads, necks, shafts, or bases of the metatarsals. Fractures of the first metatarsal occur less frequently, however, than those of the four lesser metatarsals; greater size and strength allow them to withstand significantly more trauma before a fracture is produced. Metatarsal fractures can be transverse, segmental, comminuted, oblique or spiral, compound, displaced, or undisplaced in nature. A crush injury to the dorsal aspect of the foot with resultant fractures of one or more of the three middle metatarsals seems to be the most common form of metatarsal injury.

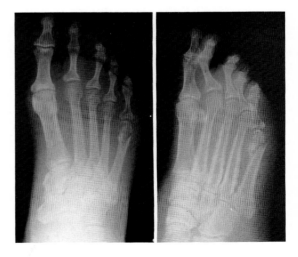

Figure 8–48. Oblique and anteroposterior views. A 56-year-old woman sustained an isolated fracture of her right fifth metatarsal head, which was treated nonoperatively with good results.

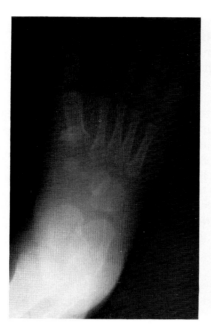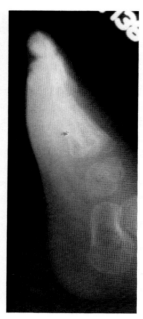

Figure 8–49. Anteroposterior and lateral views. A child had a slightly displaced fracture of the metaphyseal portion of the right first metatarsal base with some impaction of the fracture site caused by a stubbing injury.

The so-called Jones' fracture involves the proximal metaphyseal-diaphyseal junction of the fifth metatarsal and can be produced by either direct or indirect forces, with a predilection for basketball and football players. Unlike other metatarsal fractures which usually heal themselves in a reasonably short time, a Jones' fracture carries a reputation of having a high incidence of developing delayed union or non-union, and can become a source of prolonged disability. Arangio (1983) collected 106 cases of Jones' fracture from the medical literature and found a 50% incidence of non-union. Another interesting metatarsal fracture involves the base of the fifth metatarsal and is usually caused by a combination of sudden inversion of the foot and forceful contraction of the peroneus brevis muscle, which inserts into the lateral base of the fifth metatarsal and avulses it. Occasionally, direct trauma can also cause fracture of the base of the fifth metatarsal.

Another unique metatarsal fracture is the fatigue fracture, which is synonymous with March or stress fracture. The fatigue fracture usually involves the second metatarsal, less commonly the third metatarsal, and rarely the fourth metatarsal. A metatarsal stress fracture typically occurs in long-distance runners, joggers, new military recruits, and the like whose feet are subjected to prolonged and unaccustomed cyclic stresses. The metatarsal fatigue fracture that results accounts for over 50% of all fatigue fractures of the body. Fatigue fracture of the second metatarsal can occasionally take place in a foot after Keller's bunionectomy, with severe hammer toe, or after Mitchell's bunionectomy in which the first metatarsal head, which underwent osteotomy, heals in a dorsally displaced position, thus placing excessive weight-bearing stress on the second metatarsal (Figures 8–51 and 8–52).

CLINICAL SYMPTOMS AND SIGNS.   Pain, localized tenderness, swelling, ecchymosis, hematoma, crepitation, gross foot deformity with displaced metatarsal fractures, palpable step-off, and open wounds may be found in different metatarsal fractures. To identify the exact site of fracture by examination, the head

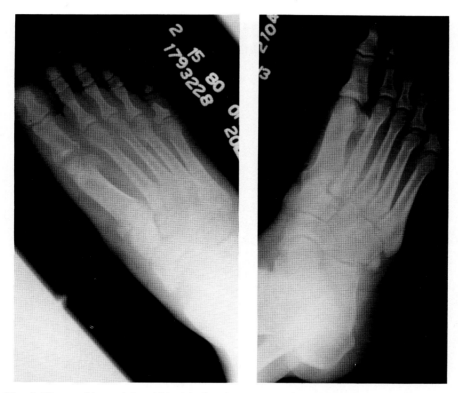

Figure 8–50. A 38-year-old man injured his right foot in a motorcycle accident. Oblique and anteroposterior views show an avulsion fracture of the medial base of the first metatarsal.

of the suspected fractured metatarsal can be grasped by the thumb and index finger of the examining physician and the metatarsal can then be manipulated. If pain, crepitation, and abnormal motion of the metatarsal are produced, a clinical diagnosis of a metatarsal fracture can be established. In contrast, a fatigue fracture tends to have an insidious onset of pain, which is usually aggravated by activity, with mild swelling, pain, and tenderness localized to the fracture site. If the symptoms of a fatigue fracture have been present for 3 to 4 weeks, a palpable thickening at the fracture site caused by callus formation may be found on careful examination.

ROENTGENOGRAPHIC MANIFESTATIONS. The majority of metatarsal fractures can be easily visualized on the anteroposterior, lateral, and oblique views of the foot. Only the lateral view, however, can clearly demonstrate the degrees of dorsal or plantar an-

gulation of these fractures. Such information is important when deciding whether a particular fracture can be treated with closed reduction and cast or whether an open reduction and internal fixation should be used. When a stress fracture is suspected, if the symptoms have been present for only a short time, the radiographic findings may be completely normal because the transverse fracture line and its associated callus formation may take 3 to 6 weeks to develop. If a radionuclide bone scan is also performed, however, it will show a significant increase in uptake at the site of the stress fracture soon after the appearance of symptoms.

In the diagnosis of an avulsion fracture of the base of the fifth metatarsal, care should be taken not to confuse the os vesalianum pedis, which is a small ossicle in the peroneus brevis tendon that is smooth and round and is usually bilateral and asymptomatic, a

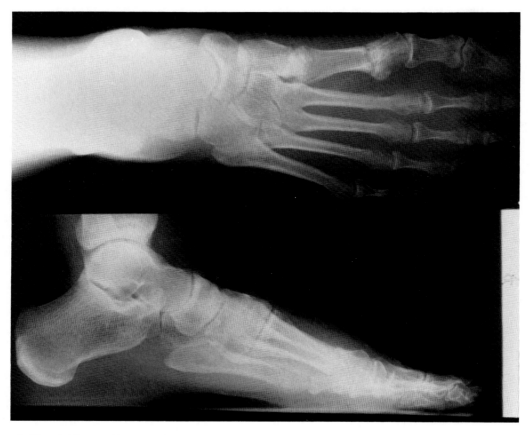

Figure 8–51. A 28-year-old woman in whom anteroposterior and lateral radiographs reveal a stress fracture of the second metatarsal caused by an improperly performed distal osteotomy of the first metatarsal. The repaired first metatarsal head healed in a dorsiflexed and medially deviated position.

true fracture of the fifth metatarsal base. Furthermore, the apophysis of the base of the fifth metatarsal, which normally fuses to the shaft of the fifth metatarsal by age 16 years, should not be mistaken for a fracture of the base of the fifth metatarsal.

TREATMENT

A. Undisplaced or minimally displaced metatarsal fractures: need only a short walking cast for 4 to 6 weeks.

B. Displaced metatarsal fractures: should be reduced by applying traction to the toes with wire finger traps and by manipulating the fracture sites into normal alignment. If

the reduced fractures are relatively stable, a short non-walking cast can be used for about 3 weeks, allowing fracture callus to form, and then a well-molded short walking cast for another 3 weeks so the fracture can consolidate. If the displaced fractures cannot be satisfactorily reduced, or if the reduced metatarsal fractures are unstable, open reduction and longitudinal K-wire fixation can be employed (Figures 8–53—8–55). The aforementioned 3-week weight-bearing walking cast routine is followed. Open reduction is particularly indicated when the fractured metatarsal is plantarly angulated, because a malunited plantarly angulated metatarsal fracture frequently produces intractable painful

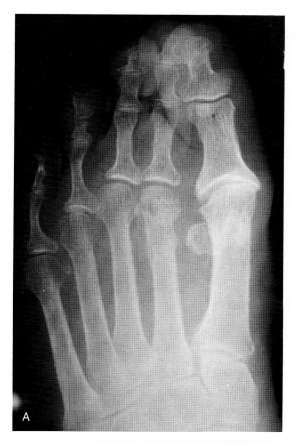

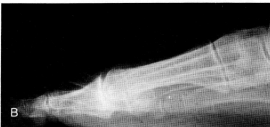

Figure 8–52. Anteroposterior (**A**) and lateral (**B**) radiographs show a stress fracture of the second metatarsal. A severe hammer toe deformity of the second toe, which resulted in excessive weight-bearing pressure on the second metatarsal head, eventually produced the fracture.

plantar callosity due to concentrated weight-bearing pressure on the prominent metatarsal head.

C. Comminuted metatarsal fractures: require a reasonable reduction and cast immobi-

lization for a long enough time so the fracture fragments can consolidate.

D. Compound metatarsal fractures: should be thoroughly irrigated, debrided, and covered. Skin care should be meticulous and, prophylactic intravenous antibiotics should be given to prevent massive skin slough and the development of osteomyelitis, both of which have disastrous consequences.

E. Displaced fracture of the first metatarsal: may require open and anatomic reduction and firm internal fixation to restore normal, major weight-bearing function (Figure 8–56). Postoperative cast immobilization is usually 8 weeks.

F. Avulsion fracture of the base of the fifth metatarsal: if the fracture is undisplaced or minimally displaced (Figure 8–57), the use of a short walking cast for 5 to 6 weeks is all that is required. If the avulsed fragment is widely separated, however, it should be anatomically reduced and fixed with a mini-bone screw, followed by the use of a short walking cast for 5 to 6 weeks. Well-established non-union of the avulsion fracture of the fifth metatarsal can be treated with excision of the non-united fragment and reattachment of the peroneous brevis tendon to the base of the fifth metatarsal. The use of a short leg cast should follow for 4 to 6 weeks to allow the tendon to become firmly attached to the bone.

G. Jones' fracture: in competitive athletes, intramedullary screw fixation may be the treatment of choice; this method is especially indicated when the injury occurs in early training. In nonathletes and recreational athletes, only cast immobilization is needed. When a well-established, painful non-union has developed in a Jones' fracture, an inlaid bone graft can be used to achieve a solid bony union (Figures 8–58— 8–61).

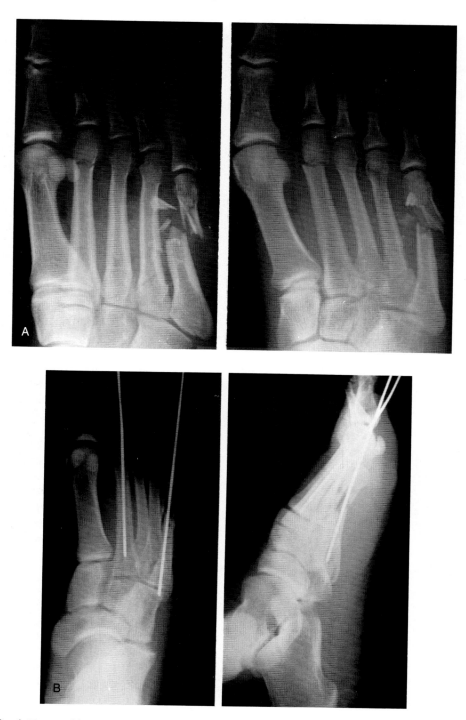

Figure 8–53. A 30-year-old man injured his right foot in an automobile accident. **A,** oblique and anteroposterior views show fractures of the second metatarsal neck and the bases of the third and fourth metatarsals, and a comminuted fracture of the shaft of the fifth metatarsal. **B,** anteroposterior and lateral views illustrate that the angulated and displaced second and fifth metatarsal fractures were successfully treated with longitudinal K-wire fixation.

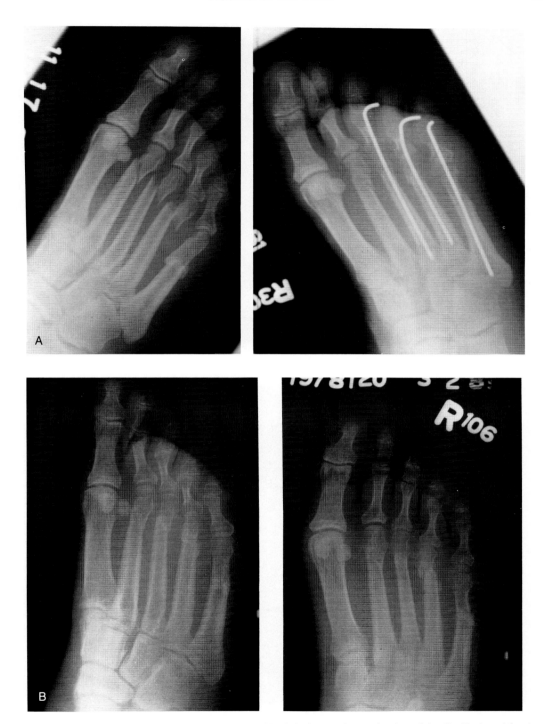

Figure 8–54. A 32-year-old man had a crush injury to his right foot and sustained a minimally displaced fracture of the second metatarsal and significantly displaced fractures of the third, fourth, and fifth metatarsals (**A,** oblique views), which required open reduction and longitudinal K-wire fixation. **B,** anteroposterior and oblique views 4 months later show good healing of the second, third, fourth, and fifth metatarsal fractures.

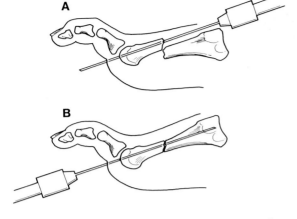

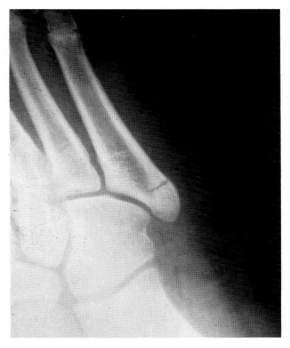

Figure 8–55. Surgical technique for reducing a displaced metatarsal fracture. **A,** drive a small K-wire longitudinally through the distal metatarsal fracture fragment to emerge through the plantar aspect of the foot. **B,** reduce the metatarsal fracture and drive the same wire in retrograde fashion into the proximal metatarsal fracture fragment to stabilize the fracture reduction.

Figure 8–57. A 13-year-old boy sustained an inversion injury to his right foot. Oblique radiograph shows an incomplete fracture of the lateral base of the fifth metatarsal where the peroneus brevis tendon inserts.

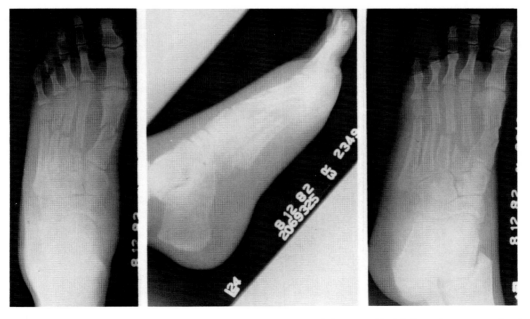

Figure 8–56. A 39-year-old factory worker sustained a severe crush injury to his left foot. Anteroposterior, lateral, and oblique views show that all five metatarsals are fractured with varying degrees of displacement. K-wire fixation of the lesser toes and a mini-bone plate fixation of the first metatarsal were eventually required.

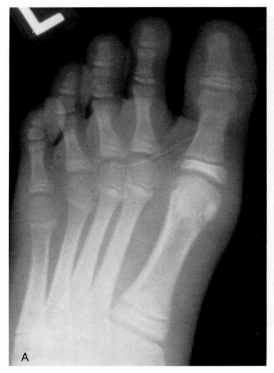
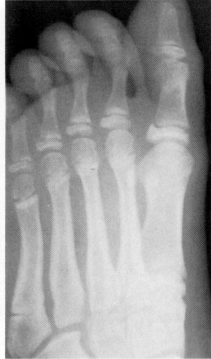

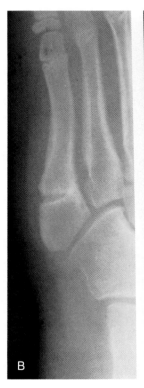
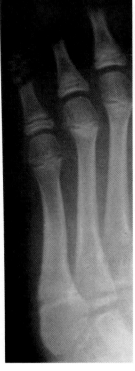

Figure 8–58. A 10-year-old girl sustained a Jones' fracture to her left foot. **A,** anteroposterior and oblique views show a transverse fracture involving the proximal metaphyseal-diaphyseal junction of the fifth metatarsal. **B,** anteroposterior and oblique radiographs 3 months later show some resorption of bone and sclerotic bone change at the fifth metatarsal fracture site, illustrating the difficulty in completely healing a Jones' fracture.

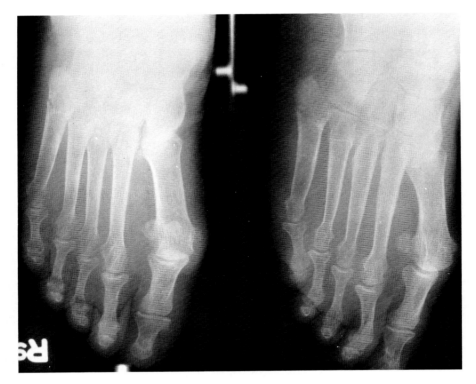

Figure 8–59. A 66-year-old woman spontaneously developed a Jones' fracture of her right fifth metatarsal. Anteroposterior and oblique views show a non-displaced transverse fracture at the metaphyseal-diaphyseal junction of the right fifth metatarsal. Note the generalized osteoporosis of the entire foot.

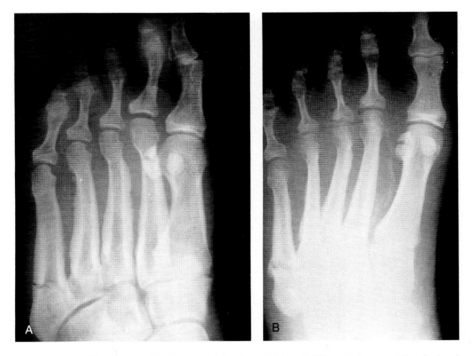

Figure 8–60. A 48-year-old man sustained a Jones' fracture of his left fifth metatarsal while playing basketball (**A,** oblique view). **B,** anteroposteriar view 10 weeks later shows callus formation at the fracture site. The patient no longer had pain at the fifth metatarsal.

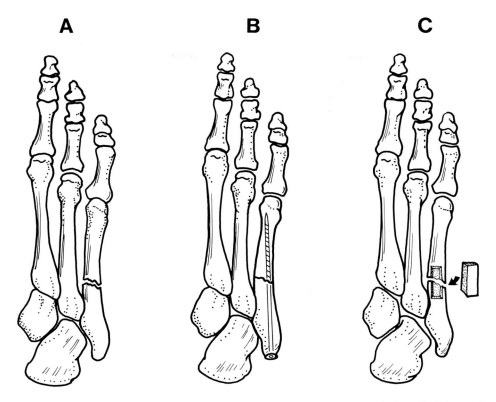

Figure 8–61. Surgical techniques for treating Jones' fracture of the fifth metatarsal. **A,** typical Jones' fracture involving the metaphyseal-diaphyseal junction of the proximal portion of the fifth metatarsal. **B,** fixation of the Jones' fracture with an intramedullary bone screw, which is a good method to use in professional athletes. **C,** treatment of an old and symptomatic Jones' fracture with an inlaid bone graft.

H. Stress fractures of the metatarsals: can be treated with avoidance of vigorous activities and the use of a metatarsal bar, metatarsal pad, or a well-molded arch support in combination with a stiff-soled shoe until the fracture is no longer symptomatic.

I. Symptomatic malunited metatarsal fractures: can be treated with a correctional osteotomy or a condylectomy to restore normal weight-bearing function and to get rid of the painful plantar callosity caused by a plantarly angulated metatarsal head, or with a simple bunionectomy eliminate a painful bunionette from a laterally deviated fifth metatarsal fracture.

REFERENCES

Fractures of the Metatarsals

1. Anderson, L.D.: Injuries of the forefoot. Clin. Orthop., *122:*18, 1977.
2. Arangio, G.A.: Proximal diaphyseal fractures of the fifth metatarsal (Jones' fracture): Two cases treated by cross-pinning with review of 106 cases. Foot Ankle, *3:*293, 1983.
3. Carp, L.: Fracture of the fifth metatarsal bone. With special reference to delayed union. Ann. Surg., *86:*308, 1927.
4. Christopher, F.: Fractures of the fifth metatarsal. Surg. Gynecol. Obstet., *37:*190, 1923.
5. Dameron, Jr., T.B.: Fractures and anatomical variations of the proximal portion of the fifth metatarsal. J. Bone Joint Surg. [Am.], *57:*788, 1975.
6. Drez, Jr., D., Young, J.C., Johnston, R.D., and Parker, W.D.: Metatarsal stress fractures. Am. J. Sports Med., *8:*123, 1980.

7. Gould, N., and Trevino, S.: Sural nerve entrapment by avulsion fracture of the base of the fifth metatarsal bone. Foot Ankle, *2:*153, 1981.
8. Irwin, C.G.: Fractures of the metatarsals. Proc. R. Soc. Lond. [Med.], *31:*789, 1938.
9. Jones, R.: Fracture of the base of the fifth metatarsal bone by indirect violent. Ann. Surg., *35:*697, 1902.
10. Kavanaugh, J.H., Brower, T.D., and Mann, R.V.: The Jones fracture revisited. J. Bone Joint Surg. [Am.], *60:*776, 1978.
11. McKeever, F.M.: Fractures of tarsal and metatarsal bones. Surg. Gynecol. Obstet., *90:*735, 1950.
12. Pritsch, M., Heim, M., Tauber, H., and Horoszowski, H.: An unusual fracture of the base of the fifth metatarsal bone. J. Trauma, *20:*530, 1980.
13. Roca, J., Roure, F., Fernandez-Fairen, M., and Yunta, A.: Stress fractures of the fifth metatarsal. Acta Orthop. Belg., *46:*630, 1980.
14. Stewart, I.M.: Jones' fracture: Fracture of base of fifth metatarsal. Clin. Orthop., *16:*190, 1960.
15. Torg, J.S., et al: Fractures of the base of the fifth metatarsal distal to the tuberosity. Classification and guidelines for non-surgical and surgical management. J. Bone Joint Surg. [Am.], *66:*209, 1984.
16. Wharton, H.R.: Fractures of the proximal end of the fifth metatarsal bone. Ann. Surg., *47:*824, 1908.
17. Whiteside, J.A., Fleagle, S.B., and Kalenak, A.: Fractures and refractures in intercollegiate athletes. An eleven-year experience. Am. J. Sports Med., *9:*369, 1981.
18. Zelko, R.R., Torg, J.S., and Rachun, A.: Proximal diaphyseal fractures of the fifth metatarsal-treatment of the fractures and their complications in athletes. Am. J. Sports Med., *7:*95, 1979.

Fractures and Dislocations of the Tarsometatarsal (Lisfranc's) Joints

INCIDENCE. Tarsometatarsal fractures and dislocations are commonly caused by high-energy trauma such as an automobile or motorcycle accident, a fall from a height, and a severe twisting injury of the foot. In a head-on automobile collision, the driver's foot is compressed in its longitudinal axis between the firewall and the front seat, and the trapezoidal shape of the metatarsal bases with their narrow sides on the plantar side, and the much weaker dorsal capsular and ligamentous structures greatly favor a dorsal dislocation of the tarsometatarsal joints. When a person falls from a horse with the foot caught in a stirrup, the weight of the falling body bends the foot at the tarsometatarsal joints and causes a lateral dislocation of all five metatarsals. In a severe twisting injury with the forefoot fixed to the ground, forceful eversion of the hindfoot can produce a dorsolateral dislocation of all five metatarsals. A forceful inversion of the same hindfoot can lead to a dislocation of only the first tarsometatarsal joint. A frequent accompaniment to this dislocation is a fracture of the base of the second metatarsal, which is deeply recessed in the three cuneiforms and is tightly bound to these structures by strong ligaments.

Classification of tarsometatarsal dislocations can thus be based on the direction of the metatarsal dislocation.

A. Homolateral dislocation: the most common form of tarsometatarsal dislocation and is caused by a forceful abduction injury of the forefoot that produces a dislocation of all five metatarsals in a dorsolateral direction (Figure 8–62). This type is frequently accompanied by a transverse fracture of the base of the second metatarsal and occasionally also a fracture of the cuboid (Figure 8–63).

B. Divergent dislocation: caused by an axial force that causes the toes to go into hyperextension and the metatarsals into acute plantar flexion, which results in rupture of all the dorsal capsules of Lisfranc's joint to produce a dorsal dislocation. If the axial load is applied between the first and second metatarsals, the first metatarsal is dislocated medially, and the four lateral metatarsals laterally, producing a so-called divergent dislocation. If the same axial force proceeds more proximally, it may also separate the first and second cuneiforms and can fracture the first cuneiform or navicular (Figure 8–64).

C. Isolated dislocation: involves one or two metatarsals and is caused by a combination of crushing and twisting forces directly or indirectly applied to the forefoot without any set pattern (Figure 8–65 and 8–66).

D. Crushing injury: produces a wide spectrum of fractures and dislocations of the

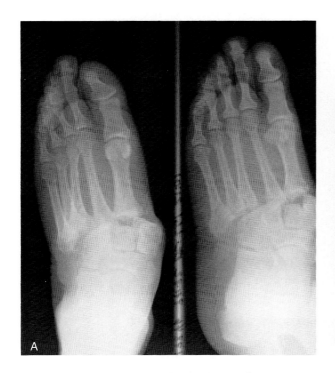

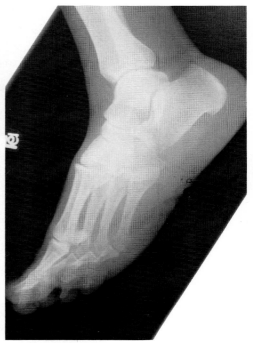

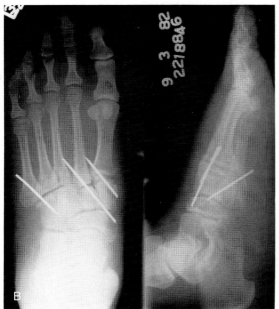

Figure 8–62. A 26-year-old man had an abduction injury to his left forefoot. **A,** oblique, anteroposterior, and lateral views show that he sustained a homolateral dislocation of all five metatarsals without fracturing the base of the second metatarsal. **B,** postoperative lateral and anteroposterior views of the same foot show anatomic reduction of the previously dislocated Lisfranc's joint.

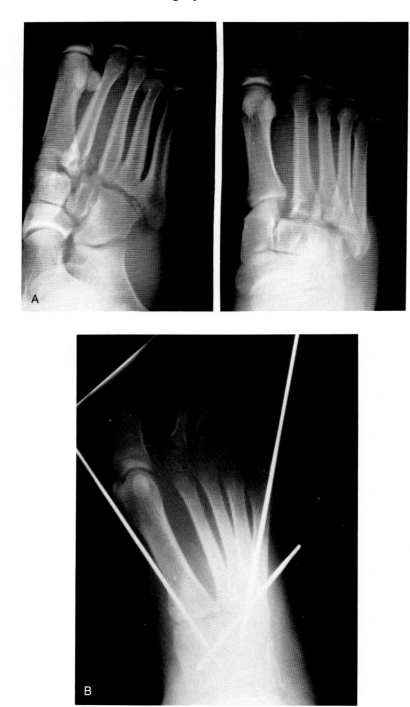

Figure 8–63. A 36-year-old man injured his right foot in an automobile accident. (**A,** oblique and anteroposterior radiographs reveal dislocation of the tarsometatarsal joints, and fractures of the bases of the second and third metatarsals and the cuboid. **B–D,** intraoperative radiographs show that the Lisfranc's dislocation has been reduced and stabilized with three K-wires; the cuboid fracture is still slightly displaced.

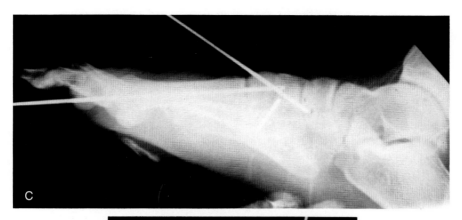

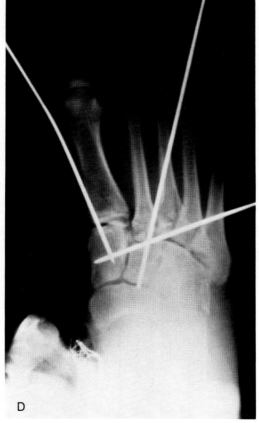

Figure 8–63. Continued.

tarsometatarsal joints and their neighboring metatarsal and tarsal bones in an unpredictable manner.

It should be noted that severe vascular injury to the foot has been known to be associated with dislocation of Lisfranc's joint, resulting in subsequent gangrene and amputation of the foot.

CLINICAL SYMPTOMS AND SIGNS. Swelling in the dorsal aspect of the foot, localized tenderness along Lisfranc's joint, production of severe pain by passively supinating and pronating the forefoot with the hindfoot

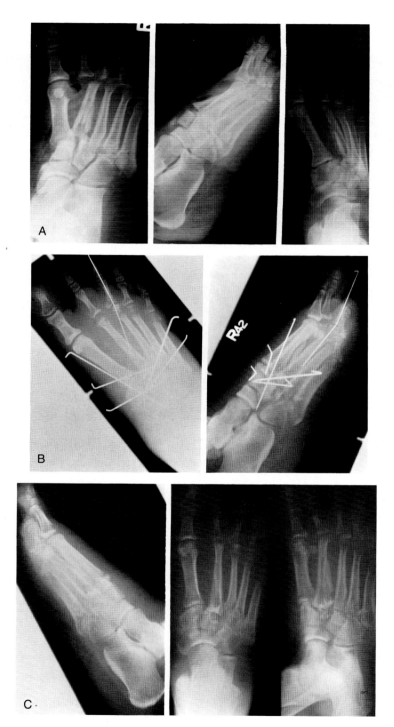

Figure 8–64. A 35-year-old woman sustained a severe injury to her right foot in an automobile accident. **A,** antero-posterior, lateral, and oblique films show dislocation of the Lisfranc's joint, subluxation of the first cuneiform-navicular joint, fractures of the first cuneiform, second metatarsal head and shaft, second cuneiform, and cuboid, and complete dislocation of the second, third, and fourth M-P joints. **B,** intraoperative radiographs reveal satisfactory reduction of all fractures and dislocations by means of multiple small K-wires. **C,** oblique, anteroposterior, and lateral views, 2 months after surgery. There is satisfactory reduction and maintenance of all fractures and dislocations.

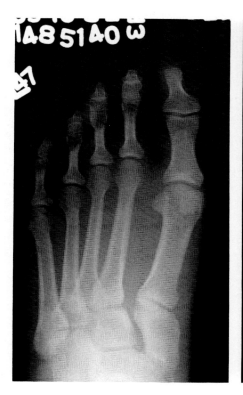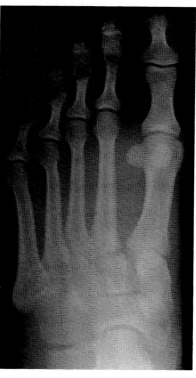

Figure 8–65. A 30-year-old man injured his left foot while playing basketball. Anteroposterior and oblique views show an isolated dislocation of the first metatarsal ray at the medial cuneiform-navicular joint, accompanied by separation of the first and second cuneiforms and a chip fracture of the medial and distal portion of the navicular produced by a shearing force.

held in a fixed position, abnormal motion at the Lisfranc's joint, shortening of the forefoot in its longitudinal axis, and broadening of the forefoot in its transverse axis are the clinical findings of a dislocation of the Lisfranc's joint. When the dislocation is of the homolateral type, a flatfoot appearance is present due to forefoot abduction and loss of the normal medial longitudinal arch of the foot. When a divergent dislocation is present, a severe metatarsus primus varus deformity is present, with a wide separation between the first and second toes.

When fractures and dislocations of the metatarsals and tarsals are associated with a Lisfranc's dislocation, pain, swelling, crepitation, abnormal motion, tenderness, and deformity are present beyond the confines of the tarsometatarsal joints. When severe vascular injury is associated with a Lisfranc's dislocation, coolness, pulselessness, sensory disturbance, and skin discoloration are the warning signs that demand immediate medical attention to prevent the development of gangrene of the foot, which usually necessitates foot amputation.

ROENTGENOGRAPHIC MANIFESTATIONS. The anteroposterior, lateral, and oblique views of the foot are required to diagnose and thus treat a Lisfranc's dislocation. In a homolateral dislocation, all five metatarsals are displaced laterally and dorsally with a transverse fracture of the base of the second metatarsal, and are no longer in alignment with their respective cuneiforms or cuboid. In a divergent dislocation, the first metatarsal ray is displaced medially and the four lateral metatarsals are displaced lat-

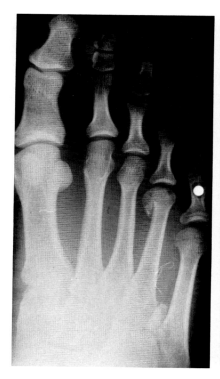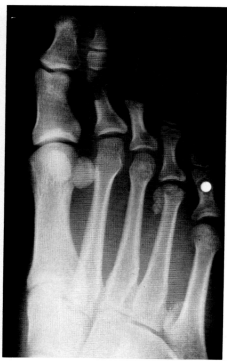

Figure 8–66. The right forefoot of a 23-year-old man was run over by the tire of a car. Anteroposterior and oblique radiographs demonstrate a fracture of the medial base and a lateral dislocation of the fifth metatarsal, accompanied by a fracture of the fourth metatarsal head. The buckshot in the fifth proximal phalanx was from a previous shotgun injury.

erally. The dislocations of the first metatarsal ray can occur at the first metatarsocuneiform joint, the first cuneiform-navicular joint with separation of the first and second cuneiforms, or at the talonavicular joint with separation of the first and second cuneiforms plus a fracture of the navicular. In an isolated dislocation of the Lisfranc's joint, only one or two metatarsals will be dislocated.

In a severe crushing injury, in addition to the dislocation of the Lisfranc's joint, fractures and dislocations of the phalanges, metatarsals, and tarsals can be variable. It should be emphasized that the roentgenographic signs of a Lisfranc's dislocation can be subtle and may be easily missed. If the following rules are carefully observed, however, the chances of overlooking a Lisfranc's dislocation are greatly minimized (Figure 8–67).

Rule 1. On the anteroposterior view of the foot, the medial margin of the base of the second metatarsal should align perfectly with the medial margin of the second cuneiform.

Rule 2. On the oblique view, the medial margin of the base of the fourth metatarsal should align with the medial margin of the cuboid.

Rule 3. On the lateral view, the metatarsal bases should never be more dorsal than their corresponding tarsal bones.

Furthermore, a Lisfranc's dislocation can undergo a spontaneous reduction. When examined radiographically, the foot appears close to normal, except for some soft tissue swelling or a hairline fracture of the second meta-

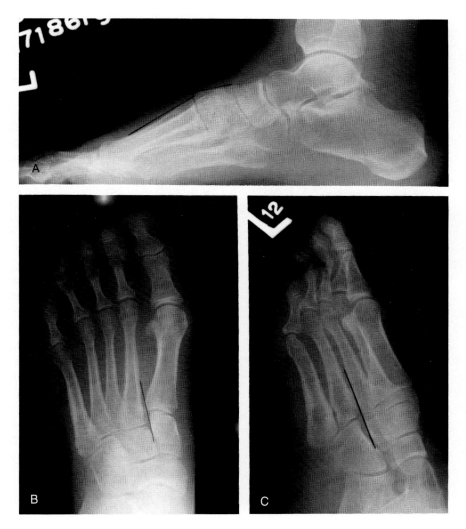

Figure 8–67. Three important anatomic landmarks commonly used to rule out the presence of a Lisfranc's dislocation. **A,** on a lateral view, the metatarsals should never rise above their corresponding tarsal bones. **B,** on an antero-posterior view, the medial border of the second metatarsal base should always line up with the medial border of the second cuneiform. **C,** on an oblique view, the medial border of the fourth metatarsal should always line up with the medial border of the cuboid.

tarsal base (Figure 8–68). Under this circumstance, radiographs taken when the foot is under stress will reveal the tarsometatarsal instability, which can then be treated properly.

TREATMENT

A. Homolateral dislocation: can be reduced by suspending the foot vertically in the air with wire finger traps and by applying downward traction to the heel manually or by placing a sling and weight around the ankle. Radiographs should be obtained with the foot in traction, and if the reduction is satisfactory and remains satisfactory after the traction is released, a well-molded short, leg cast should be worn for 6 weeks. Follow-up radiographs should be obtained at short intervals during that time to detect recurrent dislocation of these tarsometa-

316   **Surgery of the Foot**

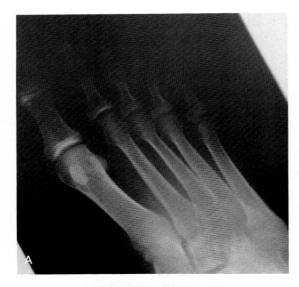

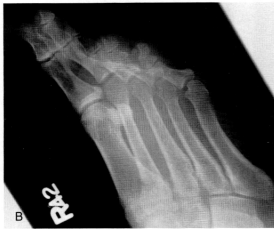

Figure 8–68. A 32-year-old man sustained a forceful abduction injury of his right foot. Anteroposterior (**A**) and oblique (**B**) radiographs show only a transverse fracture of the second metatarsal base. Physical examination revealed pain, swelling, and tenderness throughout the entire Lisfranc's joint, indicating the presence of injury to all five tarsometatarsal joints. Such an injury should be treated by a short, leg cast for 4 to 6 weeks.

tarsal joints. When the cast is removed, a well-molded arch support should be used for about 6 months.

If the tarsometatarsal joints become subluxated or dislocated after the removal of traction, they should be reduced again and

held by means of percutaneous K-wire fixation from the shafts of the first and fifth metatarsals into their respective tarsal bones. A short, leg cast should then be used for 6 weeks followed by an arch support for an additional 6 months.

B. Divergent dislocation: if only at the tarsometatarsal joints, closed reduction with traction often requires percutaneous K-wire fixation to stabilize all five metatarsals. If the dislocation of the first metatarsal ray takes place through the first cuneiform-navicular joint, maintenance of the closed reduction can be achieved by driving a K-wire from the lateral shaft of the fifth metatarsal into the cuboid, and another K-wire from the first cuneiform into the other cuneiforms in a transverse manner; the postoperative regimen is similar to that for the treatment of homolateral dislocation.

If the dislocation occurs at the medial aspect of the talonavicular joint through a transarticular fracture of the navicular, an open reduction is frequently required to reduce the navicular fracture anatomically with K-wires or a mini-bone screw. The first cuneiform can then be fixed to the second and third cuneiforms with a K-wire, and the fifth metatarsal to the cuboid with another K-wire.

C. Isolated dislocation: the one or two dislocated metatarsals can usually be reduced by closed means; K-wire fixation can be added if the dislocation is unstable after reduction.

D. Crushing injury: in addition to reducing the tarsometatarsal dislocation, the fractures and dislocations of the toes, metatarsals, and tarsals should also be treated by both closed and open methods (Figure 8–69).

E. Irreducible dislocation: usually caused by blockage by bone fragments and peroneus longus and anterior tibial tendons and frequently requires open reduction (Figure

A

B

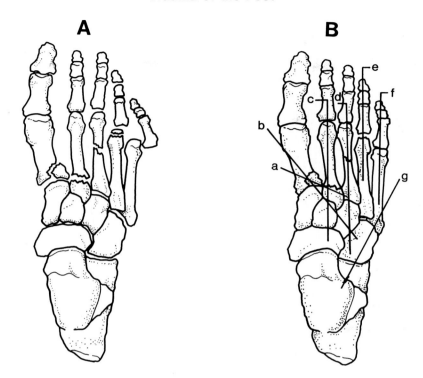

Figure 8–69. Various metatarsal and phalangel injuries that can accompany a Lisfranc's dislocation. **A,** fracture of the lateral base of the first metatarsal, transverse fracture of the base of the second metatarsal, oblique third metatarsal shaft fracture, fracture of the fourth metatarsal held in association with a dislocation of the fourth M-P joint, and lateral dislocation of the fifth M-P joint. **B,** surgical treatments of the metatarsal and phalangeal injuries with K-wires. a, fixation of the transarticular fracture of the first metatarsal base; b, stabilization of the first tarsometatarsal joint; c, stabilization of the second metatarsal fracture; d, reduction and stabilization of the third metatarsal fracture; e, excision of the loose bone fragment from the fourth M-P joint and reduction and stabilization of the fourth M-P joint; f, reduction and stabilization of the fifth M-P joint; g, stabilization of the lateral tarsometatarsal joints.

8–70). Two dorsal longitudinal incisions, one between the first and second metatarsals and the other between the fourth and fifth metatarsals, can be used to gain access to the entire Lisfranc's joint, to reduce dislocations and fractures or to perform arthrodesis of the same joint.

F. Compound Lisfranc's dislocation: in addition to reducing the tarsometatarsal dislocation, the wound should be irrigated and debrided, prophylactic intravenous antibiotic therapy should be initiated and skin care should be meticulous.

G. Lisfranc's dislocation in association with evidence of major vascular injury of the

foot: should be reduced promptly and then evaluated by careful examination in combination with evaluation by a Doppler flow meter. If the circulation of the foot is in jeopardy, vascular surgeons should be immediately consulted so to prevent the tragic consequence of the development of a gangrenous foot, which usually results in either a Syme's or a below-knee amputation, depending on the level of the nonviable skin margins.

H. Treated or untreated fractures and dislocations of Lisfranc's joint with painful degenerative arthritis: can be treated by arthrodesis of the tarsometatarsal joints by carefully resecting the arthritic joints at

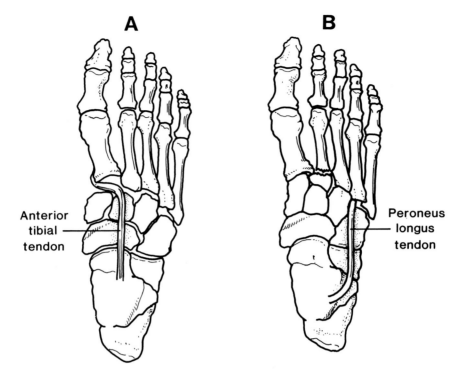

Figure 8–70. Irreducible Lisfranc's dislocation due to soft tissue interposition. **A,** interposition of the anterior tibial tendon between the first metatarsal base and the cuneiform prevents a successful closed reduction. **B,** interposition of the peroneus longus tendon between the fourth metatarsal base and the cuboid also prevents a successful closed reduction.

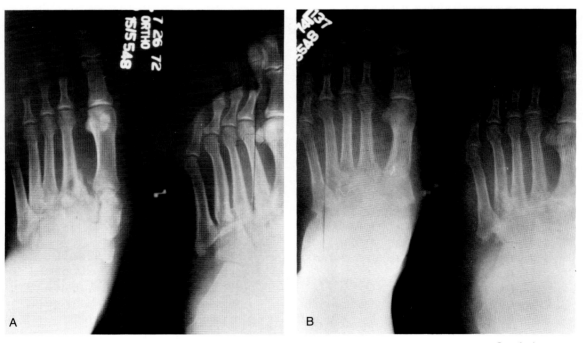

See facing page.

correct angles to restore the foot arches and the normal appearance of the foot (Figure 8–71).

REFERENCES

Fractures and Dislocations of the Tarsometatarsal Joints

1. Aitken, A.P., and Poulson, D.: Dislocations of the tarsometatarsal joint. J. Bone Joint Surg. [Am.], *45*:246, 1963.
2. Blair, W.F.: Irreducible tarsometatarsal fracture-dislocation. J. Trauma, *21*:988, 1981.
3. Cassebaum, W.H.: Lisfranc fracture-dislocations. Clin. Orthop., *30*:116, 1963.
4. Collett, H.S., Hood, T.K., and Andrews, R.E.: Tarsometatarsal fracture dislocations. Surg., Gynecol. Obstet., *106*:623, 1958.
5. DeBenedetti, M.J., Evanski, P.M., and Vaugh, T.R.: The unreducible Lisfranc fracture. Case report and literature review. Clin. Orthop., *136*:238, 1978.
6. Delsel, J.M.: The surgical treatment of tarso-metatarsal fracture-dislocations. J. Bone Joint Surg. [Br.], *37*:203, 1955.
7. Denton, J.R.: A complex Lisfranc fracture-dislocation. J. Trauma, *20*:526, 1980.
8. Engber, W.D., and Roberts, J.M.: Irreducible tarsometatarsal fracture-dislocation. Clin. Orthop., *168*:102, 1982.
9. English, T.A.: Dislocations of the metatarsal bone and adjacent toe. J. Bone Joint Surg. [Br.], *46*:700, 1964.
10. Foster, S.C., and Foster, R.R.: Lisfranc's tarsometatarsal fracture–dislocations. Radiology, *120*:79, 1976.
11. Gissane, W.A.: A dangerous type of fracture of the foot. J. Bone Joint Surg. [Br.], *33*:535, 1951.
12. Goossens, M., and DeStoop, N.: Lisfranc's fracture-dislocations: Etiology, radiology, and results of treatment. A review of 20 cases. Clin. Orthop., *176*:154, 1983.
13. Granberry, W.M., and Lipscomb, P.R.: Dislocation of the tarsometatarsal joints. Surg., Gynecol. Obstet., *114*:467, 1962.
14. Hardcastle, P.H., Reschauer, R., Kutscha-Lissberg, E., and Schoffmann, W.: Injuries to the tarsometatarsal joint. Incidence, classification and treatment. J. Bone Joint Surg. [Br.], *64*:349, 1982.
15. Hesp, W.L., Van Der Werken, C., and Goris, R.J.: Lisfranc dislocation: Fractures and/or dislocations through the tarsometatarsal joints. Injury, *15*:261, 1984.
16. Holstein, A., and Joldersma, R.D.: Dislocation of first cuneiform in tarsometatarsal fracture-dislocation. J. Bone Joint Surg. [Am.], *32*:419, 1950.
17. Jeffreys, T.E.: Lisfranc's fracture-dislocation. J. Bone Joint Surg. [Br.], *45*:546, 1963.
18. Liczner, E.M., Waddell, J.P., and Graham, J.D.: Tarsometatarsal (Lisfranc dislocation). J. Trauma, *14*:1012, 1974.
19. Lowe, J., and Yosipovitch, Z.: Tarsometatarsal dislocation: A mechanism blocking manipulative reduction. J. Bone Joint Surg. [Am.], *58*:1029, 1976.
20. Wiley, J.J.: The mechanism of tarsometatarsal joint injuries. J. Bone Joint Surg. [Br.], *53*:474, 1971.
21. Wilppula, E.: Tarsometatarsal fracture-dislocation. Acta Orthop. Scand., *44*:335, 1973.
22. Wilson, D.W.: Injury of the tarsometatarsal joints. Etiology, classification and results of treatment. J. Bone Joint Surg. [Br.], *54*:677, 1972.

Fractures and Dislocations of the Navicular, Cuneiforms, Cuboid and Midtarsal (Talonavicular and Calcaneocuboid) Joints

The three cuneiforms that articulate with the navicular, the navicular with the head of the talus, the cuboid with the anterior process of the calcaneus, and the talonavicular and calcaneocuboid joints are the anatomic structures of the midpart of the foot. As a region, their fractures and/or dislocations are among the least frequently encountered injuries of the foot. When they do happen, however, they tend to occur as a combination of multiple fractures and/or dislocations.

FRACTURES OF THE NAVICULAR

INCIDENCE. The navicular forms the keystone of the medial longitudinal arch of the foot and occupies the highest position of the same arch. Navicular fractures are relatively uncommon, and are usually caused by inversion, eversion, crushing, and axial compression forces. On an anatomic basis, all the navicular fractures can be classified into four major types (Figure 8–72).

A. Fracture of the dorsal lip of the navicular: a cortical avulsion fracture commonly

---

Figure 8–71. A 35-year-old man sustained a Lisfranc's dislocation in an automobile accident 6 months before seeing the author. **A,** oblique and anteroposterior views show marked destruction of the left tarsometatarsal joints. The patient eventually underwent fusion of all five tarsometatarsal joints of his left foot in an attempt to relieve constant foot pain and to correct the rocker-bottom foot deformity. **B,** anteroposterior and oblique views 2 years later show solid fusion of all five tarsometatarsal joints. The patient had a strong and painless foot.

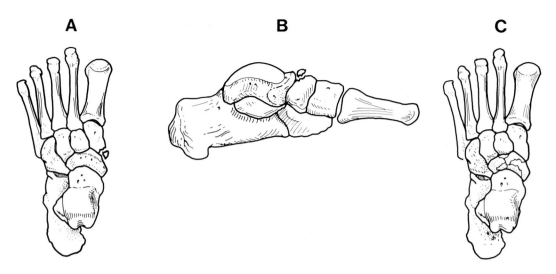

Figure 8–72.   Various fractures of the navicular and first cuneiform. **A,** a chip fracture of the proximal medial aspect of the first cuneiform, which is equivalent to a fracture of the navicular tuberosity. **B,** a fracture of the dorsal lip of the navicular. **C,** a comminuted fracture of the body of the navicular.

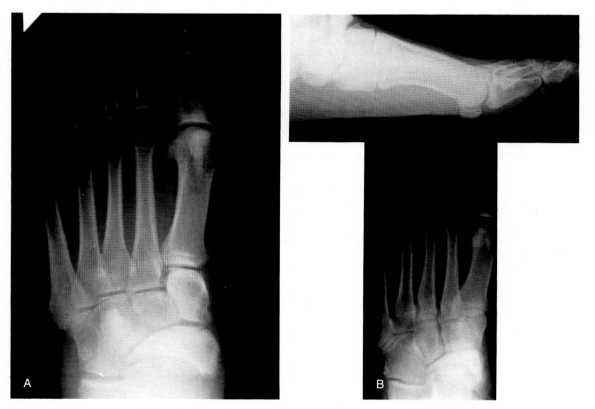

Figure 8–73.   A 42-year-old man had previously injured his left foot in an automobile accident. Anteroposterior (**A**), as well as lateral and oblique (**B**) views show osteosclerosis and flattening of the navicular and arthritic changes of the naviculocuneiform and talonavicular joints.

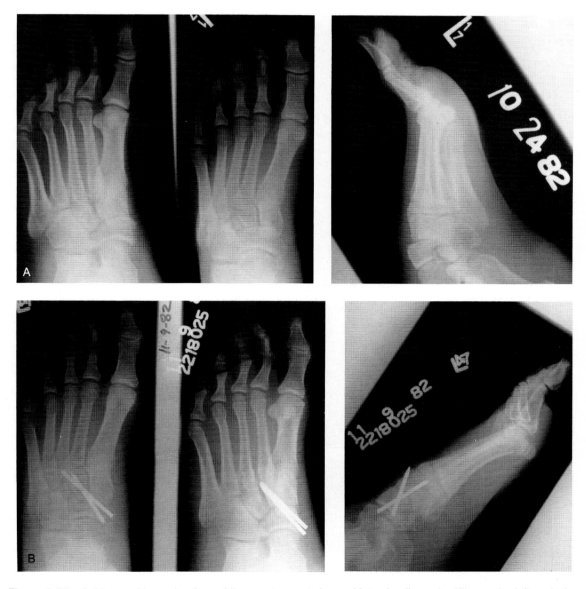

Figure 8-74. A 24-year-old man in whom oblique, anteroposterior, and lateral radiographs (**A**) reveal a left navicular fracture with some dorsal migration of the main portion of the fractured navicular. **B,** same views after surgery show an anatomic reduction of the navicular fracture and subluxation.

caused by an eversion injury with dorsi-flexion of the forefoot during which the tib-ionavicular portion of the deltoid ligament, which inserts into the dorsal lip of the na-vicular, avulses the dorsal lip.

B. Fracture of the navicular tuberosity: caused by an eversion injury of the foot with forced abduction of the forefoot. Forceful con-traction of the posterior tibial tendon, which inserts into the navicular tuberosity, avul-ses the same tuberosity.

C. Fracture of the body of the navicular: can be produced directly by dropping a heavy object on the dorsum of the foot, or indirectly by applying a longitudinal force to the medial metatarsal heads. A variety of undisplaced, displaced, and even greatly comminuted fractures of the navicular may be produced (Figures 8–73—8–75).

D. Stress fracture of the navicular: caused by prolonged and excessive cyclic stresses to the foot, and shows a definite predilection for young male athletes.

CLINICAL SYMPTOMS AND SIGNS. In dorsal lip fracture, fracture of the body, and stress fracture, pain, swelling, and tenderness are over the dorsomedial aspect of the foot at the high point of the longitudinal arch. With fracture of the navicular tuberosity, however, the swelling and tenderness are localized to the superomedial aspect of the medial longitudinal arch, and the pain is greatly aggravated by passive eversion and active inversion of the foot. When a comminuted navicular fracture has caused a dorsal displacement of a large bony fragment, if the swelling is not too severe, a bony mass may be palpated on the dorsal aspect of the foot.

ROENTGENOGRAPHIC MANIFESTATIONS. Stress fracture, tuberosity fracture, and comminuted fractures of the navicular are best demonstrated by the anteroposterior and oblique views, but the dorsal lip fracture and

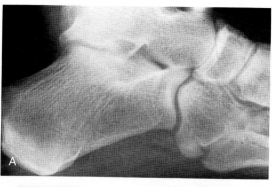
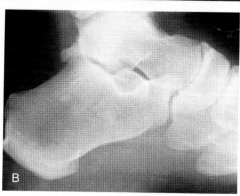

Figure 8–75. **A,** lateral view of the hindfoot shows an avulsion-type chip fracture of the dorsal lip of the navicular. Note the irregularity of the fracture line, the slight displacement of the chip fracture, and the presence of a small cuboid fracture. **B,** lateral view of a completely asymptomatic hindfoot shows the presence of an os supranaviculare, which is smooth and continuous with margins of the navicular bone and should be differentiated from a small dorsal lip fracture of the navicular.

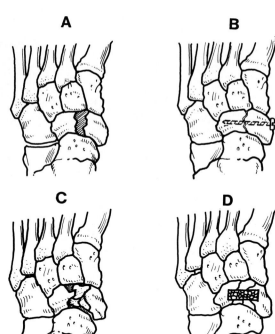

Figure 8–76. Surgical techniques for treating different fractures of the body of the navicular. **A,** simple longitudinal fracture of the body of the navicular with displacement. **B,** open reduction and fixation of the simple navicular fracture with a transverse bone screw. **C,** comminuted fracture of the body of the navicular with disruption of both the naviculocuneiform and talonavicular joints. **D,** restoration of the navicular portion of the naviculocuneiform and talonavicular articular surfaces by elevating the displaced articular surface and packing the subchondral bone defect with autogenous bone chips.

dorsal migration of a bony fragment from a comminuted navicular fracture are best seen on the lateral view. Varying degrees of soft tissue swelling on the dorsal aspect of the foot overlying the fracture site can also be seen on the lateral view. An os supranaviculare should not be mistaken for a dorsal lip fracture of the navicular, and an os tibiale externum should be differentiated from a fracture of the tuberosity of the navicular. The smooth bony outlines, bilateral nature, and lack of symptoms of these accessory ossicles are

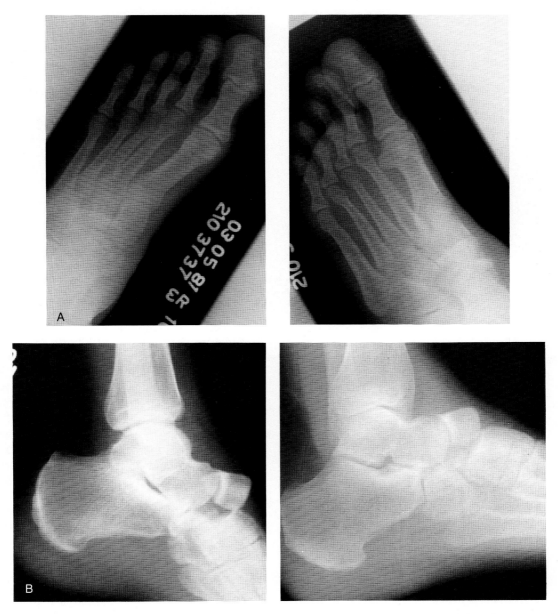

Figure 8–77. A 28-year-old man slipped on ice and sustained a severe twisting injury to his left foot. Anteroposterior and oblique (**A**) as well as oblique and lateral (**B**) views demonstrate a fracture and dislocation of the navicular, which no longer articulates with the cuneiforms.

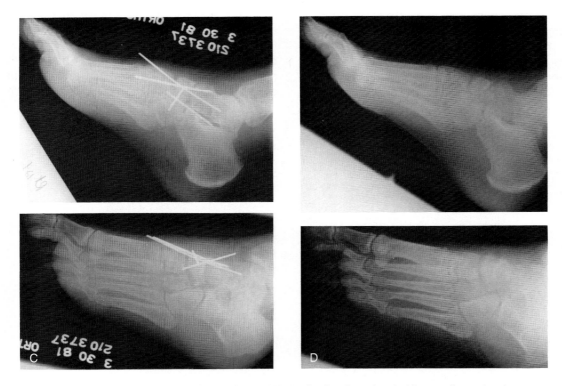

Figure 8–77. Continued. C, after open reduction and K-wire fixation, lateral and oblique radiographs show anatomic reduction of the navicular fracture and dislocation. **D,** lateral and oblique films 6 months after surgery show excellent healing of the navicular fracture and normal alignment of the talonavicular and naviculocuneiform joints.

usually distinctive enough to provide the necessary differentiation.

TREATMENT

A. Fracture of the dorsal lip of the navicular: if the fractured dorsal lip fragment is small, only immobilization in a short walking cast for 4 to 6 weeks is required. If the fracture involves more than 20% of the articular surface and is displaced, open reduction with anatomic reduction and fixation of the fractured bony fragment with a mini-bone screw should be performed; 6 weeks of cast immobilization should follow. Whenever a small dorsal lip fracture fails to become united to its parental bone and becomes symptomatic, simple surgical excision of this irritating bone chip under local anesthesia is the treatment of choice.

B. Fracture of the navicular tuberosity: if undisplaced or minimally displaced, a short walking cast for 4 to 6 weeks is all that is required. When the fractured navicular tuberosity is significantly displaced, it can be anatomically reduced and fixed to the navicular with a small bone screw. When a navicular tuberosity fracture occasionally fails to unite to its parental bone and becomes painful, it can be excised and the posterior tibial tendon should be securely anchored to the undersurface of the navicular to preserve its normal weight-bearing function.

C. Fracture of the body of the navicular: if undisplaced, a short walking cast should be used for 4 to 6 weeks. When the fracture is displaced, every attempt should be made to restore the navicular articular sur-

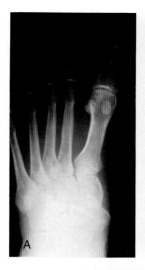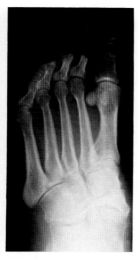

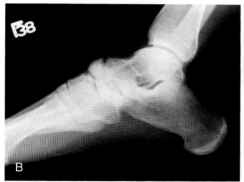

Figure 8–78. A 37-year-old man sustained a comminuted navicular fracture of his left foot 3 years before seeking medical attention because of pain. Anteroposterior and oblique (**A**) and lateral (**B**) radiographs show significant collapse, sclerosis, and some dorsal migration of the navicular. The patient was treated with a custom-made total-contact arch support, but a naviculocuneiform and talonavicular fusion with an inlaid iliac graft was eventually required.

faces that form part of the naviculocuneiform and talonavicular joints. A simple displaced fracture can be reduced and fixed with small bone screws or K-wires. A complex fracture of the navicular with severe disruption of its articular surfaces may need careful elevation of these displaced articular surfaces back into their anatomic position. The subchondral bony defect should be tightly packed with autogenous bone chips to prevent recurrent collapse

of the restored articular surfaces (Figures 8–76 and 8–77). A short, non–weight-bearing cast should also be used for the first 6 to 8 weeks, after which a short walking cast can be worn for another 4 to 6 weeks to allow the bone graft to consolidate.

Regardless of the different methods of treatment rendered, some patients with fracture of the navicular body develop painful arthritis in the talonavicular and/or naviculocuneiform joints to the extent that arthrodesis of one or both of these joints will eventually be required (Figure 8–78).

D. Stress fracture of the navicular: usually necessitates a short walking cast for about 6 weeks, after which a well-fitted arch support should be used until the fracture is no longer symptomatic.

FRACTURES AND DISLOCATIONS OF THE CUNEIFORMS AND CUBOID

INCIDENCE. Isolated fracture or dislocation of the cuneiforms or cuboid is rare, (Figures 8–79 and 8–80) due to their relatively protected anatomic sites and their intimate connections with the tarsometatarsal and midtarsal joints. Consequently, injuries of the cuneiforms and the cuboid are frequently associated with fractures and/or dislocations of the tarsometatarsal and midtarsal joints (Figures 8–81—8–85). When a powerful abduction force is applied to the forefoot, if the dislocation occurs at the tarsometatarsal joints, the anterior aspect of the cuboid can be fractured by the bases of the fourth and fifth metatarsals. If the same force caused dislocation of the midtarsal joints, however, the cuboid can be crushed between the fourth and fifth metatarsal bases and the anterior process of the calcaneus. Although extremely rare, a total dislocation of the cuboid can also take place.

If a longitudinal force is applied between the first and second metatarsals, the first cuneiform can become fractured or dislocated medially with the first metatarsal. If a crushing

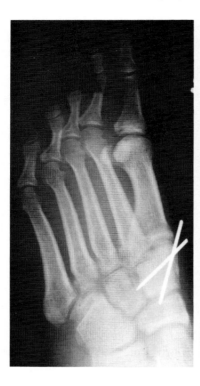 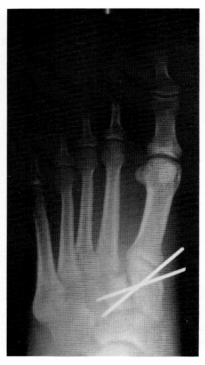

Figure 8–79. A 30-year-old man sustained a dislocation of his left first cuneiform in a basketball game. An open reduction and fixation of the first cuneiform to the second cuneiform and the navicular with two small K-wires was required (anteroposterior and oblique views).

force is applied directly to the dorsal aspect of the foot, a fracture of one or more of the three cuneiforms and the cuboid can occur, but their dislocations are unlikely due to the strong ligamentous connections between these midtarsal bones and the adjacent metatarsals, navicular, talus, and calcaneus. Isolated dislocation of the second and third cuneiforms is virtually impossible to produce, because they are securely protected on all four sides by their neighboring tarsal and metatarsal bones. The causes that produce fractures and dislocations of the three cuneiforms and the cuboid include dropping a heavy object on the dorsum of the foot, falling from a height, motor cycle or car accidents, and severe twisting injuries of the foot.

CLINICAL SYMPTOMS AND SIGNS. Pain, swelling, ecchymosis, tenderness, and hematoma over the dorsal aspect of the foot are frequently present. By holding the hindfoot in a fixed position, dorsiflexion, plantar flexion, adduction, abduction, supination, pronation, or axial compression significantly aggravate the foot pain. When a large fracture fragment has become significantly displaced or the entire bone is subluxated or dislocated, a bony prominence with or without irregular borders may be palpated if the swelling of the foot is not too great. All of the aforementioned symptoms and signs tend to be dorsal or dorsomedial when fractures and dislocations of the three cuneiforms are present, and dorsolateral when the cuboid is injured.

ROENTGENOGRAPHIC MANIFESTATIONS. Anteroposterior, lateral, and oblique views are routinely required in demonstrating fractures and dislocations of the cuneiforms and cuboid. Fractures are represented by radiolucent lines that traverse the fractured midtarsal bones, and dislocations are represented by overlapping or opening of the

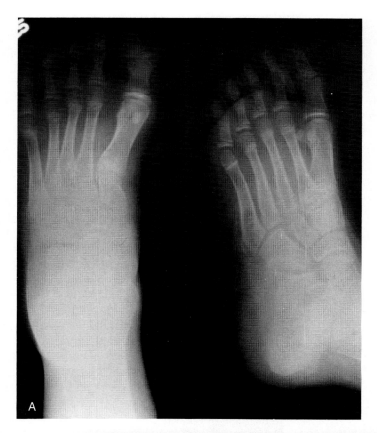

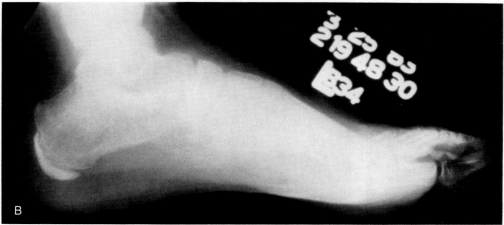

Figure 8–80. Anteroposterior, and oblique (**A**) and lateral (**B**) radiographs show a chip fracture of the lateral aspect of the left cuboid, which was caused by a twisting injury.

articular margins. In a total dislocation of the cuboid, its articulations with the lateral border of the third cuneiform, the bases of the fourth and fifth metatarsals, and the anterior process of the calcaneus are interrupted. When the first cuneiform is completely dislocated, it

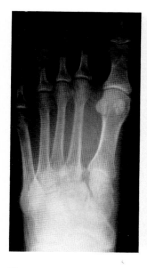
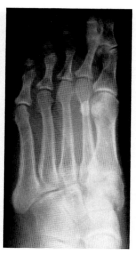

no longer articulates with the base of the first metatarsal, the medial side of the second cuneiform, and the distal articular surface of the navicular.

TREATMENT. Isolated fractures of the cuneiforms and cuboid resulting from a direct crush injury usually do not show much displacement. Therefore, all that is required is the use of a short, leg cast for 5 to 6 weeks. When injuries of these same midtarsal bones are associated with fractures or dislocations of the metatarsals or the tarsal bones of the hindfoot, a carefully evaluated surgical plan should be established before putting it into action. If the routine radiographs do not provide sufficient information, regular or computer assisted tomography should be employed to clearly delineate the exact nature of the fractures and dislocations.

When dealing with complex fractures and dislocations of the tarsometatarsal and midtarsal bones and joints, surgery should almost always proceed in a proximal to distal and medial to lateral direction due to the fact that the key structures are more proximally

Figure 8–81. A 42-year-old man injured his left foot in an automobile accident. Anteroposterior and oblique radiographs reveal separation of the bases of the first and second metatarsals as well as the first and second cuneiforms, together with an oblique fracture of the first cuneiform. This uncommon injury is most likely caused by an axial force that is applied between the first and second metatarsal heads causing the first and second metatarsals and the cuneiforms to separate. The force then proceeds medially to produce the oblique fracture of the first cuneiform.

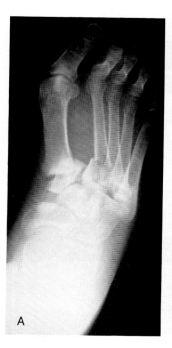
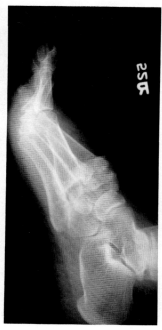
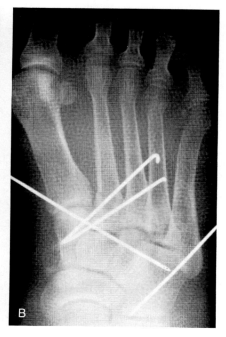

Figure 8–82. An automobile accident victim in whom oblique and lateral radiographs (**A**) show a divergent type of tarsometatarsal dislocation accompanied by a fracture and dislocation of the first cuneiform and a transverse fracture of base of the second metatarsal. The patient also had a displaced tibial fracture.

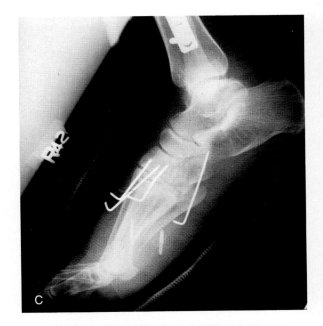

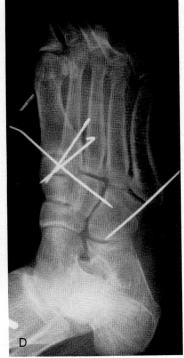

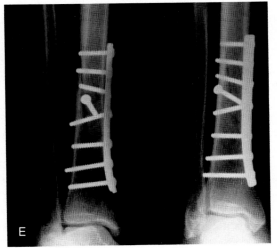

Figure 8–82. Continued. Antero-posterior (**B**), lateral (**C**), and oblique (**D**) views show satisfactory reduction of the Lisfranc's dislocation and the associated cuneiform and metatarsal fractures and dislocation. The tibial fracture was treated with a bone plate fixation (**E**).

and medially based. Dislocation of the first cuneiform or the cuboid usually requires open reduction, and these structures can be approached through a longitudinal dorsomedial or dorsolateral skin incision, respectively. After the dislocated first cuneiform or cuboid has been satisfactorily reduced, they can be fixed to their neighboring tarsal or metatarsal bones with K-wires. A short, leg cast should be used

for 5 to 6 weeks to allow the torn capsular and ligamentous structures to heal.

In a young and vigorous person, if the cuneiform or cuboid fracture has destroyed a significant portion of its articular surface, serious consideration should be given to restoring the fractured and depressed articular surface by elevating the displaced and comminuted articular surface back to its orig-

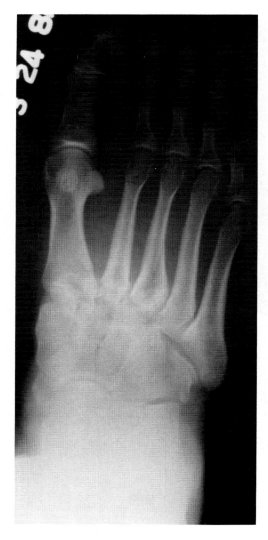

Figure 8–83. Anteroposterior radiograph shows an oblique fracture of the cuboid with involvement of the metatarsocuboid and calcaneocuboid joints caused by an abduction injury of the forefoot.

inal position, and by tightly packing the subchondral bony defect with autogenous bone chips. When painful arthritis has developed in the tarsometatarsal, calcaneocuboid, or naviculocuneiform joints, arthrodesis can provide a stiff but painless joint.

FRACTURES AND DISLOCATIONS OF THE MIDTARSAL JOINTS

INCIDENCE. The midtarsal joints, also known as Chopart's joint or transverse tarsal

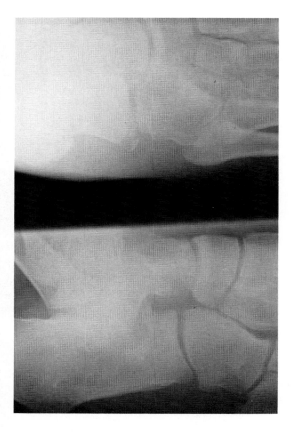

Figure 8–84. Lateral and anteroposterior radiographs of the hindfoot show chip fractures of both the calcaneus and the cuboid.

joints, consist of the talonavicular and calcaneocuboid joints, which occupy a key position in the medial and lateral longitudinal arches of the foot and act together as a single functional unit. In addition, they also act in unison with the subtalar joint in controlling the inversion and eversion of the foot. The midtarsal joints are moderately mobile when the heel is in pronation, and are relatively rigid when the heel is in supination. The small amount of motion that exists in the midtarsal joints makes them less vulnerable to fractures or dislocations, although high-energy trauma, such as car and motorcycle accidents, a fall from a height, the wheel of a heavy vehicle running over the foot, or a severe twisting injury of the foot may result in fracture or dislocation.

A comprehensive classification of the various injuries of the midtarsal joints can be

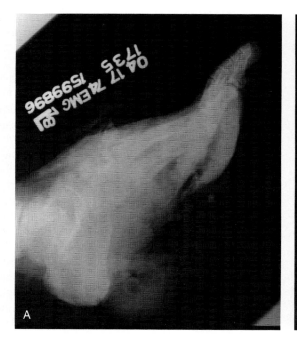
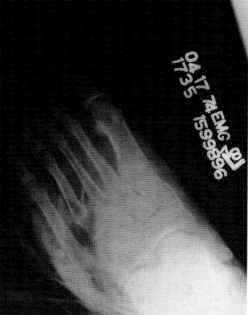

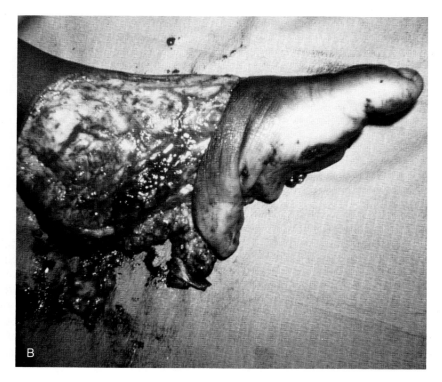

Figure 8–85. A 10-year-old boy was hit by a train. **A,** lateral and anteroposterior views of the left foot show extensive soft tissue disruption, fractures of the fourth and fifth metatarsals, and dislocation of the cuboid of the left foot. **B,** photograph taken in the emergency room shows extensive soft tissue damage of the left foot.

based on the mechanism of injury, the extent of injury, and the direction of displacement of the forefoot.

A. Medial stress injury: caused by a medially directed force that is applied to the lateral aspect of the forefoot. Sprain and medial subluxation or dislocation of the midtarsal joints is produced and can be associated with fracture of the talar head, navicular, lateral margins of the cuboid, and anterior process of the calcaneus (Figure 8–86). Occasionally, the same force can produce a so-called medial swivel dislocation in which the calcaneocuboid joint remains in-

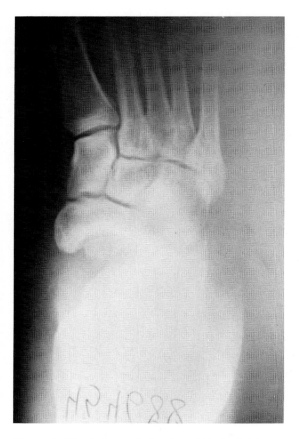

Figure 8–86. Anteroposterior view of the foot shows a medial dislocation of the two midtarsal joints (talonavicular and calcaneocuboid joints) in association with a shear fracture of the head of the talus caused by a medial stress injury with a violent force applied directly to the lateral aspect of the forefoot.

tact, but the talonavicular joint is dislocated and the subtalar joint is subluxated (Figure 8–87).

B. Lateral stress injury: caused by a laterally directed force that is applied to the medial aspect of the forefoot. Sprain and lateral subluxation or dislocation of the midtarsal joints results and can be associated with avulsion fracture of the navicular tuberosity, fracture of the anterior process of the calcaneus, compression fracture of the cuboid (the so-called "nutcracker fracture" caused by crushing the cuboid between the calcaneus and the bases of the fourth and fifth metatarsals), or less frequently, total dislocation of the cuboid (Figure 8–88). Rarely, a lateral talonavicular dislocation is not followed by a calcaneocuboid dislocation but by a subtalar subluxation to produce a lateral swivel dislocation (Figure 8–89).

C. Longitudinal stress injury: caused by an axially directed force that is applied to the metatarsal heads and is transmitted proximally along the metatarsal rays. The results are disruption of the midtarsal joints and compression of the navicular between the cuneiforms and the head of talus. Shearing forces in line with the intercuneiform joints are produced, creating different navicular fractures, fracture of the head of the talus, fracture of the cuboid, and subluxation of the calcaneocuboid joint in different combinations.

D. Plantar stress injury: caused by a plantarly directed force that is applied to the dorsal aspect of the forefoot. Sprain, plantar subluxation, or dislocation of the forefoot at the midtarsal joints are produced, which can be accompanied by avulsion fracture of the dorsum of the navicular, talus, and anterior process of the calcaneus. Rarely, purely plantar dislocation of the midtarsal joints with plantar displacement of the navicular and cuboid without any associated fractures can occur.

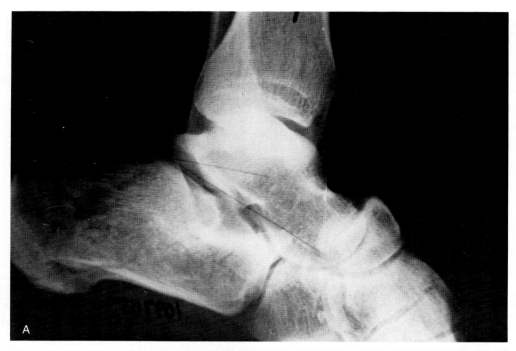

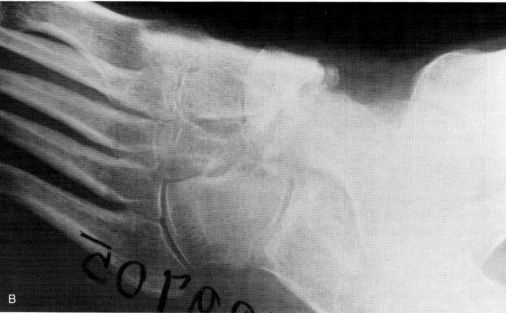

Figure 8–87. Lateral (**A**) and oblique (**B**) radiographs reveal a medial dislocation of the talonavicular joint and subluxation of the subtalar joint with the calcaneocuboid joint remaining completely intact. This unusual midtarsal injury is the so-called medial swivel dislocation in which the medial dislocation of the talonavicular joint is not followed by medial dislocation of the calcaneocuboid joint. Instead, tethered by the strong interosseous talocalcaneal ligament, the calcaneus internally rotates with the medially dislocated forefoot to cause a subtalar subluxation. If the interosseous talocalcaneal ligament also is ruptured, the calcaneus and the forefoot will be dislocated medially to produce a medial subtalar dislocation.

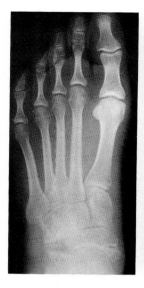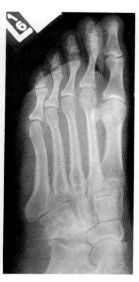

Figure 8–88. Anteroposterior and oblique radiographs demonstrate an avulsion fracture of the navicular tuberosity, fracture of the anterior process of the calcaneus, and compression fracture of the cuboid (the so-called nutcracker fracture) caused by a lateral stress injury of the midtarsal joints.

E. Crush injury: usually caused by a heavy weight that falls directly on the dorsum of the foot, producing a wide spectrum of comminuted and/or compound fractures of the midtarsal joints with varying degrees of bony fragment displacement that do not fit any particular patterns.

CLINICAL SYMPTOMS AND SIGNS. Pain, swelling, tenderness, and ecchymosis over the proximal portion of the dorsum of the foot are commonly associated with midtarsal fractures or dislocations. A severe medial stress injury produces a medial midtarsal joint dislocation with significant medial displacement of the forefoot, resulting in an acquired clubfoot-like deformity. Similarly, a severe lateral stress injury dislocates the forefoot plantarly at the midtarsal joints to produce an acquired cavus foot deformity due to the equinus position of the forefoot.

ROENTGENOGRAPHIC MANIFESTATIONS. Unless the fractures or dislocations of the midtarsal joints are obvious, they can

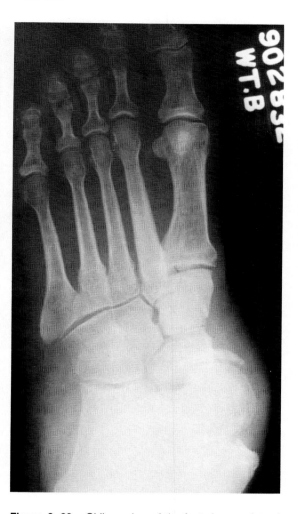

Figure 8–89. Oblique view of the foot shows a lateral dislocation of the left talonavicular joint in association with a shear fracture of the head of the talus and subluxation of the subtalar joint with the calcaneocuboid joint remaining completely intact. This uncommon injury of the midtarsal joints is called the lateral swivel dislocation, in which the lateral dislocation of the talonavicular joint is not accompanied by lateral dislocation of the calcaneo-cuboid joint. Instead, held by the strong interosseous talocalcaneal ligament, the calcaneus laterally rotates with the laterally dislocated forefoot to produce a subtalar subluxation. If the interosseous talocalcaneal ligament also is ruptured, both the calcaneus and the forefoot will be laterally dislocated to produce a lateral subtalar dislocation.

be easily overlooked by the attending trauma surgeons or emergency room physicians due to rarity of these injuries and their unfamiliarity with the subtle radiographic abnormalities

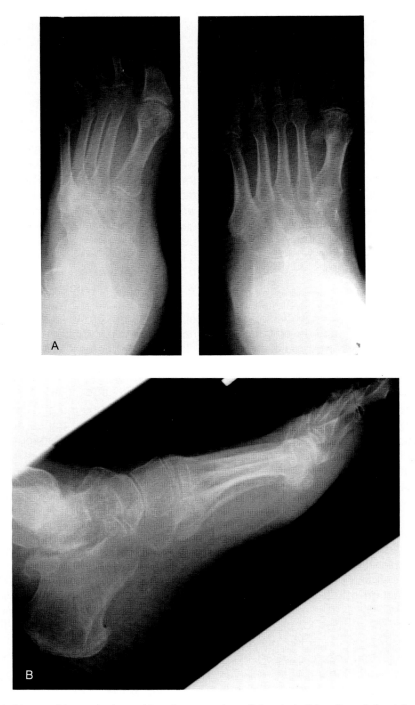

Figure 8–90. A 56-year-old man had an old and untreated medial swivel dislocation of the left midtarsal joints. Anteroposterior and oblique (**A**) and lateral (**B**) views show persistent dislocation of the talonavicular joint and subluxation and arthritic changes of the subtalar joint of the left foot, which can be treated with a triple arthrodesis.

of these rare injuries. When evaluating the radiographs of a patient with a possible midtarsal injury, the talonavicular, calcaneocuboid, and naviculocuboid articulations should be carefully checked for malalignments, and any fractures of the navicular tuberosity, dorsal lip of the navicular, talar head, anterior process of the calcaneus, or the cuboid should alert the physician to a possible midtarsal injury. When the routine radiographs are not sufficient to indicate definitively the presence of a midtarsal joint injury, regular or computer assisted tomography should be employed to confirm or rule out the presumptive diagnosis. Careful evaluation of the routine radiographs, however, should enable the physician to determine the correct mechanism of injury and to plan a proper course of treatment.

A. Medial stress injury: look for medial subluxation or dislocation of the midtarsal joints and the associated fractures of the talar head, navicular, lateral margins of the cuboid, anterior process of the calcaneus, and subluxation of the subtalar joint.

B. Lateral stress injury: look for lateral subluxation or dislocation of the midtarsal joints and the associated avulsion fracture of the navicular tuberosity, fracture of the anterior process of the calcaneus, compression fracture of the cuboid, and even total dislocation of the cuboid.

C. Longitudinal stress injury: look for disruption of the midtarsal joint, vertical fracture of the navicular in line with the intercuneiform joints, fracture of the head of the talus, and fracture of the navicular.

D. Plantar stress injury: look for plantar subluxation or dislocation of the forefoot at the midtarsal joints and the associated avulsion fractures of the dorsum of the navicular, talus, and anterior process of the calcaneus.

E. Crush injury: look for comminuted fractures of the midtarsal bones and joints with varying degrees of displacement of the fracture fragments and the associated air shadow in the soft tissue over the fracture site caused by a compound fracture.

TREATMENT.   Regardless of the direction of a midtarsal dislocation, closed reduction should first be attempted by suspending the foot vertically in the air with wire finger traps and applying a downward manual traction to the heel, or by placing a sling with attached weights around the ankle. After reduction, if the midtarsal joints are relatively stable, a well-molded short, leg cast should be applied and worn for 6 weeks. If the midtarsal joints are unstable after reduction, K-wires can be driven percutaneously from the cuboid into the calcaneus and from the navicular into the talus to maintain the reduction. A short, leg cast worn for 6 weeks provides further protection.

When a displaced fracture involves a significant portion of the articular surface of the navicular, talus, cuboid, or calcaneus, the displaced bone fragment should be reduced and held with small bone screws or K-wires in conjunction with open reduction of the associated midtarsal dislocation. In severe crush injury with a compound and comminuted fracture of the midtarsal bones and joints, copious irrigation, careful debridement, and prophylactic intravenous antibiotic administration should be carried out as soon as possible. In addition, an attempt should be made to save as much bone as possible in the compound fracture and to achieve a reasonable alignment of the fractured bony fragments so to preserve the maximal use of the injured foot. When painful traumatic arthritis has developed in the midtarsal joints and conservative treatments have failed, a triple arthrodesis, which fuses the midtarsal and subtalar joints, should be seriously considered (Figure 8–90).

REFERENCES

Fractures and Dislocations of Joints of the Midfoot

1. Brown, D.C., and McFarland, Jr., G.B.: Dislocation of the medial cuneiform bone in tarsometatarsal fracture-dislocation. A case report. J. Bone Joint Surg. [Am.], *57*:858, 1975.

2. Crossan, E.T.: Fractures of the tarsal scaphoid and the os calcis. Surg. Clin. North Am., *10:*1477, 1930.
3. Day, A.J.: The treatment of injuries to the tarsal navicular. J. Bone Joint Surg., *29:*359, 1947.
4. DeWar, F.P., and Evans, D.C.: Occult fracture-subluxation of the midtarsal joint. J. Bone Joint Surg. [Br.], *50:*386, 1968.
5. Dick, I.L.: Impacted fracture-dislocation of the tarsal navicular. Proc. R. Soc. Lond. [Med.], *35:*760, 1941.
6. Drummond, D.S., and Hastings, D.E.: Total dislocations of the cuboid bone. J. Bone Joint Surg. [Br.], *51:*716, 1969.
7. Eichenholtz, S.N., and Levine, D.B.: Fractures of the tarsal navicular bone. Clin. Orthop., *34:*142, 1964.
8. Friedmann, E.: Key graft fixation in midtarsal fracture dislocation. Am. J. Surg., *96:*81, 1958.
9. Gopal-Krishnan, S.: Dislocation of medical cuneiform in injuries of tarsometatarsal joints. Int. Surg., *58:*805, 1973.
10. Hermel, M.B., and Gershon-Cohen, J.: The nutcracker fracture of the cuboid by indirect violence. Radiology, *60:*850, 1953.
11. Holstein, A., and Joldersma, R.D.: Dislocation of first cuneiform in taro-metatarsal fracture-dislocation. J. Bone Joint Surg. [Am.], *32:*419, 1950.
12. Lehman, E.P., and Eskale, I.H.: Fracture of tarsal scaphoid; with notes on the mechanism. J. Bone Joint Surg., *10:*108, 1928.
13. Main, B.J., and Jowett, R.L.: Injuries of the midtarsal joint. J. Bone Joint Surg. [Br.], *57:*89, 1975.
14. McGlinchey, J.J.: Dislocation of the intermediate cuneiform bone. Injury, *12:*501, 1980.
15. Nadeau, P., and Templeton, J.: Vertical fracture dislocation of the tarsal navicular. J. Trauma, *16:*669, 1976.
16. Penhallow, D.P.: An unusual fracture-dislocation of the tarsal scaphoid with dislocation of the cuboid. J. Bone Joint Surg., *19:*517, 1937.
17. Pavlov, H., Torg, J.S., and Freiberger, R.H.: Tarsal navicular stress fractures: Radiographic evaluation. Radiology, *148:*641, 1983.
18. Ross, P.M., and Mitchell, D.C.: Dislocation of the talonavicular joint: Case report. J. Trauma, *16:*397, 1976.
19. Schiller, M.G., and Ray, R.D.: Isolated dislocation of the medial cuneiform bone—a rare injury of the tarsus. J. Bone Joint Surg. [Am.], *52:*1632, 1970.
20. Seymour, N.: The late results of naviculo-cuneiform fusion. J. Bone Joint Surg. [Br.], *49:*558, 1967.
21. Stark, W.A.: Occult fracture-subluxation of the midtarsal joint. Clin. Orthop., *93:*291, 1973.
22. Wilson, P.D.: Fractures and dislocations of the tarsal bones. South Med. J., *26:*833, 1933.

Fractures of the Talus

INCIDENCE. Fractures of the talus account for less than 1% of all fractures. Its dense cancellous bone is stronger than that of the navicular or calcaneus, and its anatomic location in the ankle mortise protected by the distal ends of the tibia and fibula superiorly, medially, and laterally, and by the much weaker navicular and calcaneus anteriorly and inferiorly, respectively, may explain the low incidence of talar fractures or dislocations. Nevertheless, such damage to the talus does occur and is usually caused by extension, flexion, inversion, eversion, and compression injuries of the ankle produced by automobile and motorcycle accidents, aircraft accidents, falls from heights, the fall of a heavy object on the dorsum of the foot, athletic injuries, and violent twisting injuries of the ankle.

It is of prognostic importance to note that the blood supply of the talus comes from three sources:

A. The artery of the tarsal canal from the posterior tibial artery is the major blood supply and supplies the inferior surface of the neck, medial talar wall, and most of the talar body.

B. The dorsalis pedis artery from the anterior tibial artery supplies the dorsomedial aspect of the talar neck and the talar head.

C. The communicating branch of the lateral tarsal artery and the peroneal artery gives off the artery of the tarsal sinus (sinus tarsi), which enters the talar neck in the sinus tarsi to supply the inferior part of the talar head and neck.

In summary, most of the talar body is supplied by the artery of the tarsal canal, and the talar head and neck by the dorsalis pedis artery and the artery of the tarsal sinus.

On an anatomic basis, the various fractures of talus can be classified into several categories.

A. Fracture of the head of the talus: can be produced by a medially directed force that is applied to the lateral aspect of the forefoot, a longitudinally directed force that is applied to the medial metatarsal heads, a plantarly directed force that is applied to the dorsal aspect of the foot, or a crushing force that acts directly on the talar head.

The fracture can vary from a chip fracture from an avulsion injury to a greatly displaced or comminuted fracture of the talar head that involves a significant portion of the anterior articular surface of the talus (Figure 8–91).

B. Fracture of the neck of talus: usually caused by a hyperdorsiflexion injury of the foot that causes the neck of talus to impact against the sharp leading anterior edge of distal tibia. The resulting neck fracture can be classified into four different types:

Type I: a nondisplaced fracture of the neck of the talus with low incidence of avascular necrosis of the body of the talus due to disruption of only one source of its blood supply (Figures 8–92 and 8–93).

Type II: a displaced fracture of the neck of the talus with subluxation or dislocation of the subtalar joint with a higher incidence of avascular necrosis of the body of the talus due to disruption of two and sometimes all three sources of its blood supply (Figure 8–94).

Type III: a fracture of the talar neck with dislocation of the body of the talus from both subtalar and ankle joints with an extremely high incidence of avascular necrosis of the body of talus due to disruption of all of its blood supply (Figure 8–95).

Type IV: a fraction of the neck of the talus with dislocation of the body of the talus from both the subtalar and ankle joints and subluxation or dislocation of the talonavicular joint with an extremely high incidence of avascular necrosis of the talar body to complete disruption of the blood supply.

C. Fracture of the body of the talus: produced by compression or shearing forces. There are three main types:

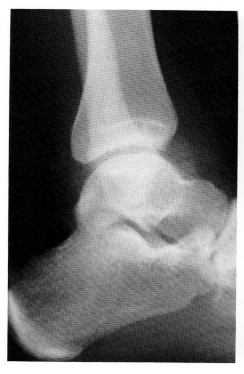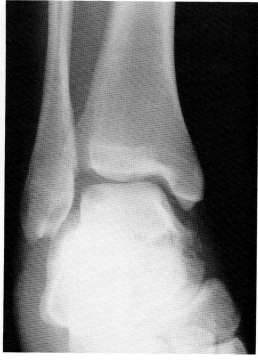

Figure 8–91. A 20-year-old man in whom lateral and anteroposterior views demonstrate a chip fracture of the dorsomedial aspect of the talar head caused by a twisting injury of the ankle.

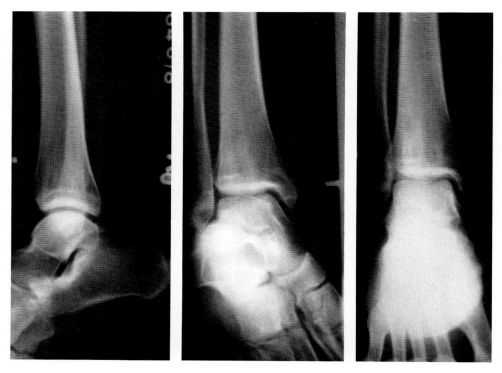

Figure 8–92. Lateral anteroposterior, and oblique radiographs show a minimally displaced fracture of the neck of the talus, which can be treated with a short non-walking cast with good result because damage to the blood supply to the body of the talus was minimal.

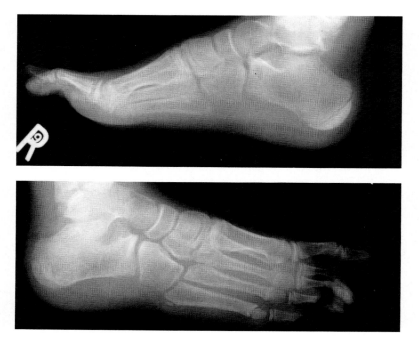

Figure 8–93. A 9-year-old boy sustained a dorsiflexion injury of his right ankle. Lateral and oblique views demonstrate a non-displaced fracture of the talar neck.

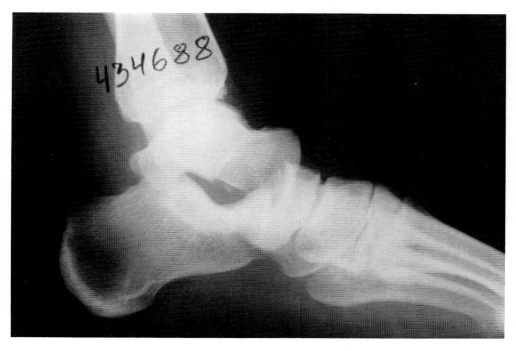

Figure 8–94. Lateral view shows a fracture of the neck of the talus associated with subluxation of the subtalar joint and dislocation of the talonavicular joint. This type of talar neck fracture is associated with a high incidence of avascular necrosis of the talar body.

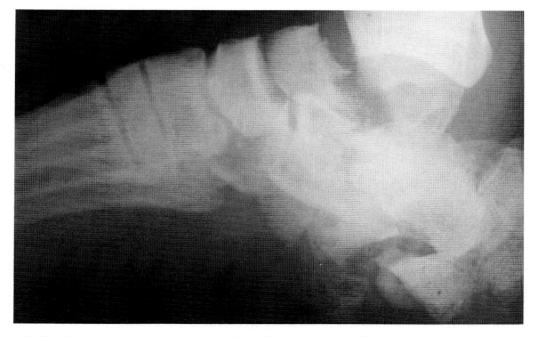

Figure 8–95. A 44-year-old man jumped from the fourth floor of a burning building and landed on his left foot. Lateral view shows a severely comminuted calcaneal fracture, a markedly displaced fracture of the neck of the talus, dislocation of the calcaneocuboid joint, and a complete inferior dislocation of the body of the talus. The long-term prognosis for this severely injured foot was poor.

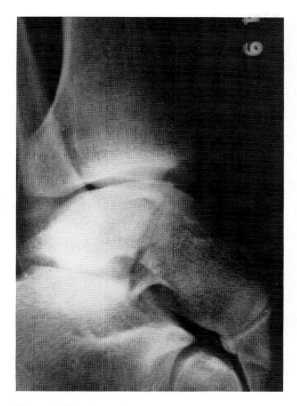

Figure 8–96. Lateral view of an ankle shows a slightly displaced fracture of the body of the talus, which should be anatomically reduced to avoid subsequent development of ankle and subtalar arthritis.

Type I: produces coronal and sagittal shearing fractures that are often displaced. This is the most common type of talar body fracture (Figure 8–96).

Type II: produces displaced compression of the talar articular surface of the ankle joint with no subluxation of the ankle or subtalar joint. This type is less common than type I.

Type III: produces a severely comminuted fracture with multiple fragments and carries an unfavorable long-term prognosis. Fortunately, type III are the least common type of talar body fractures.

D. Osteochondral fracture of the dome of talus: synonymous with intra-articular fracture of the talus, osteochondritis dissecans of the talus, flake fracture of the talus, and transchondral dome fracture of the talus. There are two main types. The midlateral talar dome fracture can be caused by an inversion and dorsiflexion injury of the ankle, producing a shallow lesion of the midlateral talar dome that is more likely to become displaced and symptomatic than the medial lesion (Figure 8–97). The posteromedial talar dome fracture can be caused by an inversion and plantar flexion injury of the ankle. Such a fracture can also occur in the absence of any apparent acute trauma to the ankle joint. The lesion tends to be deeper with less chances of becoming displaced and symptomatic than the lateral lesion (Figure 8–98).

The medial and lateral talar dome fractures can be classified into four stages:

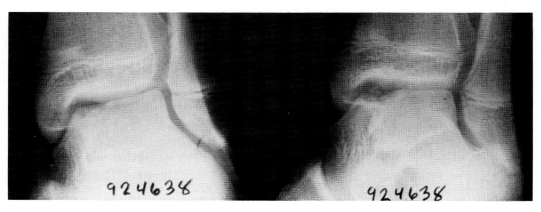

Figure 8–97. Anteroposterior and oblique ankle radiographs reveal a slightly comminuted osteochondral fracture of the medial talar dome caused by an inversion injury.

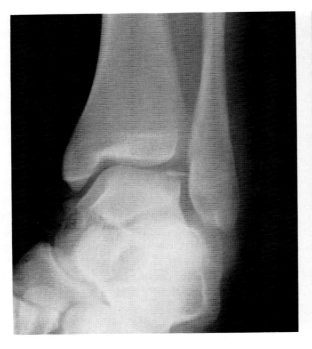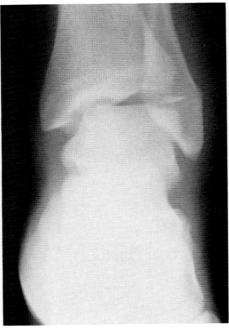

Figure 8–98. A 20-year-old man sustained an inversion injury to his left ankle. Anteroposterior and oblique radiographs demonstrate a completely displaced osteochondral fracture of the lateral dome of the talus and a slightly comminuted chip fracture to the medial aspect of the head of the talus.

Stage I: small area of subchondral bone compression.
Stage II: partial detachment of the osteochondral fragment.
Stage III: complete detachment of the osteochondral fragment to become a loose body in the ankle joint.
Stage IV: complete displacement of the osteochondral fragment to become a loose body in the ankle joint.

E. Fracture of the lateral process of talus: can involve both the posterior subtalar and fibulotalar articulations. This lesion is caused by an inversion and dorsiflexion injury of the ankle, such as a fall on a dorsiflexed and supinated foot (Figures 8–99).

F. Fracture of the posterior process of talus: can be produced by a plantar flexion injury while jumping or kicking.
CLINICAL SYMPTOMS AND SIGNS.
Swelling of the ankle joint from hemarthrosis and joint effusion is frequently associated with intra-articular fractures of the talus. Pain and tenderness tend to be in the anteromedial aspect of the ankle in fracture of the head or neck of the talus, in the depth of the ankle joint in fracture of the body of the talus, in the region of the tibiofibular syndesmosis in a midlateral talar dome fracture, behind the medial malleolus in a posteromedial talar dome fracture, in the lateral malleolar region in a fracture of the lateral process of the talus, and in the posterior aspect of the ankle in a fracture of the posterior process of the talus. Weight-bearing usually aggravates the pain and swelling, which can be relieved by rest and elevation of the affected leg. A loose osteochondral fracture of the talus cannot only cause pain and swelling of the ankle, but also can produce giving-way, catching, locking, and a grating sensation of the ankle.
ROENTGENOGRAPHIC MANIFESTATIONS. Although anteroposterior, lateral, and oblique radiographs of the ankle are routinely

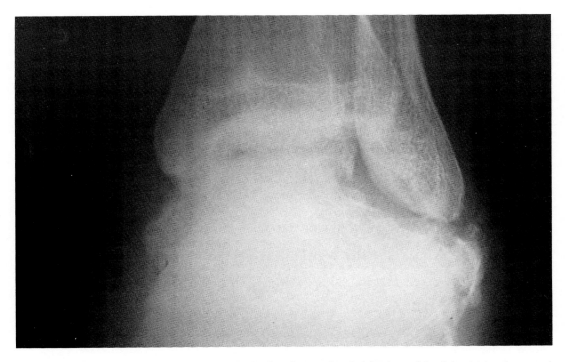

Figure 8–99. Oblique view of the ankle shows a displaced osteochondral fracture of the lateral talar dome and an associated comminuted fracture of the lateral process of the talus. Both injuries require surgical excision to regain optimal function of the ankle.

required for the diagnosis of different talar fractures, fractures of the head, neck, body, and posterior process of the talus are best seen on the lateral view. Fractures of the dome and lateral process of the talus and sagittal fracture of the body of the talus are best appreciated on the anteroposterior and oblique views. When routine ankle films are not sufficient to provide a definitive diagnosis of a talar fracture, regular and computer assisted tomography should be employed to clearly delineate the true nature of the talar fracture.

Because the displaced fractures of the neck or body of the talus have a high incidence of producing avascular necrosis of the body of the talus (Figures 8–100 and 8–101), the presence of the so-called Hawkins' sign, which is a narrow zone of subchondral osteoporosis under the talar dome that is best seen on the anteroposterior view of the ankle about 6 weeks after the fracture, virtually eliminates the diagnosis of avascular necrosis. Care

should be taken in the search for the Hawkins' sign when diagnosing major fracture, subluxation, or dislocation of the talus. It should be mentioned that an os trigonum tarsi can be easily differentiated from a fracture of the posterior process of the talus by its smooth outline and its bilateral and asymptomatic nature.

TREATMENT.

A. Fracture of the head of the talus: small avulsion fracture of the dorsal aspect of the talar head only requires the use of a short walking cast for 4 to 6 weeks. Painful non-union of a chip fracture and an old and untreated displaced avulsion fracture of the talar head can be treated by surgical excision of this symptomatic bony fragment. When the fracture involves a significant portion of the articular surface of the head of the talus, and satisfactory reduction cannot be obtained by closed

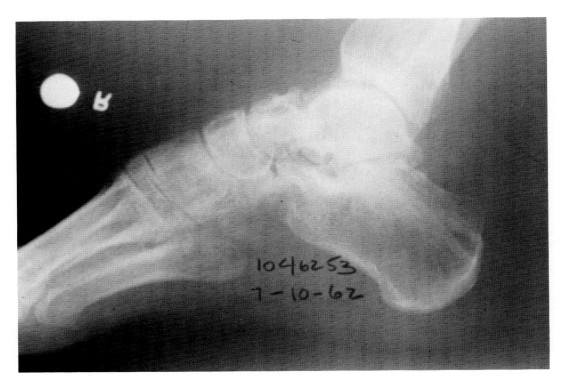

Figure 8–100. Lateral view of a foot shows a somewhat displaced and comminuted fracture of the neck of the talus associated with an osteosclerotic talar body caused by avascular necrosis.

means, open anatomic reduction and fixation of the fractured bone fragment back to the head of the talus with a small bone screw should be performed. Painful post-traumatic degenerative arthritis of the talonavicular joint can be treated with a talonavicular arthrodesis.

B. Fracture of the neck of the talus:

Type I (nondisplaced fracture of the talar neck): should be treated with a short non-walking cast for about 6 weeks to prevent displacement of the fracture. A short walking cast can then be used until a solid union has occurred.
Type II (displaced fracture of the neck of the talus with subluxation or dislocation of the subtalar joint): if a satisfactory reduction can be achieved by closed means, a short non-walking cast should be applied, and the fracture should be carefully mon-

itored until a solid union has taken place. If the talar neck fracture and the subtalar subluxation or dislocation cannot be satisfactorily reduced, open anatomic reduction with internal fixation of the fractured talar neck with a bone screw should be protected by a short non-walking cast to improve the chances of achieving a solid bony union (Figure 8–102). When a compound wound is also present, irrigation and debridement of the open wound should be performed and antibiotics should be administered systematically in addition to the reduction of the talar fracture and subluxation or dislocation.
Type III (displaced fracture of the talar neck with dislocation of the body of the talus from both the subtalar and ankle joints): often a compound fracture that requires immediate treatment of the open wound before taking care of the talar fracture and dislocation.

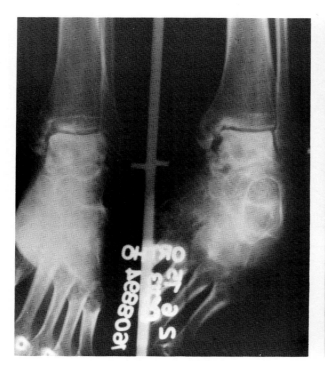 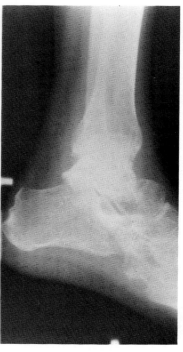

Figure 8–101. Anteroposterior, oblique, and lateral radiographs show well-established avascular necrosis of the talar body in association with a displaced talar neck fracture and arthritic changes of the ankle joint. In such a case, a Blair-type tibiotalar fusion may be required for symptomatic relief and functional improvement.

Type IV (displaced fracture of the neck of the talus with dislocation of the talar body from both the subtalar and ankle joints and subluxation or dislocation of the talonavicular joint): often an open fracture that requires thorough irrigation and debridement before reduction of the talar fracture and subtalar, ankle, and talonavicular dislocations may be performed.

It should be noted that the rate of development of avascular necrosis of the talar body in fracture of the neck of the talus is directly related to the degree of displacement of the fracture. Consequently, a number of the type II and many of types III and IV talar neck fractures will develop avascular necrosis of the talar body. If treated conservatively, these lesions may take from 1 to 1.5 years to become revascularized.

When treating avascular necrosis of the

body of the talus, the initial cast immobilization can later be replaced by a patellar-tendon-weight-bearing ankle-foot orthosis, which is lighter and is more comfortable, convenient, and hygienic to wear. When symptomatic avascular necrosis of the talar body has failed to respond to conservative treatment, a Blair-type fusion may be employed. The dead talar body is removed and the tibia is fused to the remaining head of the talus by sliding a rectangular tibial graft from the anterior surface of the distal tibia into a slot cut into the head of the talus (Figure 8–103). The apparent advantages of a Blair-type fusion over a tibiocalcaneal fusion include a normal-looking foot, no shortening, preservation of motion at the talonavicular and anterior subtalar joints, and a more physiologic relationship between foot and ankle.

When severe osteomyelitis has devel-

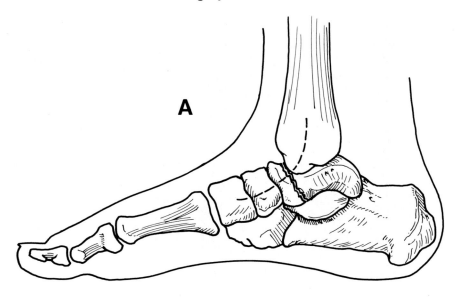

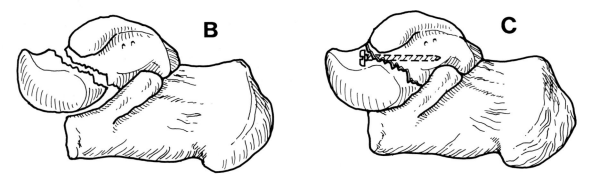

Figure 8–102. Surgical technique for reducing a displaced fracture of the neck of the talus. **A,** a curvilinear dorsomedial skin incision. **B,** exposure of the talar neck fracture. **C,** reduction of the talar neck fracture and fixation with a cancellous bone screw.

oped in a talar fracture, a tibiocalcaneal fusion is a useful salvage procedure that may eliminate the infection and provide a stable and relatively painless foot at the same time. If severe arthritis of the talonavicular and subtalar joints has been caused by a fracture of the neck of the talus, and there is no avascular necrosis of the talar body, triple arthrodesis should be seriously considered, as a means of treatment.

C. Fracture of the body of the talus:

Type I (with displaced coronal or sagittal body fracture): usually requires open anatomic reduction and internal fixation with bone screws through either a medial or lateral transmalleolar approach. A cast should be applied postoperatively and worn until bony union has taken place (Figure 8–104).

Type II (with depression fracture of the talar

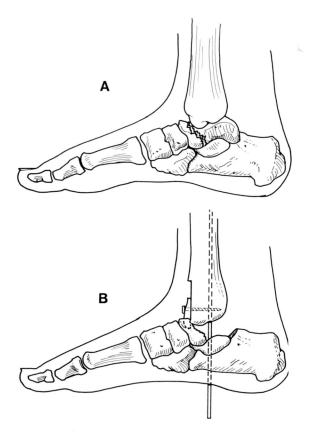

Figure 8–103. Surgical techique for a Blair-type tibio-talar fusion. **A,** talar neck fracture with vascular necrosis of the talar body. **B,** retangular anterior tibial graft has been inserted into a matching slot cut in the head of the talus. Its upper portion has been fixed to the tibia with a screw, and a Steinmann pin has been driven from the sole of the foot through the calcaneus into the distal tibia to provide extra support.

articular surface of the ankle joint): should be treated by an open reduction to elevate the depressed articular surface through an osteotomy of the medial or the lateral malleolus; the subchondral bony defect should be packed with autogenous bone chips. A short non-walking cast should be worn for several months so that the bone graft can incorporate into the fractured talus.

Type III (with severe comminution): often a compound fracture that carries a poor long-term prognosis. The initial treatment is to salvage the foot by taking good care of the open wound and grossly aligning the ankle and foot by means of a cast or some form of external skeletal fixator, and later by a patellar-tendon-weight-bearing ankle-foot orthosis. Many type III fractures, however, eventually require a tibiocalcaneal fusion.

The body of the talus contains the major part of the talar portion of the ankle and subtalar joints. Fracture of the body of the talus usually involves these two joints and subjects them to develop post-traumatic arthritis, which may require a pantalar arthrodesis for symptomatic relief and functional improvement of the affected foot and ankle.

D. Osteochondral fracture of the dome of the talus:

Stages I (small area of subchondral bone compression) *and II* (partial detachment of the osteochondral fragment): should be treated nonoperatively with initial casting and later use of a patellar-tendon weight-bearing brace, ankle corset, or well-molded arch support until healing takes place.

Stage III (complete detachment of the osteochondral fragment without displacement): should be managed nonoperatively, first with a cast, brace, ankle corset, or arch support. If symptoms persist, excision of the loose osteochondral fragment plus drilling of its osteosclerotic crater to encourage the ingrowth of fibrocartilaginous tissue into the bony defect from the medullary cavity of the talus should be performed. When the loose osteochondral fragment is large and its removal may significantly affect the integrity of the articular surface of the talar dome, an attempt should be made to drill the osteosclerotic crater with small drill bits, replace the loose osteochondral fragment, and internally fix it to the talus with multiple small stainless steel nails. Prolonged cast immobilization should follow surgery in an effort to induce a bony union.

Stage IV (complete displacement of the osteochondral fragment into the ankle joint

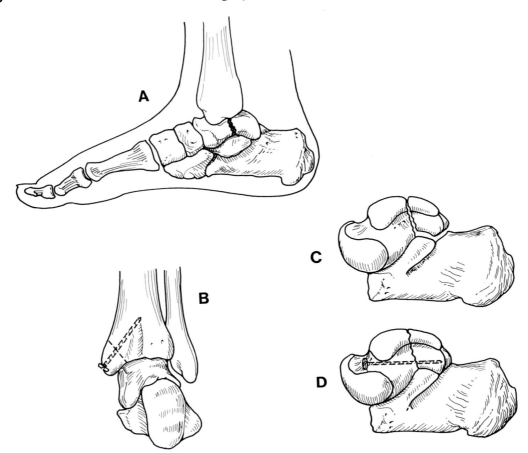

Figure 8–104.   Surgical technique for achieving an anatomic reduction of a fracture of the body of the talus. **A,** lateral view shows a fracture of the body of the talus. **B,** accurately insert a bone screw into the medial malleolus, and remove the screw before performing a medial malleolar osteotomy with a microsaw. **C,** expose the displaced talar body fracture. **D,** anatomically reduce the talar body fracture and fix it with a cancellous bone screw.

to become a loose body): the loose body should be removed by means of either an arthroscopic extraction or a surgical arthrotomy approach. A medial lesion, due to its relatively inaccessible posteromedial site, may necessitate the use of a medial malleolar osteotomy. If the transmalleolar approach is used, a bone screw should be accurately preinserted into the medial malleolus and then removed. A microsaw should be used to perform the osteotomy to sacrifice a minimal amount of bone so the affected medial malleolus can be accurately replaced and securely fixed to the tibia after the loose osteochondral fragment has been removed. In contrast, a lateral lesion can be approached easily through an anterolateral incision because of the relatively more posterior position of the distal fibula in relationship to the ankle joint and the talus. When these osteochondral fractures of the talar dome have produced severe degenerative arthritis of the ankle joint, ankle fusion may be required.

E. Fracture of the lateral process of the talus: if undisplaced or minimally displaced, a

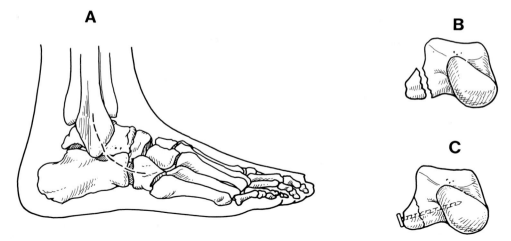

Figure 8–105. Surgical technique for reducing a displaced fracture of the lateral process of the talus. **A,** make a curvilinear incision over the lateral aspect of the ankle. **B,** expose the displaced fracture of the lateral process of the talus. **C,** anatomically reduce the fracture and fix it to the body of the talus with a cancellous bone screw.

short, leg cast should be applied and worn for 4 to 6 weeks. If the fractured fragment is large and displaced, however, open reduction and screw fixation through a slightly curved incision along the anterior border of the lateral malleolus are usually required to restore the integrity of the fibulotalar and posterior talocalcaneal articulations (Figure 8–105). Comminuted fracture and painful non-union of the lateral process of the talus often require simple surgical excision.

F. Fracture of the posterior process of talus: if small, a short walking cast should be worn for 4 to 6 weeks. If the fracture is large and displaced, open reduction and screw fixation should be performed through a longitudinal skin incision along the lateral border of the Achilles tendon. A short leg cast should then be worn for 6 weeks. Comminuted fracture and painful non-union of the posterior process of the talus frequently require surgical excision. Occasionally, a large fracture of the posterior process of the talus can produce traumatic arthritis of the posterior talocalcaneal joint, which may lead to a subtalar fusion for pain relief.

REFERENCES

Fractures of the Talus

1. Alexander, A.H., and Lichtman, D.M.: Surgical treatment of transchondral talar-dome fractures (osteochondritis dissecans). Long-term follow-up. J. Bone Joint Surg. [Am.], *62:*646, 1980.
2. Berndt, A.L., and Marty, M.: Transchondral fractures (osteochondritis dissecans) of the talus. J. Bone Joint Surg. [Am.], *41:*988, 1959.
3. Blair, H.C.: Comminuted fractures and fracture dislocations of body of the astragalus. Operative treatment. Am J. Surg., *59:*37, 1943.
4. Blom, J.M.H., and Strijk, S.P.: Lesions of the trochlea tali. Osteochondral fractures and osteochondritis dissecans of the trochlea tali. Radiol. Clin. North Am., *44:*387, 1975.
5. Boyd, H.B., and Knight, R.A.: Fractures of the astragalus. South. Med. J., *35:*160, 1942.
6. Cameron, B.M.: Osteochondritis dissecans of the ankle joint. Report of a case simulating a fracture of the talus. J. Bone Joint Surg. [Am.], *38:*857, 1956.
7. Canale, S.T., and Belding, R.H.: Osteochondral lesions of the talus. J. Bone Joint Surg. [Am.], *62:*97, 1980.
8. Canale, S.T., and Kelly, Jr., F.B.: Fractures of neck of the talus. Long-term evaluation of seventy-one cases. J. Bone Joint Surg. [Am.], *60:*143, 1978.
9. Cedell, C.A.: Rupture of the posterior talo-tibial ligament with avulsion of a bone fragment from the talus. Acta Orthop. Scand., *45:*454, 1974.
10. Cimmino, C.V.: Fracture of the lateral process of the talus. AJR, *90:*1277, 1963.
11. Coltart, W.D.: Aviator's astragalus. J. Bone Joint Surg. [Br.], *34:*535, 1952.
12. Davidson, C.D., Steel, H.D., Mackenzie, D., and Penney, J.A.: A review of twenty-one cases of trans-

chondral fractures of the talus. J. Trauma, *7:*378, 1967.

13. Davis, M.W.: Bilateral talar osteochondritis dissecans with lax ankle ligaments. Report of a case. J. Bone Joint Surg. [Am.], *52:*168, 1970.
14. Dennis, M.D., and Tullos, H.S.: Blair tibiotalar arthrodesis for injuries of the talus. J. Bone Joint Surg. [Am.], *62:*103, 1980.
15. Detenbeck, L.C., and Kelly, P.J.: Total dislocation of the talus. J. Bone Joint Surg. [Am.], *51:*283, 1969.
16. Dimon, J.H.: Isolated displaced fracture of the posterior facet of the talus. J. Bone Joint Surg. [Am.], *41:*275, 1961.
17. Dunn, A.R., Jacobs, B., and Campbell, Jr., R.D.: Fractures of the talus. J. Trauma, *6:*443, 1966.
18. Fahey, J.J., and Murphy, J.L.: Dislocations and fractures of the talus. Surg. Clin. North Am., *45:*79, 1965.
19. Fjeldborg, O.: Fracture of the lateral process of the talus. Acta Orthop. Scand., *39:*407, 1968.
20. Haliburton, R.A., Sullivan, C.R., Kelly, P.J., and Peterson, L.F.A.: The extra-osseous and intra-osseous blood supply of the talus. J. Bone Joint Surg. [Am.], *40:*115, 1958.
21. Hawkins, L.G.: Fracture of the lateral process of the talus. J. Bone Joint Surg. [Am.], *47:*1170, 1965.
22. Hawkins, L.G.: Fractures of the neck of the talus. J. Bone Joint Surg. [Am.], *52:*991, 1970.
23. Kendrick, R.E.: Tibiocalcaneal stabilization using reinforced acrylic cement as a substitute for the talus. A case report. J. Bone Joint Surg. [Am.], *66:*288, 1984.
24. Kenwright, J., and Taylor, R.G.: Major injuries of the talus. J. Bone Joint Surg. [Br.], *52:*36, 1970.
25. Johansson, J.E., Harrison, J., and Greenwood, F.A.: Subtalar arthrodesis for adult traumatic arthritis. Foot Ankle, *2:*294, 1982.
26. Kelly, P.J., and Sullivan, C.R.: Blood supply of the talus. Clin. Orthop., *30:*37, 1963.
27. Kenny, C.H.: Inverted osteochondral fracture of the talus diagnosed by tomography. A case report. J. Bone Joint Surg. [Am.], *63:*1020, 1981.
28. Kerr, T.S.: Osteochondritis dissecans of the talus. Proc. R. Soc. Lond. [Med.], *66:*517, 1973.
29. Kleiger, B., and Ahmed, M.: Injuries of the talus and its joints. Clin. Orthop., *121:*243, 1976.
30. Lemaire, R.G., and Bustin, W.: Screw fixation of fractures of the neck of the talus using a posterior approach. J. Trauma, *20:*669, 1980.
31. Letts, R.M., and Gibeault, D.: Fractures of the neck of the talus in children. Foot Ankle, *1:*74, 1980.
32. Lorentzen, J.E., Christensen, S.B., Krogsoe, O., and Sneppen, O.: Fractures of the neck of the talus. Acta Orthop. Scand., *48:*115, 1977.
33. Mannis, C.I.: Transchondral fracture of the dome of the talus sustained during weight training. Am. J. Sports Med., *11:*354, 1983.
34. Marks, K.L.: Flake fracture of the talus progressing to osteochondritis dissecans. J. Bone Joint Surg. [Br.], *34:*90, 1952.
35. McKeever, F.M.: Treatment of complications of fractures and dislocations of talus. Clin. Orthop., *30:*45, 1963.
36. Mindell, E.R., Cisek, E.E., Kartalian, G., and Dziob, J.M.: Late results of injuries to the talus. Analysis of forty cases. J. Bone Joint Surg. [Am.], *45:*221, 1963.
37. Morris, H.D., Hand, W., and Dunn, A.W.: The modified Blair fusion of fractures of the talus. J. Bone Joint Surg. [Am.], *53:*1289, 1971.
38. Mukherjee, S.K., Pringle, R.M., and Baxter, A.D.: Fracture of the lateral process of the talus. A report of thirteen cases. J. Bone Joint Surg. [Br.], *56:*263, 1974.
39. Mulfinger, G.L., and Trueta, J.: The blood supply of the talus. J. Bone Joint Surg. [Br.], *52:*160, 1970.
40. Nash, W.C., and Baker, Jr., C.L.: Transchondral talar dome fractures: Not just a sprained ankle. South. Med. J., *77:*560, 1984.
41. Naumetz, V.A., and Schweigel, J.F.: Osteocartilaginous lesions of the talar dome. J. Trauma, *20:*924, 1980.
42. Newcomb, W.J., and Brav, E.A.: Complete dislocation of the talus. J. Bone Joint Surg. [Am.], *30:*872, 1948.
43. Nisbet, N.W.: Dome fracture of the talus. J. Bone Joint Surg. [Br.], *36:*244, 1954.
44. Pennal, G.F.: Fracture of the talus. Clin. Orthop., *30:*53, 1963.
45. Penny, J.N., and Davis, L.A.: Fractures and fracture-dislocations of the neck of the talus. J. Trauma, *20:*1029, 1980.
46. Peterson, L., Goldie, I.F., and Lindell, D.: The arterial supply of the talus. Acta Orthop. Scand., *45:*260, 1974.
47. Reckling, F.W.: Early tibiocalcaneal fusion in the treatment of severe injuries of the talus. J. Trauma, *12:*390, 1972.
48. Roden, S., Tillegard, P., and Unarder-Scharin, L.: Osteochondritis dissecans and similar lesions of the talus. Report of fifty-five cases with special reference to etiology and treatment. Acta Orthop. Scand., *23:*51, 1953.
49. Shrock, R.D., Johnson, H.E., and Waters, Jr., C.H.: Fractures and fracture-dislocations of astragalus (talus). J. Bone Joint Surg., *24:*560, 1942.
50. Smith, G.R., Windquist, R.A., Allan, N.K., and Northrop, C.H.: Subtle transchondral fractures of the talar dome: A radiological perspective. Radiology, *124:*667, 1977.
51. Sneppen, O., Christensen, S.B., Krogsoe, O., and Lorentzen, J.: Fracture of the body of the talus. Acta Orthop. Scand., *48:*317, 1977.
52. Spak, I.: Fractures of the talus in children. Acta Chir. Scand., *107:*553, 1954.
53. Wray, D.G., and Muddu, B.N.: Lateral dome fracture of the talus. J. Trauma, *21:*818, 1981.
54. Yvars, M.F.: Osteochondral fractures of the dome of the talus. Clin. Orthop., *114:*185, 1976.

Subtalar Dislocation and Total Talar Dislocation

INCIDENCE. Subtalar dislocation, also known as peritalar or subastragalar dislocation, is a fairly uncommon injury. It is usually caused by violent trauma such as car and motorcycle accidents, falls from heights, and athletic injuries, with a predilection for young and middle-aged adult males and a tendency to produce an open wound. In a subtalar dislocation, both the talocalcaneal and talonavicular joints must be totally dislocated; in about 50% of cases there are associated osteochondral fractures of these two joints.

The different types of subtalar dislocation can be classified according to the direction the calcaneus and forefoot are displaced.

A. Medial subtalar dislocation: the most common type and is produced by an inversion injury of the foot (a combination of plantar flexion, adduction, and supination of the foot). The injury displaces the calcaneus and the forefoot medially with initial dislocation of the talonavicular joint, which is immediately followed by subtalar joint dislocation (Figures 8–106—8–108).

B. Lateral subtalar dislocation: the second most common type and is produced by an eversion injury of the foot (a combination of dorsiflexion, abduction, and pronation of the foot). The calcaneus and the forefoot are laterally displaced, producing compound fracture and dislocation and sometimes neurovascular injury (Figures 8–109—8–111).

C. Posterior subtalar dislocation: is quite rare and can be produced by a fall from a height with the foot in a plantar-flexed position.

D. Anterior subtalar dislocation: is extremely rare and can be produced by a fall from a height with the foot in a dorsiflexed position.

It is of interest to note that Grantham (1964) collected 225 cases of subtalar dislocation from the medical literature and found the following distribution:

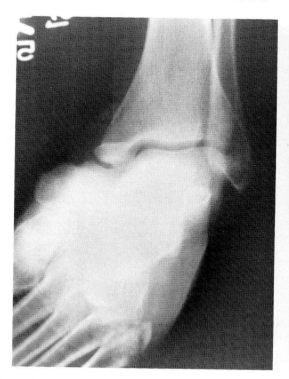
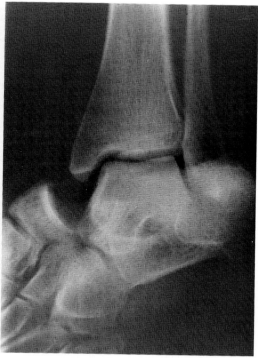

Figure 8–106. Anteroposterior and oblique radiographs of an ankle show a complete medial subtalar dislocation in association with an avulsion fracture of the base of the fifth metatarsal. The injuries were caused by a forceful contraction of the peroneus brevis muscle, which inserts into the lateral base of the fifth metatarsal.

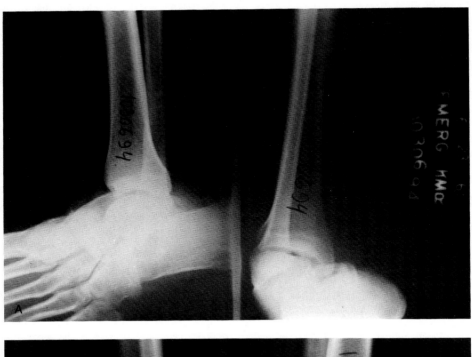

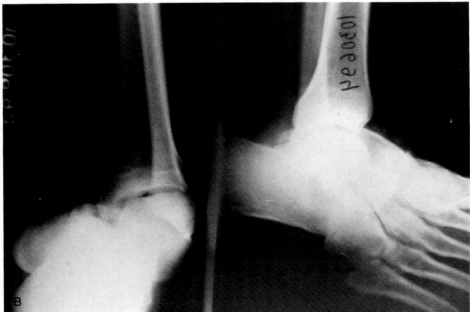

Figure 8–107. Anteroposterior and lateral (**A** and **B**) views of the ankle show a medial subtalar dislocation manifested by overlapping of the articular surfaces of the talonavicular and subtalar joints and medial displacement of the forefoot and calcaneus.

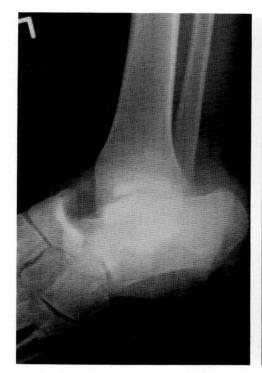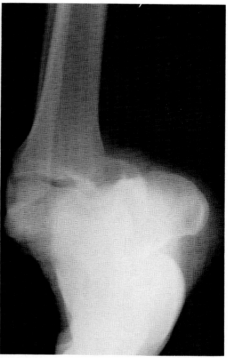

Figure 8–108. A 29-year-old man had a motorcycle accident and sustained an open medial subtalar dislocation. Lateral and oblique views reveal that the cup-shaped navicular articular surface is no longer occupied by the head of talus, and the talus and calcaneus overlap each other so much that the normal subtalar joint space is completely obliterated.

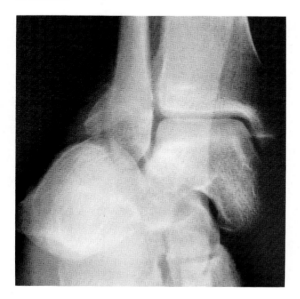

Type of Subtalar Dislocation	Number of Cases	Percent
Medial	145	80.1
Lateral	27	14.9
Posterior	6	3.3
Anterior	3	1.7

Figure 8–109. Anteroposterior radiograph shows a lateral subtalar dislocation associated with a lateral malleolar fracture. Note that the calcaneus and the forefoot are lateral to the talus.

Subtalar dislocations are violent injuries and are frequently associated with intra-articular fractures of the subtalar, talonavicular, and ankle joints; fracture of the medial and/or lateral malleolus; and fractures of the metatarsals, navicular, talus, and calcaneus (Figure 8–112). As a group, however, few subtalar dislocations develop avascular necrosis of the talus due to preservation of its important blood supply in the majority of cases.

In contrast, total dislocation of the talus occurs less frequently than subtalar dislocation, but it is caused by the same violent forces that produce subtalar dislocation, such as car

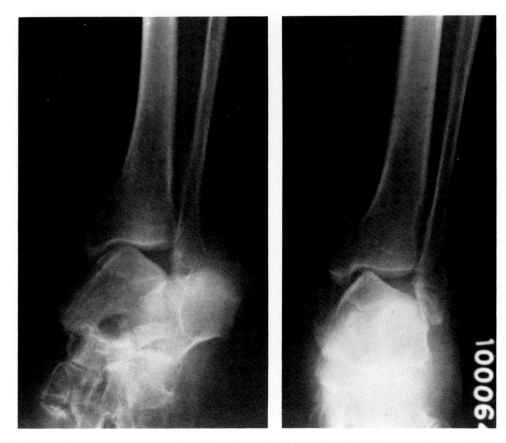

Figure 8–110. Oblique and anteroposterior ankle radiographs show a lateral subtalar dislocation in association with a medial subluxation of the ankle joint owing to rupture of the lateral collateral ligament of the ankle. This condition is the forerunner of a complete medial dislocation of the talus, can follow a lateral subtalar dislocation.

and motorcycle accidents, falls from heights, and severe twisting injuries. A total dislocation of the talus requires disruption of the ankle, subtalar, and talonavicular joints, which deprives the talus of its blood supply and is usually accompanied by an open wound, resulting in a catastrophic ankle injury. It has been suggested that subtalar dislocation is a prerequisite for the following types of total talar dislocation:

A. Lateral total dislocation: caused by a severe inversion injury of the foot that first produces a medial subtalar dislocation can be followed by a lateral total dislocation of the talus.

B. Medial total dislocation: caused by a severe eversion injury of the foot that first produces a lateral subtalar dislocation and can be followed by a medial total dislocation of the talus.

C. Anterior total dislocation: produced by a fall from a height on a plantar-flexed foot that first causes a posterior subtalar dislocation and can result in an anterior total dislocation of the talus.

D. Posterior total dislocation: produced by a fall from a height on a dorsiflexed foot that first causes an anterior subtalar dislocation and can result in a posterior total dis-

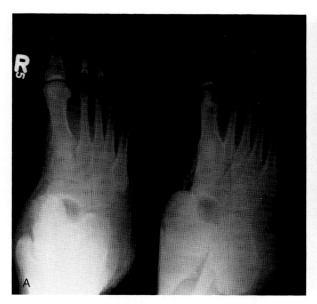 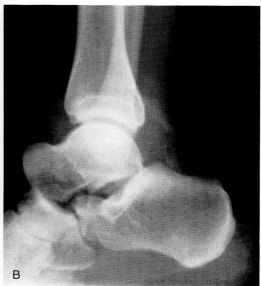

Figure 8–111. The right foot of a 30-year-old factory worker was caught by a conveyor belt. Anteroposterior and oblique (**A**) and lateral (**B**) views show an open lateral subtalar dislocation, as evidenced by lateral dislocation of both the talonavicular and talocalcaneal joints and the presence of air bubbles in the soft tissue around the ankle joint.

location of the talus. Diastasis of the ankle mortise often accompanies a posterior total dislocation of the talus (Figure 8–113).

CLINICAL SYMPTOMS AND SIGNS. In addition to the pain, swelling, ecchymosis, and tenderness commonly associated with any major fracture or dislocations, subtalar dislocation or a total dislocation of the talus is often highlighted by the presence of an open wound, marked deformity of the foot, and a relatively high incidence of neurovascular disturbances.

In a lateral subtalar dislocation, the calcaneus and the forefoot are displaced laterally, the head of the talus becomes prominent medially, and the signs of neurovascular compromise, such as coolness, skin discoloration, pulselessness, and sensory disturbance, are quite evident. In a medial subtalar dislocation, the heel and forefoot are displaced medially and the head of the talus becomes prominent laterally. In a posterior subtalar dislocation, both the heel and forefoot are displaced posteriorly and the foot appears to be shortened.

In an anterior subtalar dislocation, both the heel and forefoot are displaced anteriorly and the foot appears to be flattened.

In a total dislocation of the talus, the talus is usually displaced in a direction opposite to the displacement of the heel and forefoot, producing grotesque deformity of the ankle region and often stretching the skin around the ankle beyond its limits of elasticity. A large open wound may be produced, through which part of the talus and/or the ankle malleoli can usually be seen. The talus can be completely extruded from the wound to become a loose piece of bone outside the human body.

ROENTGENOGRAPHIC MANIFESTATIONS. In a subtalar dislocation, the talocalcaneal and talonavicular joints are completely dislocated, whereas in a total dislocation of the talus, the ankle, talonavicular, and talocalcaneal joints are completely dislocated. In a medial, lateral, posterior, or anterior subtalar dislocation, the calcaneus and forefoot are dislocated medially, laterally, posteriorly, or anteriorly, respectively. Medial and lateral

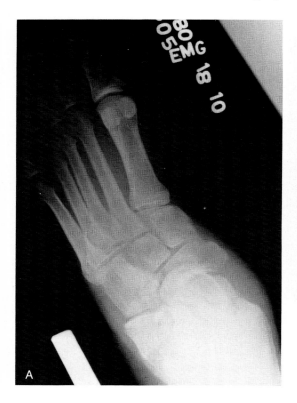

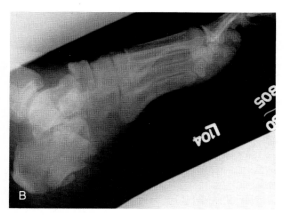

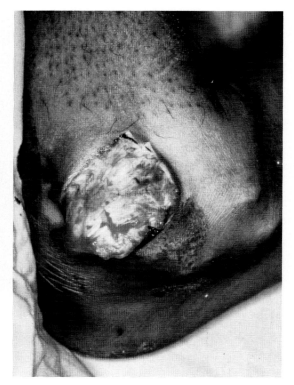

Figure 8–113. A 36-year-old man was involved in an automobile accident and sustained a total posterior dislocation of his right talus, which resulted in a diastasis of the ankle joint and perforated the skin between the Achilles tendon and the lateral malleolus, to appear at the posterolateral aspect of the ankle joint.

Figure 8–112. A 43-year-old man seriously injured his left foot in a motorcycle accident. Anteroposterior (**A**) and lateral (**B**) films demonstrate a complex subtalar dislocation in which the forefoot is dislocated medially due to dislocation of the talonavicular joint and a transverse fracture through the anterior process of the calcaneus. In addition, the body of the calcaneus is subluxated posteriorly from the subtalar joint and is associated with a severely comminuted fracture of the body of the calcaneus. Note the displaced transarticular fractures of the anterior process of the calcaneus of the lateral portion of the navicular.

subtalar dislocations are best seen on anteroposterior and oblique views, whereas anterior and posterior subtalar dislocations are best visualized on lateral radiographs. In a medial, lateral, anterior, or posterior total dislocation of the talus, the talus is situated medial, lateral, anterior, or posterior to the ankle joint, respectively, instead of in the ankle mortise. Because both subtalar dislocation and a total dislocation of the talus are often associated with an open wound, air shadow is commonly seen in the soft tissue of the ankle region near the area of the open wound. Both dislocations can be associated with diastasis of the distal tibiofibular articulation as well as fractures and/or dislocations of the malleoli, talus, calcaneus, navicular, cuboid, cuneiforms, metatarsals, and phalanges in many different combinations.

TREATMENT.   Because subtalar dislocation and total dislocation of the talus are commonly accompanied by an open wound and severe foot deformity, prompt closed reduction and meticulous wound care, with copious irrigation, careful debridement, antibiotic coverage, and tetanus shot administration, should be carried out as soon as possible to minimize the chances of developing wound infection, skin necrosis, gangrene, permanent nerve deficits, osteomyelitis, and pyarthrosis. A subtalar dislocation can usually be reduced by bending the knee and applying traction to the foot while pushing the calcaneus in the opposite direction of its dislocation. After the reduction, a short, leg cast should be worn for 3 to 4 weeks to allow the torn joint capsules and ligaments to heal before physiotherapy is initiated.

Interposition by bony or soft tissue structures, however, may prevent a successful closed reduction. These obstructive objects may include posterior tibial, peroneus longus, peroneus brevis, flexor digitorum longus, anterior tibial, extensor digitorum longus, and extensor digitorum brevis tendons or muscles; ruptured extensor retinaculum; fracture fragments from the talus, navicular, and calcaneus; and interlocking of articular marginal fractures of the talonavicular joint, which often require open reduction with or without K-wire fixation after the reduction. In addition to reducing the subtalar dislocation, all other associated fractures or dislocations of the foot should be properly treated at the same time.

Damage to the subtalar joint frequently leads to traumatic subtalar arthritis, which may eventually require a subtalar fusion; trauma-induced degenerative arthritis of both the subtalar and talonavicular joints may necessitate a triple arthrodesis for pain relief. It should be noted that subtalar dislocation is rarely associated with avascular necrosis of the talus, because the major blood supply to the talus is usually not disrupted by this dislocation.

In contrast, when a talus is completely dis-

located, all three main sources of blood supply are completely cut off, and the development of avascular necrosis of the talus is virtually a certainty. In addition, severe and uncontrollable infection of the foot that sometimes follows an open subtalar dislocation or total dislocation of the talus may require a Syme's or below-knee amputation for eradication of the infection.

It has been suggested that a completely extruded talus should be washed and replaced in the ankle joint and protected with a cast for 1 to 1.5 years to give the completely devitalized talus a chance to become revascularized. The argument against this method of treatment is that the period of 1 to 1.5 years is long, and there is no assurance whatso-

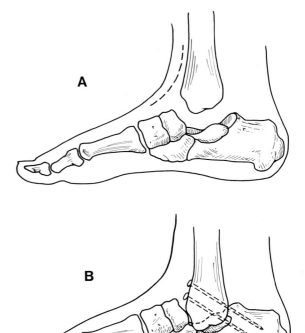

Figure 8–114. Surgical technique for performing a tibiocalcaneal fusion. **A,** make a longitudinal incision over the anterior aspect of the ankle. **B,** remove all articular cartilage from the distal tibia, fibula, and calcaneus. Tightly insert two stout cancellous bone screws from the anterior surface of the tibia obliquely into the calcaneus to hold the raw bone surfaces in intimate contact so to facilitate early bony fusion.

ever that the talar revascularization will take place at all. Two alternatives include throwing the talus away (talectomy) and performing a delayed tibiocalcaneal fusion after the open wound has properly healed (Figure 8–114). The disadvantages of talectomy include a slight shortening of the limb, possible presence of pain, and a tendency to develop a varus deformity of the ankle. Although tibiocalcaneal fusion also creates some shortening of the extremity, it produces a stable and painless foot and is therefore a logical method of treating a completely extruded total talar dislocation. Furthermore, if a completely dislocated talus is returned to the ankle joint and soon becomes infected, or subsequently undergoes progressive collapse of its body, the treatment of choice is once again a tibiocalcaneal fusion.

REFERENCES

Subtalar Dislocation and Total Talar Dislocation

1. Barber, J.R., Bricker, J.D., and Haliburton, R.A.: Peritalar dislocation of the foot. Can. J. Surg., 4:205, 1961.
2. Buckingham, Jr., W W.: Subtalar dislocation of the foot. J. Trauma, 13:753, 1973.
3. Christensen, S.B., Lorentzen, J.E., Krogsoe, O., and Sneppen, O.: Subtalar dislocation. Acta Orthop. Scand., 48:707, 1977.
4. DeLee, J.C., and Curtis, R.: Subtalar dislocation of foot. J. Bone Joint Surg. [Am.], 64:433, 1982.
5. Detenbeck, L.C., and Kelly, P.J.: Total dislocation of the talus. J. Bone Joint Surg. [Am.], 51:283, 1969.
6. Dunn, A.W.: Peritalar dislocation. Orthop. Clin. North Am., 5:7, 1974.
7. Elkhoury, G.Y., Yousefzadeh, D.K., Mulligan, G.M., and Moore, T.E.: Subtalar dislocation. Skeletal Radiol., 8:99, 1982.
8. Grantham, S.A.: Medial subtalar dislocation: Five cases with a common etiology. J. Trauma, 4:845, 1964.
9. Gross, R.H.: Medial peritalar dislocation—associated foot injuries and mechanism of injury. J. Trauma, 15:682, 1975.
10. Haliburton, R.A., Barber, J.R., and Fraser, R.L.: Further experience with peritalar dislocation. Can. J. Surg., 10:322, 1967.
11. Heppenstall, R.B., Farahvar, H., Balderston, R., and Lotke, P.: Evaluation and management of subtalar dislocations. J. Trauma. 20:494, 1980.
12. Horer, D.I., and Fishman, J.: The early treatment of peritalar dislocation. Int. Orthop., 7:263, 1984.
13. Larsen, H.W.: Subastragalar dislocation (luxatio pedia subtalo). A follow-up report of eight cases. Acta Chir. Scand., 113:380, 1957.
14. Leitner, B.: Obstacles to reduction in subtalar dislocations. J. Bone Joint Surg. [Am.], 36:299, 1954.
15. Leitner, B.: The mechanism of total dislocation of the talus. J. Bone Joint Surg. [Am.], 37:89, 1955.
16. McCurrich, H.J.: Traumatic expulsions of the astragalus. Br. J. Surg., 28:611, 1941.
17. Mitchell, J.I.: Total dislocation of the astragalus. J. Bone Joint Surg., 18:212, 1936.
18. Monson, S.T., and Fyan, J.T.: Subtalar dislocation. J. Bone Joint Surg. [Am.], 63:1156, 1981.
19. Mulroy, R.D.: The tibialis posterior tendon as an obstacle to reduction of a lateral anterior subtalar dislocation. J. Bone Joint Surg. [Am.], 37:859, 1955.
20. Newcomb, W.J., and Brav, E.A.: Complete dislocation of the talus. J. Bone Joint Surg. [Am.], 30:872, 1948.
21. Pinzur, M.S., and Meyer, Jr., P.R.: Complete posterior dislocation of the talus. Case report and discussion. Clin. Orthop., 131:205, 1978.
22. Plewes, L.W., and McKelvey, K.G.: Subtalar dislocation. J. Bone Joint Surg., 26:585, 1944.
23. St. Pierre, R.K., Velazco, A., Fleming, L.L., and Whitesides, T.: Medial subtalar dislocation in an athlete. A case report. Am. J. Sports Med., 10:240, 1982.
24. Segal, D., and Wasilewski, S.: Total dislocation of the talus. Case report. J. Bone Joint Surg. [Am.], 62:1370, 1980.
25. Shands, Jr., A.R.: The incidence of subastragaloid dislocation of the foot, with a report of one case of the inward type. J. Bone Joint Surg. [Am.], 37:859, 1955.
26. Smith, H.: Subastragalar dislocation: Report of 7 cases. J. Bone Joint Surg., 19:373, 1937.

Fractures of the Calcaneus

INCIDENCE. The calcaneus is the largest and the most commonly fractured tarsal bone that forms the posterior limb of the longtitudinal arch. It has four articular facets, three of which articulate with the undersurface of the talus, and the fourth one with the cuboid. The calcaneus is a relatively hollow bone composed of extremely vascular cancellous bone with a paucity of trabeculae and a thin cortical shell. The thick and resilient heel fat pad under the calcaneus is composed of fibroelastic adipose tissue with many vertical fibrous septa that extend from the skin of the heel to the undersurface of the calcaneus in the form of the letter U, with opening of the U firmly attached to the calcaneus.

The hydraulic action of the heel pad in cushioning the heel is severely damaged when a comminuted calcaneal fracture occurs. Falls from heights, motorcycle and automobile accidents, and twisting injuries of the foot produce the majority of the calcaneal fractures,

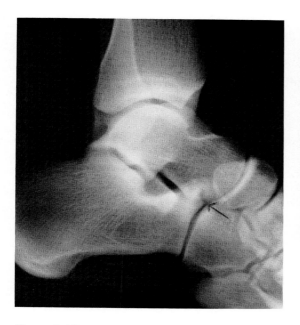

Figure 8–115. Lateral view of the hindfoot shows an avulsion fracture of the beak of calcaneus (*arrow*) where the calcaneonavicular and calcaneocuboid ligaments are attached. An inversion injury of the foot usually causes this fracture.

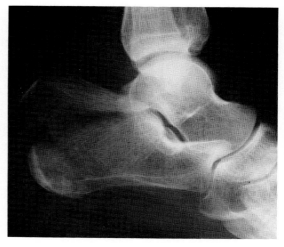

Figure 8–116. Lateral view of the hindfoot shows a displaced, horizontal, and slightly comminuted fracture of the body of the calcaneus caused by a violent contraction of the triceps surae muscle.

especially the compression type with subtalar joint involvement. Violent pulling by tendons or ligaments, however, can produce avulsion-type fractures; fracture of the anterior process of the calcaneus by the pull of the bifurcated ligament that attaches itself to the navicular and the cuboid (Figure 8–115), and fracture of the posterosuperior calcaneal tuberosity by the pull of the Achilles tendon (Figure 8–116) are typical examples.

In a typical compression fracture of the calcaneus caused by a fall from a height, because the center of the calcaneal tuberosity is situated slightly lateral to the center of the talus, the downward force placed on the talus creates a shear stress through the calcaneus, producing two primary fracture fragments: the superomedial sustentacular fragment and the inferolateral tuberosity fragment. As the shearing force continues, the sustentacular fragment, which is firmly connected with the talus by the anterior, posterior, medial, lateral, and interosseous talocalcaneal ligaments, moves downward, medially, and posteriorly;

the tuberosity fragment moves upward, laterally, and anteriorly, resulting in a decrease of the vertical height and longitudinal length of the calcaneus, and an increase in the lateral width of the calcaneal body (Figure 8–117). In addition, the lateral process of the talus splits the posterior articular facet of the calcaneus. A smaller medial part and a larger lateral part are formed, with varying degrees of comminution and impaction of the fractured articular surface into the substance of the body of calcaneus, the lateral part attaching to the tuberosity fragment and the medial part to the sustentacular fragment.

On an anatomic basis, a comprehensive classification of the various calcaneal fractures can be obtained.

A. Extra-articular calcaneal fractures: account for about 25 to 30% of all calcaneal fractures. These include fractures of the anterior calcaneal process (beak) (Figure 8–116), the posterior superior calcaneal tuberosity (Figure 8–118), the posterior inferior calcaneal tuberosity (Figure 8–119), the body of the calcaneus (Figure 8–120), and the sustentaculum tali.

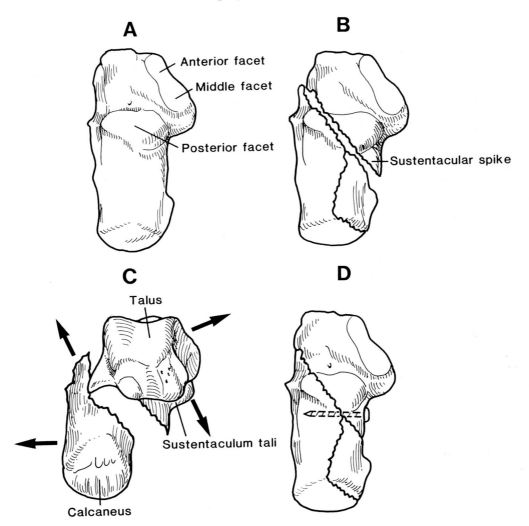

Figure 8–117. Mechanism that produces a typical intra-articular fracture of the calcaneus. **A,** top view of a calcaneus shows the anterior, middle, and posterior articular facets. **B,** an oblique fracture through the posterior articular facet and the calcaneal body is usually caused by a shearing force that acts on the sustentaculum tali through the overlying talus. The center of gravity of the talus is medial to that of the calcaneal body and is therefore responsible for producing the shear fracture. The posterior migration of the sustentacular fragment produces a shortening of the calcaneus along its longitudinal axis. **C,** medial and inferior migration of the sustentacular fragment, which is still connected to the talus, produces a decrease in the vertical height of the calcaneus, a broadening of the lateral width of the calcaneus, and depression and displacement of the fractured posterior articular facet of the calcaneus. **D,** to reduce this fracture, the sustentacular spike should be accurately matched with the corresponding triangular defect on the medial wall of the calcaneus. One or two bone screws can be used to hold the sustentacular and the tuberosity fragments together.

B. Intra-articular calcaneal fractures: account for about 70 to 75% of all calcaneal fractures. The joint depression type and the tongue type are the two most common fractures in this category, which include:

1. Non-displaced or minimally displaced fracture of the posterior talocalcaneal joint.
2. Joint depression-type fracture of the posterior talocalcaneal joint with frac-

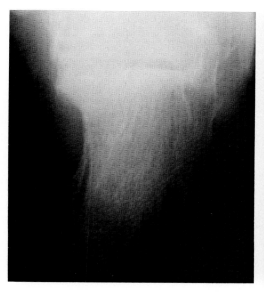
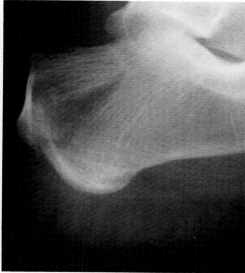

Figure 8–118. Axial and lateral views of the hindfoot show a slightly displaced avulsion fracture of the posterior superior calcaneal tuberosity caused by a forceful contraction of the triceps surae muscle. A short, leg cast with the foot in an equinus position worn for a few weeks is all that is needed to treat this fracture.

ture lines extending only a short distance behind the posterior facet.
3. Tongue-type fracture of the posterior talocalcaneal joint with long fracture lines extending to the rear of the calcaneal tuberosity.
4. Extremely comminuted fracture of the calcaneus defies any reasonable description.
5. Fracture of both the subtalar and calcaneocuboid joints.

Ten percent of calcaneal fractures are associated with compression fractures of the dorsal or lumbar spine, and 20 to 30% are associated with fractures of the spine, foot, ankle, and tibia. Although calcaneal fractures do occur in children, they differ from adult calcaneal fracture in several important ways. First, children sustain non-displaced and extra-articular fractures approximately twice as frequently as adults. Resiliency of the cartilage and supple adjacent soft tissues act as a shock absorber to vertical compression, resulting in few displaced intra-articular fractures. Second, children with calcaneal fractures have a twofold increase in the frequency of associated fractures of the extremities as adults. Third, there is a 50% reduction in the rate of

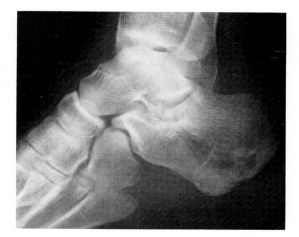

Figure 8–119. A 41-year-old man fell off a stepladder and landed on his right foot. Lateral radiograph reveals a slightly comminuted fracture of the inferior aspect of the calcaneus, with little displacement and minimal involvement of the subtalar joint. A good long-term result can be expected in such a case.

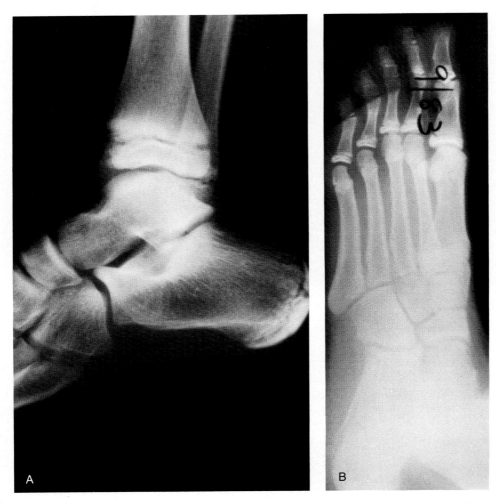

Figure 8–120. A 12-year-old boy in whom lateral (**A**) and oblique (**B**) radiographs demonstrate a minimally displaced fracture of the body of the calcaneus, which can be treated with a cast with full expectation of obtaining a good long-term result.

occurrence of axial skeletal fractures in children as in adults. Fourth, it is more difficult to recognize calcaneal fractures in children than in adults because of the minimal disturbance of the bony architecture and the high percentage of cartilage present. Fifth, as a group, calcaneal fractures in children have a better long-term prognosis than those in adults because the development of post-traumatic arthritis in the subtalar joint of children is rare.

Occasionally, a stress fracture of the calcaneus, the second most common site of stress fracture in the foot (that of the meta-tarsals is first) can occur in young military recruits or older and athletically unconditioned individuals who suddenly engage in unaccustomed and vigorous physical activities. Such a fracture usually involves the upper portion of the body of the calcaneus and can be bilateral.

CLINICAL SYMPTOMS AND SIGNS. These depend on the stages and the anatomic site of the fracture. In the acute stage, pain, tenderness, swelling, crepitation, ecchymosis, heel deformity, and skin laceration with extrusion of calcaneal bony fragment are the possible clinical findings. The point of maximal tenderness is usually anteriorly in a beak fracture, inferomedially in a posterior inferior calcaneal tuberosity fracture, superoposteriorly in a posterior superior calcaneal tuberosity fracture, in the sinus tarsi in a joint depression fracture of the posterior talocalcaneal joint, and medially in a fracture of the sustentaculum tali.

In the chronic stage, the symptoms and signs of a calcaneal fracture are the reflections of the sequelae of the initial calcaneal fracture, which can include traumatic arthritis of the subtalar and calcaneocuboid joints; lateral pain syndrome due to impingement of the peroneal tendons by the lateral broadening of the calcaneus and the medial surface of the tip of the fibula; injury of the ligaments surrounding the calcaneus, such as the tibiocal-

caneal, calcaneofibular, interosseous talocalcaneal, and medial and lateral talocalcaneal ligaments; soft tissue injury of the heel pad (Figure 8–121); and fibrosis of the ankle, subtalar, or midtarsal joints. These sequelae contribute to the unsatisfactory outcome of a calcaneal fracture. To be more specific, traumatic arthritis of the subtalar and calcaneocuboid joints causes pain in active or passive motion, tenderness, swelling, osteophyte formation at joint margins, crepitation, and limitation of range of motion of these two joints. Broadening of the calcaneus compresses the peroneal tendons against the fibula to produce a peroneal tendinitis (stenosing tenovaginitis) that is manifested clinically by pain, tenderness, and swelling over the peroneal tendons at the site where they pass from the retromalleolar groove region into the ex-

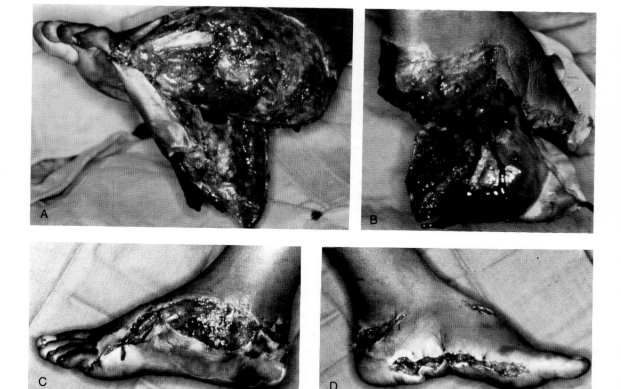

Figure 8–121. A–D, a 12-year-old boy was hit by a train and sustained a complete avulsion of his left heel pad plus part of the plantar skin of the forefoot. In spite of an attempt to save the foot, most of the heel pad turned gangrenous and the foot was subsequently amputated.

panded lateral wall of the calcaneus; a broadened heel also makes proper shoe fitting difficult. Injury of the ligamentous structures surrounding the calcaneus causes instability of the foot, especially during running or walking on uneven ground. Disruption of the fibrofatty element in the heel pad from fracture of the plantar surface of the calcaneus severely interferes with the hydraulic and cushioning function of the heel pad, resulting in chronic heel pain on weight-bearing. This pain can be further aggravated by the presence of any large bony spur on the posterior inferior calcaneal tuberosity produced by the same fracture. Periarticular fibrosis of the ankle, subtalar, and midtarsal joints diminishes their normal function and tends to place more stress on the neighboring joints, thus contributing to the premature development of degenerative arthritis of these joints.

A severe os calcis fracture may take 1 to 2 years to stabilize, and both the treating physician and the patient should patiently allow the damage to heal before unwisely rushing into radical surgical procedures. In contrast to an acute calcaneal fracture, the clinical symptoms and signs of a stress fracture of the calcaneus usually have a gradual onset, and are characterized by milder soft tissue swelling around the heel, diffuse heel pain aggravated by ambulation, tenderness of the body of the calcaneus to deep palpation, and production of heel pain with toe walking, heel walking, or resisted plantar flexion of the ankle.

ROENTGENOGRAPHIC MANIFESTATIONS.   An adequate evaluation of a calcaneal fracture should automatically include anteroposterior, lateral, oblique, and axial views of the foot and ankle. The axial view, probably the most important view, shows the site and extent of the fractures of the calcaneal body, medial and inferior displacement of the superomedial (sustentacular) fragment, the sustentacular spike, lateral widening of the calcaneus caused by impaction from fragments of the posterior talocalcaneal articular facet, and fracture and displacement of the posterior inferior calcaneal tuberosity. The lateral view, also important, demonstrates short-

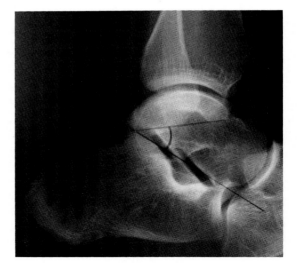

Figure 8–122.   Lateral view of the hindfoot shows the so-called tuberosity angle (Bohler's angle) formed by the two lines drawn parallel to the posterior superior border of the calcaneus and the subtalar joint.

ening in the longitudinal length and the vertical height of the calcaneus; fracture and displacement of the posterior superior calcaneal tuberosity; the nature and extent of intra-articular fractures (e.g., tongue-type or joint depression-type fractures); loss of the tuberosity angle (Bohler's angle) (Figure 8–122), which is about 30 to 35° in a normal foot; and the extent of impaction of the posterior talocalcaneal articular surface into the body of the calcaneus. The anteroposterior and oblique views are helpful to show the fracture of the anterior calcaneal process, beak fracture of the calcaneus, and fracture of the calcaneocuboid joint. It should be noted that CT scanning is useful in delineating the exact site and extent of all kind of calcaneal fractures. In addition, a peroneal synoviagram can clearly demonstrate a blockage of the radiopaque dye column at the site of symptomatic impingement of the peroneal tendons.

When a stress fracture of the calcaneus has been present for a few weeks, a band of sclerosis is present in the body of the calcaneus and is often perpendicular to the calcaneal bony trabecular pattern. A mild degree of periosteal new bone formation may also be present. If the radiographs taken soon after the onset of symptoms of a stress calcaneal fracture are completely normal, a bone scan performed simultaneously will show a definite increase in uptake in the calcaneal body at the site of the stress fracture.

TREATMENT. All undisplaced and minimally displaced extra-articular calcaneal fractures can usually be treated with a cast for a few weeks followed the use of physical therapy, gentle exercises, soaking, elastic stockings, and elevation to regain the normal function of the foot. A displaced avulsion fracture of the posterior superior calcaneal tuberosity by its calcaneal tendon, however, should be accurately reduced and fixed with a screw (Figures 8–123—8–125). A significantly displaced fracture of the posterior inferior calcaneal tuberosity may also require open reduction and screw fixation to restore the cushioning function of the thick heel pad and to prevent development of a large painful heel spur, which often requires surgical excision. Occasionally, a painful non-union occurs in an anterior beak fracture of the calcaneus, which also may require surgical excision. In contrast, numerous intra-articular calcaneal fractures require closed or open reduction.

Closed reduction usually involves relaxing the powerful gastrocnemius muscle by flexing the knee to 90°, applying traction to the heel to restore the vertical height of the calcaneus, and then exerting opposing lateral pressure to reduce the fracture-induced lateral broadening of the calcaneus. Although the axial pin method has been advocated for treating the tongue-type intra-articular calcaneal fracture, a comminuted joint depression-type calcaneal fracture may well require an open reduction to achieve an optimal result.

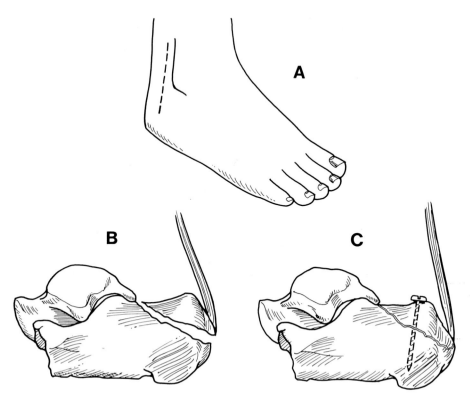

Figure 8–123. Surgical technique for reducing a displaced avulsion fracture of the posterior superior calcaneal tuberosity. **A,** make a longitudinal incision between the lateral malleolus and the lateral border of the Achilles tendon. **B,** reduce the calcaneal tuberosity fracture. **C,** fix the reduced calcaneal tuberosity with a bone screw.

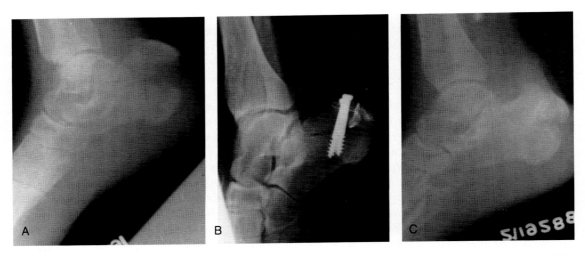

Figure 8-124. After falling down about 3 m and landing on his left heel, a 47-year-old man sustained an avulsion fracture of the upper portion of the body of the calcaneus (**A**) which was treated with open reduction and screw fixation (**B**) with a satisfactory result. **C,** 9 months later.

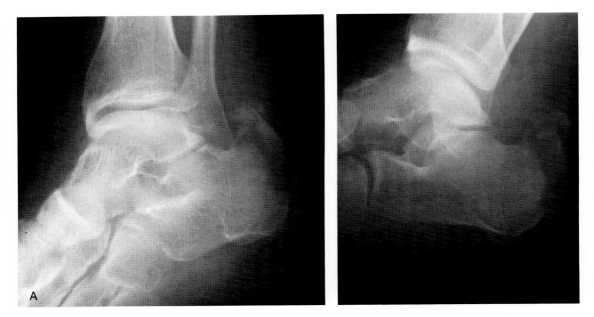

Figure 8-125. A 35-year-old woman in whom oblique and lateral views (**A**) show a comminuted avulsion fracture of the posterior superior calcaneal tuberosity, which was pulled off by the calcaneal tendon.

Figure 8-126. Surgical technique for treating a severely comminuted intra-articular fracture of the calcaneus. **A,** make a curvilinear incision along the anterior border of the fibula to the dorsolateral aspect of the foot. **B,** normal calcaneus with a full view of its three articular facets. **C,** an extremely comminuted calcaneal fracture with extensive involvement of the posterior articular facet. **D,** depressed and displaced fragments of the posterior articular facet have been elevated through a rectangular bone slot cut in the lateral aspect of the body of the calcaneus. The rectangular bone defect has been tightly filled with iliac bone chips to prevent collapse to the elevated articular surface. **E,** a reduced comminuted calcaneal fracture.

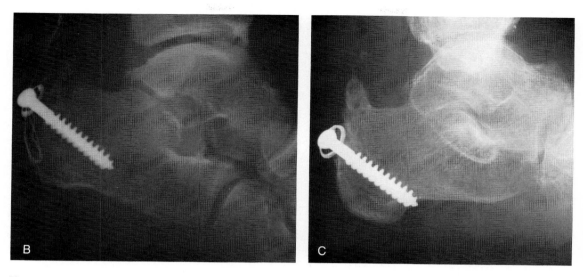

Figure 8–125. Continued. Intraoperative (**B**) and 1-year postoperative (**C**) radiographs show satisfactory reduction (**B**) and healing (**C**) of the avulsed calcaneal bone fragment.

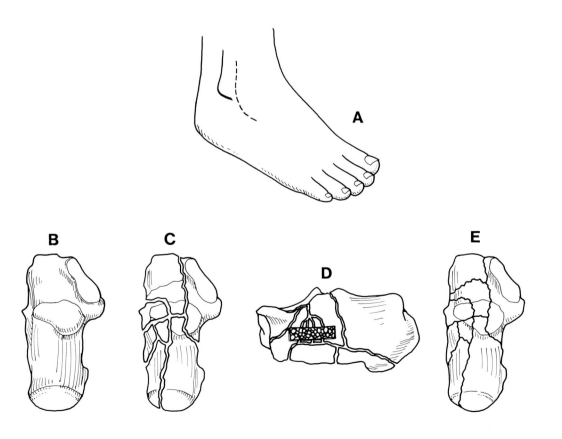

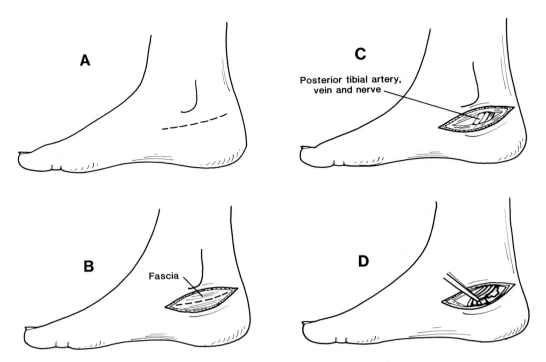

Figure 8–127. Medial approach to reduce a calcaneal fracture. **A,** make a horizontal incision midway between the tip of the medial malleolus and the bottom of the heel. **B,** horizontally incise the fascia of the foot. **C,** carefully expose and isolate the posterior tibial neurovascular bundle. **D,** retract the isolated neurovascular bundle before proceeding with the surgical reduction of the calcaneal fracture, which often requires perfect alignment of the sustentacular spike with its matching bone defect on the medial wall of the calcaneus.

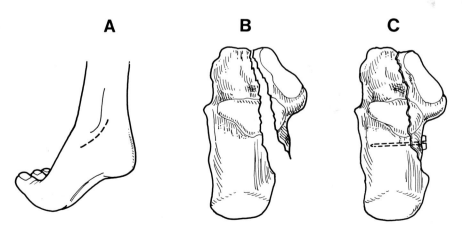

Figure 8–128. Surgical technique for treating a displaced longitudinal transarticular fracture of the calcaneus. **A,** make a curvilinear incision behind and below the medial malleolus. **B,** medial calcaneal fracture fragment goes through the posterior articular facet and carries the anterior and middle articular facets with it. **C,** displaced medial fragment has been reduced and fixed to the main portion of the calcaneus with one or two bone screws.

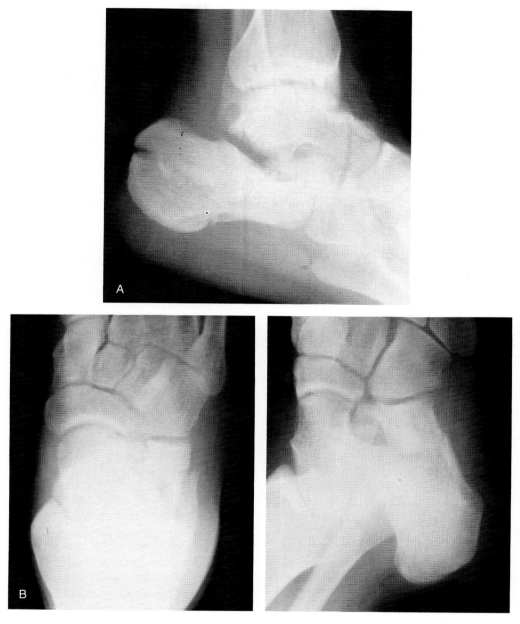

Figure 8–129. A 17-year-old high school star basketball player sustained a severe injury to his right hindfoot during a basketball game. Lateral (**A**) and anteroposterior and oblique (**B**) views reveal a severely depressed and comminuted fracture of the calcaneus with the Bohler's angle measuring about 0°. Open reduction was employed; and severely comminuted articular surface of the calcaneus was elevated and the subchondral bony defect was tightly packed with autogenous iliac bone chips through a lateral incision. The displaced sustentacular fragment was then aligned with the tuberosity fragment and fixed with a bone screw.

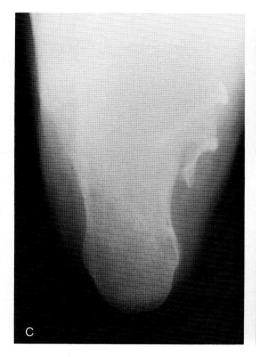
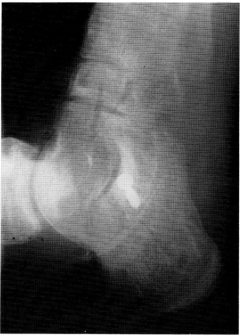

Figure 8–129. Continued. C, lateral view of the hindfoot and axial view of the calcaneus 3 months after surgery show a satisfactory reduction and healing of this complex calcaneal fracture. The patient had an excellent result and continued to pursue a career in basketball.

A slightly curved incision placed along the anterior border of the fibula enables the surgeon to gain access to the posterior talo-calcaneal joint, where the depressed and displaced articular surface can be carefully elevated and the resultant subchondral bony defect may be tightly packed with autogenous bone chips (Figure 8–126). The medial incision, in contrast, should be placed parallel to the sole and half way between the tip of the medial malleolus and the bottom of the foot. After incising the fascia of the foot and retracting the neurovascular bundle (Figure 8–127), the fracture on the medial cortex of the calcaneus can be reduced by realigning the sharp sustenaculum spike with its matching bony defect on the medial cortex of the calcaneus. In addition the upper portion of the sustentacular spike of the sustentacular calcaneal fragment is fixed to the tuberosity fragment of the calcaneus with one or two screws, thus restoring the normal longitudinal

length, vertical height, and lateral width of the calcaneus (Figures 8–128—8–130).

When a displaced fracture involves the articular surface of the anterior calcaneal process, and closed reduction fails to achieve an acceptable result, open reduction can then be employed to reduce the fracture and to fix it with a small K-wire or a small bone screw so to prevent the development of traumatic arthritis. When severe peroneal tendinitis is caused by compression of the peroneal tendons by the laterally broadened calcaneus and the fibula, significant symptomatic relief can be achieved by removing the excessive bone from the lateral surface of the calcaneus or from the inner and inferior surface of the tip of fibula at the exact site of the peroneal tendon compression.

When severe degenerative arthritis has developed in a subtalar joint after a calcaneal fracture, and conservative treatment fails to provide adequate relief, the performance of a

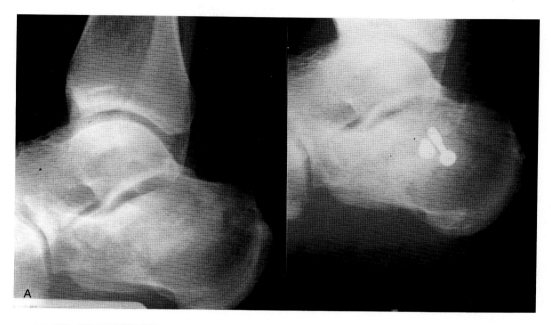

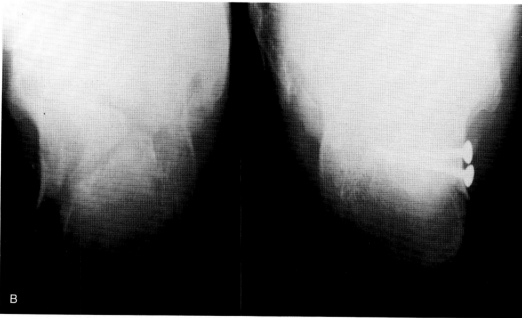

Figure 8–130. A 36-year-old man sustained a serious injury to his left calcaneus in a fall from a height. Comparison lateral (**A**) and axial (**B**) views show a rather comminuted calcaneal fracture with depression of the subtalar joint, lateral broadening of the calcaneus, and a significant decrease in the vertical height of the calcaneus preoperatively. After surgically elevating the depressed calcaneal articular surface, closely approximating the medial sustentacular fragment and the lateral tuberosity fragment together, and fixing them with two bone screws, the comparable post-operative radiographs do reveal an improvement of the Bohler's angle, restoration of the vertical calcaneal height, and a significant reduction of the trauma-induced lateral calcaneal broadening.

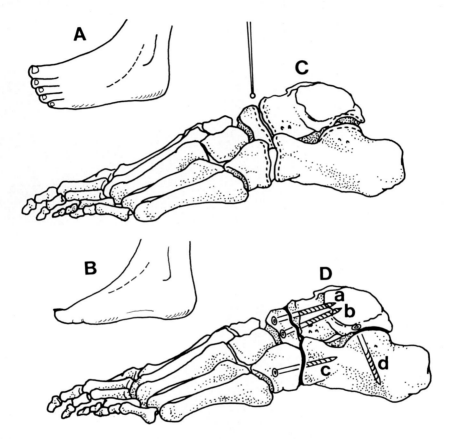

Figure 8–131. Surgical technique for performing a triple arthrodesis with cancellous bone screws. **A,** make a curvilinear incision along the anterior border of the lateral malleolus to the dorsolateral aspect of the foot, to gain access to the posterior talocalcaneal and calcaneocuboid joints as well as the lateral one half of the talonavicular joint. **B,** make a longitudinal curvilinear incision over the dorsomedial aspect of the foot to gain access to the talonavicular joint. **C,** remove all the articular cartilage from the talonavicular, calcaneocuboid, and subtalar joints with an air-driven burr. **D,** compress the opposing raw bone surfaces of the talonavicular, calcaneocuboid, and subtalar joints together with stout cancellous screws to complete the triple arthrodesis. Screws *a* and *b* fix the talonavicular joint; screw *c,* the calcaneocuboid joint; and screw *d,* the subtalar joint.

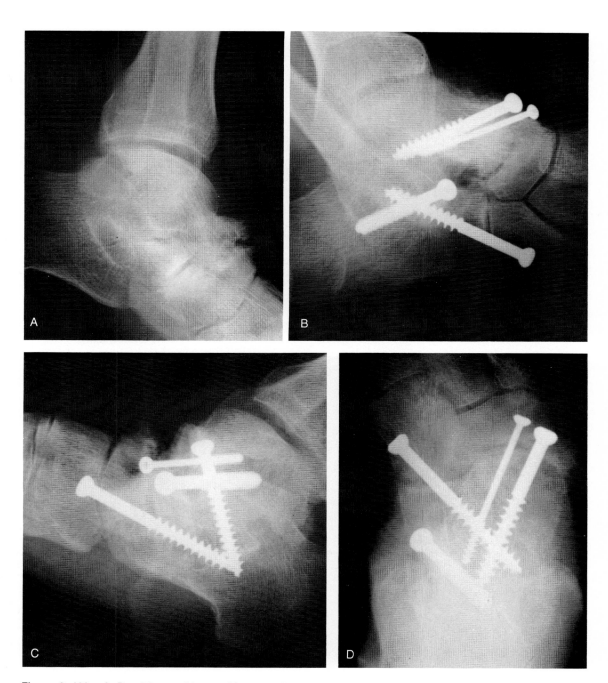

Figure 8–132. **A–D,** a 54-year-old man with severe degenerative arthritis of his right talonavicular and subtalar joints underwent a triple arthrodesis, which was performed by first denuding the midtarsal and subtalar joints and then holding and compressing the opposing raw bone surfaces together with cancellous bone screws. The triple arthrodesis healed uneventfully and the patient had a stable and painless right foot.

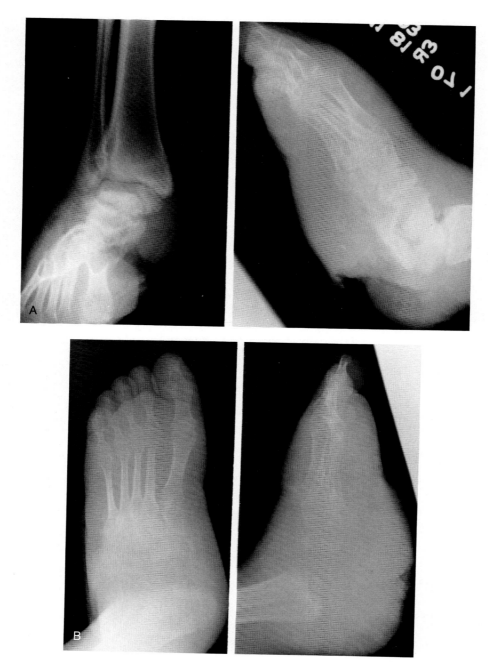

Figure 8–133. A 31-year-old woman had an old compound fracture of her left calcaneus, which was complicated by the development of a chronic osteomyelitis of the calcaneus (**A,** anteroposterior and lateral views). Several calcaneal sequestrectomies were required. **B,** subsequent anteroposterior and lateral radiographs show complete absence of the calcaneus and the talus after complete excision in an attempt to control a severe foot infection.

subtalar arthrodesis by various surgical methods should be considered. Furthermore, if the same subtalar arthritis is also associated with arthritis of the calcaneocuboid and/or talonavicular joints, a triple arthrodesis instead of a subtalar fusion is the treatment of choice. Triple arthrodesis can be performed according to various surgical techniques, among which the fixation of the surgically denuded articular surfaces of the talocalcaneal, calcaneocuboid, and talonavicular joints with stout cancellous screws appears to be easy and effective (Figures 8–131 and 8–132). Chronic osteomyelitis that follows a compound fracture of the calcaneus may require sequestrectomies, and may eventually lead to radical bone excision or foot amputation (Figure 8–133).

REFERENCES

Fractures of the Calcaneus

1. Aitken, A.P.: Fractures of the os calcis—treatment by closed reduction. Clin. Orthop., *30:*67, 1963.
2. Allan, J.H.: The open reduction of fractures of the os calcis. Am. Surg., *141:*890, 1955.
3. Anthonsen, W.: An oblique projection for roentgen examination of the talo-calcaneal joint of the calcaneus. Acta Radiol., *24:*306, 1943.
4. Bachman, S., and Johnson, S.R.: Torsion of the foot causing fracture of the anterior calcaneal process. Acta Chir. Scand., *105:*460, 1953.
5. Barnard, L.: Non-operative treatment of fractures of the calcaneus. J. Bone Joint Surg. [Am.], *45:*865, 1963.
6. Bradford, C.H., and Larsen, I.: Sprain-fractures of the anterior lip of the os calcis. N. Engl. J. Med., *244:*970, 1951.
7. Brindley, H.H.: Fractures of the os calcis: A review of 107 fractures in 95 patients. South. Med. J., *59:*843, 1966.
8. Buchanan, J., and Greer, R.B.: Stress fractures in the calcaneus of a child. A case report. Clin. Orthop., *135:*119, 1978.
9. Burdeaux, B.D.: Reduction of calcaneal fractures by the McReynold's medial approach technique and its experimental basis. Clin. Orthop., *177:*87, 1983.
10. Carothers, L.: Early mobilization in treatment of os calcis fractures. Am. J. Surg., *83:*279, 1952.
11. Chapman, H.G., and Galway, H.R.: Os calcis fracture in children. J. Bone Joint Surg. [Br.], *59:*510, 1977.
12. Christopher, F.: Fracture of the anterior process of the calcaneus. J. Bone Joint Surg., *13:*877, 1931.
13. Cotton, F.J., and Henderson, F.F.: Results of fractures of os calcis. Am. J. Orthop. Surg., *16:*290, 1916.
14. Dachtler, H.W.: Fractures of the anterior superior portion of the os calcis due to indirect violence. AJR, *25:*629, 1931.
15. Dart, D.E., and Graham, W.D.: The treatment of the fractured calcaneum. J. Trauma, *6:*362, 1966.
16. Degan, T.J., Morrey, B.F., and Braun, D.P.: Surgical excision for anterior-process fractures of the calcaneus. J. Bone Joint Surg. [Am.], *64:*519, 1982.
17. Deyerle, W.M.: Long term follow-up of fractures of the os calcis: Diagnostic peroneal synoviagram. Orthop. Clin. North Am., *4:*213, 1973.
18. Dick, I.L.: Primary fusion of the posterior subtalar joint in the treatment of fractures of the calcaneum. J. Bone Joint Surg. [Br.], *35:*375, 1953.
19. Essex-Lopresti, P.: The mechanism, reduction technique, and results in fracture of the os calcis. Br. J. Surg., *39:*395, 1952.
20. Farrow, R.C.: Peroneal release in calcaneal fractures. J. Bone Joint Surg. [Br.], *44:*961, 1962.
21. Gallie, W.E.: Subastragalar arthrodesis in fractures of the os calcis. J. Bone Joint Surg., *25:*131, 1943.
22. Gaul, Jr., J.S., and Greenburg, B.G.: Calcaneus fractures involving the subtalar joint: A clinical and statistical survey of 98 cases. South. Med. J., *59:*605, 1966.
23. Geckeler, E.O.: Comminuted fractures of os calcis. Arch. Surg., *61:*469, 1950.
24. Gellman, M.: Fracture of the anterior process of the calcaneus. J. Bone Joint Surg. [Am.], *33:*382, 1951.
25. Hall, M.C., and Pennal, G.F.: Primary subtalar arthrodesis in the treatment of severe fractures of the calcaneum. J. Bone Joint Surg. [Br.], *42:*336, 1960.
26. Hammesfahr, J.F., and Fleming, L.L.: Calcaneal fractures: A good prognosis. Foot Ankle, *1:*296, 1981.
27. Harris, R.I.: Fractures of os calcis: Treatment by early subtalar arthrodesis. Clin. Orthop., *30:*100, 1963.
28. Harty, M.: Anatomic considerations in injuries of the calcaneus. Orthop. Clin. North Am., *4:*179, 1973.
29. Hazlett, J.W.: Open reduction of fractures of the calcaneum. Can. J. Surg., *12:*310, 1969.
30. Hermann, O.J.: Conservative therapy for fractures of the os calcis. J. Bone Joint Surg., *19:*709, 1937.
31. Hopson, C.N., and Perry, D.R.: Diagnosis and treatment of calcaneal stress fractures. U.S. Navy Med., *64:*34, 1974.
32. Hopson, C.N., and Perry, D.R.: Stress fractures of the calcaneus in women Marine recruits. Clin. Orthop., *128:*159, 1977.
33. Hullinger, C.W.: Insufficiency fracture of the calcaneus: Similar to March fracture of the metatarsals. J. Bone Joint Surg., *26:*751, 1944.
34. Hunt, D.D.: Compression fracture of the anterior articular surface of the calcaneus. J. Bone Joint Surg. [Am.], *52:*1637, 1970.
35. Hunter, G.A., and James, E.T.R.: Amputation following os calcis fractures: A rare complication not previously emphasized. Orthop. Trans., *6:*480, 1982.
36. Isbister, J.F.S.C.: Calcaneo-fibular abutment following crush fracture of the calcaneus. J. Bone Joint Surg. [Br.], *56:*274, 1974.
37. James, E.T., and Hunter, G.A.: The dilemma of painful old os calcis fractures. Clin. Orthop., *177:*112, 1983.
38. King, R.E.: Axial pin fixation of fractures of the os calcis (method of Essex-Lopresti). Orthop. Clin. North Am., *4:*185, 1973.

39. Lance, E.M., Carey, Jr., E.J., and Wade, P.A.: Fractures of the os calcis: Treatment by early mobilization. Clin. Orthop., *30:*76, 1963.
40. Leabhart, J.W.: Stress fractures of the calcaneus. J. Bone Joint Surg. [Am.], *41:*1285, 1959.
41. Lindsay, W.R.N., and Dewar, F.P.: Fractures of the os calcis. Am. J. Surg., *95:*555, 1958.
42. Lowry, M.: Avulsion fractures of the calcaneus. J. Bone Joint Surg. [Br.], *51:*494, 1969.
43. Matteri, R.E., and Frymoyer, J.W.: Fracture of calcaneus in young children. Report of three cases. J. Bone Joint Surg. [Am.], *55:*1091, 1973.
44. Maxfield, J.E.: Os calcis fractures. Treatment by open reduction. Clin. Orthop., *30:*91, 1963.
45. McLaughlin, H.L.: Treatment of late complications after os calcis fractures. Clin. Orthop., *30:*111, 1963.
46. McReynolds, I.S.: Open reduction and internal fixation of calcaneal fractures. J. Bone Joint Surg. [Br.], *54:*176, 1972.
47. Miller, W.E.: The heel pad. Am. J. Sports Med., *10:*19, 1982.
48. Miller, W.E.: Pain and impairment considerations following treatment of disruptive os calcis fractures. Clin. Orthop., *177:*82, 1983.
49. Miller, W.E., and Purita, J.: Fractures of the calcaneus—open vs. closed treatment. Foot Ankle, 1:50, 1980.
50. Morris, J.M., and Blickenstaff, L.D.: Fatigue Fractures: A Clinical Study. Springfield, Charles C Thomas, 1967.
51. Nade, S., and Monalian, P.R.: Fractures of the calcaneum: A study of the long term prognosis. Injury, *4:*200, 1973.
52. Noble, J., and McQuillan, W.M.: Early posterior subtalar fusion in the treatment of fracture of the os calcis. J. Bone Joint Surg. [Br.], *61:*90, 1979.
53. O'Connell, F., Mital, M.A., and Rowe, C.R.: Evaluation of modern management of fractures of the os calcis. Clin. Orthop., *83:*214, 1972.
54. Odegard, B.: Conservative approach in treatment of fractures of calcaneus. J. Bone Joint Surg. [Am.], *37:*1231, 1975.
55. Omoto, H., Sukurada, K., Sugi, M., and Nakamura, K.: A new method of manual reduction for intra-articular fracture of the calcaneus. Clin. Orthop., *177:*104, 1983.
56. Palmer, I.: The mechanism and treatment of fractures of the calcaneus: Open reduction with the use of cancellous grafts. J. Bone Joint Surg. [Am.], *30:*2, 1948.
57. Parkes, II, J.C.: The non-reductive treatment of fractures of the os calcis. Orthop. Clin. North Am., *4:*193, 1973.
58. Pennal, G.F., and Yadav, M.P.: Operative treatment of comminuted fractures of the os calcis. Orthop. Clin. North Am., *4:*197, 1973.
59. Piatt, A.D.: Fracture of the promontory of the calcaneus. Radiology, *67:*386, 1956.
60. Pozp, J.L., Kirwan, E.O., and Jackson, A.M.: The long-term results of conservative management of severely displaced fractures of the calcaneus. J. Bone Joint Surg. [Br.], *66:*386, 1984.
61. Reich, R.S.: Subastragloid arthrodesis in treatment of old fractures of calcaneus. Surg. Gynecol. Obstet., *82:*671, 1946.
62. Resnick, D., and Goergen, T.G.: Peroneal tenography in previous calcaneal fractures. Radiology, *115:*211, 1975.
63. Roberts, N.W.: Fracture of the calcaneus. J. Bone Joint Surg. [Br.], *50:*884, 1968.
64. Rowe, C.R., Sakellarides, H., Freeman, P., and Sorbie, C.: Fractures of the os calcis—a long term follow-up study of one hundred forty-six patients. J.A.M.A., *184:*920, 1963.
65. Savoca, C.J.: Stress fractures: A classification of the earliest radiographic signs. Radiology, *100:*579, 1971.
66. Schmidt, T.L., and Weiner, D.S.: Calcaneal fractures in children. An evaluation of the nature of the injury in 56 children. Clin. Orthop., *171:*150, 1982.
67. Shannon, F.T., and Murray, A.M.: Os calcis fractures treated by non-weight-bearing exercises: A review of 65 patients. J. R. Coll. Surg. Edinb., *23:*355, 1978.
68. Simon, R., and Stultz, E.: Operative treatment of compression fractures of the calcaneus. Ann. Surg., *91:*731, 1930.
69. Soeur, R., and Remy, R.: Fractures of the calcaneus with displacement of the thalamic portion. J. Bone Joint Surg. [Br.], *57:*413, 1975.
70. Stein, R.E., and Stelling, F.H.: Stress fracture of the calcaneus in a child with cerebral palsy. J. Bone Joint Surg. [Am.], *59:*131, 1977.
71. Stephenson, J.R.: Displaced fractures of the os calcis involving the subtalar joint: The key role of the superomedial fragment. Foot Ankle, *4:*91, 1983.
72. Tanke, G.M.: Fractures of the calcaneus. A review of the literature together with some observations on methods of treatment. Acta Chir. Scand., *1:*103, 1982.
73. Thomas, H.M.: Calcaneal fracture in childhood. Br. J. Surg., *56:*664, 1969.
74. Thompson, K.R.: Treatment of comminuted fractures of the calcaneus by triple arthrodesis. Orthop. Clin. North Am., *4:*189, 1973.
75. Thompson, K.R., and Friesen, C.M.: Treatment of comminuted fractures of the calcaneus by primary triple arthrodesis. J. Bone Joint Surg. [Am.], *41:*1423, 1959.
76. Vestad, E.: Fractures of the calcaneum. Open reduction and bone grafting. Acta Chir. Scand., *134:*617, 1968.
77. Viswanath, S.S., and Shephard, E.: Dislocation of the calcaneus. Injury, *9:*50, 1977.
78. Warrick, C.K., and Bremner, A.E.: Fractures of the calcaneum. J. Bone Joint Surg. [Br.], *35:*33, 1953.
79. Whitaker, A.H.: Treatment of fractures of the os calcis by open reduction and internal fixation. Am. J. Surg., *74:*687, 1947.
80. Wilson, P.D.: Treatment of fractures of the os calcis by arthrodesis of subtalar joint. J.A.M.A., *89:*1676, 1927.
81. Winfield, A.C., and Dennis, J.M.: Stress fractures of the calcaneus. Radiology, *72:*415, 1959.
82. Zayer, M.: Fracture of the calcaneus: A review of 110 fractures. Acta Orthop. Scand., *40:*530, 1969.
83. Zeiss, C.R.: Treatment of comminuted fracture of os calcis. J.A.M.A., *169:*792, 1959.

Dislocation of the Calcaneus

INCIDENCE. Isolated dislocation of the calcaneus occurs so rarely that only a few

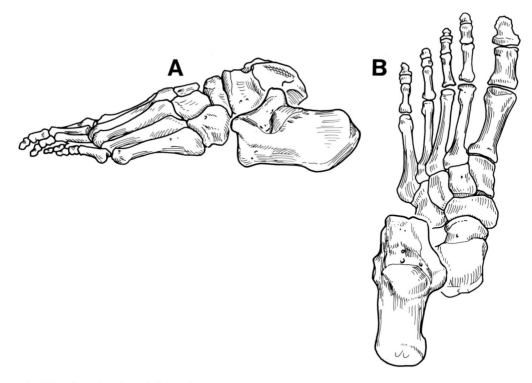

Figure 8–134. Complete lateral dislocation of the left calcaneus. **A,** lateral view shows that the lateral side of the talus is overlapped by the sustentaculum tali, and the anterior process of the calcaneus no longer articulates with the cuboid. **B,** top view shows a complete lateral dislocation of the calcaneus with its three articular facets now facing the viewer instead of hiding under the talus.

cases have been reported. The calcaneus is usually dislocated laterally with dislocation of both the talocalcaneal and calcaneocuboid joints by completely rupturing their joint capsules and associated ligaments (Figure 8–134). Violent trauma, such as a car accident and severe twisting injury of the hindfoot, are responsible for producing an isolated total dislocation of the calcaneus.

CLINICAL SYMPTOMS AND SIGNS. In addition to pain, swelling, tenderness, ecchymosis, and loss of normal function, which are frequently associated with any major dislocation of the extremities, lateral dislocation of the calcaneus produces a severe valgus heel deformity with flattening of the longitudinal arch of the foot, and may be associated with an open wound. The skin over the medial aspect of the ankle is tense and the posterior tibial nerve and blood vessels too are under ten-

sion. The entire inferomedial margin of the talus becomes quite prominent and the medial aspect of the undersurface of the talus may become palpable.

ROENTGENOGRAPHIC MANIFESTATIONS. Anteroposterior, lateral, oblique, and axial views of the ankle show that the calcaneus is laterally displaced and no longer articulates with either the talus or the cuboid. On the lateral view of the ankle, the articular surfaces of the talocalcaneal joint overlap each other; on the oblique view, the whole calcaneal portion of the subtalar joint is completely exposed. Axial view of the calcaneus shows that the entire calcaneus is inferolateral to the talus instead of directly under the talus.

TREATMENT. Closed reduction of a laterally dislocated calcaneus can be achieved by bending the knee to 90° to relax the gastrocnemius muscle and by applying traction to the dislocated calcaneus and then pushing it medially to relocate it under the talus. If postreduction radiographs show normal alignment of the subtalar and calcaneocuboid joints, a short, leg cast should be applied and worn for 4 to 6 weeks before starting on physiotherapy. If closed reduction fails to reduce the dislocation, however, an open reduction through a lateral incision can be used to reduce the dislocation. If the reduction is not stable, K-wire fixation from the neck of the talus into the calcaneus and through the calcaneocuboid joint should be employed, and a short, leg cast should be worn for 4 to 6 weeks before the K-wires are removed and physiotherapy is initiated.

When severe arthritis has developed in the subtalar joint after a total lateral dislocation of the calcaneus, subtalar fusion can provide a stiff but painless joint. If the severe arthritis involves both the subtalar and calcaneocuboid joints, a triple arthrodesis should be employed.

REFERENCES

Dislocation of the Calcaneus

1. Carey, E.J., Lance, E.M., and Wade, P.A.: Extra-articular fractures of os calcis. J. Trauma, *5:*362, 1965.
2. Ekehorn, G.: Ein fallvon isolierter luxation des calcaneus. Nord. Med. Arkiv., *1:*15, 1904.
3. Hamilton, A.R.: An unusual dislocation. Med. J. Aust., *1:*271, 1949.
4. Horand, R.: Un cas de luxatio du calcaneum en bas 'calcaneum cabre'. Lyon Med., p. 1259, 1912.
5. Parcellier, A., and Chenut, A.: Un cas de luxation du calcaneum. Rev. Orthop., *15:*418, 1912.
6. Viswanath, S.S., and Shephard, E.: Dislocation of the calcaneum. Injury, *9:*50, 1977.

9 AN ATLAS OF THE VARIOUS DISORDERS OF THE FOOT AND ANKLE REGIONS

With the exceptions of rheumatoid arthritis, gout, leprosy, diabetes mellitus, and sarcoidosis, most diseases usually do not affect the foot. However, at the Henry Ford Hospital Medical Center and its satellites in the Detroit metropolitan area, which currently handle well over 1 million patient visits per year, many unusual and extremely rare diseases of the foot have been seen over the years. The cases presented in this chapter are intended to familiarize the reader with the clinical, radiologic, and pathologic appearance of a variety of pathologic processes and deformities of the foot. In addition, a list of references is provided to guide those readers who wish to know more about a particular disease or deformity of the foot that is briefly discussed in this text.

BONE TUMORS

METASTASIS (Figures 9–1—9–4). Metastatic tumors are the malignant tumors that occur most often in the human skeleton. Breast and prostatic carcinomas are the most com-

mon metastatic tumors of bone, but carcinomas from the lung, colon, kidney, stomach, bladder, uterus, and thyroid can also metastasize to bones at a lesser frequency. The long tubular bones, large flat bones, and the vertebral column are the usual sites for metastatic carcinomas and sarcomas, but the foot and ankle region can occasionally become the site of metastasis.

CHONDROGENIC TUMORS (Figures 9–5—9–24). This group includes chondrosarcoma, chondroma (enchondroma), chondromyxoid fibroma, chondroblastoma, and osteochondroma, the main histologic features of which consist of cartilage cells in different stages of maturation and differentiation in association with a chondroid intercellular matrix. Chondrosarcoma is a malignant bone tumor with a tendency for local recurrence and late metastasis. In contrast, enchondroma, chondromyxoid fibroma, chondroblastoma, and osteochondroma are benign bone tumors that can be treated by local surgical eradication with good long-term results.

A. Chondrosarcoma (Figures 9–5—9–8): the third most common malignant bone tumor, the frequency of which is surpassed only by myeloma and osteogenic sarcoma. Chondrosarcoma has a slight predilection for male adults and usually involves the long tubular bones (femur, tibia, and humerus) and the large flat bones (ilium and scapula).

B. Chondromyxoid Fibroma (Figures 9–9—9–13): an uncommon benign cartilaginous bone tumor characterized by chondroid, fibrous, and myxoid cellular differentiation in a lobulated pattern with a definite predilection for bones of the lower extremity such as the femur, tibia, fibula, and small bones of the foot.

C. Chondroma (enchondroma) (Figures 9–14—9–17): a relatively common benign cartilaginous bone tumor. It is the most common bone tumor of the hands and feet without any particular age or sex predilection.

D. Ollier's Disease (enchondromatosis) (Figure 9–18): a polyostotic form of enchondroma that shows a strong predilection for phalanges and metacarpals of the hand and to a lesser extent for the femur, tibia, and ilium; asymmetric involvement, affecting one part of the body more severely than the other; and a tendency for chondrosarcomatous transformation.

E. Osteochondroma (exostosis) (Figures 9–19—9–21): a benign cartilaginous bone tumor and one of the most common primary bone tumors with a predilection for the lower metaphysis of the femur and the upper metaphysis of the tibia in teenagers.

F. Hereditary Multiple Exostosis (Figure 9–22): characterized by the presence of multiple osteocartilaginous exostoses and inheritance in an autosomally dominant manner. This process shows a predilection for the long tubular bones in a symmetric fashion with some tendency to undergo chondrosarcomatous transformation in time.

G. Chondroblastoma (Figures 9–23 and 9–24): a relatively unusual benign cartilaginous tumor that shows a strong predilection for the epiphyseal region of long tubular bones of adolescents, especially the lower femur, upper tibia, and upper humerus, and affects approximately twice as many male patients as female patients.

FIBROGENIC TUMORS (Figures 9–25—9–39). This classification includes fibrosarcoma, malignant fibrous histiocytoma, giant cell tumor, desmoplastic fibroma, aneurysmal bone cyst, unicameral (solitary) bone cyst, fibrous dysplasia, fibrous cortical defect, and nonossifying (nonosteogenic) fibroma, all of which share the common histologic features of fibroblastic cells and associated collagenous intercellular matrix as important constituents of their tumor tissues. Fibrosarcoma and malignant fibrous histiocytoma are malignant bone tumors that are invasive and have a high local recurrence rate and a propensity for fatal distant metastasis. Giant cell tumor should be treated as a low-grade malignant bone tumor because of its high local recurrence rate, ability to produce nonfatal and rarely fatal metastasis, and liability to undergo sarcomatous degeneration. In contrast, desmoplastic fibroma, aneurysmal bone cyst, unicameral bone cyst, fibrous dysplasia, fibrous cortical defect, and nonossifying fibroma are benign bone tumors that do not produce fatal metastasis and usually respond favorably to local surgical eradication.

A. Unicameral Bone Cyst (Figures 9–25—9–28): a relatively common benign fibrous bone tumor characterized by an attenuated cortical wall that is lined by a thin fibrous membrane containing a straw-colored or serosanguineous fluid. This process shows a proclivity for the metaphyseal and diaphyseal regions of the long tubular bones such as the humerus, femur, tibia, and fibula in the order of decreasing frequency of occurrence.

B. Giant Cell Tumor (Figures 9–29—9–32): a locally aggressive bone tumor of young adults between 20 and 40 years of age. The tumor occurs most often in the epiphyseal ends of the distal femur, proximal tibial, and distal radius with its characteristic multinucleated giant cells, the nuclei of which have a basically identical histologic appearance to those of the stromal cells.

C. Fibrous Dysplasia (Figures 9–33—9–36): a form of bone dysplasia in which normal bone is replaced by an abnormal proliferation of fibrous tissue and abnormal osteoid, resulting in marked deformities of bones. When fibrous dysplasia shows polyostotic involvement, disturbance of endocrine function, and cutaneous cafe-au-lait spots, it is known as Albright's syndrome.

D. Nonossifying (Nonosteogenic) Fibroma (Figures 9–37—9–39): a benign fibrous bone tumor that favors the long tubular bones of the lower limbs of teenagers and tends to show spontaneous healing after skeletal maturity.

OSTEOGENIC TUMORS (Figures 9–40—9–45). These tumors include osteogenic sarcoma (osteosarcoma), parosteal (juxtacortical) osteosarcoma, osteoblastoma, and osteoid osteoma. The presence of many osteoblastic cells with varying histologic features and their ability to produce new bone are the common features shared by these osteogenic tumors. Osteogenic sarcoma and parosteal osteosarcoma are malignant bone tumors with the ability to produce local bone destruction, extraosseous tumor extension, and fatal distant metastases. Osteoblastoma and osteoid osteoma are benign bone tumors that respond favorably to adequate local surgical eradication.

A. Osteogenic Sarcoma (Figures 9–40—9–41): one of the most malignant bone tumors that shows a definite predilection for the long tubular bones, especially the femur, of adolescents and young adults. Its sarcomatous connective tissue can directly produce osteoid and osseous tissue.

B. Osteoid Osteoma (Figures 9–42—9–45): a small, benign, osteoblastic and painful bone tumor with a strong predilection for the femur and tibia of teenagers and young adults.

EWING'S SARCOMA (Figures 9–46 and 9–47). A highly malignant bone tumor thought to arise from undifferentiated mesenchyme of the bone marrow, Ewing's sarcoma most commonly affects patients in their second decade of life and shows a strong proclivity for the ilium and the metaphyseal and diaphyseal regions of the long tubular bones such as the femur, tibia, fibula, and humerus.

VASOGENIC TUMORS (Figures 9–48 and 9–49). Malignant hemangioendothelioma, hemangiopericytoma, hemangioma, and lymphangioma are of this type. Malignant hemangioendothelioma and hemangiopericytoma are frankly malignant bone tumors capable of producing local destruction, extraosseous tumor extension, and fatal distal metastases. In contrast, benign hemangiopericytoma, hemangioma, and lymphangioma are benign processes and do not produce fatal metastases. Massive osteolysis, diffuse hemangiomatosis, and lymphangiomatosis, however, can cause their victims' demise by their involvement of vital visceral organs.

A. Hemangioma (Figures 9–48 and 9–49): a benign vascular bone tumor and the most common form of all the intraosseous vascular tumors. It shows a strong predilection for the axial skeleton (skull and vertebral column), particularly the vertebral bodies at the thoracolumbar junction.

MYELOMA (Figures 9–50 and 9–51). The most common primary bone tumor, myeloma is caused by neoplastic proliferation of a single clone of plasma cells, which have their origin in the primitive marrow reticulum of bones with hematopoietic red marrow, such as the spine, skull, ribs, and pelvis.

LEUKEMIA (Figure 9–52). A systemic neoplastic disease that is characterized by uncontrolled proliferation of hematopoietic cells in the bone marrow and other organs. These cells can be expected to appear in the peripheral blood during the course of the disease.

MALIGNANT SOFT TISSUE TUMORS

SYNOVIAL CELL SARCOMA (Figures 9–53—9–57). A malignant tenosynovial tumor that occurs predominantly in the extremities, particularly in the flexor surfaces of the thigh, ankle, foot, shoulder, and forearm and close to a joint.

MELANOMA (Figures 9–58—9–63). A malignant skin tumor found most frequently on the lower extremities. This process tends to metastasize to regional lymph nodes, liver, and lungs, with skeletal metastasis via the hematogenous route at a lower frequency.

FIBROSARCOMA (Figures 9–64—9–66). A fully malignant fibrogenic tumor that is usually found in the thigh, arm, forearm, buttock, and leg in the order of decreasing frequency of occurrence.

RHABDOMYOSARCOMA (Figure 9–67). A relatively common malignant myogenic tumor, the incidence of which largely depends on its histologic appearance. Pleomorphic (adult) rhabdomyosarcoma is usually found in the thigh, shoulder, and upper arm of adult patients, whereas juvenile rhabdomyosarcomas, which include embryonal, alveolar, and botryoid types, affect many different regions of the body, such as the extremities, trunk, head and neck, and genitourinary tract of children and adolescents.

LIPOSARCOMA (Figures 9–68 and 9–69). The most common malignant, soft somatic tissue sarcoma that may occur wherever adipose tissue is present, but favors the upper and lower extremities and the retroperitoneum of middle-aged or older patients.

MALIGNANT FIBROUS HISTIOCYTOMA (Figures 9–70 and 9–71). This process is a common soft tissue sarcoma and shows a predilection for the upper and lower extremities and the retroperitoneum of male patients between the ages of 50 and 70 years.

CLEAR CELL SARCOMA (malignant melanoma of soft parts) (Figures 9–72 and 9–73). A relatively uncommon soft tissue sarcoma that is usually intimately associated with tendons or aponeuroses, and shows a predilection for the extremities of young adults (between the ages of 20 and 40 years), particularly the foot, ankle, knee, thigh, and hand.

EPITHELIOID SARCOMA (Figures 9–74 and 9–75). A malignant soft tissue tumor of uncertain histogenesis that tends to occur in the hand and forearm regions of adolescents and young adults between 15 and 35 years of age, with a male to female ratio of approximately 2 to 1.

BENIGN SOFT TISSUE TUMORS AND TUMOR-LIKE CONDITIONS

XANTHOMA (GIANT CELL TUMOR OF TENDON SHEATH) (Figures 9–76—9–79). A soft, yellowish-brown benign soft tissue tumor that is usually associated with the tendons of the hands and feet, and has the ability to cause destruction of adjacent bones.

FIBROMATOSES (Figures 9–80—9–83). A family of fibrous proliferative diseases characterized by their infiltrative growth, propensity for local recurrence, and absence of metastasis. Plantar, palmar, penile, extra-abdominal, abdominal, and intra-abdominal fibromatoses and knuckle pads are examples.

LIPOMA (Figures 9–84 and 9–85). The most common benign soft tissue tumor that occurs mainly in persons over 40 years of age in the subcutaneous tissue of the shoulder, back, chest, neck, and thigh.

EPIDERMOID INCLUSION CYST (Figures 9–86—9–88). This growth is caused by displacement of live skin into deeper soft tissues, where proliferation of this ectopic skin produces a cystic subcutaneous tumor mass or, occasionally, underlying bone destruction.

NEUROFIBROMATOSIS (VON RECK-LINGHAUSEN'S DISEASE) (Figures 9–89—9–91). A hereditary and familial disorder of the supportive tissue of both the central and peripheral nervous systems that usually involves the skin. The skeleton and other systems in the body may also be affected.

RHEUMATOID NODULE (Figures 9–92 and 9–93). This process is found in about 20% of all cases of rheumatoid arthritis and is usually located in the subcutaneous tissue of the olecranon area of the elbow.

TUMORAL CALCINOSIS (Figure 9–94). A rare idiopathic disease that produces calcium salt deposit in soft tissues about joints, and most frequently affects children and adolescents with some familial tendency.

CALLUS (Figure 9–95). An accumulation of hypertrophied horny layer of squamous epithelium caused by excessive pressure on any bony prominences.

BONE DYSPLASIAS

Bone dysplasias are members of a family of interesting diseases of the skeleton with their individual predilections for the epiphyseal, physeal, metaphyseal, and diaphyseal regions of the bones.

EPIPHYSEAL DYSPLASIA (Figures 9–96—9–99).

A. Stippled Epiphyses (Dysplasia Epiphysealis Punctata or Chondrodystrophia Calcificans Congenita) (Figure 9–96): an uncommon, nonfamilial congenital disease characterized by the presence of multiple punctate opacities in the nonossified cartilage, short extremities, and varying degrees of flexion contracture of the hip, knee, and elbow joints.

B. Multiple Epiphyseal Dysplasia (Dysplasia Epiphysealis Multiplex) (Figure 9–97): a rare familial congenital disease characterized by irregular outline and density of many epiphyses, dwarfism, and stubby digits. Early onset of degenerative arthritis of many joints results.

C. Tarsal Epiphyseal Aclasia (Dysplasia Epiphysealis Hemimelica or Osteochondroma of the Epiphysis) (Figure 9–98): characterized by the unilateral presence of an osteochondroma in the epiphyseal portion of the hip, knee, or ankle joint, which usually produces cosmetic deformity and functional impairment of the affected joint.

D. Diastrophic Dwarfism (Figure 9–99): a rare congenital epiphyseal dysostosis characterized by the presence of retarded growth (dwarfism), talipes equinovarus, scoliosis, and hitchhiker's thumb, which is the most outstanding feature of this disease.

PHYSEAL (GROWTH PLATE) DYSPLASIA (Figures 9–100—9–104).

A. Achondroplasia (Figures 9–100 and 9–101): characterized by a pronounced shortness of the extremities (micromelia), enlargement of the head with a depression at the root of the nose, dwarfism, and marked disturbance of endochondral bone growth. This form is produced sporadically as a result of gene mutation or is inherited in an autosomally dominant manner.

B. Marfan's Disease (Hyperchondroplasia or Arachnodactyly) (Figure 9–102): characterized by the presence of ectopia lentis, aortic aneurysm, pectus excavatum, lanky body stature, long and tapering digits (arachnodactyly or spider legs), and rocker-bottom flatfeet.

C. Peripheral Dysostosis (Figure 9–103): a form of physeal dysostosis characterized by varying degrees of chondroectodermal dysplasia such as defective nails, defective limb bones, and aplasia and hypoplasia of short tubular bones.

D. Metaphyseal Dysostosis of Jansen (Metaphyseal Chondrodysplasia) (Figure 9–104): an extremely rare form of physeal dysplasia characterized by the presence of radiolucent and knobby metaphyseal regions caused by masses of proliferating cartilage which results from an irregular attempt to form hypertrophic cartilage.

E. Ollier's Disease (Enchondromatosis or Multiple Enchondromas): has been discussed previously.

METAPHYSEAL DYSPLASIA (Figure 9–105).

A. Osteopetrosis (Albers-Schönberg Disease or Chalk Bones) (Figure 9–105): caused by failure or inhibition of resorption of calcified chondroid and primitive bone (primary spongiosa), resulting in a generalized marble-like skeleton, stunted growth, optic nerve atrophy, deafness, facial nerve palsy, frequent occurrence of osteomyelitis of the jaw, brittle bones, myelophthisic anemia, and hepatomegaly.

B. Hereditary Multiple Exostoses (Osteochondromatosis or Diaphyseal Aclasia): has been discussed previously.

DIAPHYSEAL DYSPLASIA.

A. Osteogenesis Imperfecta (Figure 9–106): can appear sporadically as a result of gene mutation or is inherited in an autosomally dominant manner. This disease is characterized by bone fragility, slate blue sclerae, poor teeth, progressive deafness, hyperlaxity of joints, and thinness of the skin. The fundamental abnormality of this disease is most likely due to defective formation, organization, and chemical composition of the collagen in the body, resulting in disturbed endochondral and intramembranous bone formation, evidenced by the poor quality and quantity of bone.

THE MUCOPOLYSACCHARIDOSES (Figures 9–107 and 9–108). A family of related diseases caused by failure of the normal metabolic maturation of fibroblasts. This failure results in the presence of abnormal quantities of mucopolysaccharides, which interfere with the normal function and development of many body systems.

A. Morquio's Disease (Figure 9–107): a genetic disease that is inherited in an autosomally recessive manner and produces an abnormal quantity of mucopolysaccharides, which interfere with the normal growth of the skeleton; dwarfism, kyphosis, and deformities of many bones and joints result.

B. Hurler's Disease (Gargoylism) (Figure 9–108): causes skeletal deformities, mental retardation, blindness, splenohepatomegaly, and significantly increased urinary excretion of mucopolysaccharides.

MISCELLANEOUS BONE DYSPLASIA.

A. Apert's Syndrome (Acrocephalosyndactylism) (Figure 9–109): a congenital disturbance in the growth of bone and soft tissues characterized by an elongated and peaked head and various degrees of syndactylism of the hands and feet.

DISEASES OF THE JOINTS

RHEUMATOID ARTHRITIS (Figure 9–110). A systemic connective tissue disease of uncertain etiology that causes destruction of the articular and periarticular structures, especially the knees and small joints of the hands, wrists, and feet.

PSORIATIC ARTHRITIS (Figures 9–111 and 9–112). A disease complex characterized by the presence of cutaneous psoriasis and inflammatory polyarthritis and the absence of rheumatoid nodules and serum rheumatoid factor.

GOUT (Figures 9–113—9–117). A disturbance in uric acid metabolism in which an excessive amount of uric acid is produced and then is deposited in different mesenchymal tissues as sodium monourate crystals initiates an inflammatory reaction in the affected tissues. Primary gout is inherited in an autosomally dominant manner, and over 90% of cases occur in male subjects. In contrast, secondary gout is caused by excessive breakdown of nucleoproteins in diseases like polycythemia, leukemia, lymphomas, multiple myeloma, and sickle-cell anemia.

CHARCOT'S JOINT (NEUROTROPHIC ARTHROPATHY) (Figures 9–118—9–121). This disease manifests itself as severe joint destruction, swelling, instability, and loose bodies, is associated with amazingly little discomfort, and is caused by diabetic neuropathy, tabes dorsalis, congenital insensitivity to pain, leprosy, diseases of the spinal cord, and injury or inflammation of peripheral nerves.

HEMOPHILIC ARTHRITIS (Figure 9–122). This process is caused by repeated and excessive bleeding into a joint, resulting in synovial proliferation, fibrosis, and hemosiderosis, and in destruction of the articular cartilage by enzymatic degradation. Hemophilia is inherited in a sex-linked recessive manner; its etiology pertains to a deficiency of a plasma coagulation protein, antihemophilic factor (Factor VIII).

PULMONARY HYPERTROPHIC OSTEOARTHROPATHY (Figure 9–123). This condition, caused by different pulmonary diseases, is manifested clinically by clubbing of the ends of the fingers and toes, periosteal new bone formation of the long tubular bones of the extremities, and pain and swelling of joints.

SYNOVIAL CHONDROMATOSIS (OSTEOCHONDROMATOSIS) (Figures 9–124 and 9–125). A benign disease in which foci of cartilage develop in the synovial membrane of a joint. The knee joints of young or middle-aged adults are primarily affected.

PYOGENIC (SUPPURATIVE) ARTHRITIS (Figures 9–126 and 9–127). This disease is usually caused by *Staphylococcus aureus* and most often affects the knee and hip joints. Septicemia, trauma, surgery, and para-articular soft tissue and bone infections can all cause septic arthritis.

TUBERCULOUS ARTHRITIS (Figures 9–128 and 9–129). This condition is caused by an acid-fast bacillus, *Mycobacterium tu-*

berculosis, and has a predilection for the intervertebral disc space and the hip and knee joints.

INFECTIOUS DISEASES

PYOGENIC (SUPPURATIVE) OSTEO-MYELITIS (Figures 9–130—9–136). Commonly caused by *Staphylococcus aureus* that can become established in any bone by means of a hematogenous or lymphatic route, compound fracture, surgery, or direct extension of infection from the soft tissues surrounding the bone, this disease shows a predilection for the long tubular bones (e.g., femur, tibia, humerus, and radius, in descending order of frequency of occurrence) of male children under 12 years of age.

TUBERCULOSIS OF BONE (Figures 9–137—9–140). This condition is usually secondary to a tuberculous infection of the lungs, and shows a predilection for the vertebral bodies, the upper end of the femur, and the ends of long tubular bones near large joints of prepubertal children.

LEPROSY (HANSEN'S DISEASE) (Figures 9–141 and 9–142). A chronic infectious disease caused by an acid-fast bacillus, *Myobacterium leprae* (Hansen's bacillus), that principally affects the skin, certain peripheral nerves, mucous membranes of the respiratory system, and the testes. Bone changes are most apparent in the ends of the short tubular bones of the hands and feet.

CONGENITAL SYPHILIS (Figures 9–143 and 9–144). This condition is causd by a bacterium called *Treponema pallidum,* which crosses the placenta from an infected mother to her fetus. Bone syphilis most frequently involves the tibia, femur, humerus, and cranial bones.

CONGENITAL RUBELLA (GERMAN MEASLES) SYNDROME (Figure 9–145). This disease is caused by the infection of a pregnant woman by the rubella virus during the first trimester of pregnancy. A wide spectrum of abnormalities in the baby can result, which may include growth retardation, hepatosplenomegaly, thrombocytopenia, central nervous system disorders, skeletal abnormalities, cataracts, glaucoma, and congenital heart disease.

CIRCULATORY DISTURBANCES

ASEPTIC NECROSIS OF BONE (OSTEO-NECROSIS) (Figures 9–146—9–151). This process is caused by deprivation or inadequacy of the blood supply to bone, which results in bone necrosis that may or may not become revascularized with time.

A. Köhler's Disease (Figure 9–146): caused by aseptic necrosis of the tarsal navicular, which more frequently affects boys than girls (male to female ratio is approximately 3 to 1), with the average age of onset of symptoms being about 5 years for boys and 4 years for girls.

B. Freiberg's Disease (Figure 9–147): caused by aseptic necrosis of the second metatarsal head, and has a propensity to affect female adolescents with a female to male ratio of approximately 3 to 1.

C. Osteochondritis of the Sesamoid (Figure 9–148): caused by aseptic necrosis of the sesamoid, and has a definite predilection for the medial sesamoid in adolescent girls and young women.

D. Aseptic Necrosis of the First Metatarsal Head (Figure 9–149): is usually iatrogenically induced, especially after distal osteotomy of the first metatarsal for correction of hallux valgus deformity. Extensive stripping of all the soft tissue attachments from the first metatarsal head prior to the distal osteotomy is usually responsible for the subsequent development of aseptic necrosis of the first metatarsal head.

E. Aseptic Necrosis of the Body of the Talus (Figure 9–150): is the most common complication of fracture of the talar neck and has an overall incidence of between 21 and 58%.

F. Osteochondritis Dissecans of the Talus (Figure 9–151): is most likely caused by

trauma by which the lateral edge of the talus strikes the medial aspect of the lateral malleolus to produce a small osteochondral fracture of the lateral talar dome. The same lesion can also involve the medial talar dome at a lesser frequency.

ASEPTIC NECROSIS OF SOFT TISSUES (Figures 9–152—9–156). This process can be caused by freezing, heat, electricity, caustic chemicals, radiation, vascular laceration or thrombosis, and arteriosclerotic diseases.

SUDECK'S ATROPHY (REFLEX SYMPA-THETIC DYSTROPHY) (Figure 9–157) This disease is caused by a neurogenically induced vasospasm of terminal portions of the arterioles that develops in response to traumas, resulting in osteoporosis, pain, edema, tenderness, cyanosis, coldness, sweating, and stiffness of the involved extremities.

ARTERIOVENOUS FISTULA (Figure 9–158). A congenital or acquired vascular anomaly in which blood flows directly from an artery into a vein without first passing through the arteriole, capillaries, and venule.

MILROY'S DISEASE (LYMPHANGIEC-TASIS) (Figure 9–159). A familial disease in which malformation of the lymphatic system produces enlarged and edematous extremities, which in later life can take on the appearance of elephantiasis when extensive fibrosis has developed.

METABOLIC DISEASES

OSTEOMALACIA (Figure 9–160). An adult form of rickets caused by lack of vitamin D intake, diseases of the gastrointestinal tract, and renal tubular dysfunctions. The disorder is manifested clinically by hypophosphatemia, elevated serum levels of alkaline phosphatase, hypocalcemia, bone pain, increasing muscular weakness, multiple pseudofractures, muscle spasm and tenderness, loss of body height, back pain, and osteopenia, and microscopically by the presence of many wide osteoid seams that result from slow osteoid mineralization (prolonged bone formation time).

RICKETS (Figure 9–161). A condition caused by deficient vitamin D intake, diseases of the gastrointestinal tract, and renal tubular dysfunctions in children that is manifested clinically by hypophosphatemia, elevated serum levels of alkaline phosphatase, hypocalcemia, genu varum or valgum, gross enlargement of joints of the upper and lower extremities, rachitic rosary of the costochondral junction, pigeon breast, dorsal kyphosis, lumbar lordosis, waddling gait, increasing muscular weakness, generalized growth retardation, widening of epiphyseal zones with flaring, and a tuft-like configuration of the metaphyseal ends of long tubular bones. Microscopically, rickets presents with many wide osteoid seams caused by slow osteoid mineralization (prolonged bone formation time).

SCURVY (Figure 9–162). Scurvy is caused by a deficiency of vitamin C (ascorbic acid), and usually appears between 6 to 9 months of age. The disease is manifested clinically by irritability, tenderness and weakness of the lower extremities, scorbutic rosary of the ribs, pseudoparalysis, bleeding of the gums, fever, and failure to thrive. Radiological signs of scurvy include a dense metaphyseal line (white line of Frankel), lateral metaphyseal spur (Pelkan spur), a radiolucent zone immediately next to Frankel's white line (Trummerfeld's zone), cortical thinning and ground glass appearance of the diaphysis, a radiodense ring around ossification centers (Wimberger's ring), and subperiosteal bone formation due to hemorrhage.

OSTEOPOROSIS (Figure 9–163). Defined as a decrease in the amount of purely osseous tissue per unit volume of bone, osteoporosis can be produced by a variety of diseases, which include senile and postmenopausal osteoporosis, Cushing's syndrome, acromegaly, osteogenesis imperfecta, polycythemia vera, prolonged heparin therapy, Gaucher's disease, multiple myeloma, lymphomas, leukemias, systemic mastocytosis, metastases, ankylosing spondylitis, hyperparathyroidism, hepatogenic osteoporosis, hyperthyroidism, prolonged systemic steroid therapy, osteoporosis associated with ulcerative colitis, and disuse osteoporosis. Whenever bone resorption exceeds bone formation, a negative skeletal balance is created. If this bone-losing process is allowed to continue, it inevitably leads to osteoporosis.

PRIMARY HYPERPARATHYROIDISM (OSTEITIS FIBROSA CYSTICA, OR VON RECKLINGHAUSEN'S DISEASE) (Figure 9–164). Caused by parathyroid adenoma, diffuse hyperplasia of all parathyroids, and parathyroid carcinoma, this condition is characterized by hypercalcemia, hypophosphatemia, elevated serum alkaline phosphatase levels, high serum levels of parathormone, pain in the limbs and back, generalized muscle weakness, pathologic fractures, deformity of the limbs and spine, polyuria, polydypsia, renal calculi, and disseminated deossification with formation of osteolytic cystic lesions called brown tumors.

LEAD POISONING (Figure 9–165). This disease is caused by ingestion of a large amount of lead-containing materials. Clinical manifestations include abdominal cramps, encephalopathy, peripheral neuritis, anemia, increased serum levels of free erythrocyte protoporphyrin, stippling of erythrocytes, high serum levels of lead, and the presence of radiodense metaphyseal bands (lead lines).

DIABETES MELLITUS. A hereditary disease caused by defective pancreatic beta cells, which are not able to produce sufficient amounts of insulin to meet the body's metabolic needs. Dysfunction of many body systems results, which may include serious diseases like blindness, renal failure, arteriosclerosis, and peripheral neuropathy. The major foot problems caused by diabetes mellitus consist of infections, diabetic gangrene, and neurotrophic arthropathy, which have been discussed.

GOUT. This disturbance of the uric acid metabolism has been discussed previously.

CONGENITAL ANOMALIES

ABNORMALITIES OF THE TOES (Figures 9–166—9–175).

A. Adactyly (Figure 9–166 and 9–167): the absence of digits on the hand or foot. It can be in the form of complete (absence of all digits) or partial adactyly (absence of one or more digits).

B. Polydactyly (Figures 9–168—9–170): commonly occurs in the foot and may require toe amputation for cosmetic reasons or for the ease of wearing shoes. The most peripheral toe is usually amputated.

C. Syndactyly (Figures 9–171 and 9–172): usually occurs between the second and third toes and usually does not produce disability or dysfunction. Syndactyly usually involves the skin of the interdigital webspace, but can occasionally produce synostosis of the neighboring phalangeal bones.

D. Microdactyly (Figure 9–173): usually an isolated deformity that may be associated with hypoplasia of the corresponding metatarsal or adjacent phalanges. A hypoplastic digit usually does not produce symptoms and thus requires no treatment.

E. Macrodactyly (Figure 9–174): can be idiopathic or caused by neurofibromatosis, lymphangioma, and hemangioma. The condition frequently requires resection of bone and hypertrophied soft tissues to allow proper shoe fitting and to achieve a cosmetically acceptable appearance.

F. Divergent Toes (Figure 9–175): usually involves the second and third toes and may require surgical syndactylization if the digits become symptomatic.

ABNORMALITIES OF THE METATARSAL REGION (Figures 9–176—9–181).

A. Lobster Clawfoot (Congenital Split or Cleft Foot) (Figures 9–176 and 9–177): caused by the absence of two or three central digital rays of the foot, and may be associated with hallux valgus, lobster clawing of the hand, cleft palate, syndactyly, polydactyly, triphalangeal thumb, and deafness.

B. Down's Syndrome (Mongolism) (Figure 9–178): caused by trisomy 21 (three number 21 chromosomes), which produces mental retardation as well as ocular, skeletal, gastrointestinal, and other abnormalities.

C. Familial Medial Cleft of the Foot (Figure 9–179): a familial, bilaterally symmetric, longitudinal plantar skin cleft between the first and second toes that is usually completely asymptomatic and requires no treatment.

D. Multiple Metatarsal Sesamoids (Figure 9–180): can vary tremendously in number and are usually completely asymptomatic.

E. Congenital Short Metatarsal (Figure 9–181): typically involves the fourth metatarsal and produces a markedly shortened fourth digital ray. Metatarsalgia of its neighboring metatarsal heads due to loss of weight-bearing function of the shortened metatarsal may also occur.

ABNORMALITIES OF THE TARSAL AND ANKLE REGIONS (Figures 9–182—9–188).

A. Congenital Vertical Talus (Congenital Convex Pes Valgus) (Figures 9–182 and 9–183): caused by a dislocation of the talonavicular joint in which the navicular articulates with the dorsal aspect of the talus in association with soft tissue contractures of the hindfoot and midfoot, and subluxation of the midtarsal, subtalar, and ankle joints.

B. Congenital Deficiency or Absence of the Tibia (Figures 9–184—9–186): commonly associated with malformations of the ipsilateral femur, absence of one or more rays of the foot, partial absence of the fibula, and marked deformity of the ankle and foot regions.

C. Congenital Deficiency or Absence of the Fibula (Figures 9–187 and 9–188): can be associated with malformations of the femur and tibia, and is frequently accompanied by the absence of the two lateral rays and valgus deformity of the foot.

MISCELLANEOUS DISORDERS OF THE FOOT

CAFFEY'S DISEASE (INFANTILE CORTICAL HYPEROSTOSIS) (Figure 9–189). A disease of uncertain etiology that is characterized by massive subperiosteal new bone formation about the diaphyses of the long tubular bones, mandible, and clavicle in infants under 6 months of age.

SARCOIDOSIS (Figures 9–190 and 9–191). A granulomatous and inflammatory disease commonly affecting the lymph nodes, spleen, lungs, liver, and small bones of the hands and feet.

PAGET'S DISEASE (OSTEITIS DEFORMANS) (Figures 9–192 and 9–193). A chronic bone disease of unknown etiology that is characterized by its predilection for the pelvis, femur, skull, tibia, and spine of middle-aged or older males; elevation of serum alkaline phosphatase levels; thickening, osteosclerosis, and deformity of osseous structures; microscopic features of dense cement lines and a mosaic pattern, increased fibrosis of the marrow space, and an increased number of osteoclasts per unit volume of bone; liability for pathologic fractures and sarcomatous degeneration; and neural compression caused by bony enlargement or malignant degeneration.

AINHUM (DACTYLOLYSIS SPONTANEA) (Figure 9–194). An interesting dermatologic disorder of African blacks that typically involves the fifth toes of male patients in their fourth and fifth decades of life. These individuals develop a hyperkeratotic fibrous band within the epidermis of the affected toe that gradually deepens, encircles the toe, and is accompanied by ulceration and bony resorption. Autoamputation results in severe cases.

COOLEY'S ANEMIA (THALASSEMIA MAJOR) (Figure 9–195). A serious hematolytic anemia seen mainly in infants and young children that is characterized by the presence of both alpha and beta thalassemiae in which

the synthesis of the alpha and beta polypeptide chains of the hemoglobins is partially or completely suppressed. The result is progressive anemia, yellowish skin discoloration due to hemolysis, hepatosplenomegaly, stunted growth, generalized osteoporosis, and susceptibility to intercurrent infections and cardiac failure.

MANDARIN FOOT (Figure 9–196). An acquired deformity produced by tightly binding young children's feet daily to achieve severe retardation of the normal growth of these bound feet, which were regarded as signs of great beauty. This practice was commonly performed on young Chinese girls of high class or from wealthy families during the many dynasties preceding the birth of the Republic of China.

MYOSITIS OSSIFICANS PROGRESSIVA (Figure 9–197). A rare congenital disease characterized by microdactyly and progressive ossification of soft somatic tissues such as fasciae, aponeuroses, ligaments, and tendons that results in marked restriction of motion of the neck, spine, shoulders, elbows, hips, and knees and in severe disability.

CONGENITAL PSEUDARTHROSIS OF THE TIBIA (Figure 9–198). A rare disease, but one commonly associated with neurofibromatosis. The replacement of normal fracture callus by hamartomatous soft tissue at the tibial and fibular fracture sites is responsible for the persistence of pseudarthrosis, which may eventually require a Syme's amputation.

ARTHROGRYPOSIS MULTIPLEX CONGENITA (Figures 9–199 and 9–200). This condition is characterized by multiple and often symmetric joint contractures, decreased muscle mass, muscle contractures, and numerous deformities of the upper and lower extremities, which may include clubfeet, clubhands, dislocation of the hips and radial heads, subluxation or dislocation of the knees, and the absence of normal skin creases.

DERMATOMYOSITIS (Figure 9–201). An inflammatory and degenerative disease of the skin and skeletal muscles that tends to affect the proximal muscles of the extremities more frequently and severely than the distal ones. Atrophy, degeneration, fibrosis, and contracture of the involved muscles and extensive subcutaneous and periarticular calcifications result.

CALCIFIC BURSITIS OR TENDONITIS (Figures 9–202—9–204). Caused by heterotopic amorphous calcium deposits in a bursa, or in or around a tendon, calcific bursitis or tendonitis is frequently associated with localized signs of inflammation, such as pain, tenderness, swelling, redness, and warmth.

STRESS FRACTURE (Figures 9–205—9–208). A fatigue fracture that occurs in a normal bone that is subjected to excessive and repeated stress. The metatarsals, calcaneus, proximal tibial and distal femoral diaphyses, femoral neck, and pubic rami are the more common sites of stress fractures.

REFERENCES

1. Aegerter, E., and Kirkpatrick, J.A.: Orthopaedic Diseases. Philadelphia, W.B. Saunders, 1975.
2. Anderson, W.A.D., and Kissane, J.M. (eds): Pathology. 7th Ed. St. Louis, C.V. Mosby, 1977.
3. Edmonson, A.S., and Crenshaw, A.H. (eds.): Campbell's Operative Orthopaedics. 6th Ed. St. Louis, C.V. Mosby, 1980.
4. Giannestras, N.J.: Foot Disorders. 2nd Ed. Philadelphia, Lea & Febiger, 1973.
5. Greenfield, G.B.: Radiology of Bone Diseases. 3rd Ed. Philadelphia, J.B. Lippincott, 1980.
6. Hoeprich, P.D. (ed.) Infectious Diseases. 3rd Ed. New York, Harper & Row, 1983.
7. Huvos, A.G.: Bone Tumors. Philadelphia, W.B. Saunders, 1979.
8. Jaffee, H.L.: Metabolic, Degenerative, and Inflammatory Diseases of Bones and Joints. Philadelphia, Lea & Febiger, 1972.
9. Jahss, M.H. (ed.): Disorders of the Foot. Philadelphia, W.B. Saunders, 1982.
10. Jett, S., Wu, K., Duncan, H., and Frost, H.M.: Adrenalcorticoid and salicylate actions in human and canine haversian bone remodeling. Clin. Orthop., *68:*301, 1969.
11. Juhl, J.H.: Essentials of Roentgen Interpretation. 4th Ed. New York, Harper & Row, 1981.
12. Kelikian, H.: Hallux Valgus, Allied Deformities of the Forefoot and Metatarsalgia. Philadelphia, W.B. Saunders, 1965.
13. Kelley, W.N., Harris, E.D., Ruddy, S., and Sledge, C.B.: Textbook of Rheumatology. Philadelphia, W.B. Saunders, 1981.
14. Klenerman, L.: The Foot and Its Disorders. London, Blackwell Scientific Publications, 1976.
15. Lichtenstein, L.: Bone Tumors. 5th Ed. St. Louis, C.V. Mosby, 1977.
16. Lovell, W.W., and Winter, R.: Pediatric Orthopaedics. Philadelphia, J.B. Lippincott, 1978.
17. Mann, R.A. (ed.): DuVries' Surgery of the Foot. 4th Ed. St. Louis, C.V. Mosby, 1978.
18. McCarty, D.J. (ed.): Arthritis and Allied Conditions. 9th Ed. Philadelphia, Lea & Febiger, 1979.
19. Mirra, J.M.: Bone Tumors: Diagnosis and Treatment. Philadelphia, J.B. Lippincott, 1980.
20. Petersdorf, K.G., et al. (eds.): Harrison's Principles of Internal Medicine. 10th Ed. New York, McGraw-Hill, 1983.
21. Resnick, D., and Niwayama, G.: Diagnosis of Bone and Joint Disorders. Philadelphia, W.B. Saunders, 1981.
22. Robbins, S.L., and Cotran, R.S.: Pathologic basis of Disease. 2nd Ed. Philadelphia, W.B. Saunders, 1979.
23. Rosai, J.: Ackerman's Surgical Pathology. 6th Ed. St. Louis, C.V. Mosby, 1981.
24. Tachdjian, M.O.: Pediatric Orthopaedics. Philadelphia, W.B. Saunders, 1972.
25. Turek, S.L.: Orthopaedics: Principles and Their Applications. 3rd Ed. Philadelphia, J.B. Lippincott, 1977.
26. Williams, R.H. (ed.): Textbook of Endocrinology. 6th Ed. Philadelphia, W.B. Saunders, 1981.
27. Wu, K.K.: Diagnosis and Treatment of Polyostotic Spinal Tumors. Springfield, Charles C Thomas, 1982.
28. Wu, K.K.: Diagnosis and Treatment of Benign and Malignant Monostotic Tumors of the Spine. Detroit, National, 1984.
29. Wu, K., and Frost, H.M.: Bone formation in osteoporosis. Arch. Pathol. Lab. Med., *88:*508, 1969.
30. Wu, K.K., and Guise, E.R.: Metastatic tumors of the foot. South. Med. J., *71:*807, 1978.
31. Wu, K.K., and Guise, E.R.: Chondrosarcoma of the foot: A report of the three new cases plus a review of the medical literature. Orthopedics, *1:*380, 1978.
32. Wu, K., Jett, S., and Frost, H.M.: Measurement and evaluation of intracortical and cortical-endosteal bone formation in senile and postmenopausal osteoporosis. J. Bone Joint Surg. [Am.], *49:*796, 1967.
33. Wu, K., Jett, S., and Frost, H.M.: Bone resorption rates in ribs in physiological senile and postmenopausal osteoporosis. J. Lab. Clin. Med., *69:*810, 1967.
34. Wu, K., Schubeck, K.E., Frost, H.M., and Villaneuva, A.: Haversian bone formation rates determined by a new method in a mastodon and in human diabetes mellitus and osteoporosis. Calcif. Tissue Int., *6:*205, 1970.
35. Wyngaarden, J.B., and Smith, L.H. (eds.): Cecil Textbook of Medicine. 16th Ed. Philadelphia, W.B. Saunders, 1982.

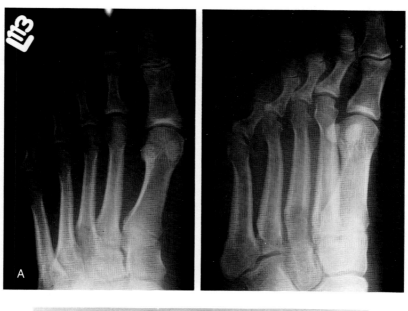

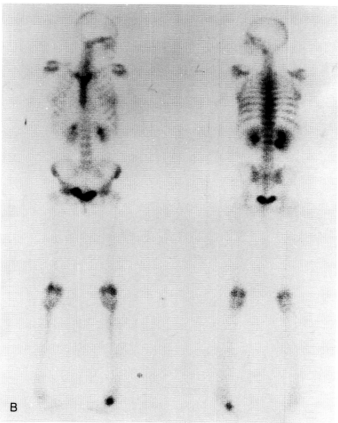

Figure 9–1. A 40-year-old woman, who was a heavy smoker for 25 years, had a constant ache in the dorsal aspect of her left foot for 3 to 4 weeks. **A,** anteroposterior and oblique radiographs of her left foot show an osteolytic lesion in the base of the third metatarsal without any periosteal reaction. **B,** bone scan shows markedly increased radionuclide uptake in the left metatarsal region.

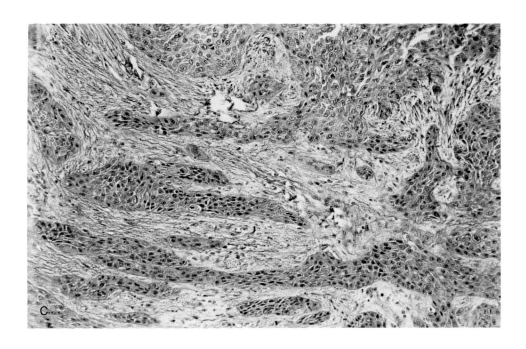

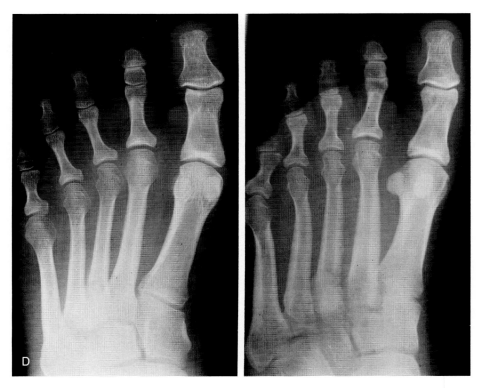

Figure 9–1. Continued. C, frozen section analysis of the third metatarsal lesion revealed squamous cell carcinoma (175×, H.&E.). The primary site was subsequently found to be the lungs. **D,** after thorough curettage of the lesion, the bony defect was filled with methylmethacrylate bone cement.

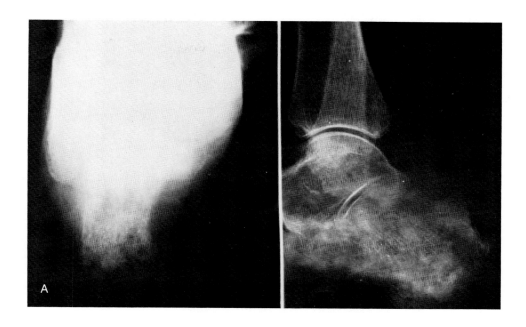

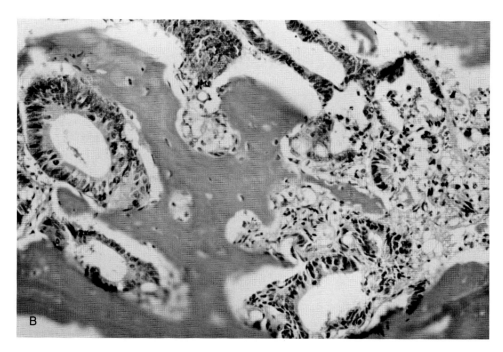

Figure 9-2. A 79-year-old man had increasing pain and swelling of his right heel for 3 months. Radiographs of his right hindfoot (**A,** axial and lateral views) show diffuse destruction of the whole calcaneus caused by (**B**) a metastatic adenocarcinoma (300×, H.&E.) of cecal origin. (From Wu, K.K., and Guise, E.R.: Metastatic tumors of the foot. South. Med. J., *71*:807, 1978, with permission).

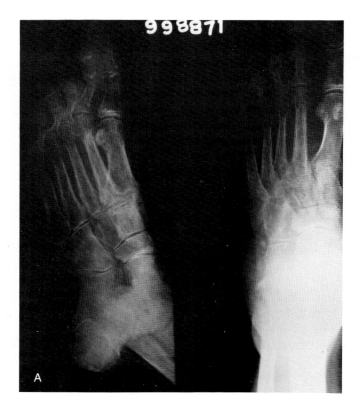

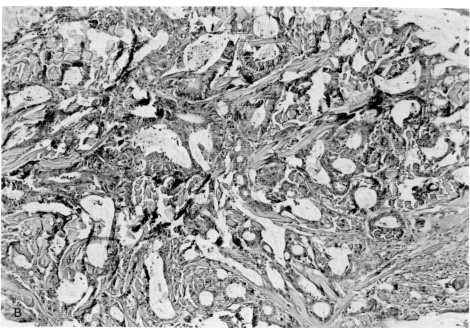

Figure 9–3. A 71-year-old man had pain and swelling of his left ankle for several months. Oblique and anteroposterior views show a generalized mottled appearance of the left talus. Subsequent biopsy (**B**) revealed the presence of a metastatic carcinoma (105×, H.&E.) with its origin in the sigmoid colon. (From Wu, K.K., and Guise, E.R.: Metastatic tumors of the foot. South. Med. J., *71*:807, 1978, with permission.)

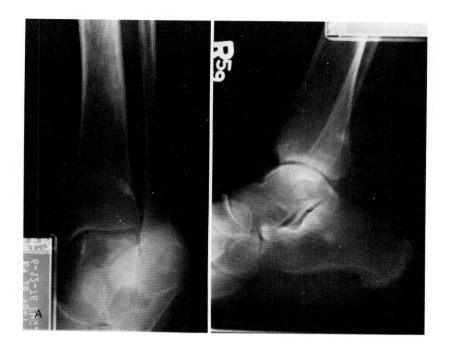

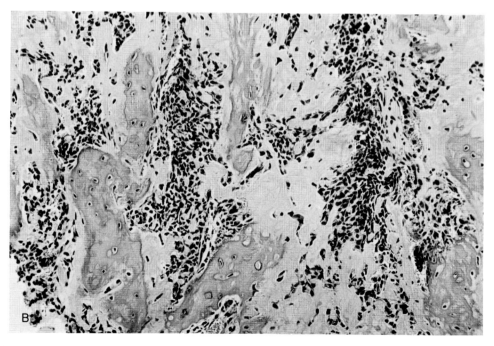

Figure 9–4. A 43-year-old man had osteoblastic metastatic lesions in his right distal tibia, talus, and calcaneus, (**A,** mortise and lateral views) the origin of which was in a right humeral osteogenic sarcoma (**B,** 100×, H.&E.). (From Wu. K.K., and Guise, E.R.: Metastatic tumors of the foot. South. Med. J., *71*:807, 1978, with permission.)

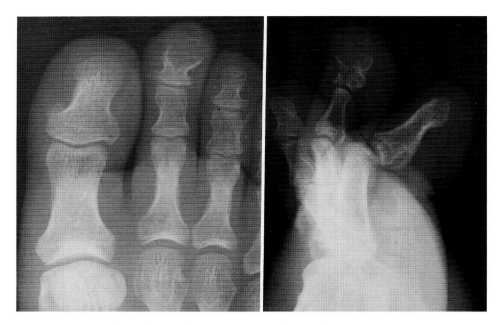

Figure 9–5. A 36-year-old man had increasing pain and swelling of his right second toe for 3 to 4 months. Anteroposterior and lateral radiographs of the forefoot show soft tissue swelling, cortical expansion and destruction, and extension of the tumor tissue into the soft tissue at the tip of second toe caused by a chondrosarcoma. Amputation of the second toe was required. (From Wu, K.K., and Guise, E.R.: Chondrosarcoma of the foot: A report of three new cases plus a review of the medical literature. Orthopedics, *1*:380, 1978, with permission.)

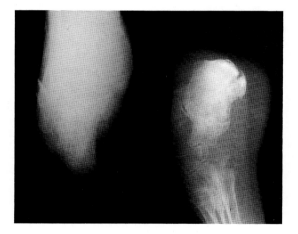

Figure 9–6. A 53-year-old woman had increasing pain and swelling of her left heel for the past ten months. Axial and lateral views of the hindfoot show diffuse and mottled destruction of the calcaneus, an accompanying pathologic fracture through the calcaneal tuberosity, and soft tissue swelling caused by a chondrosarcoma. A below-knee amputation was required. (From Wu, K.K., and Guise, E.R.: Chondrosarcoma of the foot: A report of three new cases plus a review of the medical literature. Orthopedics, *1*:380, 1978, with permission.)

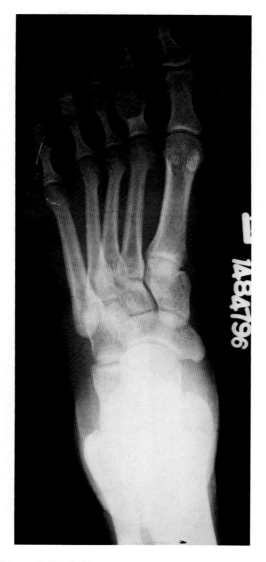

Figure 9–7. A 22-year-old woman complained of pain and swelling of her left second toe for 2 months. Radiography revealed marked cortical expansion and trabecular destruction of the left second proximal phalanx caused by a chondrosarcoma. The tumor was treated by amputation of the second toe. (From Wu, K.K., and Guise, E.R.: Chondrosarcoma of the foot: A report of three new cases plus a review of the medical literature. Orthopedics, *1*:380, 1978, with permission.)

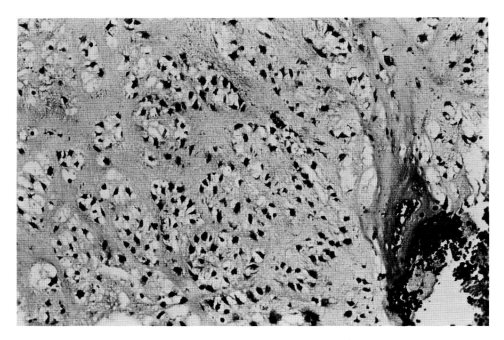

Figure 9–8. Photomicrograph (175×, H.&E.) showing the typical features of a chondrosarcoma: hypercellularity, pleomorphic and plump nuclei, hyperchromatism, and many doubly nucleated lacunae.

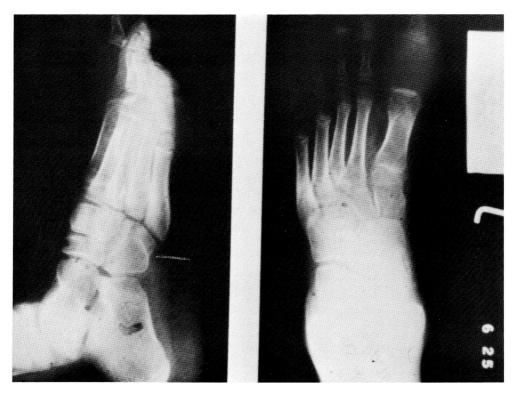

Figure 9–9. A 10-year-old girl had a chondromyxoid fibroma in the proximal phalanx of her left great toe, which produced complete destruction of the whole bone.

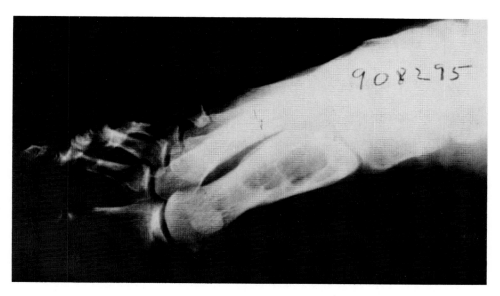

Figure 9–10. A 23-year-old man had a chondromyxoid fibroma in his right first metatarsal, which produced a loculated radiographic appearance with a thin osteosclerotic rim around the lesion.

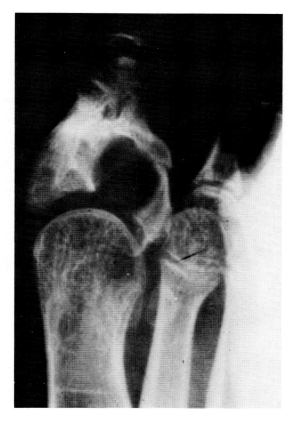

Figure 9–11. An 11-year-old boy had a chondromyxoid fibroma in the proximal phalanx of his right great toe, which produced a round, punched-out lesion in the proximal portion.

399

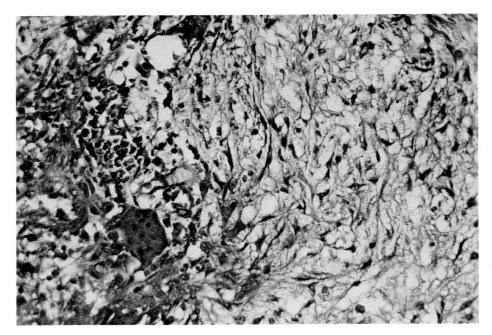

Figure 9–12. Photomicrograph (450×, H.&E.) showing a myxomatous area on the right and a somewhat fibrous area on the left with a multinucleated giant cell, some of the typical histologic features of a chondromyxoid fibroma.

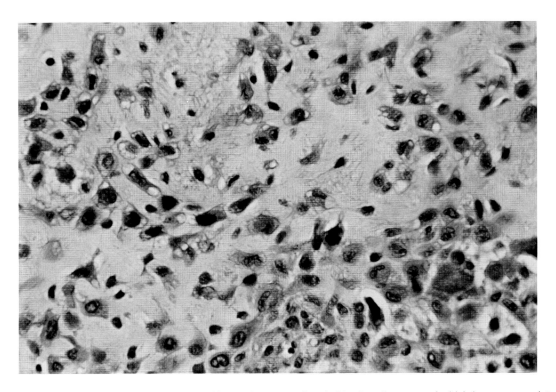

Figure 9–13. Photomicrograph (450×, H.&E.) showing many chondroblastic cells, some of which have a vacuolated cytoplasm and the beginning of formation of cartilaginous lacunae, which are common features of many chondrogenic tumors.

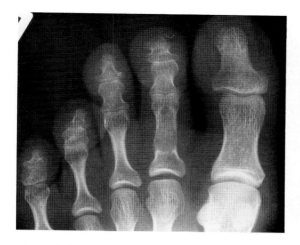

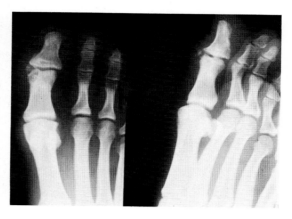

Figure 9–14. A 35-year-old man had an asymptomatic enchondroma in the proximal phalanx of his left second toe that was discovered accidentally. Note the stippled calcification and the cortical erosion and expansion produced by this cartilaginous tumor.

Figure 9–15. A 25-year-old man sought medical attention because of a small hard lump on the dorsomedial aspect of his right great toe, which proved to be a chondroma.

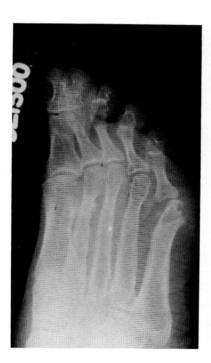

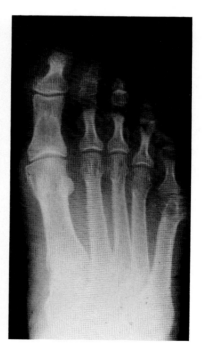

Figure 9–16. A 43-year-old man had an enchondroma in the right fifth metatarsal head. The tumor produced enlargement of the fifth metatarsal head and symptoms and signs similar to those of tailor's bunion.

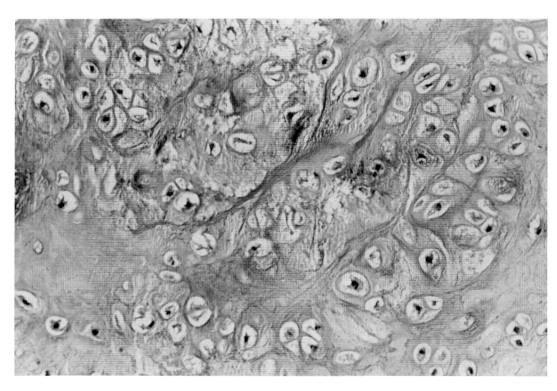

Figure 9–17. Photomicrograph (160×, H.&E.) shows the typical features of an enchondroma: low cellularity, small nuclear size, lack of pleomorphism and doubly nucleated lacunae, and absence of sarcomatous giant cells.

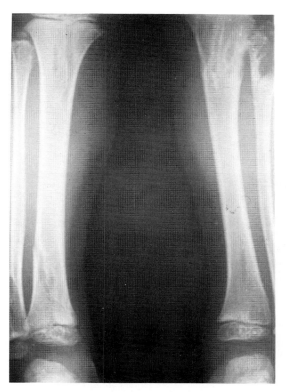

Figure 9–18. Anteroposterior view of a 7-year-old boy with Ollier's disease shows asymmetric radiolucent streaks in both the proximal and distal tibial and fibular metaphyseal regions caused by columns of ectopic cartilaginous tissue in these areas.

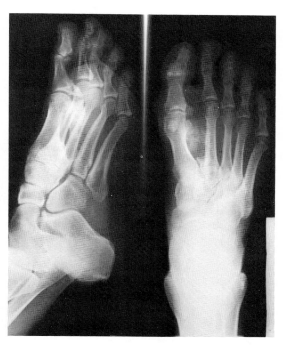

Figure 9–19. A 33-year-old woman developed a large and painful callus on the plantar aspect of her right foot under the lateral sesamoid. Oblique and anteroposterior radiographs reveal large exostosis of the lateral sesamoid, which was surgically excised.

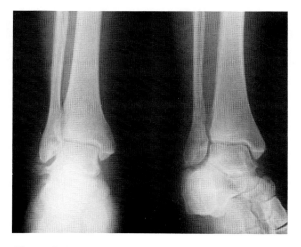

Figure 9–20. A 40-year-old man sought medical attention because of a painful lump in the left lateral malleolar area. Anteroposterior and mortise views revealed an osteochondroma arising from the lateral aspect of the talus.

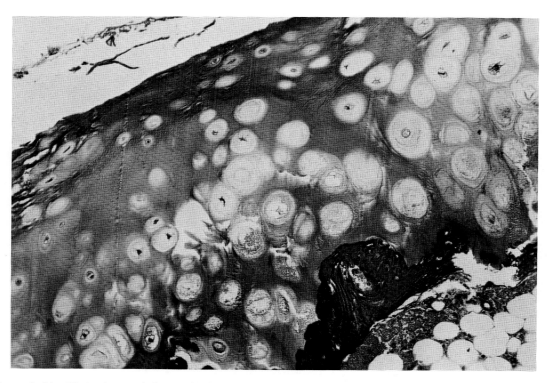

Figure 9–21. Photomicrograph (175×, H.&E.) shows a benign-looking cartilaginous cap covering some trabecular bone and bone marrow, all of which are typical histologic features of an osteochondroma.

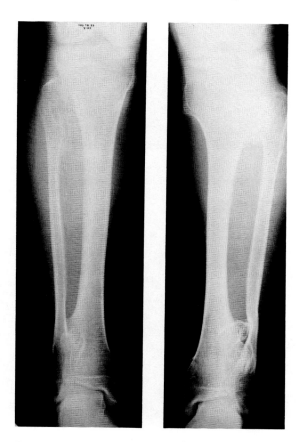

Figure 9–22. A 16-year-old youth had hereditary multiple exostoses as evidenced by multiple and symmetric osteocartilaginous exostoses in the metaphyseal regions of the upper and lower tibiae and fibulae.

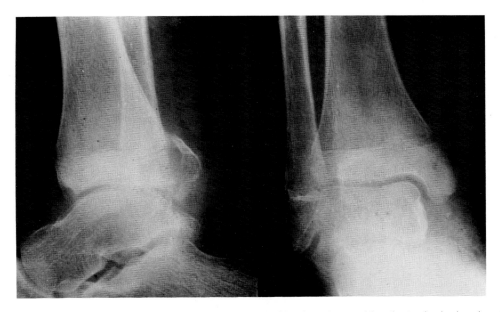

Figure 9–23. Anteroposterior and lateral radiographs of the ankle of a 14-year-old patient, who had a chondroblastoma in the posterior aspect of the distal tibial epiphysis that produced some expansion and a pathologic fracture in the involved area.

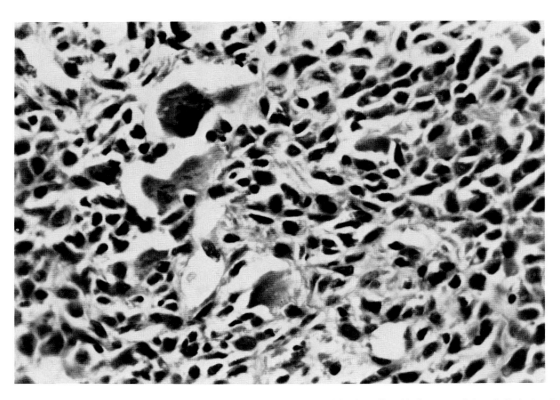

Figure 9–24. Photomicrograph (400×, H.&E.) shows many chondroblastic cells with large nuclei and distinct cytoplasmic borders and a few benign-looking multinucleated giant cells; all are typical histologic features of chondroblastoma.

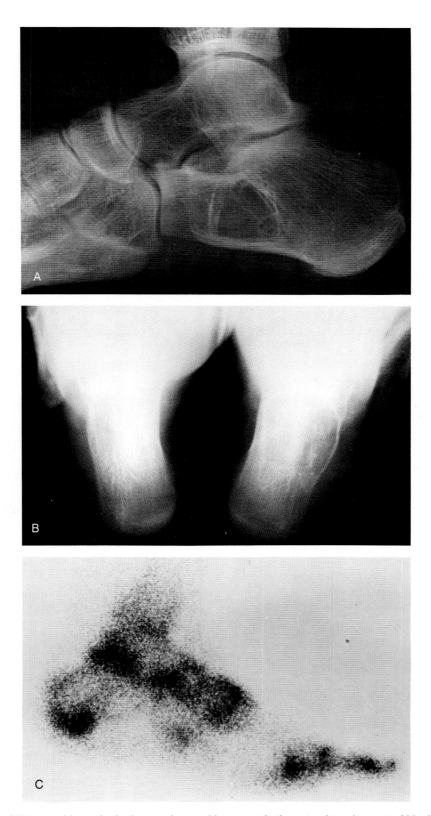

Figure 9–25. A 31-year-old man had a large unicameral bone cyst in the anterolateral aspect of his right calcaneus. The condition was successfully treated with curettage and autogenous bone graft. **A,** lateral view; **B,** axial view. **C,** bone scan shows no uptake of the radionuclide, suggesting the benign nature of this bone lesion.

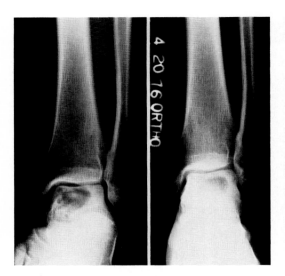

Figure 9–26. A 25-year-old man had pain in his right ankle for about 3 to 4 months. He was found to have a unicameral bone cyst in his right talus, which was treated with curettage and autogenous iliac bone graft with excellent results.

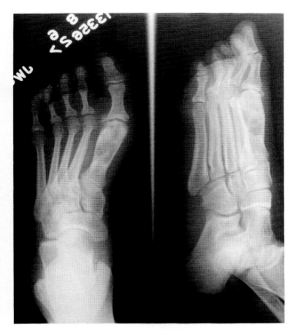

Figure 9–27. A 33-year-old woman had pain in her left first metatarsal for about 6 months. Anteroposterior and oblique radiographs show a loculated lesion causing expansion and cortical thinning of the distal two thirds of the first metatarsal. Subsequent biopsy revealed the presence of a unicameral bone cyst, which was successfully treated with curettage and autogenous iliac bone graft.

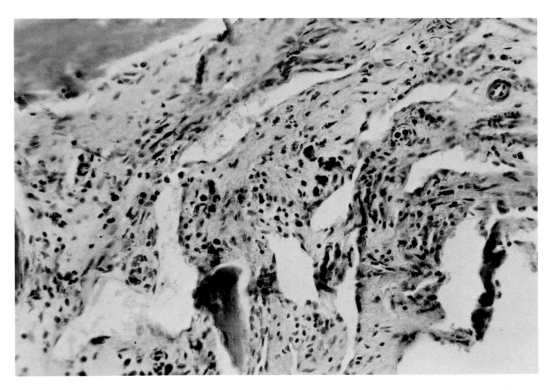

Figure 9–28. Photomicrograph (450×, H.&E.) shows some benign-looking fibrous tissue in association with scattered bone spicules and a few giant cells.

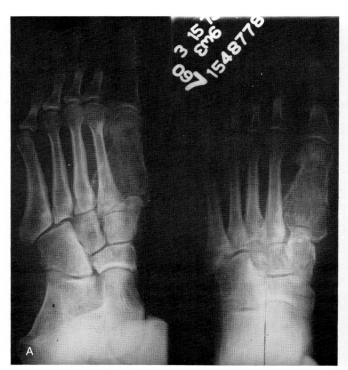

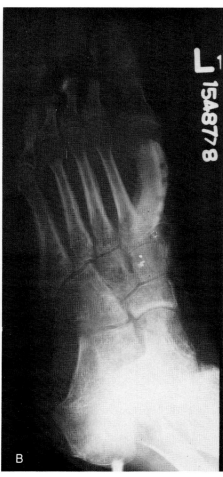

Figure 9–29. A 35-year-old patient had a giant cell tumor of the left first metatarsal. Anteroposterior and oblique views revealed extensive destruction of the proximal two thirds of the first metatarsal, which was treated with resection of the proximal portion of the first metatarsal plus insertion of a bicortical iliac bone graft. **B,** 1 year later, there is nice incorporation of the bicortical iliac graft and no evidence of tumor recurrence.

410

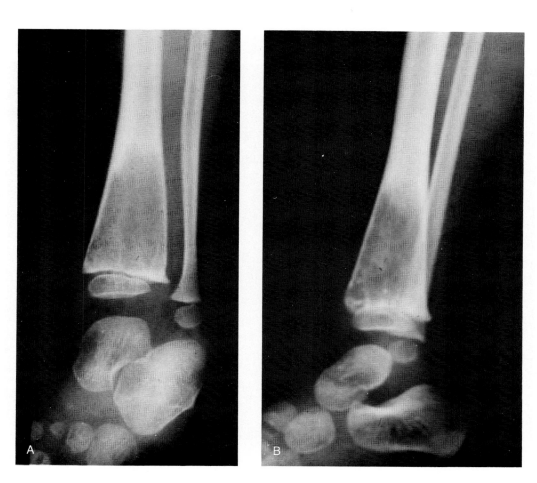

Figure 9–30. An 8-year-old boy in whom oblique (**A**) and lateral (**B**) ankle films show a large osteolytic lesion involving the entire distal metaphyseal region of the tibia. A giant cell tumor, which rarely involves immature skeleton, was found to be the cause.

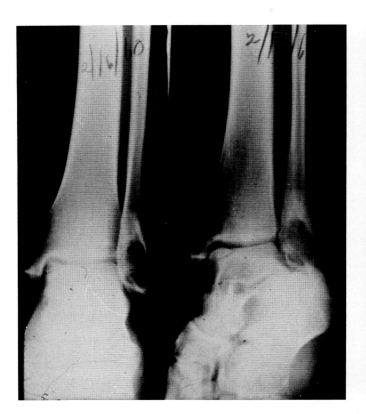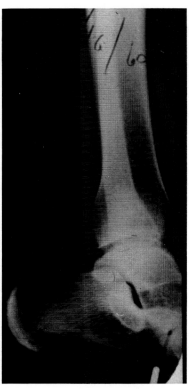

Figure 9–31. A 39-year-old man in whom anteroposterior, oblique, and lateral views of the ankle show an osteolytic lesion occupying the terminal portion of the left distal fibula, which was found to be giant cell tumor.

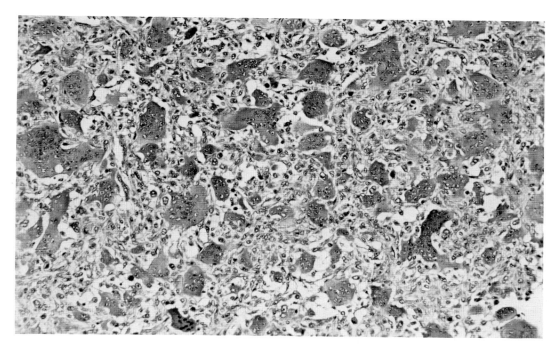

Figure 9–32. Photomicrograph (175×, H.&E.) demonstrates numerous multinucleated giant cells, the nuclei of which are similar to those of the stromal cells.

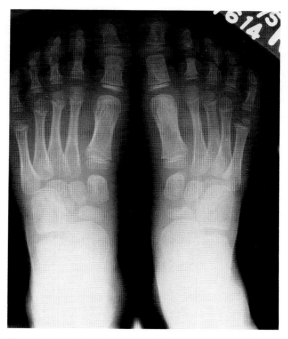

Figure 9–33. A 7-year-old child had polyostotic fibrous dysplasia. Anteroposterior view shows three lesions with a ground-glass appearance and a thin osteosclerotic rim in the right first metatarsal and the proximal and distal phalanges of the right great toe.

413

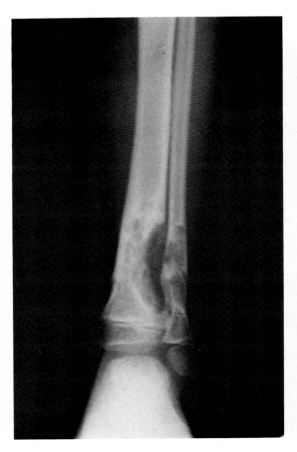

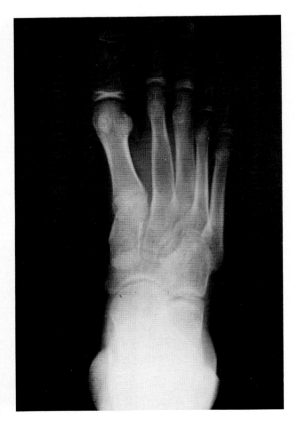

Figure 9–34. A 9-year-old girl in whom an anteroposterior radiograph of the distal tibia shows a destructive lesion involving the metaphyseo-diaphyseal region of the distal tibia and fibula caused by a fibrous dysplasia.

Figure 9–35. A 9-year-old girl in whom an anteroposterior view of the foot shows slight expansion of the second and third metatarsal shafts caused by the presence of Albright's syndrome, which includes polyostotic fibrous dysplasia, endocrine dysfunction, and cutaneous cafe-au-lait spots.

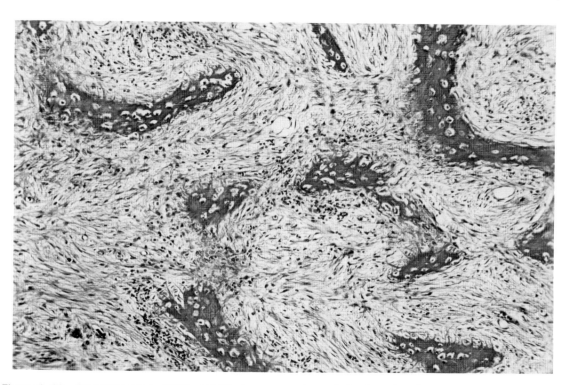

Figure 9–36. Photomicrograph (175×, H.&E.) shows several peculiarly shaped curlicues of metaplastic bony tra-beculae surrounded by whorled bundles of fibroblastic cells with a moderate amount of intercellular collagen fibers.

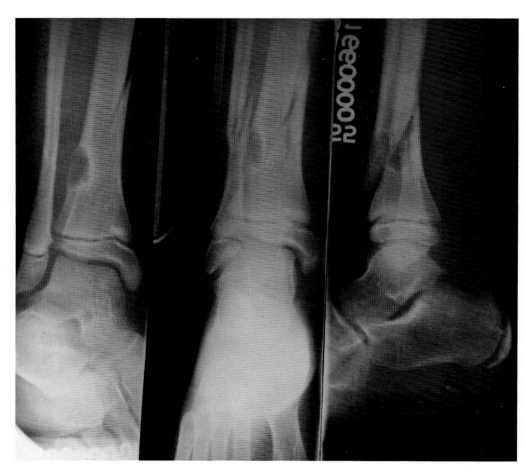

Figure 9–37. A 12-year-old boy had a nonossifying fibroma in his left tibia. Mortise, anteroposterior, and lateral views demonstrate the resultant pathologic tibial fracture.

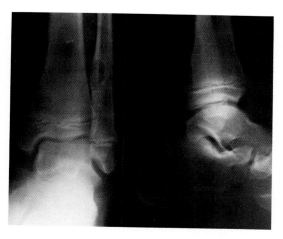

Figure 9–38. A 13-year-old girl had a nonossifying fibroma in her right distal fibula (anteroposterior and lateral views). The fibroma was completely asymptomatic and was accidentally discovered.

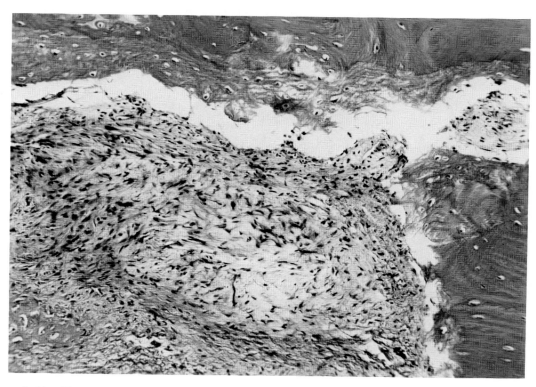

Figure 9–39. Photomicrograph (175×, H.&E.) shows the benign-looking fibrous tissue of a nonossifying fibroma. Note the small piece of immature metaplastic bone at lower left.

417

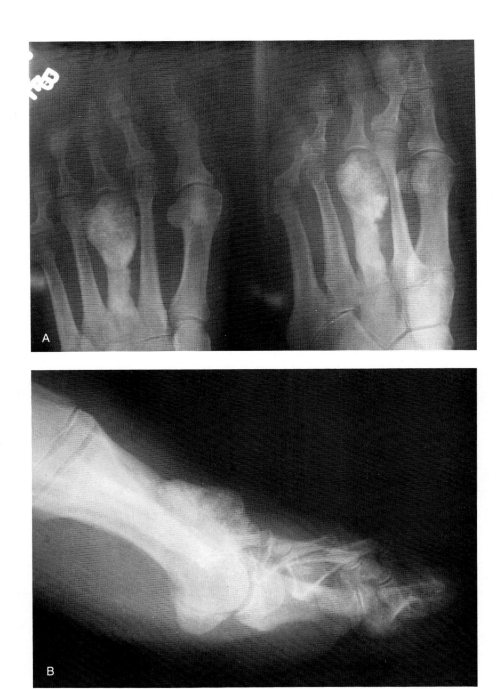

Figure 9–40. A 63-year-old woman had pain and swelling of her left forefoot for several weeks. Anteroposterior and oblique (**A**) and lateral (**B**) radiographs show great enlargement and osteosclerosis of the distal one half of the left third metatarsal, accompanied by periosteal new bone formation, on the proximal and medial aspect of the same bone caused by an osteogenic sarcoma. A below-knee amputation was required.

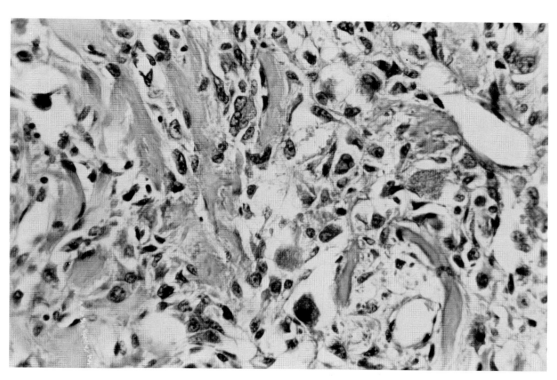

Figure 9–41. Photomicrograph (450×, H.&E.) shows many pleomorphic malignant osteoblastic cells in association with bone tumor formation.

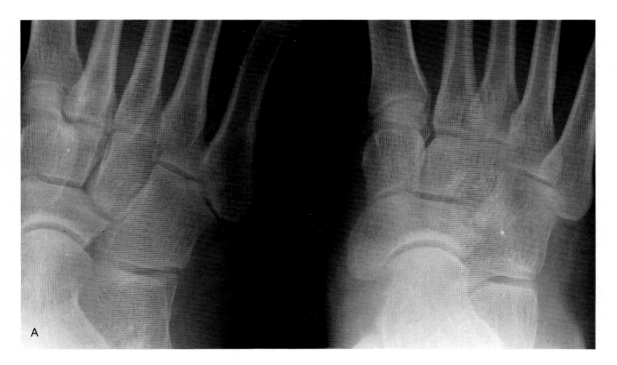

A

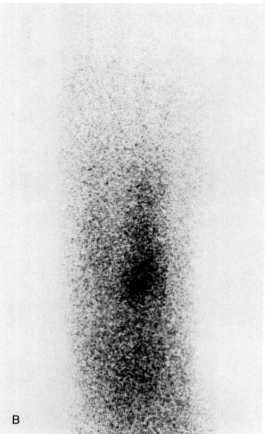

B

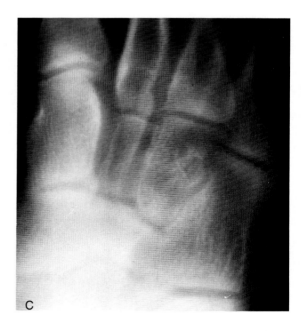

C

Figure 9–42. A 37-year-old woman complained of intermittent pain in the dorsal aspect of her right foot for 4 months. Oblique and anteroposterior radiographs (**A**) show a small, faintly radiopaque lesion in the right third cuneiform bone. **B,** bone scan shows increased radionuclide uptake in the right third cuneiform region. **C,** tomography clearly shows a radiolucent nidus surrounded by a zone of osteosclerosis in the right third cuneiform.

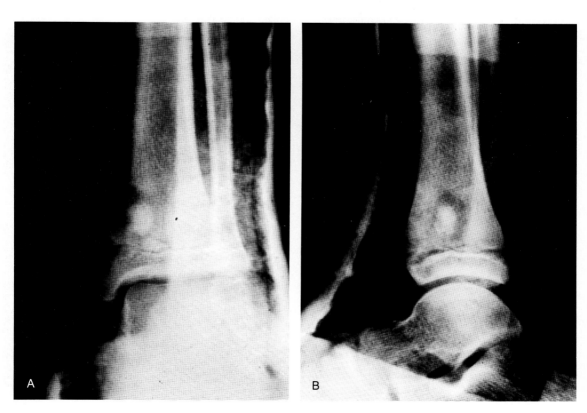

Figure 9–43. A 13-year-old boy had pain in his right ankle for 4 to 5 months. Anteroposterior (**A**) and lateral (**B**) films demonstrate a densely radiopaque nidus in the distal tibial metaphyseal region, which was subsequently found to be an osteoid osteoma.

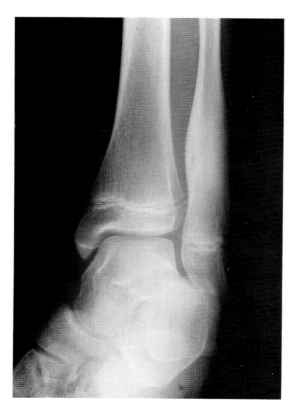

Figure 9–44. A 12-year-old girl had pain in her left lower leg for 3 months that tended to be worse at night and was relieved by the ingestion of aspirin. Radiography revealed great thickening of the inner cortex of her left distal fibula with a small radiolucent zone in the center of the fibular osteosclerosis that proved to be an osteoid osteoma.

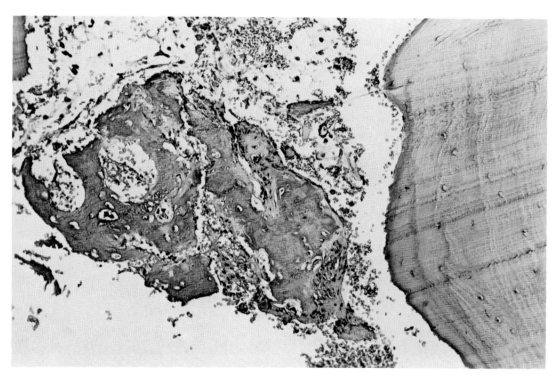

Figure 9–45. Photomicrograph (175×, H.&E.) of a specimen taken from the nidus of an osteoid osteoma shows highly vascular osteogenic granulation tissue (left) and mature lamellar bone (right).

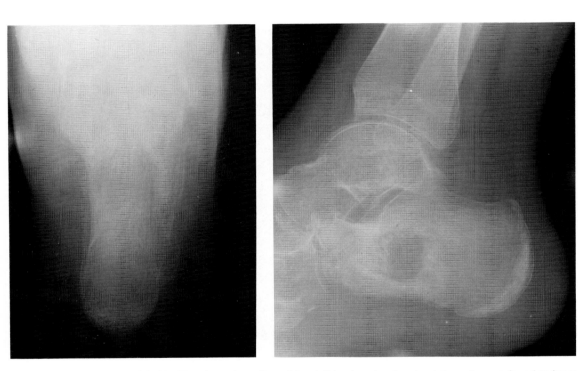

Figure 9–46. A 13-year-old girl with pain and swelling of her left heel region for about 5 weeks was found to have a calcaneal Ewing's sarcoma. On the axial and lateral views, note the bone destruction and prominent periosteal bone formation caused by the tumor.

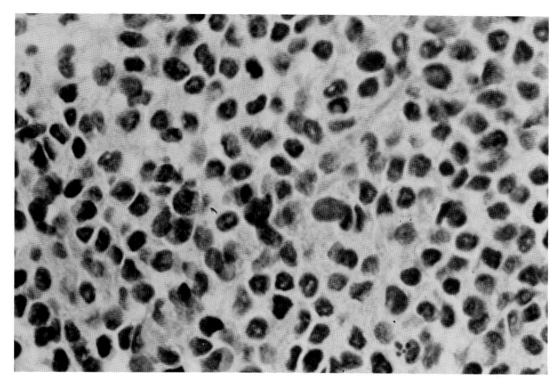

Figure 9–47. Photomicrograph (600×, H.&E.) shows many Ewing's sarcoma cells with round and smoky nuclei and indistinct cytoplasmic borders.

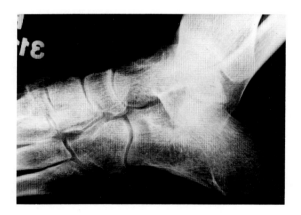

Figure 9–48. A 46-year-old patient had a hemangioma on the neck portion of the left talus. Note the semilunar destruction in the upper portion of the neck of the talus associated with a thin rim of osteosclerosis.

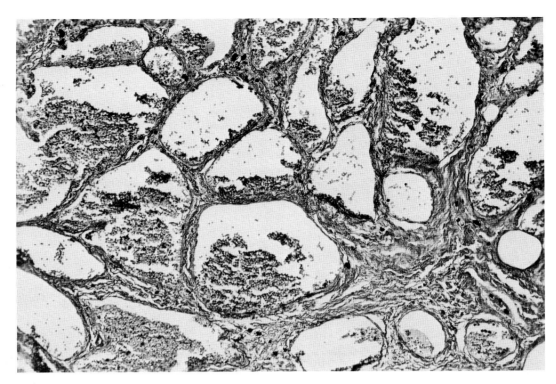

Figure 9–49. Photomicrograph (150×, H.&E.) shows many endothelially lined vascular spaces containing many blood cells, the basic features of hemangioma.

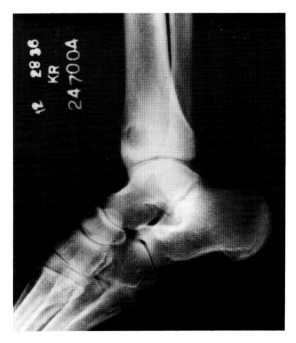

Figure 9–50. A 42-year-old patient had a painful osteolytic tibial lesion with surrounding osteosclerosis, which was found to be myeloma by open biopsy. Myeloma rarely produces osteosclerotic bone change.

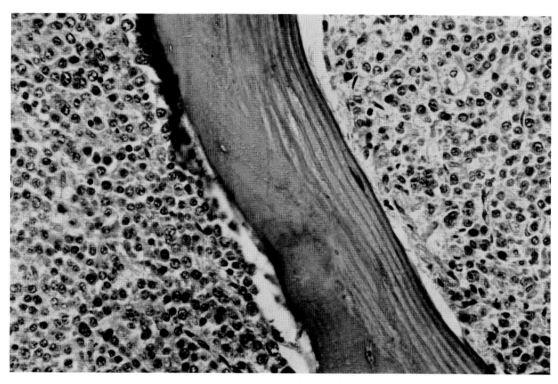

Figure 9–51. Photomicrograph (250×, H.&E.) shows many round myeloma cells with peripheral condensation of nuclear chromatin, producing the so-called wheel-spoke or clock-face appearance, and an abundance of cytoplasm.

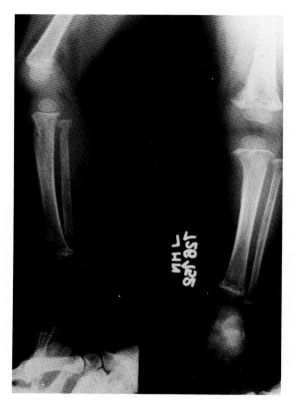

Figure 9–52. A 4-year-old child with acute lymphocytic leukemia. Lateral and anteroposterior views show an irregular radiolucent line transversely across the femoral and tibial metaphyseal regions caused by infiltration of leukemic cells into these areas.

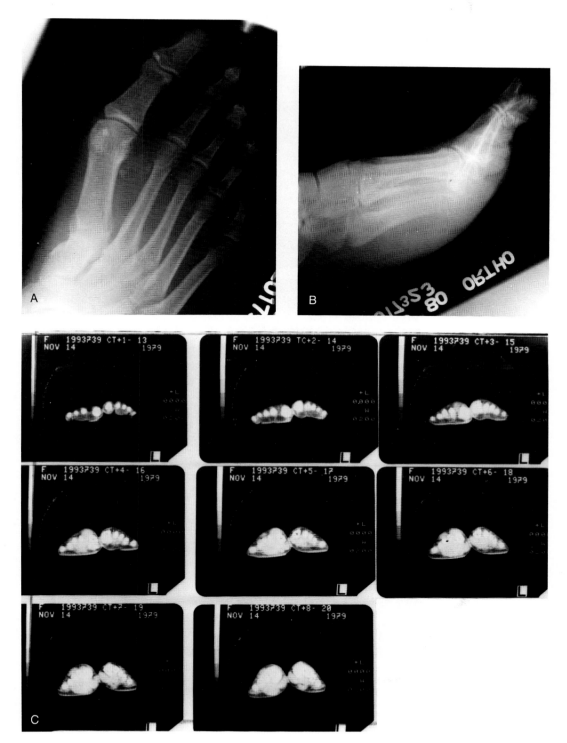

Figure 9–53. A 35-year-old man had a painful and swollen right foot for 6 weeks. Anteroposterior (**A**) and lateral (**B**) radiographs show soft tissue swelling in the plantar aspect of the forefoot plus some soft tissue calcification in the first intermetatarsal region. **C,** CT scan shows a large soft tissue tumor in the plantar aspect of the right forefoot with tumor extension to the dorsal aspect through the intermetatarsal space.

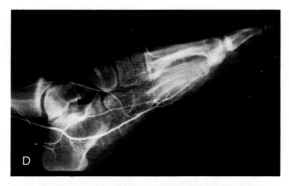

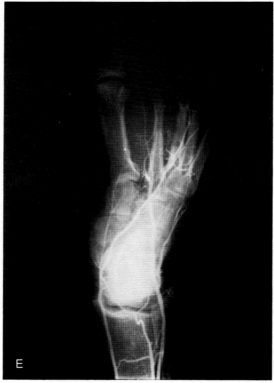

Figure 9–53. Continued. Arteriography (**D** and **E**) shows increased vascularity and neovascularization in the plantar aspect of the forefoot where the synovial sarcoma was located.

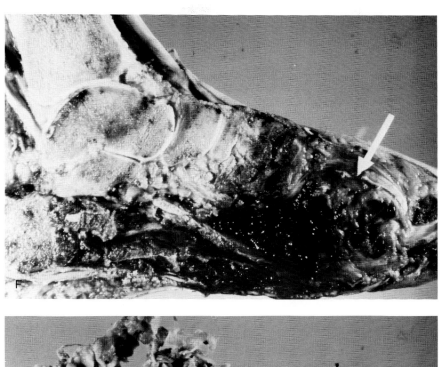

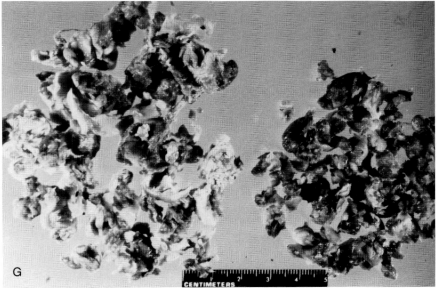

Figure 9–53. Continued. **F,** sagittal section of the amputated foot. There is extensive infiltration of the dorsal and plantar aspects of the forefoot by the synovial sarcoma tissue and diffuse necrosis and hemorrhage in the tumor tissue (*arrow*). **G,** pieces of synovial sarcoma tissue, show their fibrotic nature and lack of strong cohesiveness.

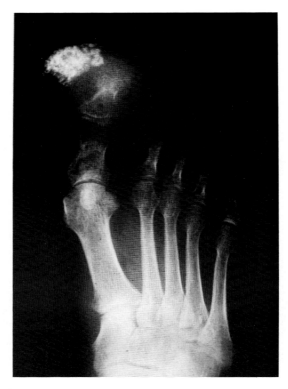

Figure 9–54. A 41-year-old man had a synovial sarcoma in the terminal portion of his right foot. Note the large radiopaque area caused by calcification in the tumor tissue.

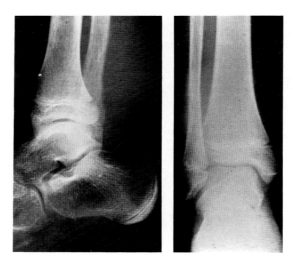

Figure 9–55. A 12-year-old girl with a painless swelling in the posterolateral aspect of her left ankle for 2 to 3 months was found to have a synovial sarcoma. Lateral and anteroposterior radiographs demonstrate the slightly radiopaque fusiform tumor mass behind the distal portion of the fibula as well as the tumor-induced bone erosion along the posterior border of the distal fibula.

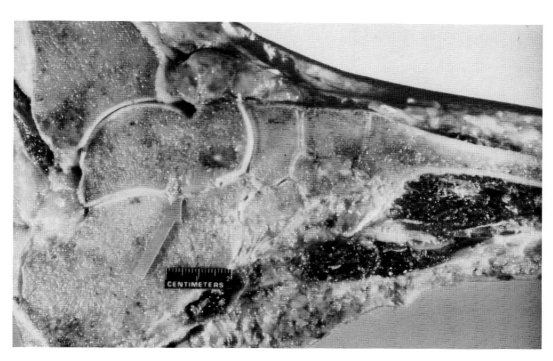

Figure 9–56. Midsagittal section of an amputated foot. A small synovial sarcoma is seen on the dorsal aspect of the ankle joint (*arrow*). Note the lobulated appearance of the tumor tissue, the tumor pseudocapsule surrounding the tumor, and the close relationship between the undersurface of the tumor and the head of talus and the superior surface of the navicular.

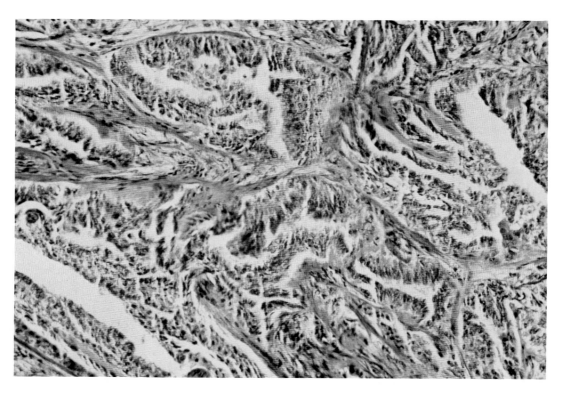

Figure 9–57. Photomicrograph of a synovial sarcoma (128×, H.&E.) shows a typical biphasic cellular pattern that includes many cuboidal and columnar cells (synovioblasts or synoviocytes) forming gland-like structures, and spindle-shaped fibroblastic cells with cigar-shaped nuclei running between these pseudoglandular structures.

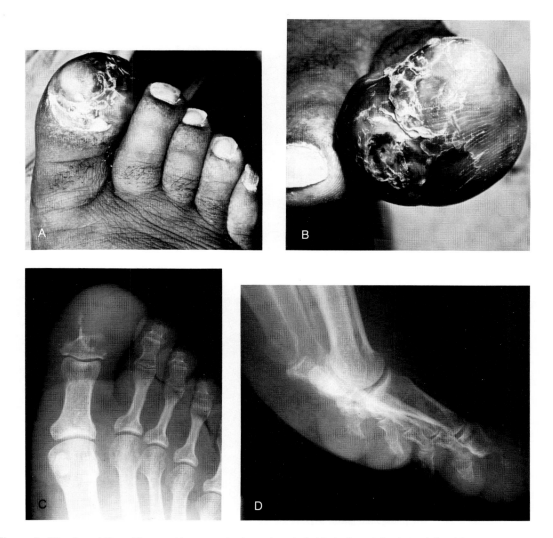

Figure 9–58. **A** and **B,** a 40-year-old woman had an ulcerated skin lesion at the lateral tip of her great toe caused by a melanoma. Anteroposterior (**C**) and lateral (**D**) radiographs show destruction of the terminal portion of the distal phalanx of the great toe caused by intraosseous invasion of the melanoma.

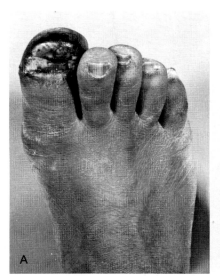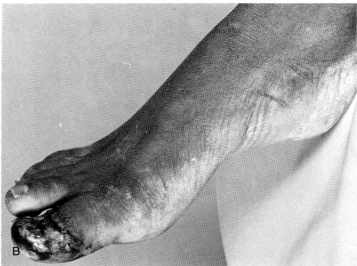

Figure 9–59. A 24-year-old man had a subungual melanoma of his right great toe (**A** and **B**), which had metastasized to his right inguinal lymph nodes.

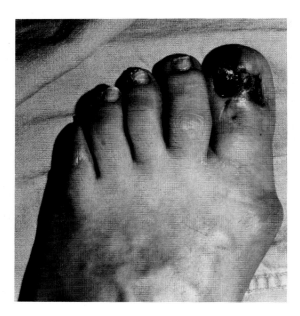

Figure 9–60. A 42-year-old man had a subungual melanoma of his left great toe that caused complete detachment of his left great toenail and deep black discoloration of the nailbed.

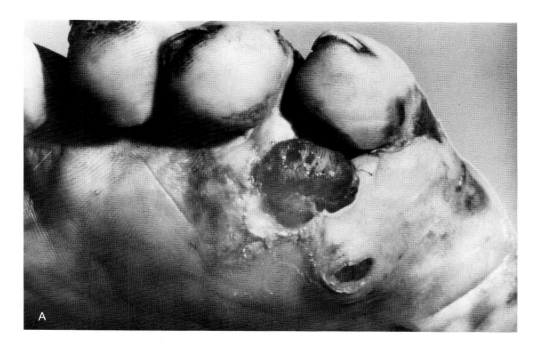

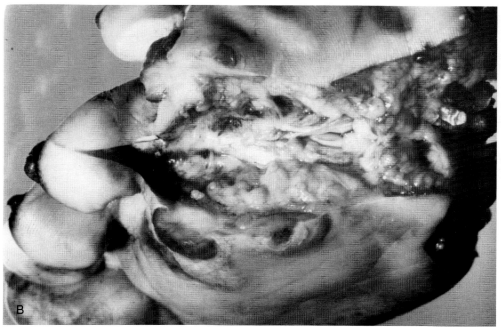

Figure 9–61. **A** and **B,** amputated left foot of a 39-year-old man shows an ulcerated melanoma in the plantar aspect of the fourth intermetatarsal region that extended into the deep soft tissues.

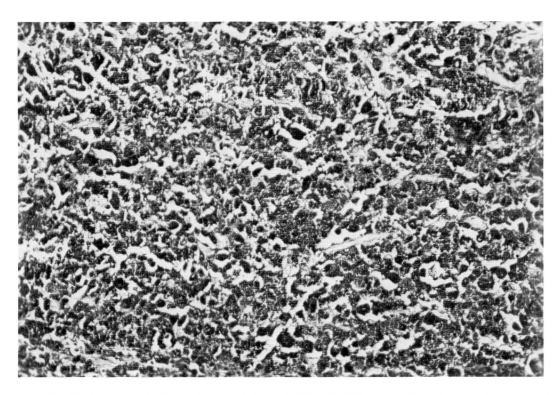

Figure 9–62. Photomicrograph of a melanoma of the foot (175×, H.&E.) shows all the tumor cells are so full of intracellular melanin that their cellular details are completely obliterated.

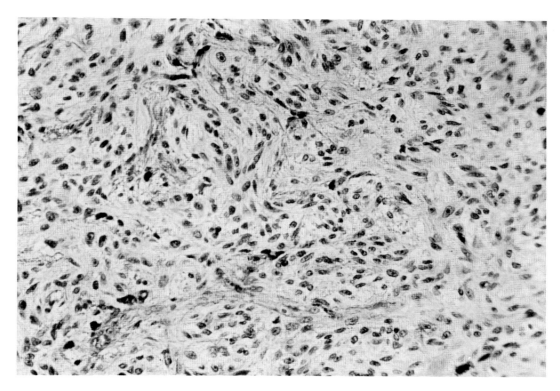

Figure 9–63. Photomicrograph of a melanoma (215×, H.&E.) shows the presence of many cells with round or elongated nuclei and prominent nucleoli. Only a few cells contain intracellular melanin pigment.

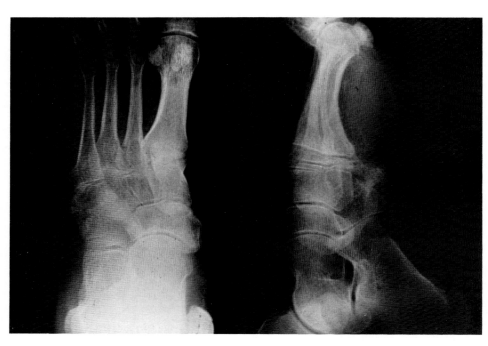

Figure 9–64. A 55-year-old man had a slowly enlarging mass in the plantar aspect of his left forefoot for 6 months. Anteroposterior and lateral radiographs show a slightly radiopaque fusiform mass occupying the plantar aspect of the left forefoot, which was found to be a fibrosarcoma by open biopsy.

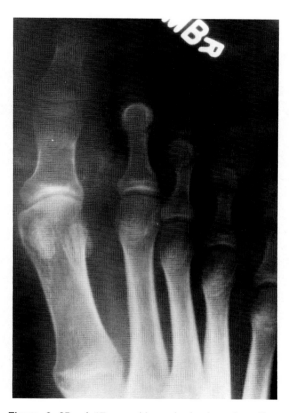

Figure 9–65. A 17-year-old man had pain and swelling in the base of his right great toe for several months. Anteroposterior view of the forefoot shows swelling and patches of radiopacity around the basal portion of the proximal phalanx of the right great toe. Subsequent biopsy revealed the presence of a fibrosarcoma.

441

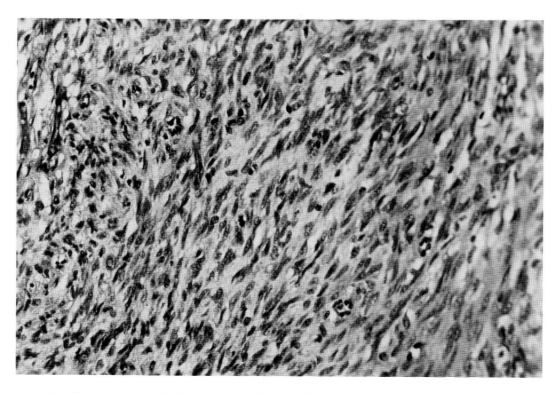

Figure 9–66. Photomicrograph of a fibrosarcoma (450×, H.&E.) shows intertwining bundles of fibroblastic cells with some cellular pleomorphism and occasional mitotic figures.

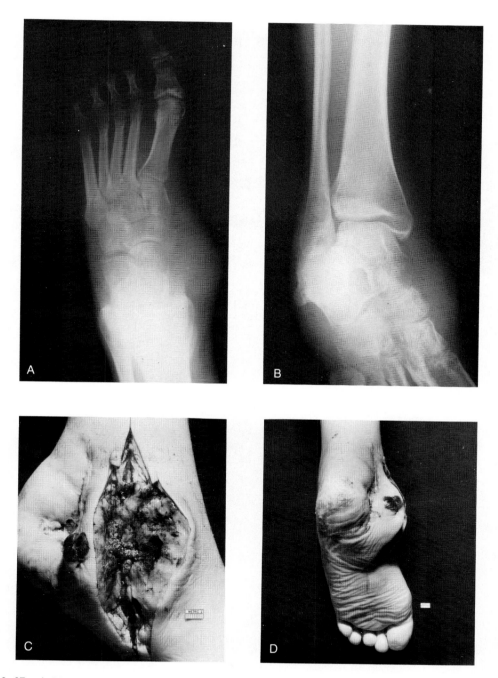

Figure 9–67. A 24-year-old woman had a growing tumor in the medial aspect of her left ankle for several weeks. Foot (**A**) and ankle (**B**) radiographs show a large soft tissue mass in the medial aspect of the ankle without any detectable intralesional calcification. **C** and **D,** amputated left foot shows skin ulceration in the medial aspect of the ankle caused by the rhabdomyosarcoma and the lobulated and hemorrhagic appearance of the tumor tissue.

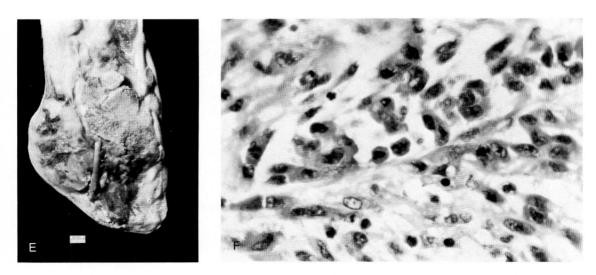

Figure 9–67 Continued. **E,** a midcoronal section shows infiltration of tumor tissue deep into the plantar arch of the foot. **F,** photomicrograph of a rhabdomyosarcoma (900×, H.&E.) shows many pleomorphic rhabdomyoblasts with large nuclei, abundant cytoplasm, and distinct cytoplasmic borders. Note the strap-shaped or racquet-shaped configuration and the tandem arrangement of some of the nuclei of these tumor cells.

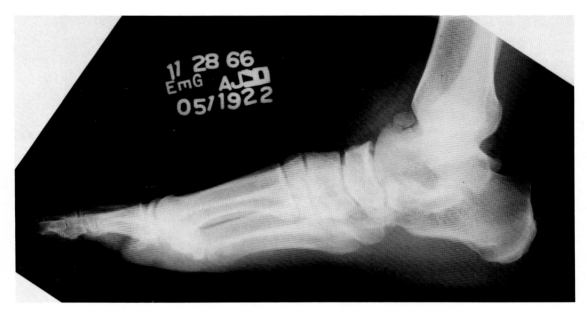

Figure 9–68. A 50-year-old man had a painless mass over the dorsal aspect of his right ankle for many months. Subsequent biopsy revealed the tumor to be liposarcoma, which was surgically excised.

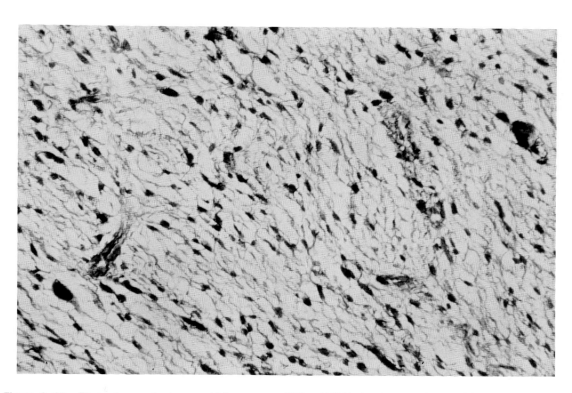

Figure 9–69. Photomicrograph of a myxoid liposarcoma (250×, H.&E.) shows some pleomorphism of the tumor cell nuclei, which are several times the nuclear size of a lipocyte; a myxomatous intercellular matrix; and several cells with large and hyperchromatic nuclei.

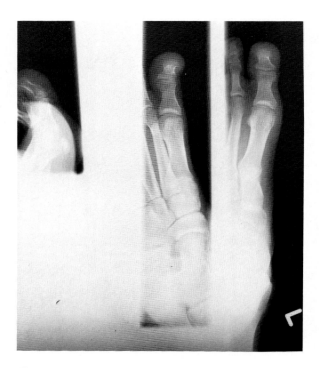

Figure 9–70. A 43-year-old man had a painful and swollen left great toe for several weeks. Radiography shows only some soft tissue swelling. Subsequent biopsy revealed the presence of a malignant fibrous histiocytoma, which required amputation of his great toe.

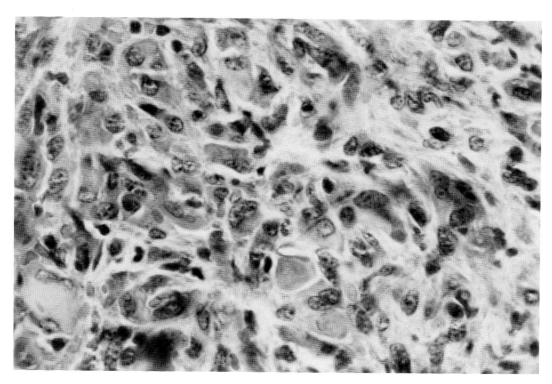

Figure 9–71. Photomicrograph (900×, H.&E.) shows many histiocytic cells with variation in the size and shape of their nuclei, a moderate amount of cytoplasm, and prominent nucleoli, all typical microscopic features of malignant fibrous histiocytoma.

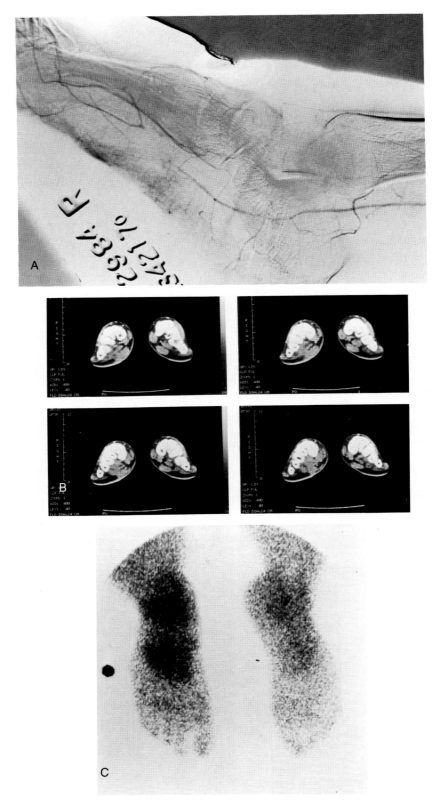

Figure 9–72. A 23-year-old woman had a palpable mass in the plantar aspect of her right foot. **A,** arteriography shows some increased vascularity in the plantar region caused by the presence of a clear cell sarcoma. **B,** CT scan shows a soft tissue tumor in the plantar aspect of the foot with distortion of the normal soft tissue anatomy. **C,** bone scan shows increased radionuclide uptake in both the right metatarsal and tarsal regions.

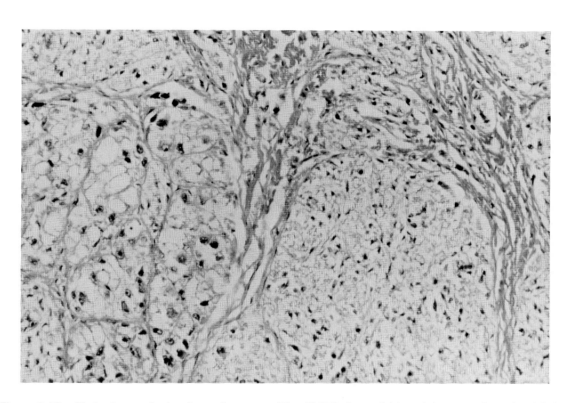

Figure 9–73. Photomicrograph of a clear cell sarcoma (88×, H.&E.) shows division of the tumor tissue into lobules by fibrous septa, prominent vesicular nuclei with a large single nucleolus, and the many typical pale-staining tumor cells.

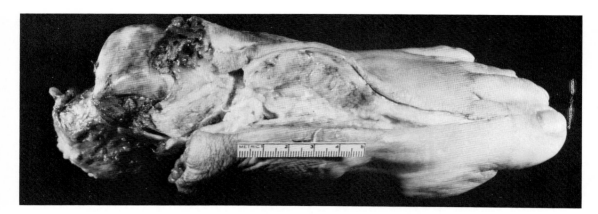

Figure 9–74. Amputated left foot from a 25-year-old woman with an epithelioid sarcoma shows the dorsal position of the tumor directly over the tarsometatarsal region with small foci of hemorrhage in the tumor tissue.

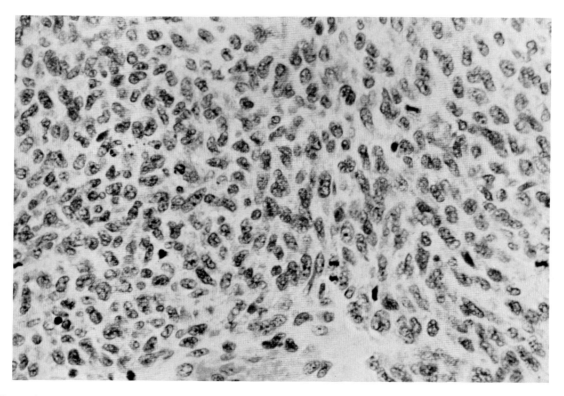

Figure 9–75. Photomicrograph of an epithelioid sarcoma (312×, H.&E.) shows the presence of many pale-looking, round, and short oval tumor cells that are similar in appearance to the epithelioid cells of biphasic and pseudoglandular tenosynovial sarcomas, but lack the long cigar-shaped cells universally present in monophasic spindle cell tumors, and the tubular or pseudoglandular structures prominently present in biphasic and pseudoglandular tenosynovial sarcomas. Note the presence of several mitotic figures.

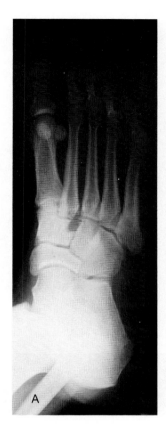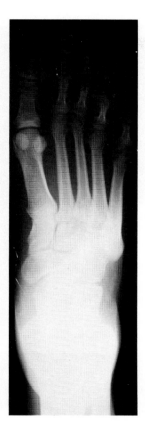

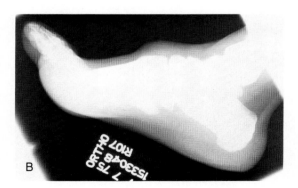

Figure 9–76. A 45-year-old woman with a giant cell tumor of tendon sheath. Oblique and anteroposterior (**A**) and lateral (**B**) views show a large soft tissue swelling over the dorsal aspect of the tarsal bones as well as destruction of the second and third cuneiforms and the adjacent bases of the second and third metatarsals.

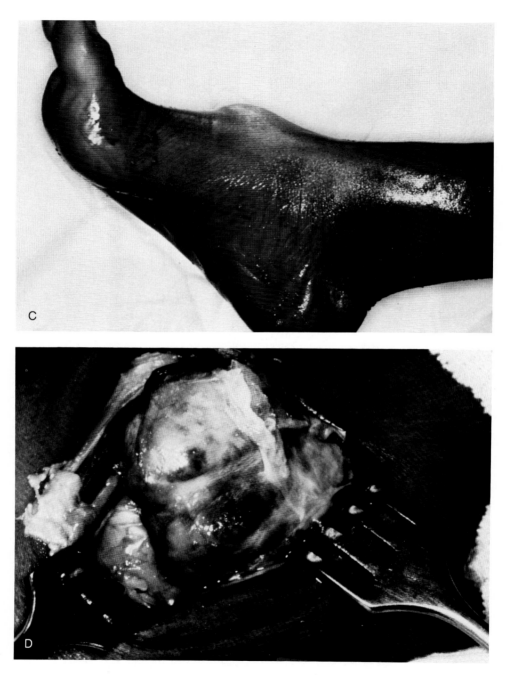

Figure 9–76. Continued. **C** and **D,** intraoperative photographs of the xanthoma show its dorsal position and a lobulated configuration with deeply pigmented spots.

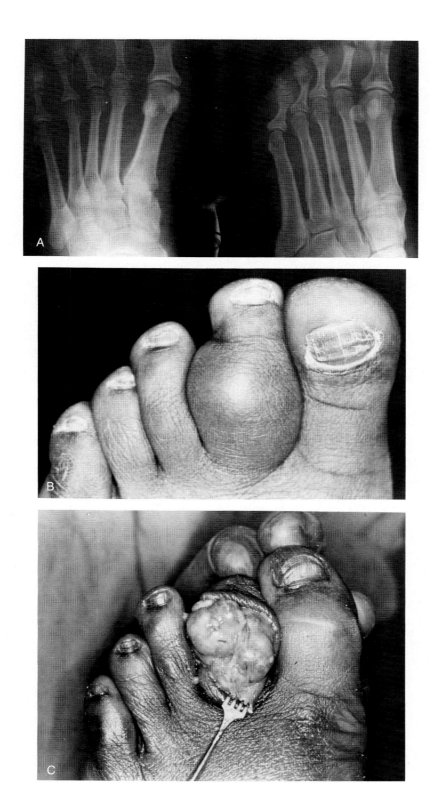

Figure 9–77. A 40-year-old woman had a xanthoma in her left second toe. **A,** Anteroposterior and oblique films show diffuse soft tissue swelling of the second toe. **B** and **C,** intraoperative photographs show a fusiform enlargement of the left second toe caused by a lobulated xanthoma.

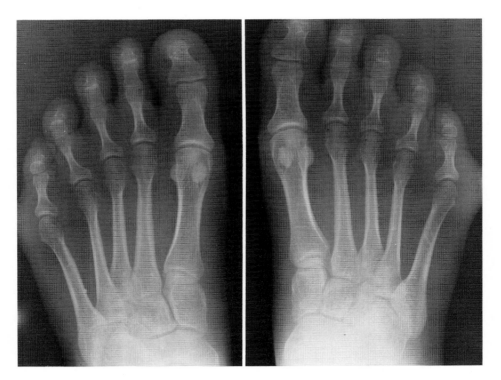

Figure 9–78. A 22-year-old woman had a xanthoma on the lateral aspect of the fifth M-P joints of her feet. This bilateral symmetric presence of xanthoma is rare.

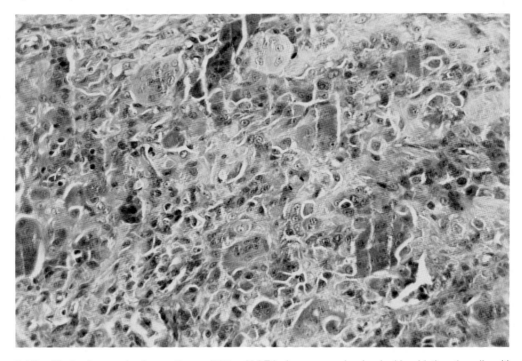

Figure 9–79. Photomicrograph of a xanthoma (390×, H.&E.) shows many benign-looking histiocytic cells with round and pale-looking nuclei in which a prominent nucleolus can usually be seen. Note the presence of many multinucleated giant cells, the nuclei of which are virtually identical to those of stromal cells.

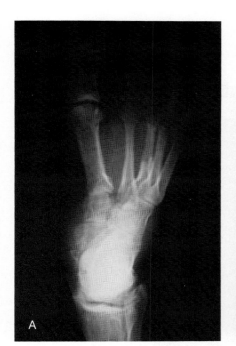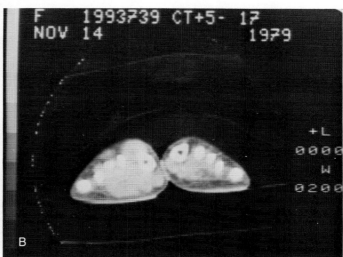

Figure 9–80. A 45-year-old woman had a large tumor in the plantar aspect of her right foot. **A,** Anteroposterior view revealed a large soft tissue density occupying almost the entire metatarsal region. **B,** CT scan shows the presence of tumor tissue in both the plantar and dorsal aspect of the right foot, which produced significant separation between the first and second metatarsals.

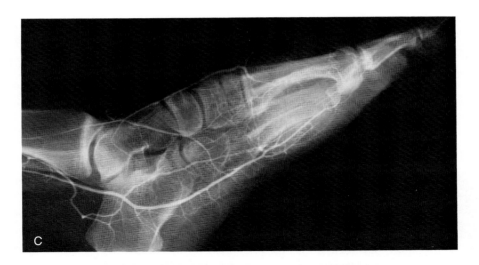

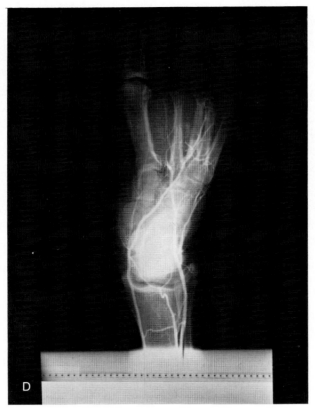

Figure 9–80. Continued. **C** and **D,** arteriograms demonstrate fairly high vascularity of the soft tissue tumor, suggestive of its possibly malignant nature.

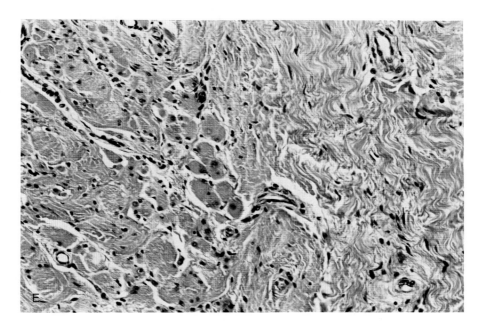

Figure 9–80. Continued. **E,** biopsy specimen (160×, H.&E.) shows invasion of many intrinsic muscles of the foot by a benign-looking fibrous tissue with a large amount of collagen. This finding is compatible with the tissue diagnosis of fibromatosis in spite of its malignant clinical appearance.

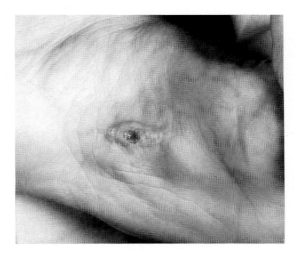

Figure 9–81. A 51-year-old woman had a large, symptomatic plantar fibromatosis excised from her left foot. Two years later, she developed a keloid at her plantar skin incision site plus a recurrence of her plantar fibromatosis in essentially the same location.

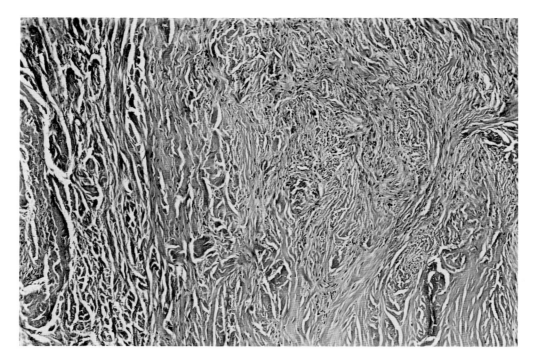

Figure 9–82. Tissue taken from a mature area of a plantar fibromatosis (105×, H.&E.) shows dense collagenous fibers in association with small and pyknotic fibroblastic cells.

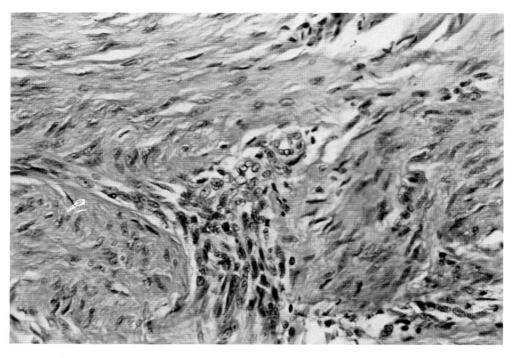

Figure 9–83. Tissue taken from a soft nodular area of a plantar fibromatosis (320×, H.&E.) shows that the nuclei of fibroblastic cells are slightly plump and have some degree of variation of size and shape, with an occasional mitosis—findings that are suggestive of a low-grade fibrosarcoma. Thus it is important to know exactly where the tissue comes from and to correlate that knowledge with the microscopic findings before arriving at the final diagnosis.

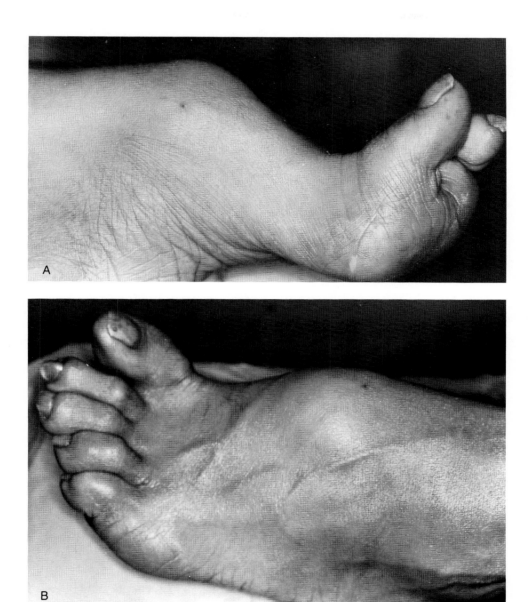

Figure 9–84. A 34-year-old woman had a large lipoma on the dorsal aspect of her left foot (**A** and **B**), that made it difficult for her to wear oxford-type shoes with laces.

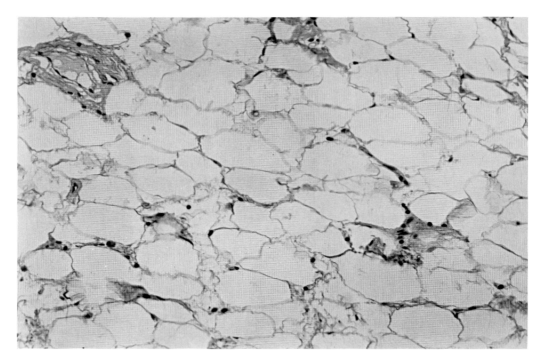

Figure 9–85. Photomicrograph of a lipoma (160×, H.&E.) shows many interconnecting mature fat cells (lipocytes) with peripheral and pyknotic nuclei.

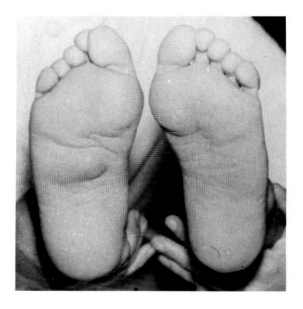

Figure 9–86. A 44-year-old woman sustained a puncture wound of the plantar aspect of her right foot. The injury apparently caused subcutaneous implantation of epithelial tissue, which resulted in the formation of a large epidermoid inclusion cyst several months later.

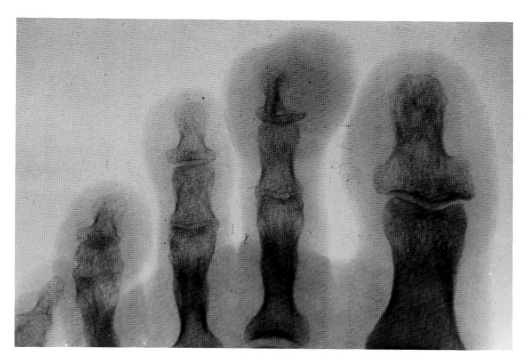

Figure 9–87. A 54-year-old man had an epidermoid inclusion cyst of his left second toe that produced a large swelling on the medial aspect of the distal portion of the second toe and a saucer-shaped erosion on the medial aspect of the distal phalanx of the same toe.

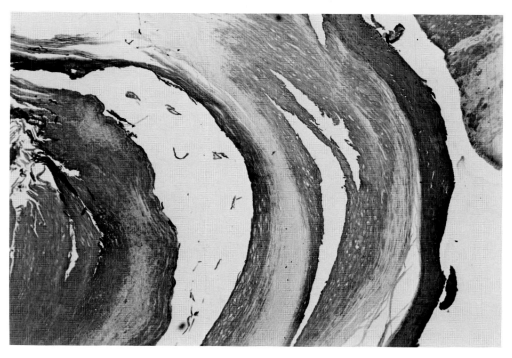

Figure 9–88. Photomicrograph of an epidermoid inclusion cyst (90×, H.&E.) shows a layer of live epithelium with cells (right) covered by several thick layers of dead keratinized tissue (left).

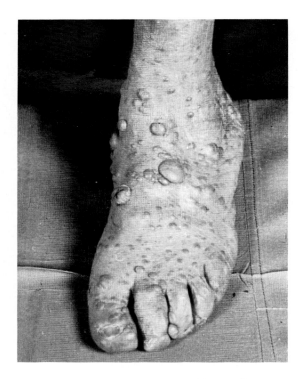

Figure 9–89. A 38-year-old man with neurofibromatosis had numerous cutaneous neurofibromas of various sizes.

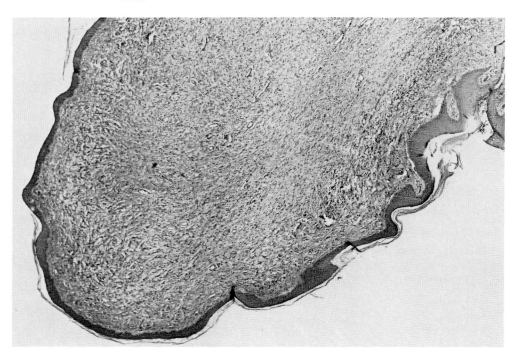

Figure 9–90. Longitudinal section through a cutaneous neurofibroma (52×, H.&E.) (molluscum fibrosum) shows its relatively high cellularity and vascularity.

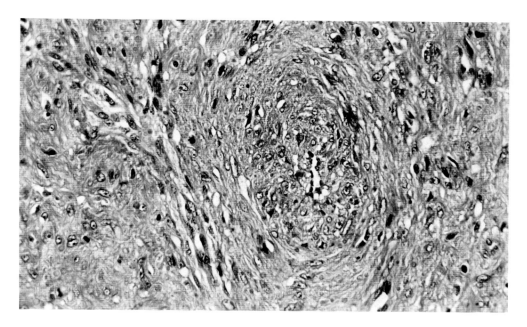

Figure 9–91. Photomicrograph of a cutaneous neurofibroma (390×, H.&E.) shows the formation of an organoid structure by the tumor cells.

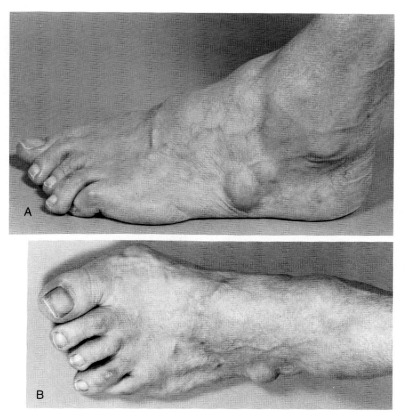

Figure 9–92. A 53-year-old woman with a long history of rheumatoid arthritis had two rheumatoid nodules on the lateral aspect of her left foot (**A** and **B**). The nodules were surgically excised.

463

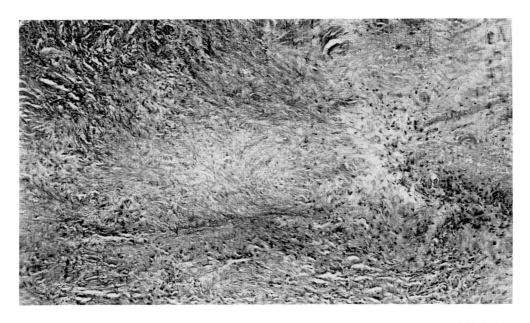

Figure 9–93. Photomicrograph of a rheumatoid nodule (105×, H.&E.) shows a central area of fibrinoid necrosis surrounded by chronic inflammatory and fibroblastic cells and fibrosis.

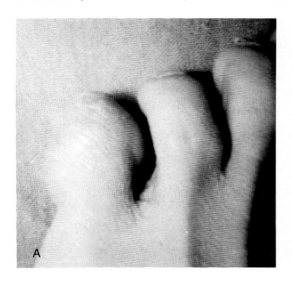

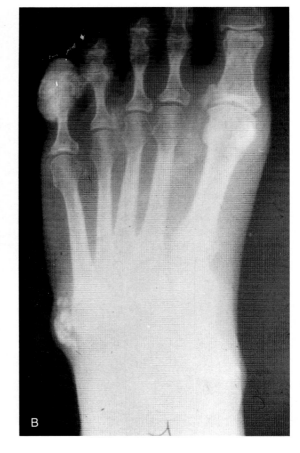

Figure 9–94. A, A 37-year-old woman had a grossly enlarged left fifth toe caused by a tumoral calcinosis. **B,** anteroposterior view shows calcium salt deposits in the fifth toe, lateral aspect of the first M-P joint, lateral aspect of the base of the fifth metatarsal, distal portion of the second toe, and the first, second, and third intermetatarsal spaces.

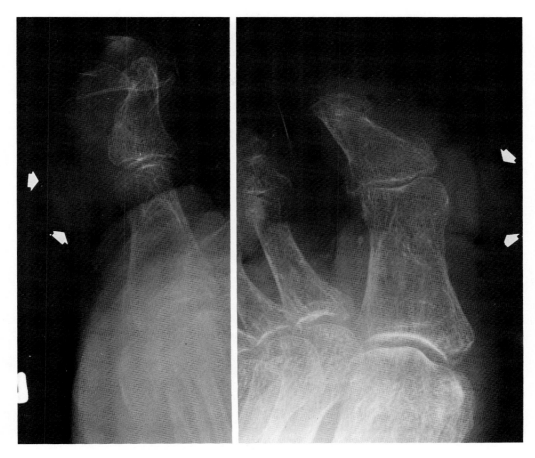

Figure 9-95. A 93-year-old man in whom anteroposterior and lateral radiographs of the left great toe reveal a large soft tissue mass (*arrows*) on the plantar aspect of the interphalangeal joint caused by a large callus of the plantar skin.

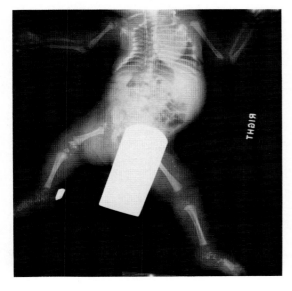

Figure 9-96. Whole-body radiographs of a newborn baby with stippled epiphyses shows multiple small calcification foci in the epiphyseal regions. Note the irregularity and punctate calcification of the tarsal bones.

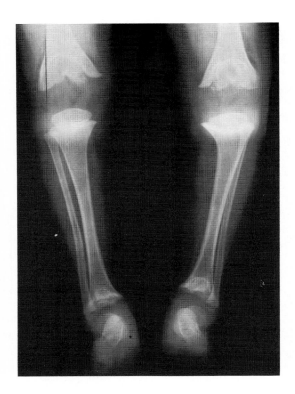

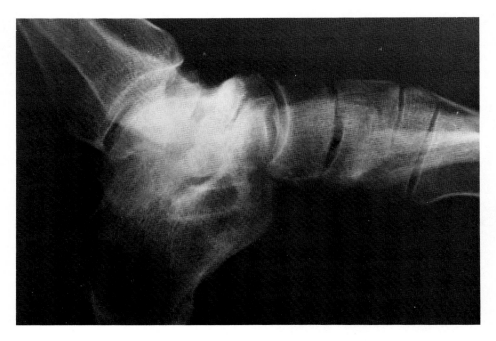

Figure 9–97. A child with multiple epiphyseal dysplasia in whom an anteroposterior view shows the epiphyses to be irregular, dense, and invaginated into their neighboring diaphyses.

Figure 9–98. A 20-year-old man with tarsal epiphyseal aclasia had an osteochondroma arising from the superior neck portion of his left talus. The tumor caused constant irritation of the left ankle joint and was treated with surgical excision.

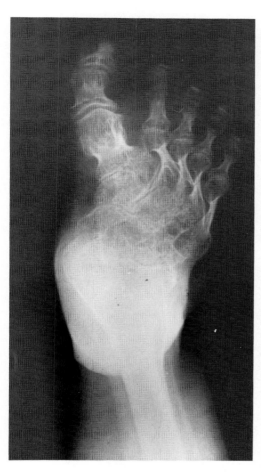

Figure 9–99. A 32-year-old woman had diastrophic dwarfism. Anteroposterior views of the right foot show the presence of talipes equinovarus with peculiar and stubby metatarsals and phalanges.

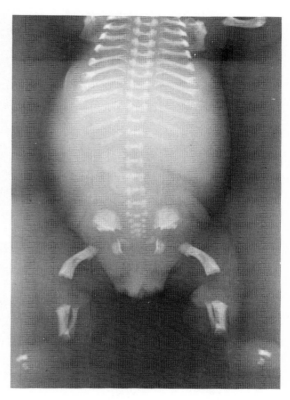

Figure 9–100. A newborn with severe congenital achondroplasia in whom a whole body radiograph shows marked underdevelopment of the iliac bone with small sacrosciatic angles, marked reduction of the interpedicular distance of the lumbar spine, and short and stubby long and short tubular bones. Note that the length of the feet is greater than that of the tibia or femur.

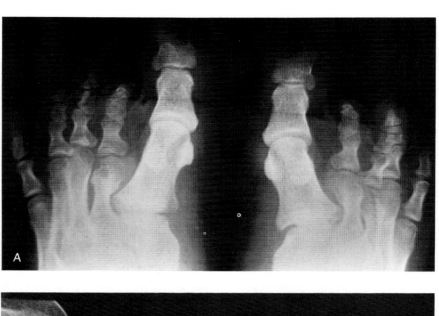

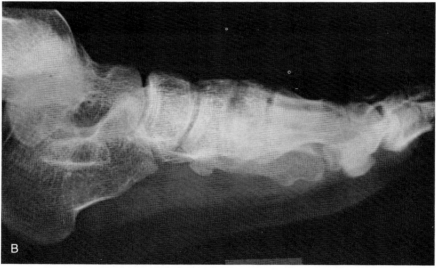

Figure 9–101. A 27-year-old man with achondroplasia in whom anteroposterior (**A**) and lateral (**B**) views of the feet show the short and stubby appearance of all the metatarsals and phalanges.

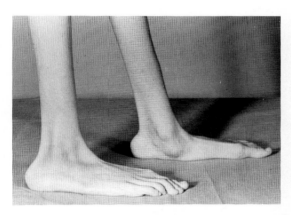

Figure 9–102. An 18-year-old woman with Marfan's syndrome. Note the long and narrow feet with long digits, which are commonly known as arachnodactyly (spider legs), and the severe planovalgus deformity (rocker-bottom deformity) of both feet.

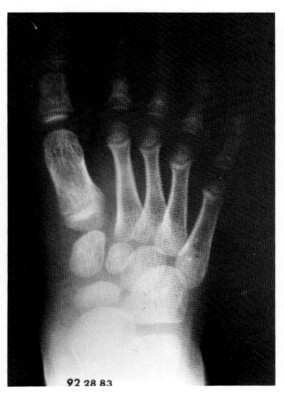

92 28 83

Figure 9–103. A patient with peripheral exostosis in whom an anteroposterior view of the foot reveals ball-in-socket appearance of the epiphyses and progressive brachydactyly from the metatarsals to the distal phalanges.

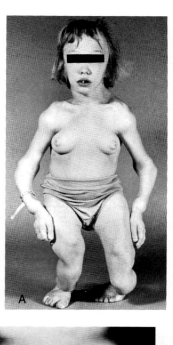
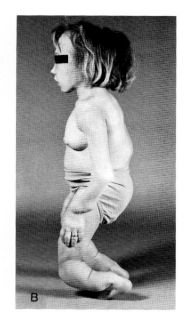
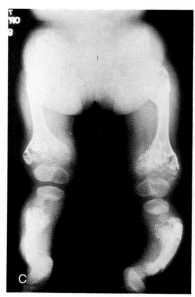
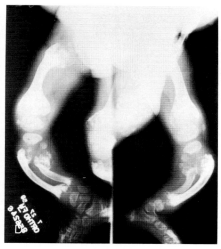
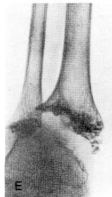
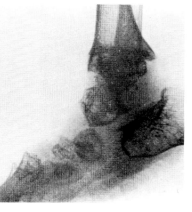

470

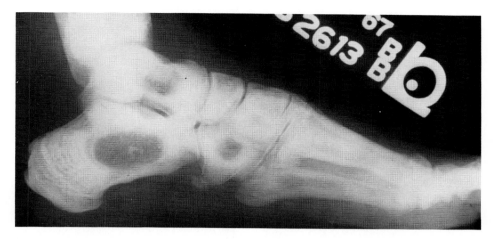

Figure 9-105. A 20-year-old man with osteopetrosis in whom lateral films of the left foot show that all the foot bones are dense and osteosclerotic except for their relatively radiolucent central portions.

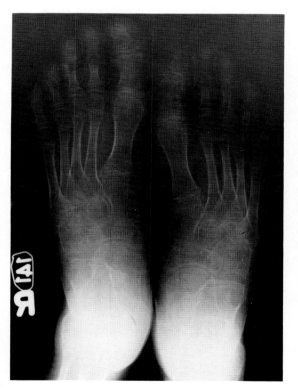

Figure 9-106. A 10-year-old boy with osteogenesis imperfecta in whom an anteroposterior view shows marked osteopetrosis of all foot bones with thin cortices and greatly diminished thickness and number of bony trabeculae.

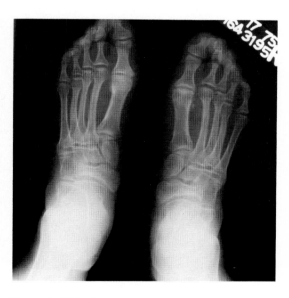

Figure 9-107. An 18-year-old patient had Morquio's disease. Anteroposterior film reveals irregularity and flattening of all metatarsal heads, which may dispose them to premature development of osteoarthritis.

Figure 9-104. **A** and **B,** a young woman with metaphyseal dysostosis of Jansen shows an immature face, widely spaced and exophthalmic eyes, markedly dwarfed stature, extremely short lower extremities, flexion contracture of the hip and knee joints producing a monkey-like stance or squat, and marked pronation of both feet. **C-E** , anteroposterior and lateral radiographs taken when the patient was a child show a peculiar cupping of the metaphyseal regions with lytic areas of irregular streaking and stippled calcification in association with anterior and lateral bowing of both legs.

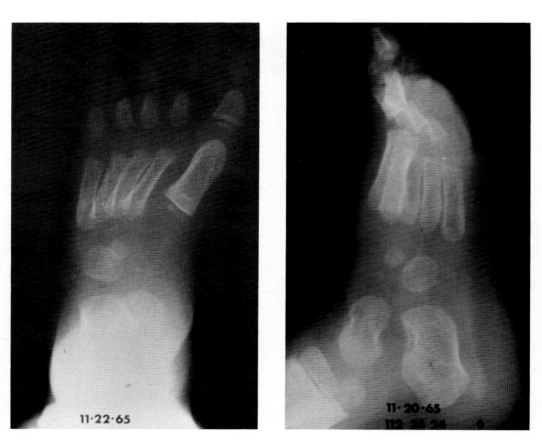

Figure 9–108. A child with Hurler's syndrome in whom anteroposterior and lateral radiographs show the metatarsals and phalanges are coarsely trabeculated, short and stubby, and tapered in a conical fashion.

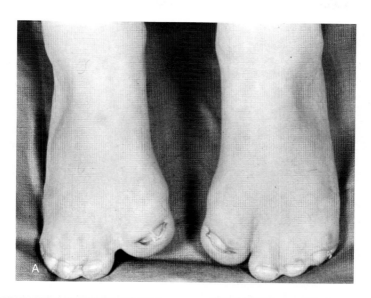

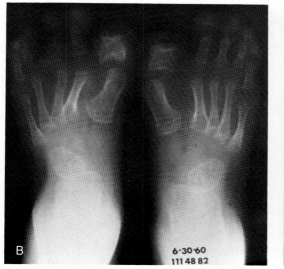
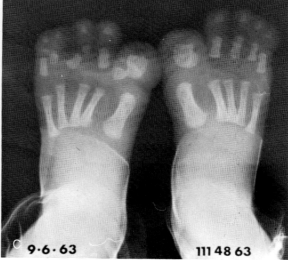

Figure 9–109. A, a child with Apert's syndrome had syndactylism of all 10 toes. **B,** anteroposterior radiograph shows absence of the distal phalanges of both great toes and the middle phalanges of several lesser toes. **C,** anteroposterior view, 3 years later. An exostosis has developed on the lateral basal portion of the proximal phalanx of the left great toe.

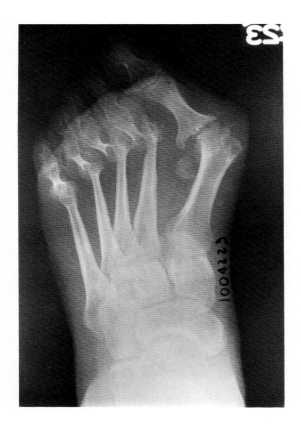

←

Figure 9–110. A 49-year-old woman had a long history of rheumatoid arthritis. Anteroposterior film shows severe hallux valgus, marked valgus deformity of all five toes, degeneration and subluxation or dislocation of all five M-P joints, and lateral migration of the medial and lateral sesamoids, all of which are typical foot deformities associated with rheumatoid arthritis.

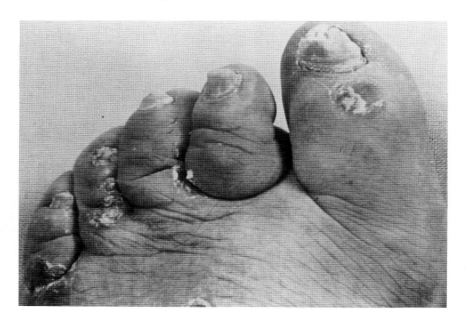

Figure 9–111. A 49-year-old woman with a long history of psoriasis had multiple psoriatic skin lesions and marked thickening and deformity of the toenails, particularly the great toenail.

474

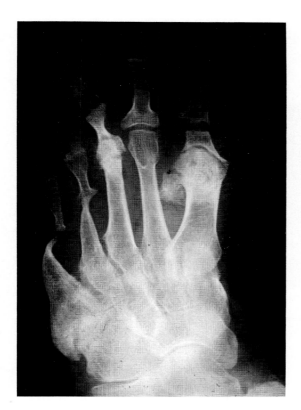

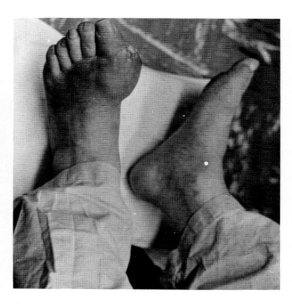

Figure 9–113. A 53-year-old man with a long history of gout had a large swelling in the first M-P joint region. A large deposit of urate was the cause which produced a draining sinus at the distal portion of the swelling.

Figure 9–112. A 55-year-old man with psoriatic arthritis in whom an anteroposterior radiograph shows marked tapering and resorption of the distal ends of the fourth and fifth metatarsals, destruction of the head of the proximal phalanx of the great toe and the bases of the fourth and fifth proximal phalanges, dislocation of the third M-P joint, degeneration of the first M-P and the metatarsocuboid joints, and lateral subluxation and degeneration of the lateral sesamoid bone.

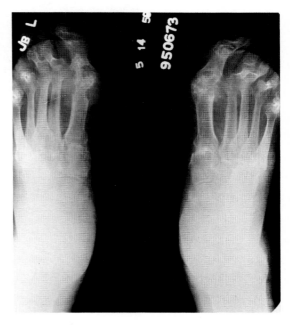

Figure 9–114. A 55-year-old man in whom an anteroposterior view reveals destruction of the first M-P joints and the heads of the first metatarsals by urate deposits.

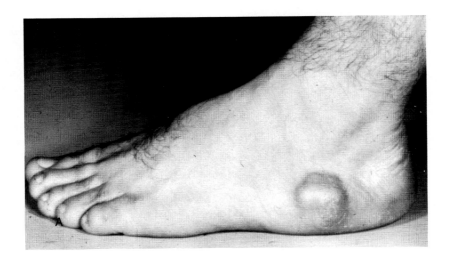

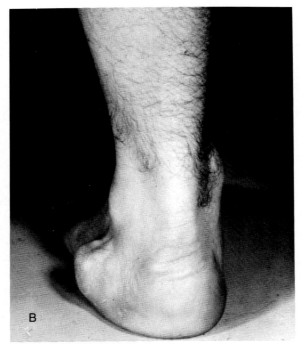

Figure 9–115. **A** and **B,** a 42-year-old man with gout had a mass over the lateral aspect of the inframalleolar area caused by a urate tophus. Surgical excision of the tophus was required for the patient to wear a shoe in comfort.

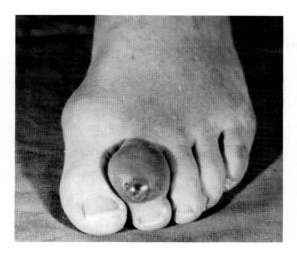

Figure 9–116. A 49-year-old man had a large urate tophus on the dorsal aspect of his left second toe. The urate deposit caused pain whenever he wore shoes and it was surgically excised.

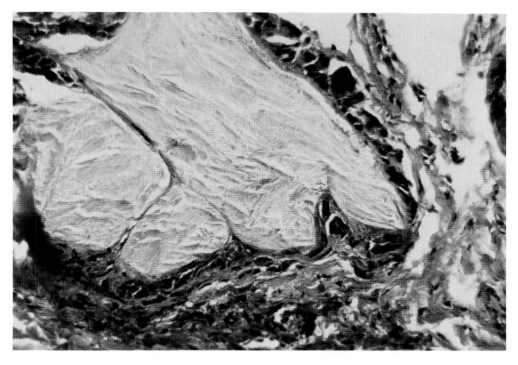

Figure 9–117. Photomicrograph of a gouty tophus (390×, H.&E.) shows urate crystals surrounded by giant cells, histiocytes, and fibroblasts, a typical picture of giant cell foreign body reaction.

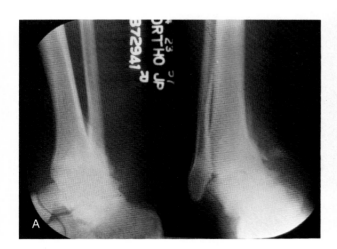 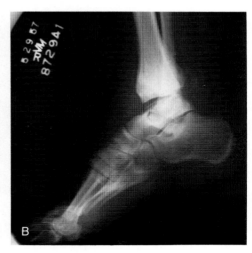

Figure 9–118. A 44-year-old man with tabes dorsalis in whom anteroposterior and oblique (**A**) and lateral (**B**) radiographs show severe destruction, swelling, instability, and loose body formation of his right ankle joint.

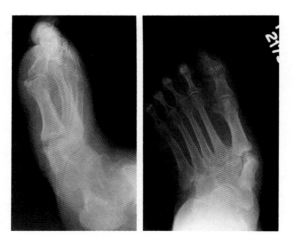

Figure 9–119. A 50-year-old woman with a long history of diabetes mellitus in whom lateral and anteroposterior films show marked rocker-bottom deformity and lateral subluxation of the metatarsotarsal joints. The deformity and subluxation were caused by severe deterioration of the metatarsotarsal joints secondary to diabetic peripheral neuropathy.

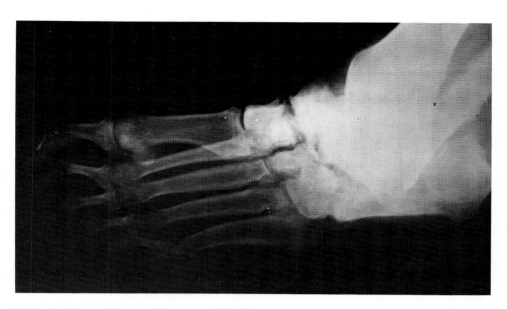

Figure 9–120. A 53-year-old man with neurotrophic arthropathy of his left foot, (oblique view) had severe degeneration and osteosclerosis of the left midtarsal joints, which will inevitably lead to a rocker-bottom flatfoot owing to the collapse of the longitudinal arch.

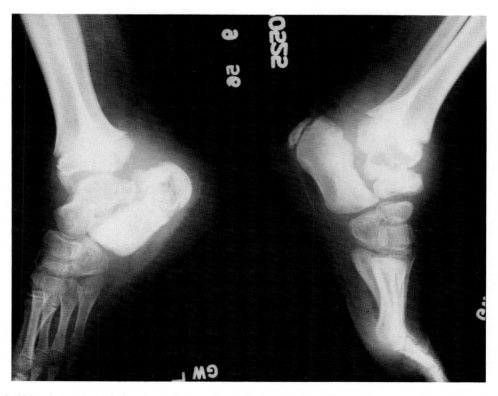

Figure 9–121. A 4-year-old girl with meningomyelocele had marked swelling and degeneration of her ankle joints and fragmentation of the right talus and left calcaneus (lateral views).

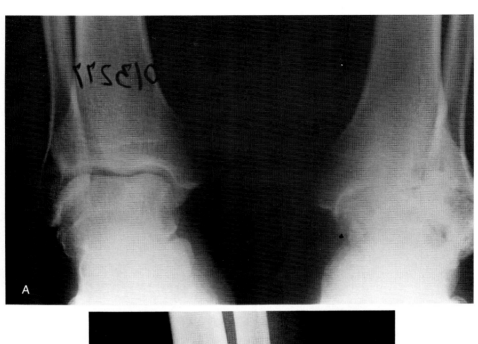

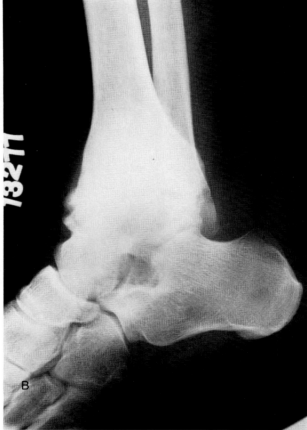

Figure 9–122. An 18-year-old man with hemophilia in whom anteroposterior and oblique (**A**) and lateral (**B**) radiographs show almost complete obliteration of the left ankle joint space owing to years of repeated and excessive hemorrhage into the joint.

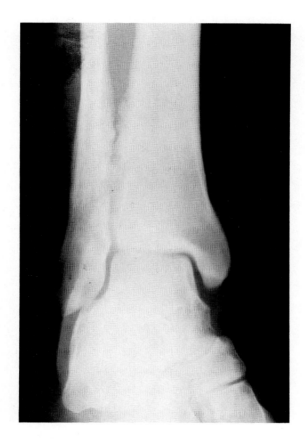

Figure 9–123. A 35-year-old man with pulmonary metastases from a poorly differentiated liposarcoma of the thigh in whom anteroposterior views show periosteal new bone formation of the distal tibial and fibular region.

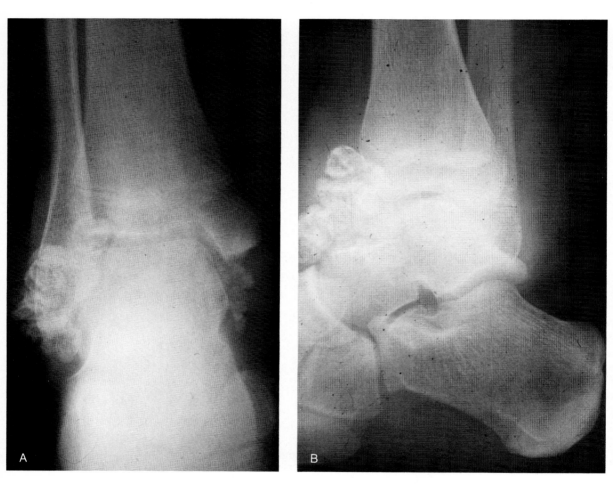

Figure 9–124. A 15-year-old boy in whom anteroposterior (**A**) and lateral (**B**) radiographs show many loose bodies in the left ankle joint caused by a synovial chondromatosis.

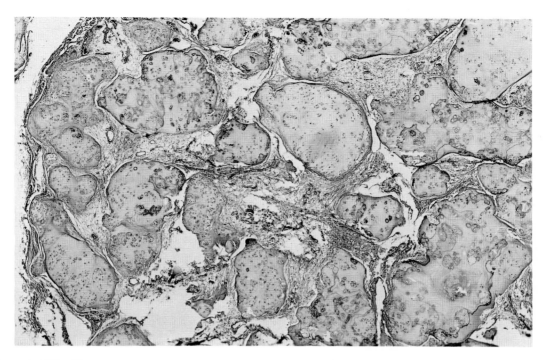

Figure 9–125. Photomicrograph of a synovial chondromatosis (28×, H.&E.) shows many individual lobules of cartilage tissue containing chondrocytes in their individual lacunae.

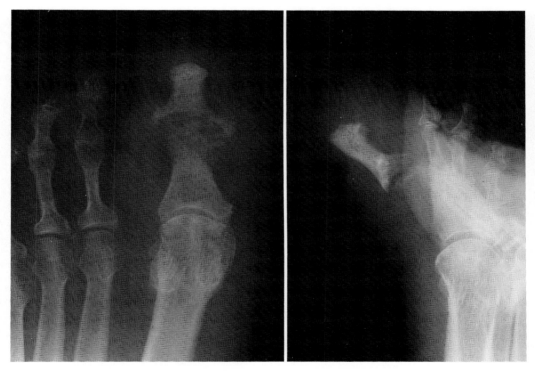

Figure 9–126. A 53-year-old man with diabetes mellitus in whom anteroposterior and lateral radiographs show destruction of the interphalangeal joint of the great toe accompanied by marked soft tissue swelling caused by a staphylococcal arthritis.

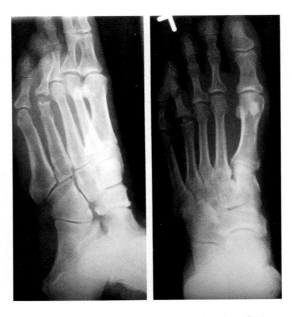

Figure 9–127. A 43-year-old woman in whom oblique and anteroposterior radiographs show destruction of the fourth M-P joint caused by septic arthritis, which developed after a fourth metatarsal osteotomy for the treatment of severe metatarsalgia.

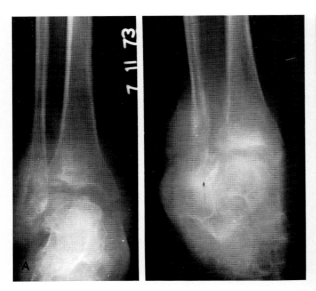

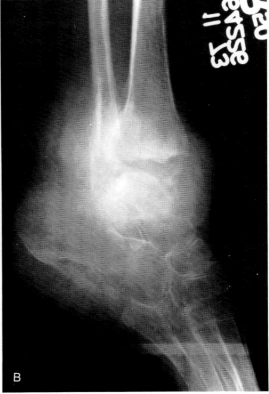

Figure 9–128. A 47-year-old man with tuberculosis of his right ankle joint in whom anteroposterior and oblique (**A**) and lateral (**B**) radiographs show marked swelling and destruction of the ankle joint, severe osteoporosis of the foot bones, and periosteal bone reaction of the distal fibula and tibia.

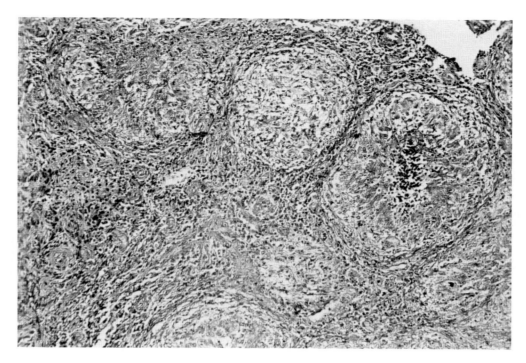

Figure 9–129. Photomicrograph of synovial tissue (175×, H.&E.) removed from a tuberculous joint shows formation of several granulomas in which chronic inflammatory cells (lymphocytes and plasma cells), epithelioid cells, fibroblasts, and Langerhans giant cells can be seen.

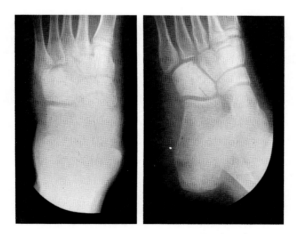

Figure 9–130. An 11-year-old boy developed osteomyelitis of his left cuboid bone after stepping on a rusty nail that penetrated the cuboid bone. On anteroposterior and oblique views, note the extensive osteosclerosis plus the small foci of radiolucency of the cuboid bone.

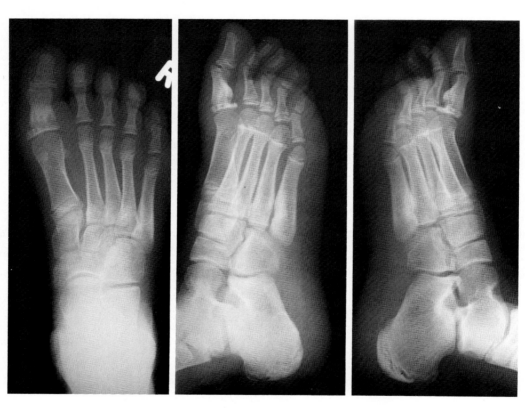

Figure 9–131. A 12-year-old boy in whom anteroposterior and oblique views reveal an osteomyelitis of the proximal phalanx of the right great toe with a radiolucent metaphyseal zone followed by an osteosclerotic diaphyseal zone.

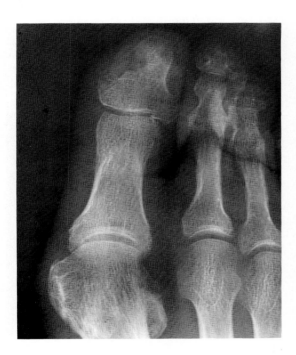

Figure 9–132. A 52-year-old man had an ingrown toe-nail of the medial border of his right great toenail. Infection eventually spread to the underlying distal phalanx to cause an osteolytic lesion with some mild osteosclerosis around the focus of bone destruction.

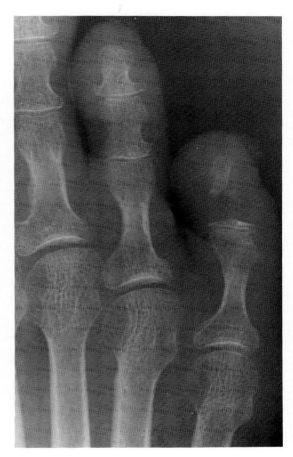

Figure 9–133. A 62-year-old man sustained a crush injury to his right fifth toe that caused osteomyelitis, manifested radiologically by destruction of the base of the distal phalanx and the distal two thirds of the middle phalanx of the right fifth toe.

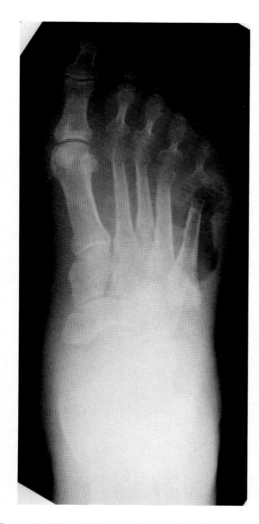

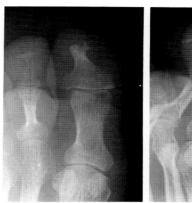
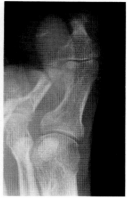

Figure 9–135. A 67-year-old man with diabetes mellitus for many years developed osteomyelitis of his left second toe, which caused complete destruction of the distal phalanx and partial destruction of the middle phalanx.

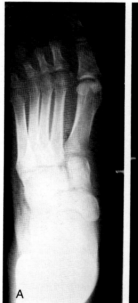
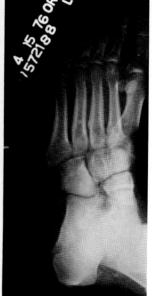

Figure 9–134. A 66-year-old man with diabetes mellitus in whom an anteroposterior radiograph shows gas around the right fifth metatarsal caused by an *E. coli* gas gangrene of the right foot. A below-knee amputation was eventually required.

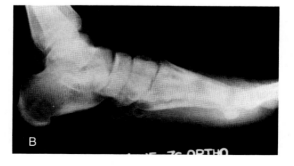

Figure 9–136. A 48-year-old man with severe diabetes mellitus in whom anteroposterior and oblique (**A**) and lateral (**B**) views show the presence of gas gangrene in the tarsometatarsal region of the left foot caused by the bacterium *E. coli*.

488

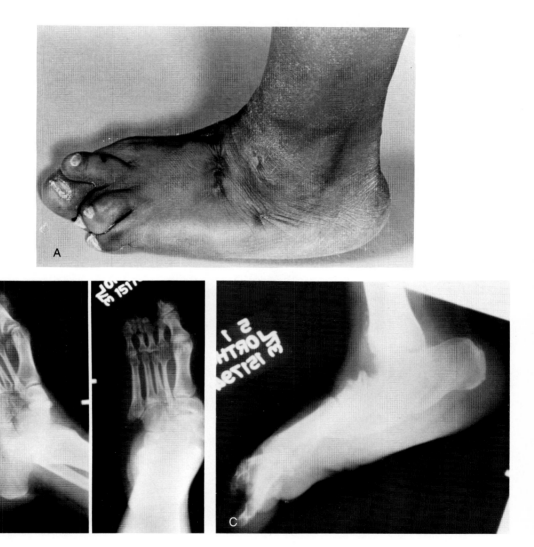

Figure 9–137. A 52-year-old man had tuberculosis of the left foot as a young man. **A,** scars on the dorsal aspect of the left foot were the sites of draining sinuses when the tuberculous infection was active. Oblique and anteroposterior (**B**) and lateral (**C**) films show arthritic changes of the tarsal joint, rocker-bottom foot deformity, and deformity of the navicular and cuneiform bones caused by the old tuberculous infection.

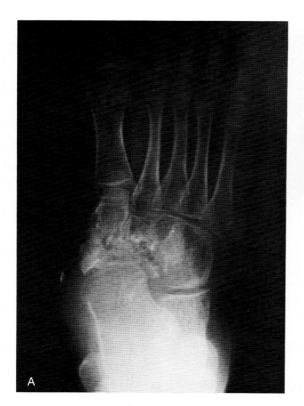

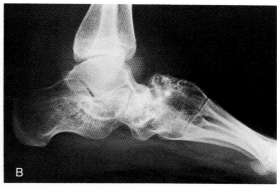

Figure 9–138. A 56-year old woman had tuberculosis of her right foot. Anteroposterior (**A**) and lateral (**B**) radiographs reveal extensive necrosis of the right tarsal navicular bone and destruction of the naviculocuneiform and talonavicular joints.

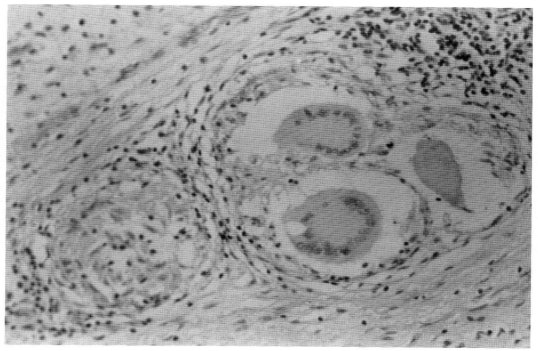

Figure 9–139. Photomicrograph of a tuberculous osteomyelitis (250×, H.&E.) shows many chronic inflammatory cells (lymphocytes and plasma cells), fibroblasts, and two large Langerhans giant cells, with their nuclei arranged in a circular or horseshoe-shaped manner.

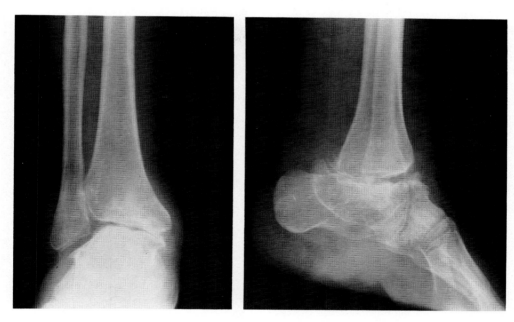

Figure 9–140. A 56-year-old woman had tuberculosis of the left ankle region at age 3 years. Anteroposterior and lateral radiographs show almost complete destruction of the left talus, with the tibia articulating directly with the calcaneus and navicular.

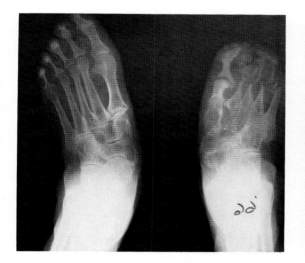

Figure 9–141. A 53-year-old patient with Hansen's disease in whom an anteroposterior film shows marked tapering of the three middle metatarsals and varying degrees of bone thinning and resorption of the phalanges of the right foot.

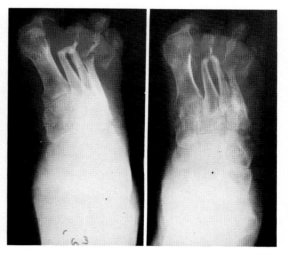

Figure 9–142. A patient with Hansen's disease had oblique and anteroposterior radiographs that reveal extensive resorption of the three middle metatarsal heads, complete disappearance of the fifth ray, and marked thinning and resorption of the phalangeal bones.

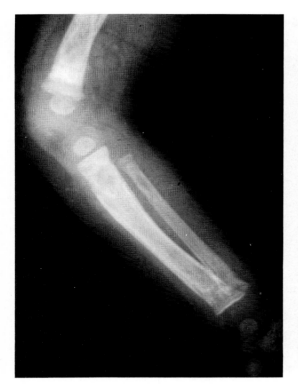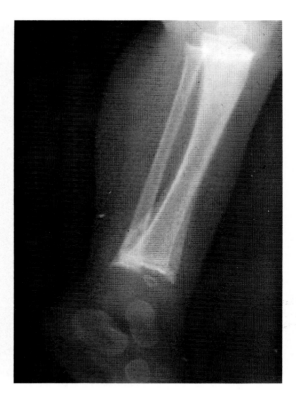

Figure 9–143. A lateral radiograph of the lower leg of a newborn baby with congenital syphilis shows a transverse, irregular radiolucent zone across the metaphyseal regions of the proximal and distal tibia and distal femur caused by the replacement of normal metaphyseal bone by syphilitic granulation tissue.

Figure 9–144. Radiograph of the lower leg of a newborn baby with congenital syphilis (lateral view) shows a narrow radiolucent line transversely across the metaphyseal region plus marked periosteal new bone formation around the distal portion of the tibia.

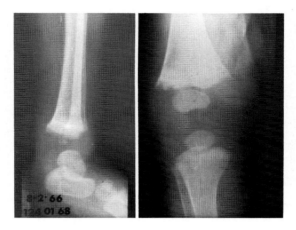

Figure 9–145. Lateral view of the ankle and anteroposterior view of the knee of a newborn baby with congenital rubella syndrome show narrow zones of alternating lucency and sclerosis in the metaphyses in association with irregular density and contour of the zone of provisional calcification.

492

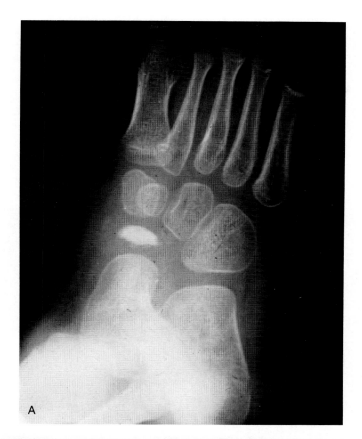

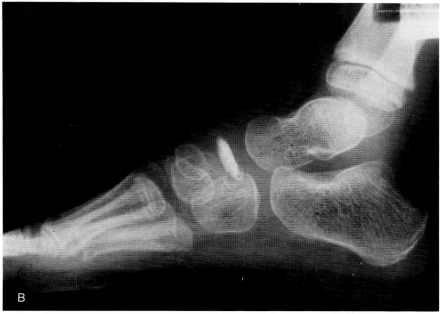

Figure 9–146. A 5-year-old boy had pain and swelling in the dorsal aspect of the right foot caused by Köhler's disease. Anteroposterior (**A**) and lateral (**B**) views show flattening and marked osteosclerosis of the tarsal navicular accompanied by some soft tissue swelling over the necrotic bone.

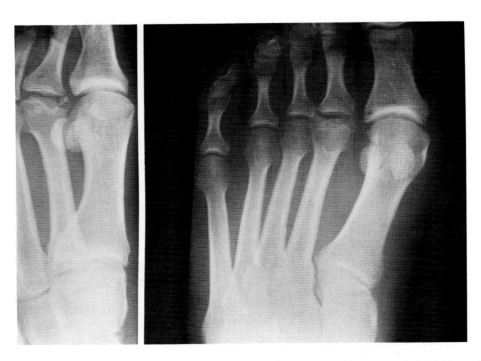

Figure 9–147. A 15-year-old girl with Freiberg's disease in whom oblique and anteroposterior radiographs reveal flattening, enlargement, irregularity, and loose body formation of the left second metatarsal head.

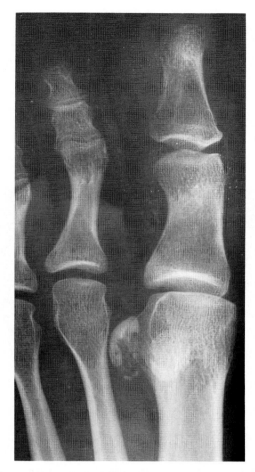

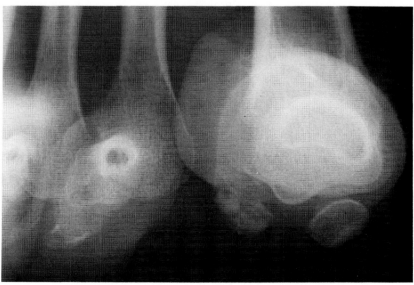

Figure 9–148. A 20-year-old woman had aseptic necrosis of the left lateral sesamoid bone. Oblique and sesamoid views show fragmentation and osteosclerosis of the lateral sesamoid bone.

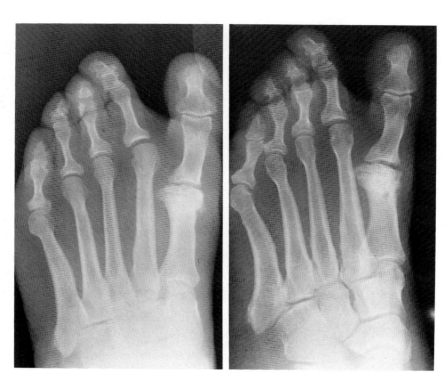

Figure 9–149. A 42-year-old woman underwent a bunion operation and developed aseptic necrosis of the left first metatarsal head. Anteroposterior and oblique radiographs show marked shortening of the first metatarsal as well as irregularity, flattening, and osteosclerosis of the first metatarsal head owing to aseptic necrosis.

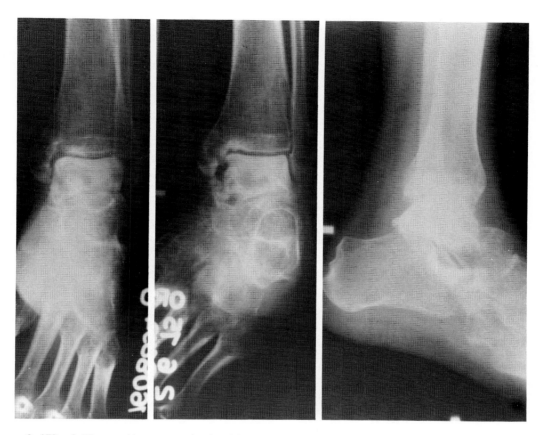

Figure 9–150. A 35-year-old man sustained a right talar neck fracture. Anteroposterior, oblique, and lateral views demonstrate osteosclerosis and cystic changes in the body of talus caused by aseptic necrosis.

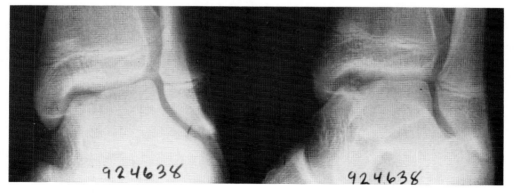

Figure 9–151. A 14-year old boy had aching and swelling of the right ankle. A small bony defect in the medial talar dome, caused by osteochondritis dissecans, was noted on anteroposterior and oblique radiographs.

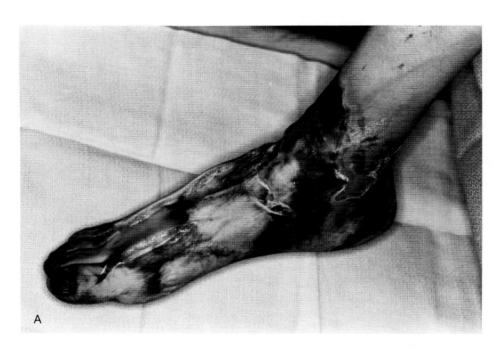

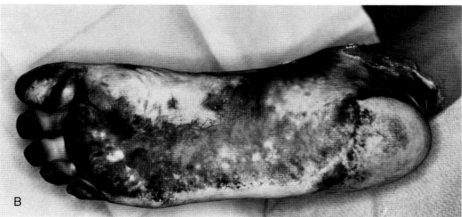

Figure 9–152. A and **B,** a 53-year-old man with epilepsy lost consciousness for at least 1 hour in a bathtub with his right foot directly under running hot water. Extensive soft tissue necrosis and an anesthetic foot resulted, which subsequently required a below-knee amputation.

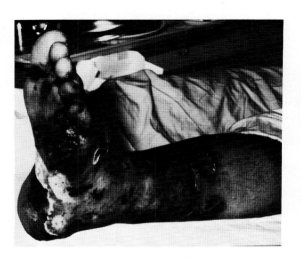

Figure 9–153. A 43-year-old factory worker sustained a severe burn to the lateral aspect of his left ankle and foot when molten iron was accidentally poured on his foot.

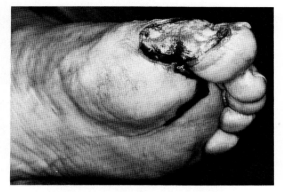

Figure 9–154. A 48-year-old man lost a large piece of skin from the medial aspect of his left toe when he accidentally touched a high-tension wire.

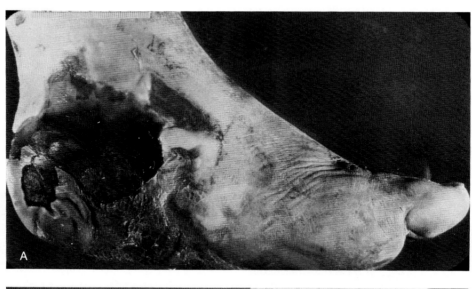

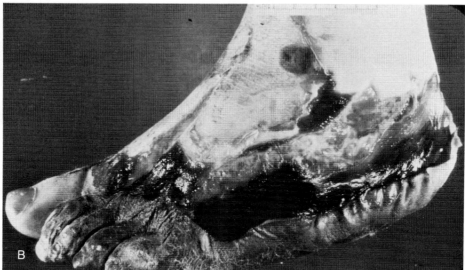

Figure 9–155. **A** and **B**, a 52-year-old man with peripheral arteriosclerotic vascular disease developed extensive dry gangrene of his left foot. A below-knee amputation was required.

500

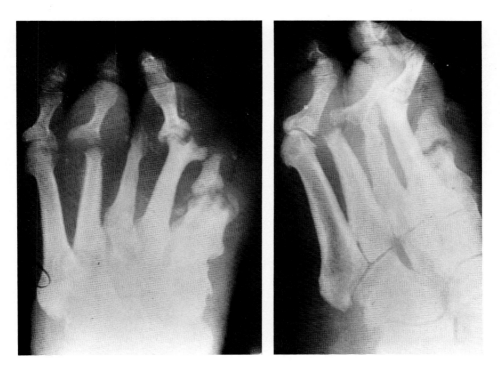

Figure 9–156. A 53-year-old man with diabetic peripheral neuropathy and peripheral vascular disease in whom anteroposterior and oblique radiographs show the absence of the great toe and the third toe, which were amputated owing to the development of dry gangrene.

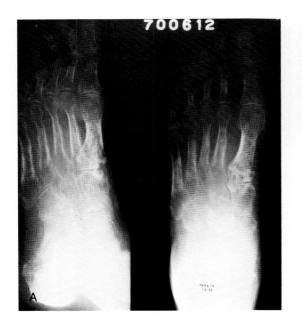

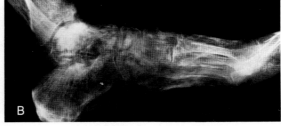

Figure 9–157. A 40-year-old man developed Sudeck's atrophy of his left foot after a left knee injury. Anteroposterior and oblique (**A**) and lateral (**B**) films show extensive spotty osteoporosis of the foot bones.

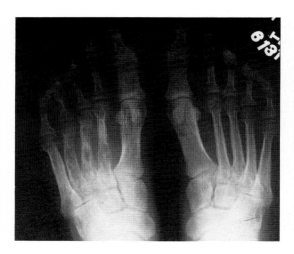

Figure 9–158. A 36-year-old man sustained a shrapnel wound to the plantar aspect of his left foot. The injury resulted in the formation of an arteriovenous fistula of the plantar arch manifested by a fullness of the plantar surface accompanied by distended superficial veins. Note the diffuse osteoporosis of the bones of the left foot, which can result from the increased blood flow through the foot brought about by the fistula.

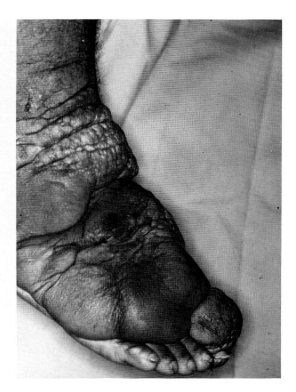

Figure 9–159. A 33-year-old woman with Milroy's disease had extensive elephantiasis-like skin changes of the right foot produced by extensive fibrosis in the lymphatic malformation of the involved extremity.

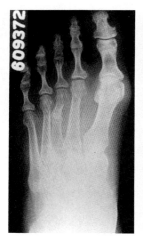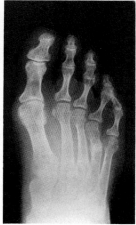

Figure 9–160. A 44-year-old man with severe osteomalacia in whom an anteroposterior radiograph shows generalized osteopenia of both feet plus symmetric fractures of the third metatarsals.

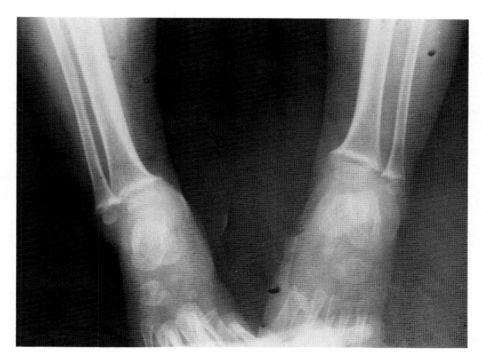

Figure 9–161. A young child with Fanconi's syndrome (hypophosphatemic rickets with aminoaciduria, acidosis, and renal glucosuria). Anteroposterior view shows flaring and a tuft-like configuration of the metaphyseal ends of both distal tibiae and fibulae in association with a transverse radiodense white line in the same area.

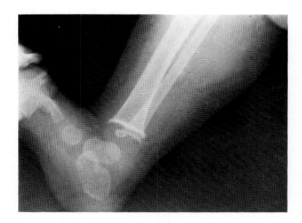

Figure 9–162. An 8-month-old baby with scurvy in whom a lateral radiograph shows tranverse radiodense lines at the ends of the distal tibial and fibular metaphyses (Frankel's white line), metaphyseal spur (Pelkan spur), a radiolucent zone adjacent to Frankel's white line (Trummerfeld's zone), cortical thinning and ground glass appearance of the tibial and fibular diaphyses, and radiodense rings around the distal tibial epiphysis and tarsal bones (Wimberger's rings).

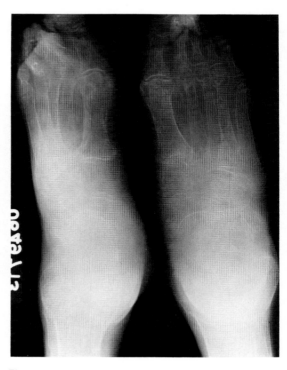

Figure 9–163. A 55-year-old man with systemic mastocytosis in whom an anteroposterior view shows marked osteoporosis of all the bones in both feet.

503

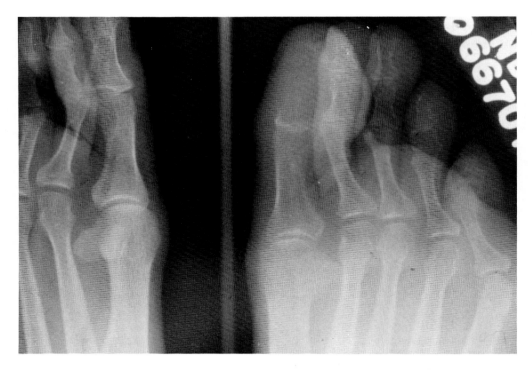

Figure 9–164. A 40-year-old man had primary hyperparathyroidism. Anteroposterior radiograph shows generalized demineralization of the foot bones plus almost complete destruction of the distal phalanx of the right great toe which was caused by a hyperparathyroidism-induced brown tumor.

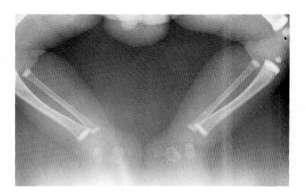

Figure 9–165. Lower extremities of a very young child with lead poisoning. Radiograph shows radiodense lead lines across the femoral, tibial, and fibular metaphyseal regions and formation of thin radiopaque rings around the calcanei and tali.

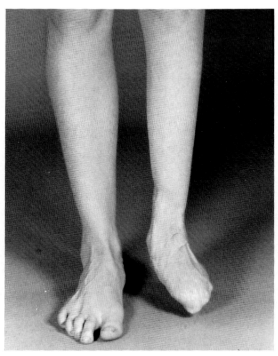

Figure 9–166. A 17-year-old youth had complete adactyly of his left foot, plus some shortening of the left femur and atrophy of the left lower extremity.

504

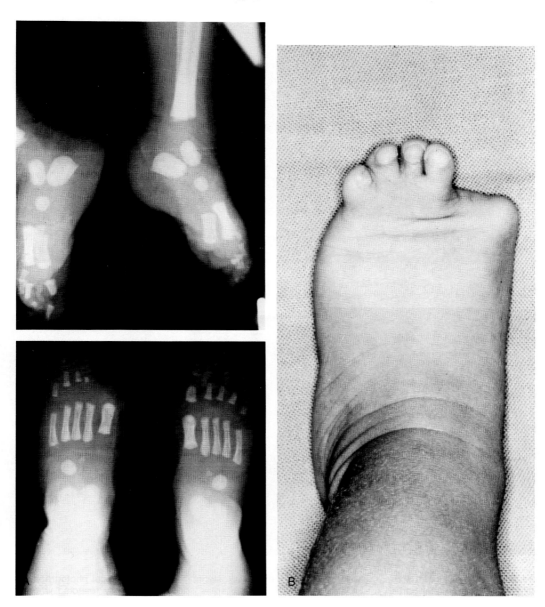

Figure 9–167. A child with partial adactyly. Radiographs (**A**) and clinical photograph (**B**) demonstrate the absence of the left great toe.

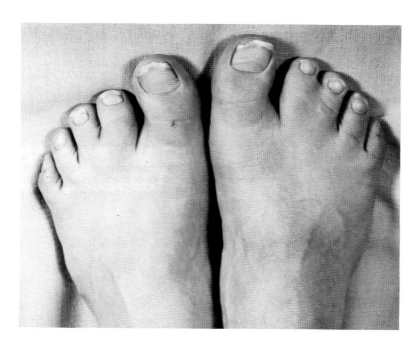

Figure 9–172. A boy had syndactyly of his right second and third toes, which was completely asymptomatic and did not produce much disfigurement. No treatment was required.

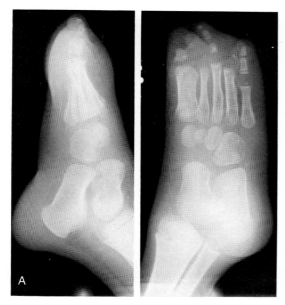

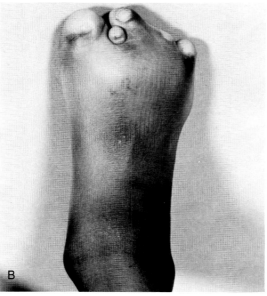

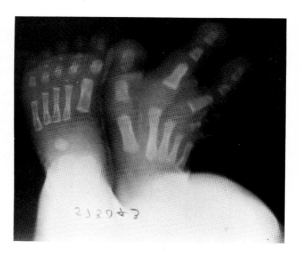

Figure 9–174. Anteroposterior radiograph of a new-born baby demonstrates a grossly enlarged right foot, especially the second and third toes. Bone and soft tissue surgery was required to improve the cosmetic appearance of the foot and for ease of shoe fitting.

Figure 9–173. Radiographs (**A**) and a clinical photograph (**B**) of a young patient with microdactyly of the right second toe, adactyly of the right fourth toe, and hypoplasia of the right great toe.

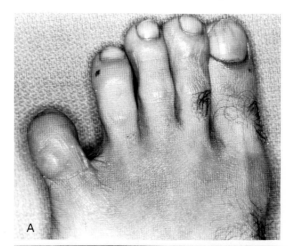

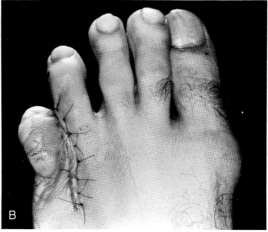

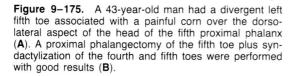

Figure 9–175. A 43-year-old man had a divergent left fifth toe associated with a painful corn over the dorsolateral aspect of the head of the fifth proximal phalanx (**A**). A proximal phalangectomy of the fifth toe plus syndactylization of the fourth and fifth toes were performed with good results (**B**).

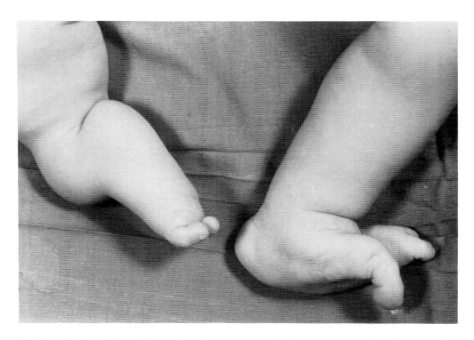

Figure 9–176. A newborn baby had lobster claw deformity of the left foot caused by the absence of the second and third digital rays, and absence of the tibia and the three medial digital rays of the right foot.

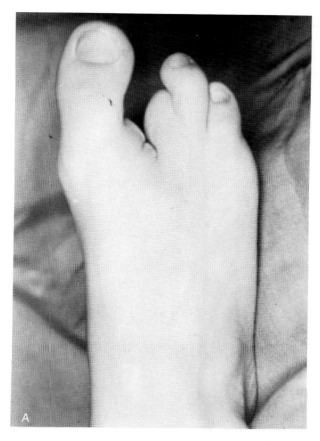

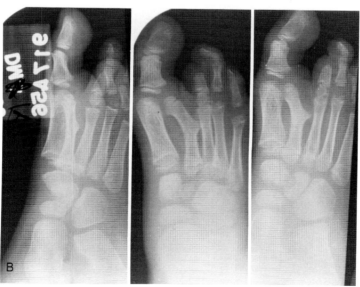

Figure 9–177. **A,** a young man had a pseudo-lobster claw deformity of his right foot caused by the absence of the second toe and a lack of the two distal phalanges of the third toe. **B,** oblique and lateral radiographs.

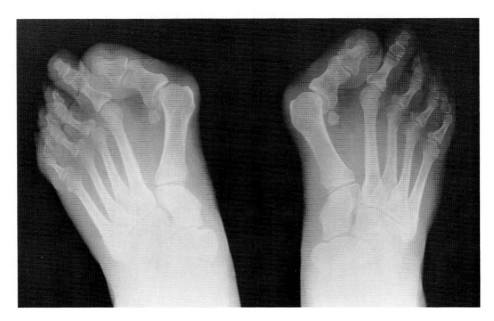

Figure 9–178. A 28-year-old patient with Down's syndrome in whom an anteroposterior radiograph shows marked metatarsus primus varus in association with severe hallux valgus and complete dislocation of the medial and lateral sesamoidometatarsal joints.

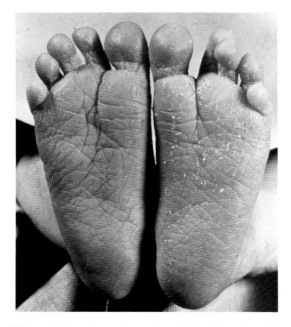

Figure 9–179. A newborn baby with familial median cleft of the foot had bilateral, symmetric longitudinal plantar skin clefts between the first and second toes.

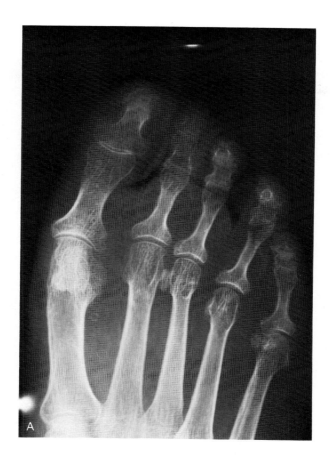

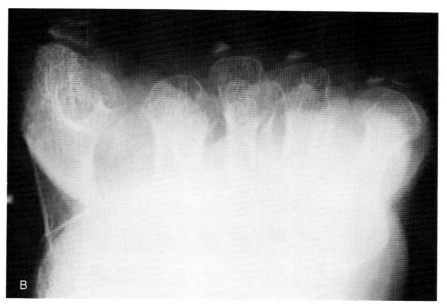

Figure 9–180. A 50-year-old man in whom anteroposterior (**A**) and axial (**B**) views show four sesamoid bones associated with the heads of the third, fourth, and fifth metatarsals.

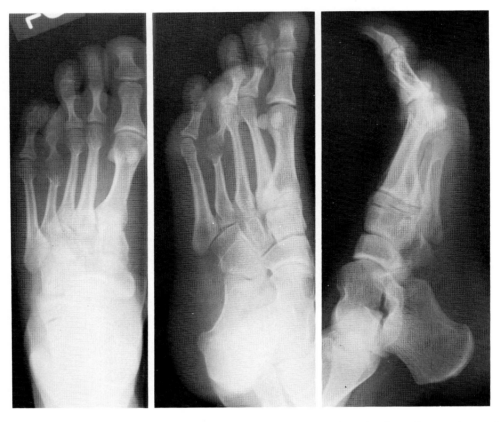

Figure 9–181. A 39-year-old woman in whom anteroposterior, oblique, and lateral radiographs reveal a greatly shortened left fourth metatarsal, which makes the fourth toe look very short.

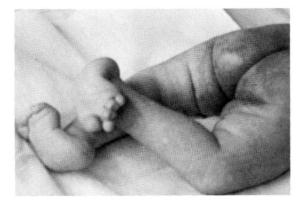

Figure 9–182. A newborn baby had bilateral vertical tali of her feet, which produced a rocker-bottom configuration of the plantar surfaces and marked valgus position of both heels.

514

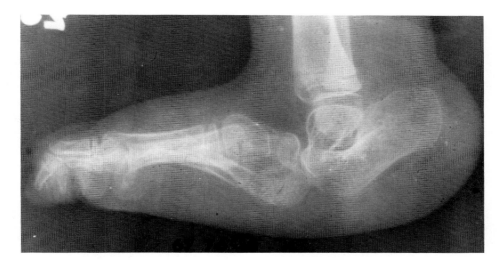

Figure 9–183. A young patient with congenital vertical talus had dislocation of the talonavicular joint, marked equinus deformity of the calcaneus, and complete loss of the longitudinal arch of the foot, producing a so-called rocker-bottom flatfoot (lateral view).

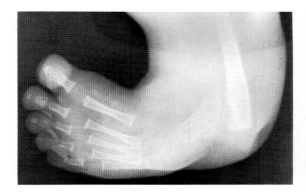

Figure 9–184. Lateral view of an ankle shows absence of the tibia associated with severe varus deformity of the foot.

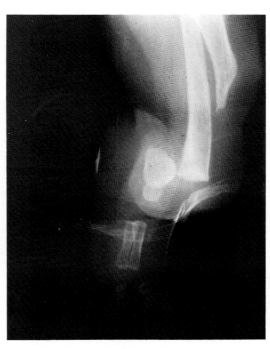

Figure 9–185. A newborn baby with absence of the distal tibia in whom a lateral view shows complete dislocation of the ankle joint with the foot parallel to the longitudinal axis of the fibula, and absence of the three medial rays of the foot.

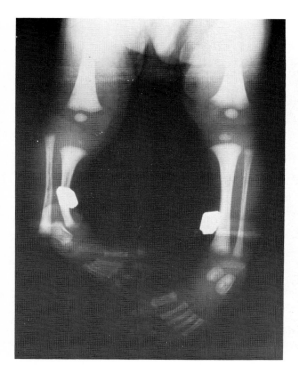

Figure 9–186. Anteroposterior view of the lower extremities of a newborn baby shows dysgenesis of the distal portion of the right tibia accompanied by a shortened right leg, diastasis of the right distal tibiofibular articulation, subluxation of the right ankle joint, and marked varus deformity of the right foot.

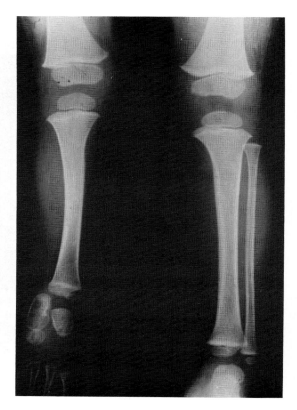

Figure 9–187. A child with complete absence of the right fibula in whom an anteroposterior film reveals significant shortening of the right femur and tibia, and lateral subluxation of the right ankle joint.

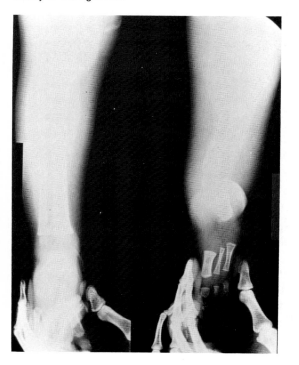

Figure 9–188. A newborn baby with complete absence of the left fibula in whom an anteroposterior radiograph shows shortening of the left lower extremity, lateral subluxation of the left ankle joint, and absence of the two lateral rays of the left foot.

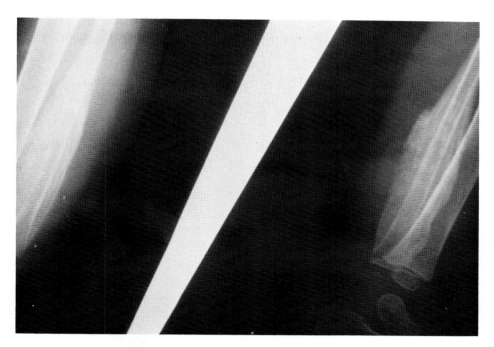

Figure 9–189. A 4-month-old baby had a painful and swollen left lower leg. Lateral views of the ankle show marked subperiosteal bone formation of the left distal fibula caused by Caffey's disease.

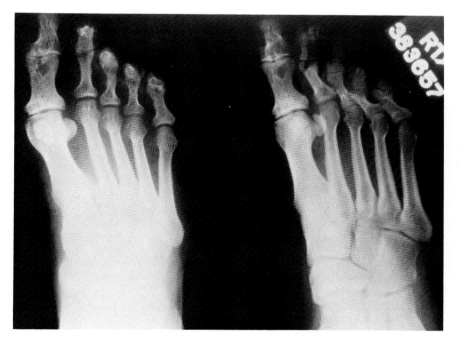

Figure 9–190. A 46-year-old man with sarcoidosis in whom anteroposterior and oblique radiographs show multiple osteolytic lesions in the phalanges of the right foot caused by sarcoidosis.

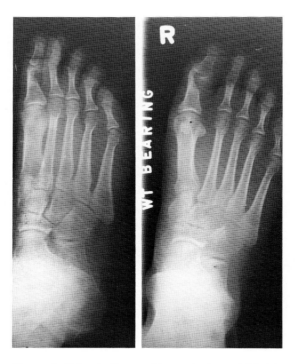

Figure 9–191. A 42-year-old man had a painful right toe. Oblique and anteroposterior films reveal destruction of the lateral aspect of the head of the first proximal phalanx. A diagnosis of sarcoidosis was made by open biopsy.

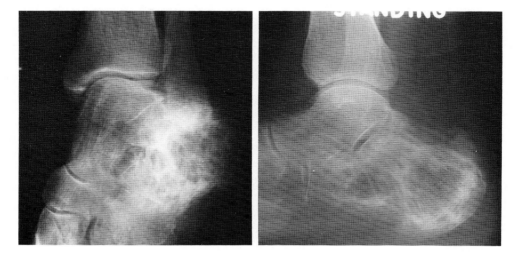

Figure 9–192. A 53-year-old man had Paget's disease of his left calcaneus. Oblique and lateral views show a mixture of osteolytic and osteoblastic bone changes in the calcaneus caused by the random and simultaneous formation and resorption processes in the same bone.

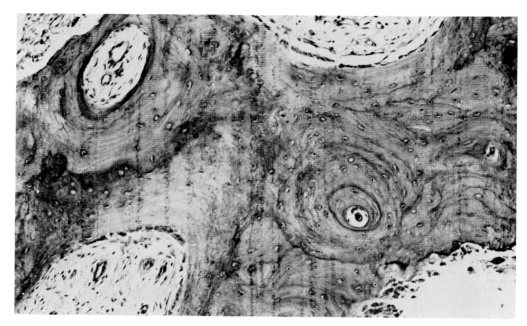

Figure 9–193. Photomicrograph of Paget's disease of bone (175×, H.&E.) shows dense cement lines and a mosaic pattern of bone accompanied by increased intramedullary fibrosis and numerous osteoclasts.

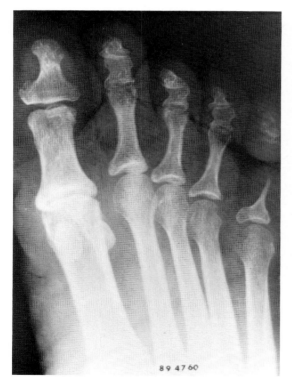

Figure 9–194. A 48-year-old man with ainhum of his right fifth toe in whom an anteroposterior radiograph shows marked resorption and tapering of the fifth proximal phalanx.

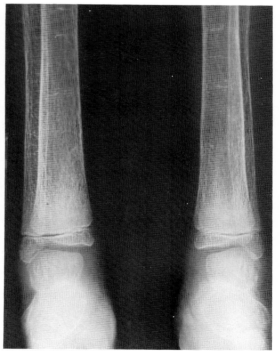

Figure 9–195. A 10-year-old boy with Cooley's anemia in whom an anteroposterior view reveals extreme osteoporosis and some coarsening of the trabecular pattern of the distal tibiae and fibulae and the tarsal bones, caused by a chronic negative skeletal balance (excessive bone resorption over formation).

519

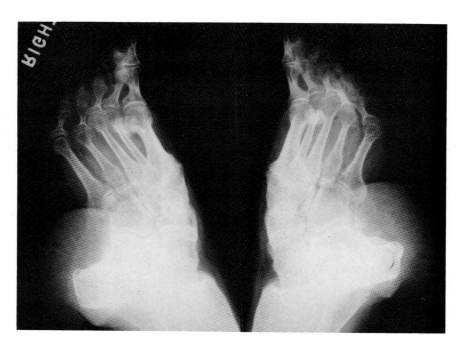

Figure 9–196. A 70-year-old Chinese woman with Mandarin feet in whom lateral radiographs show marked shortening and cavus deformity of both feet, with the heel pads shaped like two large oranges.

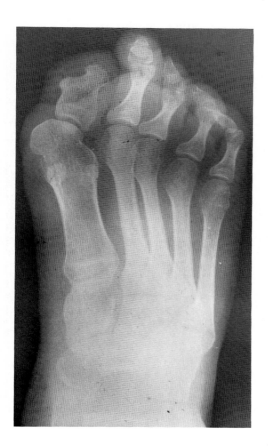

Figure 9–197. A 20-year-old man with myositis ossificans progressiva in whom an anteroposterior radiograph demonstrates hallux valgus deformity and shortening of the great toe, and fusion of the proximal phalanx of the great toe with the first metatarsal.

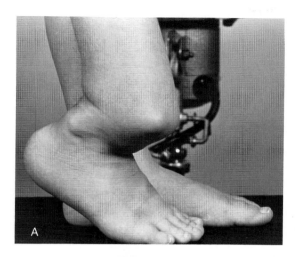

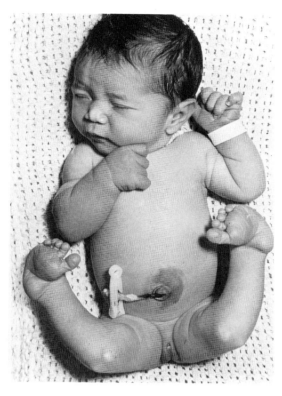

Figure 9–199. A newborn baby with arthrogryposis multiplex congenita had bilateral dislocation of both hips and knees and bilateral clubfeet.

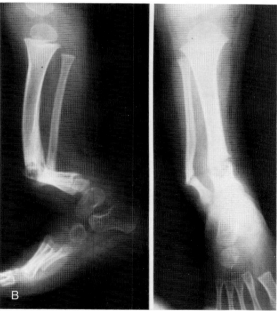

Figure 9–198. A 4-year-old boy had an acute anterior angulation of the right tibia caused by pseudarthrosis of the tibia and fibula (**A**). Lateral and anteroposterior radiographs (**B**) show pseudarthrosis of both the tibia and fibula with no detectable fracture callus formation.

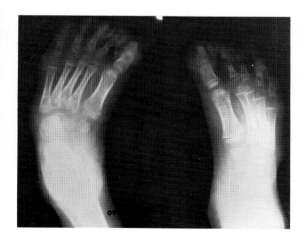

Figure 9–200. A 2-year-old girl with arthrogryposis multiplex congenita had been treated since birth. Anteroposterior radiograph shows there is still varus deformity of both feet, requiring continued treatment.

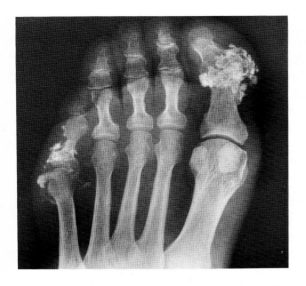

Figure 9–201. A 63-year-old woman had a long history of dermatomyositis. Anteroposterior view shows calcification around the interphalangeal joint of the great toe and the M-P joint of the fifth toe.

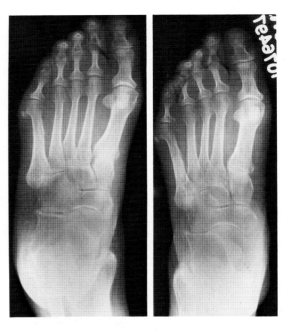

Figure 9–203. A 49-year-old woman had a symptomatic tailor's bunion of her left foot. Oblique and anteroposterior views show a calcified bursa over the tailor's bunion.

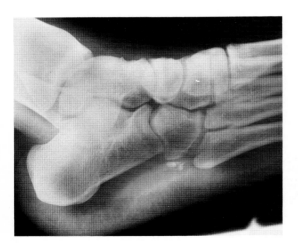

Figure 9–202. A 44-year-old man with calcific tendonitis of the right peroneus brevis tendon in whom an oblique view shows calcification of the tendon near its insertion into the lateral base of the fifth metatarsal.

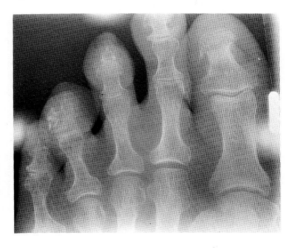

Figure 9–204. A 50-year-old man had a painful corn over the dorsolateral aspect of the DIP joint of his left fourth toe. Anteroposterior radiograph demonstrates calcification of an adventitious bursa between the overlying corn and the underlying exostosis.

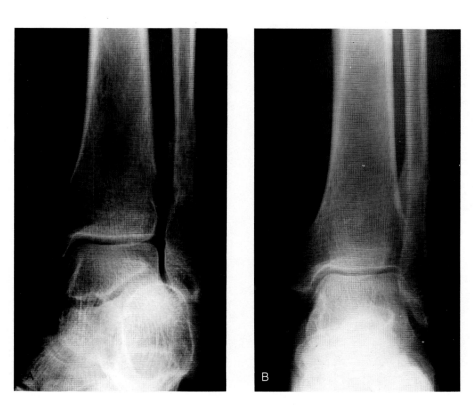

Figure 9–205. A 65-year-old man started playing 18 holes of golf daily soon after he retired from a sedentary job. **A,** anteroposterior radiograph shows marked periosteal bone formation in association with some osteolysis in the supramalleolar portion of the fibula, suggesting the presence of a malignant bone tumor. **B,** same view, 3 weeks later, shows consolidation and an orderly fusiform configuration of the periosteal bone formation around the distal fibula. These findings indicate a process of fracture healing.

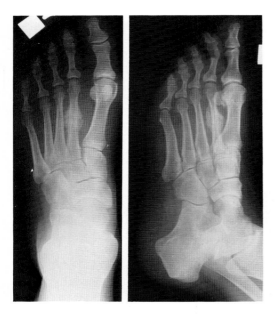

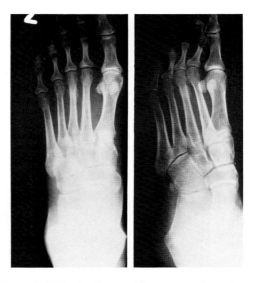

Figure 9–206. A 56-year-old woman developed pain in her left second metatarsal 3 weeks after joining a jogging club. Anteroposterior and oblique radiographs reveal abundant callus formation around the shaft of the second metatarsal caused by a stress fracture.

Figure 9–207. A 49-year-old man experienced metatarsalgia of his left foot 2 weeks after joining a tennis club. Oblique and anteroposterior views show periosteal new bone formation around a stress fracture of the third metatarsal neck.

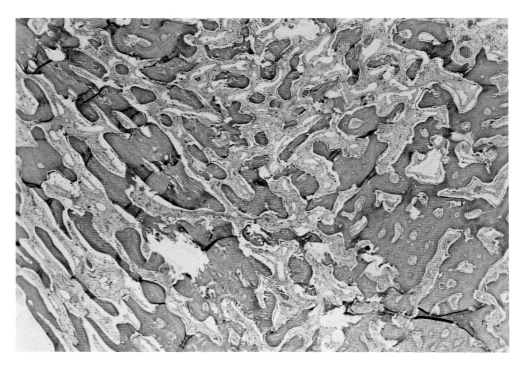

Figure 9–208. Photomicrograph of callus removed from a fracture (125×, H.&E.) shows many newly formed bony trabeculae in association with benign-looking, osteogenic interstitial tissue.

INDEX